HANDBOOK OF

PEDIATRIC

CONSTRAINT-INDUCED MOVEMENT THERAPY (CIMT)

A Guide for Occupational Therapy and Health Care
Clinicians, Researchers, and Educators

Edited by SHARON LANDESMAN RAMEY, PhD;
PATTY COKER-BOLT, PhD, OTR/L; and
STEPHANIE C. DeLUCA, PhD

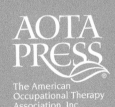

AOTA PRESS

The American
Occupational Therapy
Association, Inc.

AOTA Centennial Vision

We envision that occupational therapy is a powerful, widely recognized, science-driven, and evidence-based profession with a globally connected and diverse workforce meeting society's occupational needs.

Mission Statement

The American Occupational Therapy Association advances the quality, availability, use, and support of occupational therapy through standard-setting, advocacy, education, and research on behalf of its members and the public.

AOTA Staff

Frederick P. Somers, *Executive Director*
Christopher M. Bluhm, *Chief Operating Officer*

Chris Davis, *Director, AOTA Press*
Ashley Hofmann, *Development/Production Editor*
Victoria Davis, *Production/Digital Editor*

Beth Ledford, *Director, Marketing*
Jennifer Folden, *Marketing Specialist*
Amanda Fogle, *Marketing Specialist*

American Occupational Therapy Association, Inc.
4720 Montgomery Lane
Bethesda, MD 20814
Phone: 301-652-AOTA (2682)
TDD: 800-377-8555
Fax: 301-652-7711
www.aota.org
To order: 1-877-404-AOTA or store.aota.org

Disclaimers

This publication is designed to provided accurate and authoritative information in regard to the subject matter covered. It is sold or distributed with the understanding that the publisher is not engaged in rendering legal, accounting, or other professional service. If legal advice or other expert assistance is required, the services of a competent professional person should be sought.

—*From the Declaration of Principles jointly adopted by the American Bar Association and a Committee of Publishers and Associations*

It is the objective of the American Occupational Therapy Association to be a forum for free expression and interchange of ideas. The opinions expressed by the contributors to this work are their own and not necessarily those of the American Occupational Therapy Association.

ISBN: 978-1-56900-346-6
Library of Congress Control Number: 2013947540

Cover design by Debra Naylor, Naylor Design, Inc., Washington, DC
Text design by Judy Myers, Graphic Design, Alpine, CA
Composition by Maryland Composition, Laurel, MD
Printed by Automated Graphic Systems, Inc., White Plains, MD

DEDICATION

We dedicate this book to the primary mentors who have shaped our professional careers by emphasizing, above all, three things:
- To pursue innovation,
- To challenge and then advance knowledge about what really makes a difference in the lives of children with disabilities, and
- To collaborate with others in ways that transcend conventional boundaries.

Our primary mentors treated us from early on as if we were their peers and would succeed in whatever we pursued. They exemplify for us ideal role models.

Sharon Landesman Ramey dedicates this book to Gene (Jim) P. Sackett, PhD, Professor Emeritus, Psychology, University of Washington.

Patty Coker-Bolt dedicates this book to Maralynne D. Mitcham, PhD, OTR/L, FAOTA, Professor and Assistant Dean, College of Health Professions, Medical University of South Carolina.

Stephanie DeLuca dedicates this book to Sharon Ramey, PhD, Distinguished Research Scholar of Human Development, Virginia Tech Carilion Research Center; Professor of Psychology, Virginia Tech, and Professor of Psychiatry and Behavioral Medicine, Virginia Tech Carilion School of Medicine.

CONTENTS

section I — THEORY AND HISTORY OF CIMT FOR CHILDREN WITH CEREBRAL PALSY 1

COLLABORATION AND COORDINATION WITH FAMILIES AND OTHER PROFESSIONALS 247

FUTURE FOR RESEARCH, POLICY, AND PRACTICE. . 265

Flash Drive **Items on the Flash Drive**

- Daily Therapy Log for P–CIMT
- Parent Report Log Used During an mP–CIMT Program for an Infant

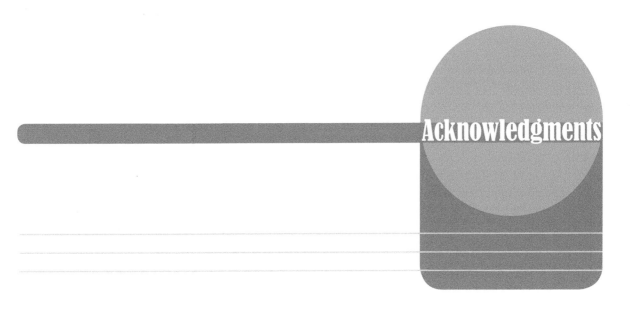

Acknowledgments

The opportunity to serve as editors of a first and landmark handbook is a true honor and a tremendous learning experience. The three of us share a sense of immense gratitude to each contributing author and to the American Occupation Therapy Association (AOTA) for its enthusiastic support at all stages of this endeavor. Above all, as the handbook has progressed, we have learned firsthand about the immense diversity, competency, and high engagement and caring of practitioners, educators, and scientists globally concerning the topic of pediatric constraint-induced movement therapy (P–CIMT) and the pursuit of evidence-based practices to benefit children with neuromotor challenges.

Specifically, we want to acknowledge the groundbreaking research findings and decades of contribution in the field of adult CIMT by both Steve L. Wolf at Emory University and Edward Taub at the University of Alabama at Birmingham. They truly helped establish the stage for the highly productive past 15 years of research and clinical applications related to pediatric populations.

The idea for this book emerged in many places, but we extend particular thanks for four individuals who deserve special mention for taking action, propelled by their own clinical passion and experience: Teressa Reidy, Erin Naber, Dory Ainsworth Wallace, and Mary Rebekah Trucks. They are ones who first engaged us and helped to introduce the idea to AOTA. They wholeheartedly supported an even broader vision for the book that expanded the scientific and clinical topics and embraced the international community with its many substantive contributions. We are fortunate that each has contributed as authors to the final handbook. We also extend a big thank you to Karen Echols, who provided many ideas that shaped this volume and who frequently reminded us to "keep things practical."

At AOTA, many people offered tangible and intangible support. Chris Davis, Director of AOTA Press, shared ideas; organized a highly effective production and editing team; sought peer reviews for the entire book; and contributed creatively to this endeavor, including plans for follow-up activities that will offer additional support and updates to those who read and use this handbook in clinical practice, to prepare next-generation practitioners, and to provide timely, science-driven, ongoing professional learning and continuing education for those already in the field. Chris fully embraced the idea that a handbook designed primarily for practitioners could also be valuable for parents and advocacy groups as well as researchers. We already have begun to think about preparing a second edition when there is an even stronger body of evidence to answer the uncertainties that are identified in this first edition. Victoria Davis and Ashley Hofmann worked closely with us to contract with authors, delicately balance how to avoid redundancy or duplication across chapters while creating chapters that can "stand on their own," to promote the use of common terms with clear definitions, and to check the accuracy of information and citations across chapters.

When a handbook such as this embraces a topic that is fundamentally multidisciplinary and that engages practitioners from different countries (where the terms used to describe treatment approaches often vary considerably), this sometimes appeared to be a daunting task. The contributing authors worked diligently and responsively with AOTA and us, often accommodating our many requests for changes and clarification. Throughout all stages, Laura Bateman at the Virginia Tech Carilion Research Institute supplied our team with her strong organizational skills, attention to detail, assistance with figures and tables, and a can-do attitude about a multitude of tasks that come with editing a volume that involves working with 23 authors!

Finally, the *Handbook of Pediatric Constraint-Induced Movement Therapy (CIMT): A Guide for Occupational Therapy and Health Care Clinicians, Researchers, and Educators* would not have been possible without the children and their families, who, along with their local practitioners, were open-minded and willing to participate in the research studies that constitute the foundational evidence that supports P–CIMT. What has been learned from documenting the histories of literally hundreds of children and families now helps to inform others about what works best and for whom and when. The global rehabilitation community has actively exchanged findings and continues to work vigorously and cooperatively to further advance our field.

Truly,

—*Sharon Landesman Ramey*
Patty Coker-Bolt
Stephanie DeLuca

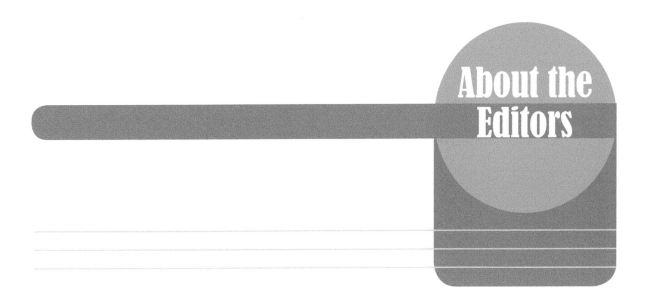

About the Editors

Sharon Landesman Ramey, PhD, is Distinguished Research Scholar of Human Development at the Virginia Tech Carilion Research Institute (VTCRI) and Professor of Psychology at Virginia Tech and Professor of Psychiatry and Behavioral Medicine at the Virginia Tech Carilion School of Medicine. Trained as developmental psychologist, she has been engaged in pioneering work in the development and testing of many theory-informed, innovative treatments for children with developmental disabilities since the early 1970s. In the mid-1990s, while serving as the Founding Director of the Civitan International Research Center at the University of Alabama at Birmingham (UAB), Dr. Ramey was the principal investigator on the first randomized controlled trial of pediatric CIMT (working with Stephanie Deluca, Karen Echols, and Edward Taub) and launched the UAB Pediatric Neuromotor Research Clinic. Her key areas of scientific inquiry and interest include behavioral teratology, school readiness, transition to adulthood, health disparities, and brain development throughout the lifespan. Currently, Dr. Ramey co-directs the VTCRI Neuromotor Research Clinic in Roanoke, Virginia. Her primary focus is on research in the specialty area of Implementation Science with the goal of advancing our understanding of critical factors associated with timely and effective translation of scientific discoveries into mainstream clinical and community-based practice. She has more than 225 publications.

Patty Coker-Bolt, PhD, OTR/L, is an Associate Professor in the Department of Health Professions, Division of Occupational Therapy at the Medical University of South Carolina (MUSC). She has worked with children with disabilities for over 20 years as a special education teacher and pediatric occupational therapist. Her work in pediatric CIMT started in 2001 when she collaborated with fellow faculty to develop a camp-based constraint therapy program staffed by occupational and physical therapy students enrolled in educational programs at MUSC. During the past decade, Dr. Coker-Bolt has investigated the effects of constraint therapy for infants younger than age 1 year and the outcomes of camp-based constraint therapy programs through grant-funded studies. She continues to train future therapists on evidence-based CIMT models and to speak at national and international conferences.

Stephanie C. DeLuca, PhD, is a developmental psychologist who works to advance pediatric rehabilitation treatments. Her research interests include the relative efficacy of differing therapies that have been scientifically evaluated and validated, the effects of therapeutic dosages on patient outcomes and the documentation of therapy-induced neuroplasticity in response to therapeutic efforts. In collaboration with Ramey, Echols, and Taub, she developed a pediatric CIMT that initially proved to be efficacious in a crossover randomized clinical trial and later in a three-site randomized clinical trial. She served as lead author on a manual for ACQUIREc therapy, a signature form of pediatric CIMT. In 2013, she joined the Virginia Tech Carilion Research Institute as director of its Neuromotor Research Center, which is dedicated to delivering on the promise of evidence-based neurorehabilitation. Dr. DeLuca also holds a faculty appointment at the Jefferson College of Health Sciences, where she helps prepare the next generation of occupational therapists and rehabilitation scientists.

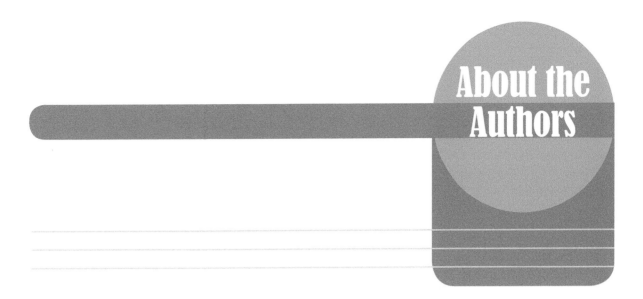

About the Authors

Sarah Blanton, PT, DPT, NCS, is Assistant Professor of Rehabilitation Medicine at Emory University School of Medicine, Division of Physical Therapy, and has been a project coordinator for two multi-site, National Institutes of Health (NIH) funded national clinical trials: the EXCITE (Extremity Constraint Induced Therapy Evaluation) and the ICARE (Interdisciplinary Collaborative Arm Rehabilitation Evaluation) randomized clinical trials. She has a specialty certification in neurology through the American Board of Physical Therapy and helped initiate the Emory Constraint-Induced Therapy Clinic.

Roslyn N. Boyd, PhD, MSc (PT), BSc (Anatomy), Pgrad (Biomechanics), is a pediatric physiotherapist with a doctorate in neuroscience. She is the founder and scientific director of the Queensland Cerebral Palsy and Rehabilitation Research Centre at the University of Queensland. She has led several randomized clinical trials of upper-limb rehabilitation for children with congenital hemiplegia funded by the National Health and Medical Research Council of Australia. These matched-pairs randomized clinical trials have compared modified CIMT directly to bimanual training (INCITE 368500), intensive block training with a distributed model (COMBIT 1003887), and recently a very early action observation training study for infants (UPBEAT 110104292). Her doctoral students and researchers have published numerous clinimetric reviews of outcome measures for children with cerebral palsy.

Jane Case-Smith, EdD, OTR/L, BCP, FAOTA, is Professor and Chair of the Division of Occupational Therapy at the Ohio State University (OSU) School of Health and Rehabilitation Sciences in Columbus. A primary focus of her research has been on interventions to improve children's hand skills and handwriting. Dr. Case-Smith is the senior editor for the textbook *Occupational Therapy for Children,* now in its 6th edition (with a 7th edition being finalized), and has written numerous chapters and articles on hand skill development, families, and evidence-based practice. Dr. Case-Smith was the clinical site principal investigator for a randomized controlled trial of constraint induced movement therapy for preschool-age children (along with Stephanie DeLuca, Richard Stevenson, and Sharon Ramey) that compared the effects of different dosage levels and recently completed a pilot study of CIMT with infants in collaboration with the occupational therapists at Nationwide Children's Hospital in Columbus. She served as editor for *OTJR: Occupation, Participation, and Health* from 2008 to 2011. Dr. Case-Smith has reviewed grants for the NIH and received numerous honors, including the President and Provost's Award for Distinguished Faculty Services at OSU (2012).

Patty Coker-Bolt, PhD, OTR/L, is Associate Professor in the Department of Health Professions, Division of Occupational Therapy at the Medical University of South Carolina (MUSC). She has worked with children with disabilities for over 20 years as a special education teacher and pediatric occupational therapist. Her work in pediatric CIMT started in 2001 when she collaborated with fellow faculty to develop a camp-based constraint therapy program staffed by occupational and physical therapy students enrolled in educational programs at MUSC. During the past decade, Dr. Coker-Bolt has investigated the effects of constraint therapy for infants younger than age 1

XIV HANDBOOK OF PEDIATRIC CONSTRAINT-INDUCED MOVEMENT THERAPY (CIMT)

year and the outcomes of camp-based constraint therapy programs through grant-funded studies. She continues to train future therapists on evidence-based CIMT models and to speak at national and international conferences.

Stephanie C. DeLuca, PhD, is a developmental psychologist who works to advance pediatric rehabilitation treatments. Her research interests include the relative efficacy of differing therapies that have been scientifically evaluated and validated, the effects of therapeutic dosages on patient outcomes, and the documentation of therapy-induced neuroplasticity in response to therapeutic efforts. In collaboration with Ramey, Echols, and Taub, she developed a pediatric CIMT that initially proved to be efficacious in a crossover randomized clinical trial and later in a three-site randomized clinical trial. She served as lead author on a manual for ACQUIREc therapy, a signature form of pediatric CIMT. In 2013, she joined the Virginia Tech Carilion Research Institute as director of its Neuromotor Research Center, which is dedicated to delivering on the promise of evidence-based neurorehabilitation. Dr. DeLuca also holds a faculty appointment at the Jefferson College of Health Sciences, where she helps prepare the next generation of occupational therapists and rehabilitation scientists.

Ann-Christin Eliasson, PhD, obtained her doctorate in neurophysiology from the Karolinska Institute in 1994. During her doctoral training, she studied the motor control of hand function in children with cerebral palsy. She became the first Professor of Pediatric Occupational Therapy in Sweden in 2008. Dr. Eliasson is known for her work on hand function and motor control in children with cerebral palsy that extends from experimental research on force regulation of precision grip and its relation to brain lesion to the development of assessment tools and new interventions. In 2000, she began to develop the approach for using CIMT in young children with cerebral palsy in Sweden and has published several studies on the findings. Dr. Eliasson is affiliated with the Department of Women's and Children's Health, Karolinska Institutet and the Astrid Lindgren Children's Hospital, and Habilitation and Health, both in Stockholm, Sweden.

Stacy L. Fritz, PT, PhD, received her master of science in physical therapy from the University of Kentucky and her doctorate in rehabilitation science from the University of Florida. She is a licensed physical therapist and serves as Assistant Professor and Director of the Physical Therapy Program at the University of South Carolina. Her main research focus is intensive interventions for individuals with chronic neurological disability and the use of walking speed as a vital sign. Her work is funded by the NIH, Department of Defense, American Heart Association, and the Robert Wood Johnson Foundation. She has published in a variety of peer-reviewed journals, including *Stroke, Clinical Gerontologist, Physical Therapy Journal, Journal of Neurologic Physical Therapy, Journal of Geriatric Physical Therapy, Archives of Physical Medicine and Rehabilitation,* and *Neurorehabilitation and Neural Repair.* She has presented locally and internationally on stroke rehabilitation.

Andrew M. Gordon, PhD, is a professor in the Movement Science program at Teachers College, Columbia University, where he has been on the faculty since 1995. He received his MS in Exercise Science from Penn State University and a PhD in Neurophysiology and Pediatrics from the Karolinska Institute in Stockholm. He was then was a postdoctoral fellow in physiology at the University of Minnesota Medical School. In 2001 his group was the first to publish a study about CIMT in children with hemiplegia. In 2004, they developed Hand–Arm Bimanual Intensive training. More than 180 children have participated in this research treatment program. His current work focuses on applying research-based knowledge toward developing evidence-based therapeutic interventions. He has published more than 100 peer-reviewed papers and has had funding from NIH, the National Science Foundation, and private foundations.

Valentina Intagliata, MD, is a native of North Carolina, where she attended the University of North Carolina at Chapel Hill for her undergraduate education, and then went on to pursue a medical degree at Wake Forest University School of Medicine. During her pediatric residency training at the University of Virginia (UVA), she realized her passion for caring for children with neurodevelopmental disabilities. Dr. Intagliata recently completed a fellowship in developmental pediatrics at the Kluge Children's Rehabilitation Center and has been involved with several projects relating to children with cerebral palsy, including constraint therapy, growth, and feeding. She joined the pediatric faculty at UVA in the summer of 2013.

Tasos Karakostas, MPT, PhD, is Associate Director at the Clinical Motion Analysis Center and the Rehabilitation Institute of Chicago and a research scientist at the Ann and Robert H. Lurie Children's Hospital of Chicago He received his doctorate in biomedical engineering from the College of Engineering at The Ohio State University and then earned a master's degree in physical therapy at Texas Tech University. His work involves investigating different aspects of gait, either as an outcome function of different interventions or as a means to identify biomechanical parameters for intervention using neuromusculoskeletal modeling or experimental data collection. During the past few years, he has investigated the effects of pediatric CIMT on walking gait under different conditions. Some of the results of this funded scientific inquiry, which is founded on the principles of corticoplasticity, are presented in this volume.

Erik C. King, MD, MS, is an attending pediatric orthopaedic surgeon in the Division of Orthopaedic Surgery and Sports Medicine at Ann and Robert H. Lurie Children's Hospital of Chicago and Associate Professor of Orthopaedic Surgery at Northwestern University's Feinberg School of Medicine. He is co-director and orthopaedic consultant to the Brachial Plexus Palsy Program at Lurie Children's Hospital. In addition, he serves as a medical consultant for upper-extremity motion analysis in the Motion Analysis Center at the Rehabilitation Institute of Chicago. His clinical interests include congenital and traumatic disorders of the upper extremity.

Reggi Lutenbacher, MS, OTR/L, is an occupational therapist with Intensive Occupational Therapy, an ACQUIREc Therapy Model, University of Alabama (UAB) at Birmingham. She is a 2001 graduate from UAB, receiving a master's degree in occupational therapy. She has spent the past decade applying the ACQUIREc therapy protocol in direct patient treatment. She assisted in developing and implementing the Level II Student Training Program at her facility in addition to training and supervising students throughout their clinical rotations.

Noelle Moreau, PT, PhD, is a physical therapist with doctoral training in biomechanics and postdoctoral training in ultrasonography of muscle architecture. Dr. Moreau's research focuses on the neuromuscular mechanisms underlying abnormal muscle function in people with cerebral palsy and the development of effective rehabilitation strategies to enhance muscle function, activity, and participation. She currently is Assistant Professor in the Department of Physical Therapy at Louisiana State University Health Sciences Center.

Erin Naber, PT, DPT, is a senior physical therapist at Kennedy Krieger Institute. She has worked in the Constraint-Induced Movement Therapy and Bimanual Intensive Therapy program since 2007. She has publications describing outcomes of supported gait training and pediatric CIMT.

Sharon Landesman Ramey, PhD, is Distinguished Research Scholar of Human Development at the Virginia Tech Carilion Research Institute (VTCRI) and Professor of Psychology at Virginia Tech and Professor of Psychiatry and Behavioral Medicine at the Virginia Tech Carilion School of Medicine. Trained as developmental psychologist, she has been engaged in pioneering work in the development and testing of many theory-informed, innovative treatments for children with developmental disabilities since the early 1970s. In the mid-1990s, while serving as the Founding Director of the Civitan International Research Center at the University of Alabama at Birmingham (UAB), Dr. Ramey was the principal investigator on the first randomized controlled trial of pediatric CIMT (working with Deluca, Echols, and Taub) and launched the UAB Pediatric Neuromotor Research Clinic. Her key areas of scientific inquiry and interest include behavioral teratology, school readiness, transition to adulthood, health disparities, and brain development throughout the lifespan. Currently, Dr. Ramey co-directs the VTCRI Neuromotor Research Clinic in Roanoke, Virginia. Her primary focus is on research in the specialty area of Implementation Science with the goal of advancing our understanding of critical factors associated with timely and effective translation of scientific discoveries into mainstream clinical and community-based practice. She has more than 225 publications.

XVI   HANDBOOK OF PEDIATRIC CONSTRAINT-INDUCED MOVEMENT THERAPY (CIMT)

Teressa Garcia Reidy, MS, OTR/L, is Senior Pediatric Occupational Therapist at Kennedy Krieger Institute. She has worked in the Constraint-Induced Movement Therapy and Bimanual Intensive Therapy Program since 2006. She has presented at state, national, and international conferences on a variety of topics, including evidence-based practice, pediatric constraint-induced movement therapy, traumatic brain injury, and occupationally based outcome measures. She has written several publications on the topic of pediatric CIMT.

Leanne Sakzewski, PhD, BOccThy, is a Translating Research into Practice Fellow at the National Health and Medical Research Council and is a pediatric occupational therapist with a doctorate in clinical medicine. Dr. Sakzewski has led a large systematic review of all nonsurgical interventions for children with hemiplegia published in *Pediatrics* and was awarded the American Academy of Cerebral Palsy prestigious Gayle Arnold Award for her doctoral work on the INCITE trial. She has published several landmark clinimetric reviews on the psychometric properties of measures relevant for measuring outcomes of children with hemiplegia.

Richard D. Stevenson, MD, is Professor of Pediatrics and Chief of Developmental Pediatrics and Medical Director of the Kluge Children's Rehabilitation Center and Research Institute at the University of Virginia School of Medicine. He is board-certified in pediatrics and neurodevelopmental disabilities. Dr. Stevenson is currently first vice president of the American Academy for Cerebral Palsy and Developmental Medicine. His primary research has focused on secondary health conditions in children with cerebral palsy. His efforts have been directed toward determining how secondary conditions (e.g., malnutrition, osteoporosis, aspiration, chronic pain) affect the health, functional abilities, social participation, and quality of life of children with cerebral palsy and their families. He was the principal investigator of the North American Growth in Cerebral Palsy Project, a multicenter, region-based study of growth and nutritional status, and has participated in several multicenter trials. Recent funding efforts have focused on CIMT for hemiplegia and practice-based evidence research (comparative effectiveness) in the multidisciplinary care of children with cerebral palsy. He is a co-principal investigator on an NIH multisite randomized clinical trial of CIMT in young children with unilateral cerebral palsy.

Mary Rebekah Trucks, MS, OTR/L, is a Senior Therapist at the Virginia Tech Carilion Research Institute Neuromotor Research Clinic in Roanoke, Virginia. She has 13 years of experience in the research and clinical application of pediatric CIMT and was part of the University of Alabama at Birmingham Pediatric Neuromotor Clinic since its inception in 1998. She assisted in developing the clinical applications of ACQUIREc therapy and pediatric CIMT and has trained numerous therapists in this approach. She has presented at several state and national occupational therapy association meetings.

Dory Ainsworth Wallace, MS, OTR/L, is currently a Senior Therapist at the Virginia Tech Carilion Research Institute Neuromotor Research Clinic in Roanoke, Virginia. She has been an occupational therapist since 2003, practicing in a variety of settings from school systems to a skilled nursing facility. The majority of her career, however, was spent at the Pediatric Neuromotor Clinic at the University of Alabama at Birmingham. For 8 years, she assisted in the clinical implementation of the ACQUIREc therapy protocol, supervised other treating therapists, and trained other professionals in the ACQUIREc protocols. She has presented at both state and national occupational therapy association meetings.

Steven L. Wolf, PhD, PT, FAPTA, FAHA, is a Professor in the Department of Rehab Medicine and a Medicine Professor in the Department of Cell Biology at Emory University School of Medicine, a Professor of Health and Elder Care at the Nell Hodgson Woodruff School of Nursing at Emory University, and a Senior Research Scientist at the Atlanta VA Rehab R&D Center. Dr. Wolf received his bachelor's degree in biology from Clark University, his physical therapy certificate from Columbia University, master's degree in physical therapy from Boston University, and doctorate in neurophysiology from Emory University. He has defined the selection criteria for the application of electromyography biofeedback to restore upper-extremity function among chronic patients with stroke. These findings became the inclusion criteria for most CIMT stroke studies. He recently completed his role as principal investigator for the NIH–funded EXCITE trial, the first multicenter, Phase III, upper-extremity stroke rehabilitation study funded by NIH. He has served in multiple administrative and leadership capacities for the American Physical Therapy Association and for groups associated with the promotion of research and clinical service within neurorehabilitation. He is the recipient of numerous awards for his research and clinical contributions.

Michelle L. Woodbury, PhD, OTR/L, is Assistant Professor in the Department of Health and Rehabilitation Science and Division of Occupational Therapy, Medical University of South Carolina. Dr. Woodbury received a bachelor's degree in occupational therapy from Elizabethtown College in Elizabethtown, Pennsylvania, and was a full-time neurorehabilitation occupational therapist for 12 years before receiving a doctorate in rehabilitation science from the University of Florida. She was involved with several adult CIMT research projects, published a secondary analysis of EXCITE data, and co-developed a pediatric CIMT day camp. Her current research is focused on the development and clinical implementation of meaningful measurement tools and effective rehabilitation programs to promote upper-extremity recovery in those with neurological injury or disease.

LIST OF FIGURES, TABLES, EXHIBITS, CASE EXAMPLES, AND APPENDIXES

FIGURES

TABLES

EXHIBITS

CASE EXAMPLES

APPENDIXES

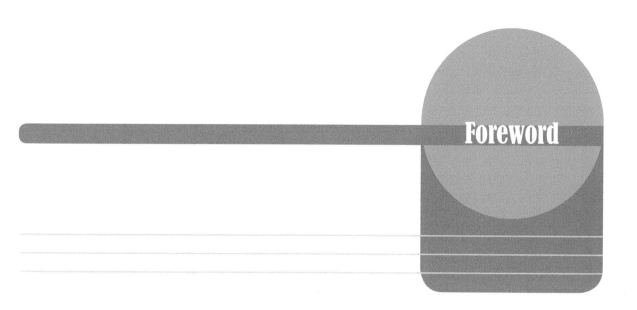

Cerebral palsy (CP) is not a disease; it is a group of disorders with varying causes, clinical phenotypes, levels of severity, and associated problems. As early as 1843, Dr. William Little described a condition with lower- and upper-extremity contractures that became known as "Little's disease." He recognized the role of the central nervous system and that the condition usually resulted from an identifiable onetime event, such as a difficult birth. In 1889, the renowned physician Sir William Osler popularized the term *cerebral palsy* in his book, *The Cerebral Palsies of Children.*

To distinguish CP from progressive conditions that present with similar initial neurological manifestations but worsen over time (e.g., leukodystrophy, mitochondrial disorder), the definition of CP that evolved restricted its application to nonprogressive lesions of the brain. Still, neurologists did not like the term *CP* because of its wide variability and non-specificity. They preferred *static encephalopathy.* Other practitioners gradually adopted the same term but for a different reason: Insurance companies began rejecting CP as a reimbursable diagnosis. Soon, *static encephalopathy* was being widely used as an insurance code for CP and other brain disorders, such as autism and even developmental delay.

It has become increasingly and definitively clear in recent years that CP is anything but a static disorder. The brain continues to mature in function and organization (the best that it can) in spite of injury. This has become evident due to the emergence of sophisticated imaging techniques, such as diffusion tensor imaging, functional magnetic resonance imaging, and magnetoencephalography. The challenge for the health care practitioner is enhancement of this naturally occurring reparative phenomenon with evidence-based treatment. One promising therapeutic approach is constraint-induced movement therapy (CIMT).

Following preliminary animal work by Taub (1980), Ostendorf and Wolf (1981) reported that forced use of the affected limb in adults post stroke resulted in persistently improved motor control. Similarly, CIMT was shown to be effective for children with asymmetric motor impairment associated with CP (Taub, Ramey, DeLuca, & Echols, 2004). The majority of studies of CIMT in children have demonstrated a positive effect, but there has been continuing consideration of the type and duration of constraint, the importance of bimanual training, and cost–benefit issues. An intriguing and important question still to be answered is, What is the optimal age or ages for receiving CIMT? On one hand, is there an age beyond which CIMT is no longer highly effective? On the other hand, could restraint of a limb, even temporarily, have a deleterious effect on an infant brain, which is normally reorganizing ipsilateral and crossover corticospinal tracts (i.e., the brain's main conduits to the peripheral motor nerves)?

Some of the most exciting recent research developments illustrate a relationship between clinical improvement in extremity use and changes in brain function and structure following CIMT. Sutcliffe, Gaetz, Logan, Cheyne, and Fehlings (2007) were the first to demonstrate cortical reorganization after CIMT in a child with hemiplegia. Understanding what is occurring in the brain as a result of therapies such as CIMT may be helpful in achieving the most natural and therefore optimal results. Ultimately, improvements in activities of daily living, reduction of frustration, participation in age-appropriate activities, and enhanced quality of life are the most important outcomes of CIMT.

As CIMT for children becomes widely accepted and implemented for children with CP and related neuromotor disorders, it is imperative that practitioners have a comprehensive grasp of its theory and practice. This volume by Ramey, Coker-Bolt, and DeLuca explores and elucidates the diverse and important strands of knowledge regarding pediatric CIMT (P–CIMT). It will be useful to practitioners in a wide array of fields: occupational therapy, physical therapy, medicine, nursing, psychology, education, and administration. The book reflects well the international clinical and research partnerships that have brought P–CIMT to its current level of maturity.

This *Handbook of Pediatric Constraint-Induced Movement Therapy (CIMT)* is a valuable, and perhaps mandatory, resource for anyone who intends to use, prescribe, or provide this therapeutic technique. It also is a strong scientific history for those interested in pursuing future research in pediatric rehabilitation, CP, and neuroplasticity.

—James A. Blackman, MD, MPH
Medical Director
Cerebral Palsy International Research Foundation
Professor of Pediatrics Emeritus
University of Virginia

REFERENCES

Osler, W. (1889). *The cerebral palsies of children: A clinical study from the infirmary for nervous diseases, Philadelphia.* London: H. K. Lewis.

Ostendorf, C. G., & Wolf, S. L. (1984). Effect of forced use of the upper extremity of a hemiplegic patient on changes in function. *Physical Therapy, 61,* 1022–1027.

Sutcliffe, T. L., Gaetz, W. C., Logan, W. J., Cheyne, D. O., & Fehlings, D. L. (2007). Cortical reorganization after modified constraint-induced movement therapy in pediatric hemiplegic cerebral palsy. *Journal of Child Neurology, 22,* 1281–1287.

Taub, E. (1980). Somatosensory deafferentation research with monkeys: Implications for rehabilitation medicine. In L. P. Ince (Ed.), *Behavioral psychology in rehabilitation medicine: Clinical applications* (pp. 371–401). New York: Williams & Wilkins.

Taub, E., Ramey, S. L., DeLuca, S., & Echols, K. (2004). Efficacy of constraint-induced movement therapy for children with cerebral palsy with asymmetric motor impairment. *Pediatrics, 113,* 305–312. PMID: 14754942

SHARON LANDESMAN RAMEY, PhD; PATTY COKER-BOLT, PhD, OTR/L; and STEPHANIE C. DeLUCA, PhD

Introduction

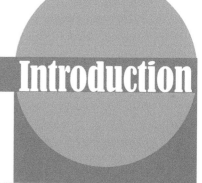

The *Handbook of Pediatric Constraint-Induced Movement Therapy (CIMT)* is possible because of the decades of basic and clinical research that have informed the development and application of a new set of therapy practices that produce positive and sustainable benefits for children with asymmetrical upper extremity (UE) impairments. In a period of about 15 years, pediatric constraint-induced movement therapy (P–CIMT) has transformed from a highly promising practice showing impressive gains in a few reported case studies to one that has been proven efficacious (to varying degrees with a variety of outcome measures) in multiple clinical trials throughout the world.

The initial skepticism from clinicians about whether such a highly intensive form of therapy, combined with constraint, would be feasible to adopt in clinical practice or modify for use in school and home settings has shifted to a fairly high level of current enthusiasm. This enthusiasm often is amplified after practitioners receive training in P–CIMT techniques and then observe firsthand how rapidly children with moderate and even severe forms of hemiparesis can acquire new and improved UE skills. Many experienced pediatric rehabilitation specialists (e.g., occupational therapists, physical therapists, pediatric physiatrists, early education interventionists) report that P–CIMT produces changes of a type and magnitude that were unprecedented in their years of providing therapy in traditional settings at traditional (low) dosages. One physical therapist, a leader in establishing community and home-based early intervention services for children with developmental disabilities and a pioneer in shaping pediatric practices in her community, shared her direct experiences with providing a 6-hour-per-day, 21-consecutive-day protocol of P–CIMT that used full-arm, semi-rigid casting on the less-impaired UE. She told us,

All of these years I really believed I was helping "my children" a lot. The children I worked with always seemed to be getting better. Their parents were very appreciative of what I did for their children and for them. I used a lot of different techniques from what I learned in graduate school and from attending professional meetings and reading the practice journals. Most of what I did could be considered under the broad label of *neurodevelopmental treatment (NDT)* that was almost universally adopted by all pediatric therapists (and continued even after strong research in the 1980s showed it did not produce measurable benefits). Like most of my colleagues, I described my practice as "eclectic," meaning that I used every technique possible to help a given child. I think that over the decades I developed a clinical sensitivity that allowed me to adjust what I offered to each child so that he or she would progress as best as possible.

Now after I have seen the benefits of P–CIMT myself, I realize what I did before was far less beneficial than I thought. Truthfully, I had never, ever seen young children with severe hemiparesis change *that much and so fast.* Some of the children who received P–CIMT started with almost no voluntary movements and no functional activities with their hemiparetic arm and hand. After only 3 weeks of daily treatment, these children could complete some important daily tasks with a lot of voluntary control. All of the children I worked with had a very positive response, and not a single one was a "non-responder." P–CIMT has radically changed my expectations for how much progress a child can make! I also think the children have a fresh view of themselves, knowing how much progress they can make with their own hard work. (The therapy *is* hard work.) In the past, these children never saw such large changes in so short a time period, even when they really "tried hard." With P–CIMT, using a highly structured approach that provides immediate and specific feedback to children, through the shaping activities and repetitive practice, they experience amazing progress. The parents and teachers also now see a much brighter future for the children after they changed so much. I think that P–CIMT has raised the expectations bar to a much higher level than what I had been taught was possible.

In retrospect, I had become fairly set in my ways, although I did not realize it. It is only because I tried this new approach and saw the results for myself that I now appreciate how important it is for all pediatric therapists to remain open-minded and receptive to trying things. For sure, P–CIMT is very different from what most of were taught and what we were practicing. My dream is that the scientific results really get shared with all therapists in ways that they can understand and translate into accurate and successful practice.

Indeed, this handbook has been prepared to help fulfill that dream of sharing what has been learned, throughout the world, by those who have developed, tested, evaluated, and refined P–CIMT.

PURPOSE OF THE HANDBOOK

The purpose of this handbook is to provide an integrative history about CIMT that includes the major research findings, the theoretical underpinnings of CIMT, practical guidelines for practitioners and health care providers, and peer-reviewed information for students preparing to be pediatric practitioners and educators.

Collectively, the scientific findings provide strong support for P–CIMT as a treatment strategy that can—and often does—produce measurable benefits to children with impairment in use of their UEs. This book is timely. We seek to present current, state-of-the-art findings balanced by the perspectives of practitioners who work directly with children in a wide array of clinical, community, educational, and home settings. We also present the thoughtful caution of scientists who realize there are still many important questions to be

answered about what comprises the optimal CIMT protocol for individual children.

Worldwide, hundreds of practitioners have read about and tried to implement, as best as they can, their own versions of P–CIMT. We estimate that P–CIMT, often in a partial and less-intensive form, has now been delivered to thousands of children. Further, preservice education and training programs throughout the world now include information about CIMT as part of graduate education to prepare pediatric rehabilitation therapists; increasingly, inservice and continuing education programs are offered on P–CIMT. We responded to the request to bring together, in a single volume, content written by P–CIMT's leading contributors. This peer-reviewed handbook offers up-to-date summary information that provides a solid framework for understanding the principles and practice of P–CIMT.

Two themes recur throughout this handbook: First, pediatric rehabilitation is a dynamic field that seeks and benefits from active inquiry and exchange of information among basic scientists, practitioners, clinical investigators, program administrators, and families. For some, the rapid infusion of new knowledge and the expectation (the new norm) that clinical treatment protocols will continually need to be revised to produce better functional outcomes and quality of life is exciting. For others, this can be challenging, particularly when there is no reliable primary source of information readily available to assist in this ongoing adaptation within clinical practice. Second, recognizing that many forms of promising and evidence-backed strategies to improve children's functional outcomes and quality of life exist complicates making clinical decisions.

Recently, the National Research Council (NRC; 2011) at the National Academy of Sciences advanced a new model that is termed *precision medicine*. For our field, we advance the proposition that precision therapy can be a new model in which there is strong endorsement for implementing practices that have generated solid, but not yet definitive, evidence. At the same time, precision practice embraces making further refinements to maximize individualization of therapy. We conclude that the evidence is sufficient to endorse responsible, informed application of P–CIMT for many children by using a variety of proven protocols. We simultaneously endorse the high-priority need for expansion of scientific investigation to improve our ability to deliver precision therapy to children worldwide. Indeed, every author contributing to this handbook has endorsed this dual conclusion about P–CIMT: It has tremendous promise on the basis of realized benefits and has many unanswered questions about how to further refine and individualize P–CIMT, alone and in combination with many other therapeutic approaches, to achieve the greatest benefits possible for children with neuromotor impairments.

Our primary goals in preparing this handbook were to

- Review the history of the development of P–CIMT, a direct extension and adaptation of a treatment originally developed to help adults labeled as *chronic stroke patients* who seemed to reach plateaus in their recovery of prior normal function;
- Lay the theoretical groundwork for understanding the components of P–CIMT and intensive therapy programs;
- Provide a medical and clinical context for understanding the needs and development of children with cerebral palsy (CP) and related conditions resulting in hemiparesis;
- Offer a vision about neuroplasticity as a process across the lifespan that can be stimulated by and help support evidence-based rehabilitation practices;
- Share the practical details about the major forms of P–CIMT that have been developed and tested in clinical research studies, so therapists and families can understand the current available choices;
- Discuss promising alternative and complementary rehabilitation treatments for hemiparesis, so decisions about when and for whom P–CIMT should be recommended can take place within the context of a much broader picture about intervention options;
- Identify highly salient research priorities for strategic investment, so the field can effectively lobby for and collaborate around the issues that will significantly affect the health and well-being of children with hemiparesis; and
- Raise awareness about the bigger health care policy world that influences the treatment options and choices made by clinicians and families.

The *Handbook of Pediatric Constraint-Induced Movement Therapy (CIMT)* gives the field a balanced and comprehensive set of papers specifically designed to support well-informed use of P–CIMT in all practice settings with a wide range of children. This text also serves to train future practitioners in the theory and practice of P–CIMT.

For third-party payers and for early interventionists who require clear support for selecting and covering the costs of particular occupational therapy and physical therapy interventions, this publication provides ample evidence from scores of peer-reviewed journal articles that is compared and synthesized by the contributing authors.

Highly practical ideas abound in this text, with many suggestions about how to adapt P–CIMT to settings that have limited therapy resources and services. With this, parents can gain understanding of P–CIMT and become more knowledgeable about it as one of the treatment options to consider for their children at different stages in their lives.

Collectively, this publication demonstrates how the evolution of P–CIMT as an emerging practice that attracted scientists and therapists worldwide can serve as a model developing future innovative therapy interventions for our rehabilitative health care and educational systems that serve children and conducting multidisciplinary scientific inquiry that moves a field from basic science discoveries into full translational research with active monitoring of widespread clinical application in diverse community settings.

PRECISION THERAPY: A NEW VISION FOR PEDIATRIC REHABILITATION

In this handbook, precision practice is a construct that identifies a new era that is driven by the dynamic intersection between scientific discovery and rapid, effective, and individualized therapy. In an era of precision practice, all of the individuals engaged in making diagnoses, recommending treatments, delivering treatments, and monitoring treatment effects would be guided by up-to-date, trustworthy scientific findings that increasingly are refined "precisely" for the needs of different individuals at different times in their lives and under different environmental situations. Precision practice represents how practitioners and patients can truly individualize treatments and how others can benefit (i.e., knowledge accrual) by sharing their results of the outcomes that are detected when alterations are made in delivering varied treatments to individuals. Rather than relying solely on firsthand clinical experiences and distant reading and interpretation of scientific findings, patients and practitioners can learn from what happens to others and be able to actively monitor their responses to treatments so that adjustments can be made to maximize benefits and prevent any negative (i.e., iatrogenic) consequences.

The NRC (2011) released a landmark report, *Toward Precision Medicine: Building a Knowledge Network for Biomedical Research and a New Taxonomy of Disease,* that proposed that the field of medicine could be dramatically advanced by establishing a new shared data network to integrate emerging research findings (primarily about molecular discoveries) about diseases with clinical data about individual patients with the explicit goals of

- Developing a more accurate classification of diseases,
- Enhancing specificity of evidence-based treatment recommendations, and
- Improving patient outcomes.

The newly proposed shared data network was envisioned as something that could enable scientists to obtain direct patient information during treatment while fully protecting their rights to privacy, confidentiality, and anonymity. Such a network was characterized further as allowing basic science and clinical data to converge at the point of care, in contrast to research information remaining largely in academia.

As editors of this volume, we were deeply moved by and felt a true connection with what Dr. Susan Desmond-Hellman, the co-chairperson of the committee that authored this report, said in a National Academies (2011) press release,

> Currently, a disconnect exists between the wealth of scientific advances in research and the incorporation of this information into the clinic. . . . In addition researchers don't have access to comprehensive and timely information from the clinic. . . . Overall, opportunities are being missed to understand, diagnose, and treat diseases more precisely, and to better inform health care decisions.

This is exactly what we were seeing as major disconnects in the field of pediatric rehabilitation.

All too often, rehabilitation practitioners do not receive timely, sufficiently complete, or clinically useful findings that they can translate into direct practice improvements in their clinical care for children with neuromotor disorders. Similarly, many scientists engaged in research studies impose (with a solid rationale) strict controls over the eligibility criteria for enrolling children in clinical trials and then they deliver the innovative treatment under "nearly ideal conditions" to test its efficacy. This control can lead to a situation in which the new research evidence is quite trustworthy (i.e., reliable and valid) but often quite limited when it comes to being translated into routine clinical practice. This is because many patients with a given condition, such as hemiparetic CP, are likely to differ in ways from the relatively homogeneous samples enrolled in the randomized controlled trials. These differences may be small (e.g., slightly older or younger, slightly more or less impaired), but frequently the differences are large and many (e.g., much different in their age, having serious co-morbid conditions, receiving pharmacological or surgical interventions close to or during the treatment period).

In addition, when practitioners in existing clinics and rehabilitation environments seek to adapt new research findings into their current practices, they often encounter many of practical challenges that the researchers failed to consider or are beyond the practitioners' control to change. Clearly, efforts to bridge this gap between practitioners and scientists need to be more vigorous, systematic, and monitored for their effectiveness. What excited us the most when we learned about the NRC report about how precision medicine could operate over time was that it would be an evolving and actively sustained system, well-suited to systematic study and open sharing of what has been learned.

Therefore, we propose a parallel effort for the field of evidence-driven pediatric rehabilitation. Our proposal to move in the direction of what we have named *precision practice* is not identical to that proposed for medicine (i.e., it is unlikely to be as linked to molecular discoveries about individual differences, but a time may come when more precise neuroimaging of the brain as it actually functions could lead be more precise tailoring of diagnoses and treatments). Precision practice would be driven by the same recognized gap and strive to reach the same goal of providing more patients with appropriately individualized treatments that improve their health and well-being. In Figure I.1, we illustrate a model for our field that would establish a network that engages leading scientists and clinicians worldwide in sharing data that will permit rapid accumulation of new knowledge, while engaged in ongoing delivery of therapy and continued research on high-priority issues that need resolution.

Figure I.1 illustrates a proposed system that offers rapid and open exchange of emerging information related to P–CIMT, alone and in combination with other therapies and services. Undoubtedly, many vital details and strategies to adequately vet new knowledge for accuracy, clarity, and relevance would need to be tried and then evaluated and refined, but moving our field forward as we strive to realize precision therapy is compelling and urgently needed.

Figure I.1 represents a translational systems framework to develop an evidence-based treatment taxonomy. This system incorporates information from research findings and clinical observations—in clearly defined, well-operationalized terms—that become available through the knowledge network and information resources. The framework permits contributions from and use by the interrelated fields relevant to P–CIMT and children with neuromotor disabilities, ranging from pediatric neurology, developmental pediatrics, behavioral pediatrics, physiatry and rehabilitation medicine, general pediatrics, and psychiatry to the specialty fields that often provide the long-term supports and direct therapies, including occupation therapy, physical therapy, psychology, speech and communication therapy, and education. Indeed, this systems framework provides a place for almost all of the information that is contained in this handbook.

HOW THIS HANDBOOK IS ORGANIZED

This handbook is divided into four sections:
- Section I. History and Theory of CIMT for Children With Cerebral Palsy
- Section II. Clinical Applications, Protocols, and Individualization
- Section III. Collaboration and Coordination With Families and Other Professionals
- Section IV. Future for Research, Policy, and Practice.

Figure I.1 PRECISION PRACTICE: A TRANSLATIONAL SYSTEMS FRAMEWORK INTEGRATING CURRENT RESEARCH, PEDIATRIC REHABILITATION APPROACHES, AND P–CIMT.

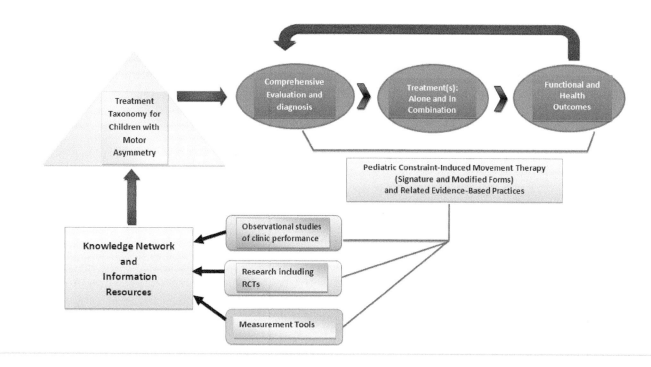

Section I provides historical context for understanding the origins of CIMT as initially developed for adult stroke patients (Chapter 1, "History and Development of CIMT for Adults With Stroke") and then adapted for and tested in pediatric populations (Chapter 2, "Pediatric CIMT: History and Definition"). Background information critical to the theory and practice principles guiding CIMT as applied in pediatric practice (Chapter 3, "Applying Occupation and Motor Learning Principles in Pediatric CIMT: Theoretical Foundations and Conceptual Framework") is complemented by an overview of the clinical issues related to children with CP (Chapter 4, "Motor Development and Physical Growth in Children With Cerebral Palsy") and how muscle and skeletal adaptations occur in this clinical population (Chapter 5, "Muscle Structural Adaptation in Cerebral Palsy and Relationship to Function"). Section I concludes with a chapter that addresses vital issues about how to assess UE functioning and the effects of P–CIMT on outcomes (Chapter 6, "Assessment Tools to Measure Upper-Limb Function and Impact of Therapy").

Section II focuses on the clinical applications and key issues that practitioners face in identifying children likely to benefit from P–CIMT and individualizing treatment protocols for diverse clinical pediatric groups. The first chapter in this section (Chapter 7, "Operationalizing Pediatric CIMT: Guidelines for Transforming Basic Principles and Scientific Evidence Into Clinical Practice for Individual Children")

provides an organizational framework for understanding the major classification scheme for different forms of P–CIMT, specifically delineating whether the therapy qualifies as signature or traditional P–CIMT, modified P–CIMT, or alternative P–CIMT. Chapter 7 also advocates adopting standard terminology to describe the components of P–CIMT and describes a framework for measuring the fidelity of implementation (i.e., the degree to which P–CIMT as actually provided to individual children adheres to the treatment protocol or intended therapy plan). Chapter 8, "ACQUIREc Protocol: What We Have Learned From a Decade of Delivering a Signature Form of Pediatric CIMT"; Chapter 9, "Alternative Pediatric CIMT: Understanding the How and Why of Clinical Variations in Pediatric CIMT"; and Chapter 10, "Group-Based Models of Pediatric CIMT: Special Camps, School-Based Treatment, and Home Environment Models," provide many clinical details and case histories about particular forms or protocols of P–CIMT to help practitioners and families make informed decisions that are grounded in both scientific evidence and practical clinical experience.

Chapter 11, "Adapting Pediatric CIMT for Children with Acquired Brain Injury, Brachial Plexus Palsy, Hemispherectomy, and Related Conditions," offers many ideas about how to individualize P–CIMT for certain distinctive clinical groups on the basis of actual case histories. Similarly, Chapter 12, "Novel and Complementary Therapy Strategies: Critical Issues and Opportunities for Combining With Pediatric CIMT," and Chapter 13, "Intensive Bimanual Training Approaches to Upper-Extremity Rehabilitation in Children With Cerebral Palsy," cover topics about other therapy approaches that are highly promising and may complement or be combined with P–CIMT, some of which already have supportive evidence about their efficacy. The concluding chapter for this section (Chapter 14, "Beyond Upper-Extremity Benefits of Pediatric CIMT: Reported Changes in Gait and Other Neuromotor Skills") addresses the possibility that P–CIMT contributes to improvements in areas that extend beyond the primary targeted therapy goals of improving UE function and movement. Although the documented "spillover effects" primarily concern lower-extremity changes, Chapter 14 raises an intriguing possibility about how therapy can trigger neuroplasticity (i.e., changes in the central nervous system) that influences other domains of development, health, and engagement.

Section III addresses a central topic that all pediatric practitioners recognize and incorporate into their treatment plans for children: How to work well with parents and other professionals who also care for and serve the same children. Because P–CIMT is highly distinctive and potentially demanding for families and children, this topic warrants thoughtful incorporation into the delivery of P–CIMT. In addition, the theoretical foundations of P–CIMT underscore that maintaining and even enhancing the benefits of P–CIMT rely on the extent to which children use their new and improved skills in their everyday routines and lives. Chapter 15, "Working With Families and Therapy Teams to Maximize Pediatric CIMT Benefits" also contains parent perspectives and a mother's detailed, compelling account of her son's journey with P–CIMT. Thus, to realize the maximal benefits of P–CIMT, practitioners seek to engage parents and other professionals in effectively understanding and delivering practice and routines.

Finally, Section IV looks forward by identifying some of the most urgent research topics that warrant new scientific studies to provide strong data to resolve areas where clinical uncertainties remain and to offer further innovations to promote the delivery of "precision practice" to all children with hemiparesis and related neuromotor conditions (Chapter 16, "Research Priorities: Understanding and Transcending the Limits of Current Knowledge to Inform Best Practices in Pediatric CIMT"). In addition to hypothesis-driven research for rigorous clinical trials, this chapter also considers the importance of further advances in assessment, understanding implementation science (i.e., how to rapidly and effectively put into practice and community settings those interventions proven to improve children's outcomes), and policy change.

The handbook concludes with an appendix that contains a rich repository of information about original research articles in peer-reviewed journals concerning the effects of P–CIMT, and a flash drive contains several useful forms.

HOW TO USE THIS HANDBOOK

We asked authors to write their contributions focused on a primary topic or issue. As such, each chapter can be read on its own. However, most authors struggled with wanting to write more about many of the topics addressed in other chapters, because they see them as closely intertwined (in some situations, we did restrict the range and length of the chapters to avoid excessive duplication). Another approach to the handbook is to study the chapters in order, starting with history and theory and then moving to the pragmatic issues from measurement and health concerns and unanticipated positive effects (i.e., spillover effects to gait and other functional domains) to in-depth presentation of a variety of clinical applications that have demonstrated measurable benefits by applying some or all of the elements of the "traditional" CIMT originally developed for treating adults with chronic stroke. The final section looks ahead and outlines the horizon for future research and a consideration of the policy and reimbursement issues that are an inescapable part of the reality of providing treatment services.

P–CIMT is an exciting treatment approach, approaching a solid evidence base but still with notable debates and uncertainties about what constitutes the optimal therapy format for individual children over the course of development. We hope this handbook will be a valuable resource for practitioners, scientists, students, parents, and policymakers. Above all, we are deeply appreciative of the substantial work and service of the authors and their colleagues who have made this handbook a reality.

CONCLUSION

Finally, we share an observation that relates to the choice of the cover photograph for this handbook, which shows a group of energetic children charging ahead. Clearly, the lives of these children are embedded socially—they are going to school, and their arms and hands and body posture all are naturally integral to their success. The occupations of children include learning, playing, taking care of themselves, and participating in social relationships. In this photograph, no single child is identified as "the one with a disability," nor is there a display of the hard work that children have done to be as accomplished as they are in their everyday lives. Rather, we think that the forward movement and energy of this photograph capture the goals of pediatric rehabilitation: to help every child fulfill his or her potential and to maximize engagement in the full range of important and personalized activities of childhood en route to becoming independent, contributing, and healthy adults.

REFERENCES

National Academies. (2011). *Report calls for creation of a biomedical research and patient data network for more accurate classification of diseases, move toward "precision medicine"* [Press release]. Retrieved from http://www8.national academies.org/onpinews/newsitem.aspx?recordid=13284

National Research Council, Committee on a Framework for Development of a New Taxonomy of Disease. (2011). *Toward precision medicine: Building a knowledge network for biomedical research and a new taxonomy of disease.* Washington, DC: National Academies Press.

section I

Theory and History of CIMT for Children With Cerebral Palsy

MICHELLE L. WOODBURY, PhD, OTR/L;
STACY L. FRITZ, PT, PhD; SARAH BLANTON, PT, DPT, NCS;
and STEVEN L. WOLF, PhD, PT, FAPTA, FAHA

History and Development of CIMT for Adults With Stroke

CHAPTER HIGHLIGHTS

- Definition of constraint-induced movement therapy (CIMT)
- History and development of CIMT
- Theoretical foundation of CIMT
- CIMT and other task-oriented upper-extremity rehabilitation approaches
- Defining CIMT outcomes
- Choosing the appropriate outcome measures
- Practicality of CIMT methods
- Alternative methods of CIMT
- Reimbursement options.

KEY TERMS

Active ingredients
Adaptive task practice
Bimanual task practice
Cortical motor representations
Deafferentation
Dendritic branching
Excitability
EXCITE multisite randomized clinical trial
Forced use
Interhemispheric inhibition
Learned nonuse
Mirror neuron system
Modified CIMT
Neuroplasticity
New skill
Repetitive task practice
Shaping
Signature form of CIMT
Skill training
Synapse growth
Synaptic responses
Task-oriented training
Unimanual task practice

Historically, constraint-induced movement therapy (CIMT) has been a rehabilitation approach for adults with stroke (Ostendorf & Wolf, 1981; Taub et al., 1993; Wolf, Lecraw, Barton, & Jann, 1989; Wolf et al., 2006). More recently, it has become a useful approach for improving functional arm and hand movement abilities in children with hemiplegia caused by cerebral palsy (DeLuca, Case-Smith, Stevenson, & Ramey, 2012), traumatic brain injury (Cimolin et al., 2012), or hemispherectomy (de Bode, Fritz, Weir-Haynes, & Mathern, 2009).

This chapter explores the history and development of CIMT for adults with stroke, discusses how CIMT is similar to and different from other upper-extremity (UE) therapeutic interventions, explores how the treatment effect of CIMT is defined on the basis of assessments

3

chosen to measure outcomes, and introduces novel modes of CIMT service delivery. Although CIMT has historical roots in neuroscience (Franz, Scheetz, & Wilson, 1915; Knapp, Taub, & Berman, 1963; Wolf & Binder-MacLeod, 1983), psychology (Taub et al., 1994), and motor learning (Ostendorf & Wolf, 1981; Page, Boe, & Levine, 2013; Wolf, Blanton, Baer, Breshears, & Butler, 2002; Wolf et al., 1989), it is currently applied by an interprofessional team, including occupational therapy practitioners (Page et al., 2013), who share a common goal to improve an adult or pediatric client's ability to successfully use his or her *paretic* (i.e., neurologically weaker) arm to accomplish daily activities in meaningful home and community contexts.

WHAT IS CIMT?

CIMT is a rehabilitative strategy to increase functional use of the paretic UE through repetitive and adaptive task practice while the nonparetic UE is restrained (Taub et al., 1993; Wolf, 2007; Wolf et al., 1989). **Adaptive task practice,** or **shaping,** involves breaking down a task into several smaller, more manageable components to improve the client's overall efficiency in learning the task. The **signature form of CIMT** involves wearing a constraint mitt on the nonparetic UE for 90% of waking hours over a 14-day period. During this time, the client participates in up to 6 hours of daily training for 10 weekdays with the paretic UE (Taub & Morris, 2001; Wolf et al., 2006).

The results of many CIMT studies provide exciting evidence that motor recovery of the affected UE can occur in adults with mild to moderate levels of UE movement impairment after stroke—that is, in people who retain some residual, purposeful movement of the paretic UE (Corbetta, Sirtori, Moja, & Gatti, 2010; Duncan, 1997; Kunkel et al., 1999; Miltner, Bauder, Sommer, Dettmers, & Taub, 1999; Morris, Crago, DeLuca, Pidikiti, & Taub, 1997; Shi, Tian, Yang, & Zhao, 2011; Sirtori, Corbetta, Moja, & Gatti, 2010; Taub & Morris, 2001; Wolf et al., 2006). Most research to date, however, has included heterogeneous samples, which may mask the improvement of certain subgroups. Nevertheless, several studies have shown that delivery of this intensive intervention to stroke survivors who are at least 3 months post stroke (Wolf et al., 2006) may be the most appropriate approach because some evidence suggests that a 3-hour version of CIMT may not be as effective as traditional therapy in the first few weeks after a stroke (Dromerick et al., 2009).

Research findings also indicate that, in general, people with higher levels of motor ability before CIMT tend to demonstrate greater improvements with CIMT than those with lower motor ability (Fritz, Light, Patterson, Behrman, & Davis, 2005; Taub, Crago, & Uswatte, 1998). For example,

the ability to release a mass flexion grasp pretreatment is a predictor of improved motor performance after CIMT (Fritz et al., 2005). More research into selection criteria for therapy participation should be carefully conducted to determine the circumstances and attributes that define those neurological patients who best respond to this intervention.

HISTORY AND DEVELOPMENT OF CIMT

The theoretical foundation of CIMT can be traced to the early 1900s, when experimental findings demonstrated that motor disabilities experienced by monkeys rendered hemiplegic by pyramidal tract lesions were accentuated through disuse, or what Franz et al. (1915) labeled "uncared-for paralyses." Evidence of recovery was seen when the unimpaired upper limb was immobilized to "compel" the animal to use the paretic limb (Ogden & Franz, 1917). Return of function was thought to be attributable to behavioral recovery and possible reorganization of cortical neural networks governing limb movement (i.e., cortical neuroplasticity; Ogden & Franz, 1917).

From the 1960s through the 1980s, a series of experiments was conducted on primates who underwent **deafferentation**— that is, disruption of the sensory nerve—of one forelimb (Knapp et al., 1963; Morris et al., 1997; Taub et al., 1993). After surgery, the animals had great difficulty using the deafferented limb because movements were clumsy. Attempts to use the limb to feed or climb failed; thus, the animals exhibited **learned nonuse** of that extremity, or nonuse of the affected limb because of a conditioned suppression of movement (Russo, 1995; Taub, Uswatte, & Pidikiti, 1999).

These early studies involving deafferented primates led to a testable hypothesis in humans with stroke. Studies investigated the effects of **forced use,** in which the nonparetic limb of a person with stroke was immobilized over several days, forcing the person to use only the paretic limb during daily activities (Ostendorf & Wolf, 1981; Wolf et al., 1989). Forced use was different from CIMT because it did not involve any specified one-on-one training or provision of adaptive task practice or shaping. Rather, it engaged the person in **repetitive task practice,** or continuous efforts to execute functional movements using the paretic limb for extended time periods (Wolf et al., 1989, 2002). Tasks practiced were relevant and valued by the participant, undertaken in familiar environments, and periodically reassessed.

The primary premise of the signature CIMT protocol is that restraint of the nonparetic arm after stroke-related neural injury necessitates use of the paretic arm to perform activities. The most recent systematic review and meta-analysis (Corbetta et al., 2010; Sirtori et al., 2010) of CIMT offered a gestalt perspective. This review, which included 755 participants from 18 different studies between 1966 and 2010, found a moderate increase (standardized mean difference = 0.44) in UE motor function after CIMT (Corbetta et al., 2010; Sirtori et al., 2010). In all likelihood, this review found only moderate effects as a result of either the diversity of the sample or the heterogeneity of changes after CIMT—that is, some people may show a lot of improvement and others little to none. Future CIMT studies should seek to more clearly describe the participants who respond to the therapy and those who do not, allowing adult or pediatric practitioners to use CIMT with clients for whom it is expected to be most effective.

THEORETICAL FOUNDATION OF CIMT

The theoretical construct of CIMT is based on both behavioral theory (learned nonuse) and activity-dependent **neuroplasticity,** or the ability of the central nervous system (CNS) to reorganize its structures and networks in response to an activity. The capability for neuroplasticity is ongoing after neural injury; thus, functional improvements can occur immediately and many years after a neurological insult. Correspondingly, time since stroke (>6 months and beyond) is not a necessary predictor of success with CIMT, making this therapy very promising for those who experience long-term UE limitations post stroke (Fritz et al., 2006; Wolf et al., 2010).

Intensive practice of functional tasks, a main feature of CIMT, is believed to cause changes in the size and **excitability** (i.e., probability that neurotransmitters will be released) of the representation of the paretic UE within the primary motor cortex, with resultant functional improvement (Liepert, Bauder, Miltner, Taub, & Weiller, 2000; Liepert et al., 1998; Liepert, Uhde, Graf, Leidner, & Weiller, 2001; Sawaki et al., 2008; Taub et al., 1999; Wittenberg et al., 2003). Adult neuroimaging studies, however, demonstrate a fair amount of variability in the outcomes of CIMT as a result of location of the lesion, corticospinal tract involvement, or changes in brain architecture. The relationship among brain structure, neuroplastic changes, and functional return warrants further investigation (Wittenberg & Schaechter, 2009).

Clear definitions of and studies validating CIMT's active ingredients are critical to continued advancements in understanding how the intervention reverses nonuse and facilitates activity-dependent neuroplasticity (Whyte, 2009). **Active ingredients** are one or more fundamental parameters or essential aspects of a program that are critical for facilitating positive outcomes. Two often-cited features of CIMT thought to be active ingredients are repetitive task practice and adaptive task practice (Wolf, 2007).

REPETITIVE TASK PRACTICE

One way to engage a client in repetitive task practice is through application of a constraint (e.g., mitt, sling) that restricts use of the less affected UE. This constraint forces use of the paretic limb in daily activities by preventing object grasp and manipulation with the less-affected limb (Wolf et al., 1989). Importantly, the constraint itself is not imbued with special properties but simply represents one technique to promote repetitive task practice (Taub et al., 1998; Wolf, 2007).

The importance of repetitive task practice as a driver of beneficial neuroplasticity is strongly supported by contemporary neuroscience. For example, in neurologically healthy people, extensive practice of specific arm and hand movements alters **cortical motor representations** (i.e., evidence of activation in the primary motor cortex), causing the cortical neural territories representing the practiced movement to expand. Alternately, cortical neural territories representing nonpracticed movements do not expand and might even shrink (Cohen, Brasil-Neto, Pascual-Leone, & Hallett, 1993; Liepert et al., 2000).

Similarly, animal models have shown the following results of repetitive task practice throughout motor cortical areas corresponding to repetitively practiced movements:

- Altered motor representations
- Increased **dendritic branching,** or slender, thread-like extensions of the cytoplasm of a neuron that are capable of being stimulated by a neurotransmitter
- Increased **synapse growth,** or establishment of connections between nerve cells and other nerve cells and between nerve cells and muscles and glands
- More efficient **synaptic responses,** or transmission of messages between synapses.

These findings suggest possible mechanisms of activity-dependent reorganization of neural pathways (Jones, Kleim, & Greenough, 1996; Kleim et al., 1997; Nudo, Milliken, Jenkins, & Merzenich, 1996). In rat and primate models of cortical stroke, UE motor representation loss was prevented and cortical reorganization was promoted with repetitive limb use (Kleim, Jones, & Schallert, 2003; Nudo, Plautz, & Frost, 2001).

In humans with stroke, imaging studies showed that task-practice rehabilitation programs increased the excitability of the damaged hemisphere, altered motor cortex topology, and contributed to the restoration of balanced interhemispheric facilitation or inhibition (Harris-Love, Morton, Perez, & Cohen, 2011). Consistent with Wolf and colleagues' (1989) concepts of forced use, repetitive use of the more affected UE may "force" activation of neural circuitry that the person had not been using or was only minimally using, thereby inducing reorganization or strengthening of neural adaptations that in turn enhance the use of that circuitry and the behaviors dependent on it.

ADAPTIVE TASK PRACTICE

Although repetitive use of a limb induces neuroplasticity in structures and networks within regions supporting motor control, the greatest neuroplastic changes are associated with the generation and repetition of new skills rather than repetition of existing skills. In a classic series of studies, Nudo and colleagues (1996) showed that training a primate to retrieve a food pellet by using a novel pattern of forelimb and digit coordination increased the size of cortical representational areas for the trained limb. In contrast, repeating an already-known limb coordination pattern did not alter the cortical representational area (Plautz, Milliken, & Nudo, 2000). In a rat model of stroke, Kleim, Barbay, and Nudo (1998) demonstrated that systematically increasing the difficulty of a reaching task resulted in reorganization of movement representations within the motor cortex, whereas repeating the task without increasing difficulty had no effect on cortical motor maps.

Findings such as these suggest that motor reorganization is dependent on the content of practice sessions; that is, if practice sessions require successful performance of a behavioral task involving acquisition of a new skill, called **skill training** (Plautz et al., 2000), then task-related cortical reorganization will occur. In contrast, if practice sessions require repetition without skill training, then little or no cortical reorganization will occur (Plautz et al., 2000). Plautz and colleagues defined a **new skill** as a task-specific movement pattern that is not part of a current behavioral repertoire.

Adaptive task practice, or shaping (Taub et al., 1994), provided during CIMT represents one method of skill training. Based on behavioral conditioning principles, CIMT is designed to reverse limb nonuse by enabling and rewarding successful task performance (Taub et al., 1994). To shape a behavior, a multistep functional task is first segmented into its one- or two-step components, and participants then practice each task component individually and ultimately in a continuous sequence. Positive feedback is provided to reinforce successful limb use (Taub et al., 1994). For example, in the **Extremity Constraint-Induced Therapy Evaluation (EXCITE) multisite randomized clinical trial** that tested the efficacy of CIMT for 222 adults who were 3 to 6 months post stroke (Wolf et al., 2006), researchers implemented adaptive task practice by providing positive feedback to participants about the results of their practice attempts after every 10 trials of up to 30 seconds duration, as well as continuous feedback throughout. Tasks were made progressively more difficult by modifying aspects of each task to challenge each participant's motor capabilities.

The appropriate dosage (i.e., amount and timing) of repetitive versus adaptive task practice was also explored in the EXCITE trial design because the amount of time on each type of practice varied according to each participant's level of motor impairment (Wolf et al., 2007). For example, participants in the high-functioning group (those with at least 20° voluntary wrist, thumb, and finger extension) were encouraged to spend half of their time in repetitive and half in adaptive task practice. Participants in the low-functioning group (those with 10° voluntary wrist, thumb, and finger extension) were encouraged to spend a third of their time in repetitive and two-thirds in adaptive task practice (Winstein et al., 2003). The study results demonstrated that the time spent in adaptive practice yielded better Wolf Motor Function Test (WMFT) outcomes compared with the time spent in repetitive practice for high- but not for low-functioning participants. Instead, low-functioning participants showed a trend toward improvement with increased time spent in repetitive task practice (Wolf et al., 2007). These data suggest that the nature of the intervention should be considered as it relates to clients' levels of impairment.

Shaping is a key feature of signature CIMT, but other forms of skill training have been incorporated into UE rehabilitation programs. For example, the Accelerated Skill Acquisition Program (Winstein et al., 2013) addresses motor skill relearning, rather than reversal of limb nonuse, by coupling task-specific practice of increasingly difficult tasks with mitigation of specific physical impairments (e.g., weakness, incoordination). Throughout this process, the person with stroke is engaged in a collaborative (i.e., Socratic decision-making and problem-solving) process to enhance self-directed behavior and motivation for limb use (Winstein & Wolf, 2009).

CIMT AND OTHER TASK-ORIENTED UE REHABILITATION APPROACHES

Accumulated evidence linking repetition and skill training to neuroplasticity has led to contemporary task-oriented training approaches to motor rehabilitation (Shumway-Cook & Woollacott, 2011). **Task-oriented training** is based on the idea that motor rehabilitation after stroke is fundamentally a process of relearning how to move; thus, the client is engaged as an active participant in a dynamic motor skill relearning process (Carr & Shepherd, 2000). A client is presented with a clear functional goal (e.g., set a table, unload a dishwasher, wrap a gift) requiring the use of visual, perceptual, cognitive, and motor systems as he or she uses problem solving to achieve the goal (Guadagnoli & Lee, 2004; Timmermans, Spooren, Kingma, & Seelen, 2010). The client repeatedly practices strategies for reaching, grasping, manipulating, and transporting real objects during meaningful activity sequences. Each practice trial provides information to the client (i.e., feedback), which forms the basis for strategizing the next attempt (Boyd & Winstein, 2006). For example, a client may attempt to reach toward and grasp a spoon. If he is successful, he may use the same movement strategy again. If he is not successful, he may realize that a new movement strategy is needed.

Over the course of practice sessions, task demands are optimally progressed according to the client's capability. This progression is critical to prevent a failure of motor learning if tasks become overly simple or too difficult (Guadagnoli & Lee, 2004).

COMPARISON OF TRADITIONAL AND CONTEMPORARY APPROACHES

Contemporary task-oriented training approaches are conceptually dissimilar from traditional neuromuscular reeducation rehabilitation approaches, many of which are still widely used in stroke rehabilitation clinics today (Wolf et al., 2002). These traditional approaches were based on theoretical models of the CNS that postulated that sensory input was a prerequisite for motor output and that normal movement resulted from cortical control over spinal-level reflexes (Jackson, Taylor, Holmes, & Walshe, 1931).

The traditional approaches strove to reduce abnormal muscle activity by providing specific sensory input to clients, who were largely passive recipients of afferent (i.e., sensory) input provided in the form of specialized rehabilitation techniques or modalities. Advocates of these approaches assumed that sensory input was required to facilitate (or inhibit) underlying neurophysiological processes that were thought to limit motor control and functional ability (Bobath & Chartered Society of Physiotherapy, 1971; Brunnstrom, 1956). Although such techniques may ameliorate some impairments (e.g., reduce edema, increase joint mobility or stability), they do not adequately engage the client in repetitious attempts to produce his or her own movements (i.e., voluntary motor drive), which is critical to elicit motor relearning (Lotze, Braun, Birbaumer, Anders, & Cohen, 2003).

In contrast, contemporary task-oriented training rehabilitation approaches view rehabilitation as an active process in which the client, given his or her internal neural and muscular deficits, relearns how to interact with the external environment to meet and overcome the demands of functional activities (Schmidt & Lee, 1999). The World Health Organization's (WHO's) *International Classification of Functioning, Disability and Health* (*ICF;* WHO, 2001) framework shows the difference in treatment foci: Traditional approaches address *ICF* body function and structure domains, whereas task-oriented therapies address *ICF* activity and participation domains.

CONTEMPORARY TASK-ORIENTED APPROACHES

Contemporary task-oriented rehabilitation approaches include not only CIMT but also forced-use interventions, in which the client engages the paretic limb in task practice without specific applications such as shaping (Wolf, 2007), and programs using innovative technologies such as robots (Mehrholz, Hadrich, Platz, Kugler, & Pohl, 2012) and virtual reality (Laver, George, Thomas, Deutsch, & Crotty, 2012). A newly expanding research frontier involves the development of multimodality rehabilitation programs that combine task-oriented training with other methods such as pharmacological interventions or brain stimulation. For example, the combination of task practice and brain stimulation (either repetitive transcranial magnetic stimulation [Celnik, Paik, Vandermeeren, Dimyan, & Cohen, 2009] or transcranial direct-current stimulation [Bolognini et al., 2011]) seems to enhance the effects of each intervention by itself. Like CIMT, all of these task-oriented therapies emphasize interactive problem solving during repetitive goal-directed movement practice.

INNOVATIVE THERAPIES AND NEW TECHNOLOGIES

A reasonable criticism of CIMT is that the majority of poststroke clients do not meet the minimum motor ability needed for inclusion in the EXCITE trial—that is, the ability to initiate at least 20° of wrist extension and at least 10° of finger and thumb extension. These criteria were derived by Wolf and Binder-MacLeod (1983), who estimated that only 20% to 25% of people achieve this amount of recovery after stroke. Without this level of motor skill, clients are unable to independently practice tasks that require reach, grasp, and manipulation of objects.

Exciting innovative therapeutic techniques such as mirror therapy (Thieme, Mehrholz, Pohl, Behrens, & Dohle, 2012), action observation (Ertelt et al., 2007), and mental practice (Page, Szaflarski, Eliassen, Pan, & Cramer, 2009) may enable such task practice for clients with limited reaching and grasping abilities. These therapies engage a client in either observing or imagining himself or herself performing functional tasks to engage the **mirror neuron system,** which activates the identical musculature and neural structures that would be active if the client were physically performing the same tasks (Lafleur et al., 2002; Ramachandran & Altschuler, 2009). Mirror neurons fire both when a person acts and when a person observes the same action performed by another; they may be important for understanding the actions of other people and for learning new skills by imitation.

In addition, new technologies, such as robot-assisted therapy, can help more severely impaired people perform goal-directed reaching tasks. In a recent multicenter randomized trial of robot-assisted therapy, Lo and colleagues (2009) showed that participants with severe-to-moderate impairment gained the same amount of voluntary UE movement with robot-assisted therapy as with an equally dosed intensive rehabilitation regimen provided by a therapist.

These results speak to the important point that new technologies are not intended to replace practitioner-provided treatment but instead offer the opportunity to safely achieve a large number of movement repetitions during therapy. Indeed, current rehabilitation programs may be vastly underdosed in terms of the number of movement repetitions per day (Lang, MacDonald, & Gnip, 2007). Therefore, technology-assisted therapies may extend therapy by enabling independent practice sessions during therapy off hours or at home.

IMPAIRMENT-ORIENTED APPROACHES

In recent years, several research groups have raised the possibility that more severely impaired people, specifically those who do not have enough ability to reach, grasp, or manipulate objects, require therapy sessions focused on improving the movement components needed for task performance (i.e., an impairment-oriented approach) rather than improving task performance itself (i.e., CIMT; Cirstea, Ptito, & Levin, 2003; Platz, 2004). For example, Platz et al. (2009) studied an impairment-oriented training approach that specifically addressed body function impairments relevant to functional task performance. Compared with conventional therapy, this approach improved voluntary movement in people with severe stroke (Platz et al., 2009). Similarly, Corti, McGuirk, Wu, and Patten (2012) demonstrated that for people with moderately severe motor impairment, therapy focused on reducing agonist weakness by means of dynamic resistive strength training resulted in greater movement skills than a comparably dosed task-practice regimen.

In addition, Ellis, Sukal-Moulton, and Dewald (2009) showed that a progressive shoulder abduction loading paradigm enabled people with moderate to severe UE motor impairment to increase their ability to reach forward and sideways across the reaching workspace. Furthermore, several research groups have shown that intensive task practice with trunk restraint improved shoulder–elbow interjoint coordination for reaching compared with task practice without trunk restraint (Combs et al., 2012; Woodbury et al., 2009; Wu, Chen, Lin, Chao, & Chen, 2012). Importantly, these and other impairment-oriented approaches differ from traditional neuromuscular reeducation approaches in that they address impairments within the context of functional task practice, a value shared by contemporary versions of the traditional approaches (Levin & Panturin, 2011).

UNIMANUAL TASK PRACTICE VS. BIMANUAL TASK PRACTICE

A longstanding debate in the UE literature is the benefit of **unimanual task practice** (practicing tasks with primarily one hand, as in CIMT) compared with **bimanual task practice** (practicing tasks with two hands). One reason for this debate is emerging evidence that suggests the influence of **interhemispheric inhibition (IHI)** on motor function of the paretic UE. *IHI* is a well-documented physiological phenomenon that occurs between the brain's two hemispheres in which one hemisphere works to inhibit certain responses from the other (Takeuchi et al., 2008; Takeuchi, Tada, Toshima, Matsuo, & Ikoma, 2009). After damage to one hemisphere, as with a stroke, the lesioned hemisphere is less able to communicate with the intact hemisphere. This communication normally involves inhibitory inputs and outputs between hemispheres to maintain an interhemispheric balance of neural excitability. However, after stroke, the lesioned hemisphere is less able to provide inhibitory inputs to the nonlesioned hemisphere, and conversely, the inhibitory outputs from the nonlesioned hemisphere to the lesioned hemisphere are unimpeded (Stoykov & Corcos, 2009; Takeuchi et al., 2008, 2009).

Unimpeded inhibitory outputs from the nonlesioned to the lesioned hemisphere alter the overall balance of neural excitability by reducing the excitability of the lesioned hemisphere. Therefore, in addition to the neural damage in the lesioned hemisphere caused by the stroke itself, the functions of the lesioned hemisphere are further impaired because of excessive IHI from the intact hemisphere, both of which may be the reasons for poststroke UE paresis.

CIMT may promote recovery of balanced interhemispheric excitability in two ways. First, intensive rehabilitation programs focused on repetitive use of the paretic UE, such as CIMT, increase excitability of the lesioned hemisphere. Second, restricting the use of the nonparetic UE may decrease neural excitability in the nonlesioned hemisphere. However, some researchers have suggested that a bimanual UE intervention may be more advantageous than CIMT, because it generates excitability and inhibitory signals simultaneously in both hemispheres (Stinear & Byblow, 2004), which may facilitate bilateral transfer of motor skills (i.e., transfer of motor skill from the nonparetic UE to the paretic UE; Ausenda & Carnovali, 2011).

However, bimanual task practice may also increase neural activity of the already overactive nonlesioned hemisphere (Renner, Woldag, Atanasova, & Hummelsheim, 2005). It is likely that bimanual and unimanual task practice have different effects on activity-dependent neuroplasticity (Whitall et al., 2011). Thus, it is important that future studies seek to parse the interaction of neuroplasticity, type of therapy intervention, and other stroke-related (e.g., lesion location, lesion size) or person-specific factors (e.g., age, comorbidities).

Taken together, these results suggest that CIMT is an appropriate unimanual intervention for moderately to mildly impaired people—that is, those who have the movement abilities to interact with functional objects. Clients who have not yet developed a repertoire of movement behaviors that enable task practice may benefit more from impairment-focused interventions to address movement components underlying task performance. In addition, bimanual task practice may also improve UE movement functions, albeit through different neural mechanisms than those involved in CIMT.

DEFINING CIMT OUTCOMES

Task-oriented approaches assume learning-dependent functional recovery and reversal of learned nonuse, which is measured in terms of the client's ability to perform functional tasks (Taub et al., 1993). Hence, CIMT outcomes are measured at the *ICF* (WHO, 2001) activity and participation levels. Regarding the nature of the CIMT therapeutic effect, Morris et al. (1997) wrote,

> the most dramatic changes are not in the ability to use the affected upper extremity when requested to do so as on a test or in a therapy setting, but rather in the amount of use to which the affected limb is actually put in the life situation—a parameter that might be termed actual amount of use. (p. 43)

The original CIMT outcome measurement toolbox included Emory Motor Test (Wolf et al., 1989; now called WMFT; Morris et al., 1997; Morris, Uswatte, Crago, Cook, & Taub, 2001), Arm Motor Ability Test (AMAT; Kopp et al., 1997), Motor Activity Log (MAL; Taub et al., 1998), and Actual Amount of Use Test (AAUT; Taub et al., 1993).

WOLF MOTOR FUNCTION TEST

The WMFT was established to measure the effect of forced-use therapy on limb function for daily living tasks (Morris et al., 1997; Wolf et al., 1989). The assessment consists of 15 task performance items and 2 strength items. The performance items are sequentially ordered to initially require single-joint proximal reaching movements without object grasping (e.g., place forearm on table, place forearm on box) and then to require multiple-joint proximal and distal movements for reaching and grasping functional objects (e.g., lift a soda can, fold a towel). Task performance items are timed and rated on a 6-point functional ability scale (0 = *nonuse* to 5 = *normal;* Morris et al., 2001).

ARM MOTOR ABILITY TEST

The AMAT (Kopp et al., 1997) was developed to augment information gained from the WMFT. Whereas the WMFT items include only discrete movement tasks, the AMAT tests the ability to carry out more complex multistep movement tasks similar to those encountered in real-life situations (e.g., dial the phone, don a sweater, unscrew a jar lid). The original assessment comprised 16 items, each having one to three movement segments involving contributions from proximal or distal segments of the affected limb. Task performance was timed and also rated on a functional ability and quality of movement scale (0 = *nonuse* to 5 = *normal*), on which higher scores indicate greater arm motor ability.

MOTOR ACTIVITY LOG

The MAL (Taub et al., 1998) provides information about how the person perceives his or her motor function while performing activities of daily living (ADLs). In its original version, the MAL consisted of 30 items, each of which is a common ADL task (e.g., opening a car door, carrying a glass of water, tying shoes). For each item, the client reports "how often" the activity was performed with the more affected arm and hand and "how well" each activity was performed on a 6-point rating scale (0 = *nonuse* to 5 = *normal*). Item scores are summed; higher scores indicate greater client-reported arm motor ability (Taub et al., 1998).

ACTUAL AMOUNT OF USE TEST

The AAUT (Taub et al., 1993) is a measure of spontaneous arm use rather than arm use during an instructed testing session. For this assessment, a client is unknowingly videotaped while he or she is presented with opportunities, but not specific instructions, to use the affected limb. For example, during conversation, the interviewer hands the client an object to see which limb the client naturally uses to receive the object. The assessment is scored from the videotape. Amount of arm use is rated on a 3-point scale (0 = *nonuse* to 2 = *normal*), and quality of arm movement is rated on a 6-point scale (0 = *nonuse* to 5 = *normal*); higher scores represent greater arm use (Chen, Wolf, Zhang, Thompson, & Winstein, 2012). Although the AAUT represents an objective and unobtrusive measure of spontaneous arm use, a recent investigation into its psychometrics suggests that it may not be sensitive enough to detect treatment effects (Chen et al., 2012).

SUMMARY OF CIMT OUTCOME MEASURES

Studies of CIMT have shown that it enables people to perform tasks more quickly, as defined by the WMFT, and improves client-reported arm use, as defined by the MAL (Wolf et al., 2006). However, neither the WMFT nor the MAL quantifies the movement strategies used to accomplish tasks. Kinematic analyses have shown that although CIMT enables more efficient motor planning (Caimmi et al., 2008; Wu, Lin, Chen, Chen, & Hong, 2007), it may exaggerate compensatory movement patterns and thereby reduce movement efficiency (Massie, Malcolm, Greene, & Thaut, 2009; Woodbury et al., 2009).

Wolf et al. (2011) examined WMFT items that could not be completed after the EXCITE trial to identify what movement components the participants did *not* acquire during therapy. The results revealed that after CIMT, participants had ongoing deficits in performing tasks requiring shoulder joint rotations, pronation and supination movements, and manipulation of objects of variable sizes. Knowledge of how specific motor behaviors are affected by treatment is needed to establish clear guidelines for new therapies and refinements of existing therapies to determine which clients can best benefit from this application.

CHOOSING THE APPROPRIATE OUTCOME MEASURES

As CIMT and other task-oriented training strategies move forward, considerable thought must be given to the choice of outcome measures. This very important decision-making process is required because the interpretation of treatment effect, subsequent treatment decisions, and quantification of the treatment's cost-to-benefit ratio depend on the quality and relevance of the outcome measures.

The measurement tools chosen to define an intervention's outcome must relate to the attributes of the clients being studied (e.g., well-defined impairments and limitations) and must directly connect to the underlying purposes of the intervention (i.e., what is expected to change and for whom the intervention is appropriate or not appropriate). The choice of appropriate outcome measurement tools may be especially important for more severely impaired people with stroke who do not have enough motor skill to reach, grasp, or manipulate objects. For these clients, the original CIMT assessments (e.g., MAL, AAUT, WMFT, AMAT) may not be appropriate because the items are too difficult, thus their baseline performance and possible gains from the intervention cannot be detected with these tools. In this case, choosing outcome tools measuring at the *ICF* (WHO, 2001) body function domain may be advised. For example, the Fugl-Meyer Upper Extremity Assessment (FMA–UE; Fugl-Meyer, Jääskö, Leyman, Olsson, & Steglind, 1975) and the Action Research Arm Test (ARAT; Lyle, 1981) are widely used to measure movement impairment. The FMA–UE assesses clients' ability to perform 30 voluntary shoulder, elbow, wrist, and hand movements on a 3-point rating scale (0 = *unable* to 2 = *normal performance*), and the ARAT assesses clients' ability to perform 19 items assessing grasp, grip, pinch,

and gross arm movement using a 4-point rating scale (0 = *unable* to 3 = *normal performance*).

Two studies (Pang, Harris, & Eng, 2006; Winstein et al., 2004) clearly showed that selecting appropriate outcome measures is important. Winstein and colleagues tested the immediate and long-term effects of two stroke rehabilitation outcomes in participants stratified by stroke severity. Results showed that participants with mild impairment made statistically greater improvements on an assessment of activity performance compared with participants with more severe impairment. However, when measured with an assessment of motor impairment (i.e., FMA–UE), all participants (across all impairment levels) demonstrated statistically significant improvement. Pang and colleagues (2006) tested the effects of a community-based exercise program for persons with chronic poststroke arm movement impairment. Results showed that more severely impaired clients demonstrated statistically significant FMA–UE change scores but no change in WMFT scores. Moderately impaired clients had concurrent changes in both assessments, and the least severely impaired clients demonstrated little increase in FMA–UE scores but showed statistically significant WMFT change scores.

These studies demonstrate the importance choosing which assessments to use to measure the outcomes of a rehabilitation program. If an assessment is chosen that measures outcomes in the *ICF* (WHO, 2001) activity or participation domains, the effect of the treatment on a subgroup of clients with more severe impairment may be hidden. Hence, identifying the most appropriate outcome measures for the level of client impairment is central to reaching accurate conclusions about the effects of a treatment.

PRACTICALITY OF CIMT METHODS

Although CIMT is a promising intervention for UE motor recovery, some have criticized the practicality of the methodology and the limitations of the signature form of CIMT (Dettmers et al., 2005; Page, Sisto, Levine, & McGrath, 2004; Reiss, Wolf, Hammel, McLeod, & Williams, 2012; Sterr et al., 2002; Taub, Lum, Hardin, Mark, & Uswatte, 2005; Wolf, 2007; Wu, Chen, Tang, Lin, & Huang, 2007). For example, CIMT requires proper allocation of time and personnel, both of which are costly. Reimbursement for the multiple hours of treatment required for CIMT may be challenging. In fact, 61% of clinicians stated that managed care payers were "somewhat unlikely" to "very unlikely" to reimburse for CIMT, and 75% said it would be "difficult" to "very difficult" to implement CIMT in their clinic (Daniel, Howard, Braun, & Page, 2012).

The feasibility of a long intervention such as CIMT must also be evaluated from the client's perspective. Research demonstrates that only 32% of adult participants actually comply with the recommended voluntary constraint (restriction) schedule (i.e., wearing the mitt 90% of awake hours; Schaumburg, Pierce, Gaffney, & Gershkoff, 1999), and 68% of adult participants appeared not to be interested in participating in the signature form of CIMT (Daniel et al., 2012; Page, Sisto, Levine, Johnston, & Hughes, 2001). Therefore, various alternatives to improve or modify the CIMT protocol have been investigated.

ALTERNATIVE METHODS OF CIMT

MODIFIED CIMT

The most well-known alternative to the signature version of CIMT is **modified CIMT (mCIMT),** originally described by Steven Page (an occupational therapist) and colleagues (2001, 2013). mCIMT is different from signature CIMT because it includes 30-minute training sessions, 3 days per week for 10 weeks, with shorter constraint times of 5 hours a day during each weekday (Page et al., 2004). Many variations on the methodology of mCIMT have been explored ranging from 30 minutes to 3 hours of treatment a day for 2- to 10-week periods with various restraint periods (Barzel et al., 2009; Lin, Wu, Wei, Lee, & Liu, 2007; Page & Levine, 2007; Richards, Gonzalez Rothi, Davis, Wu, & Nadeau, 2006; Shi et al., 2011; Smania et al., 2012; Sterr et al., 2002; Wu, Chen, et al., 2007). Despite the variation among these protocols, all the interventions are often referred to as *mCIMT* or *distributed CIMT*.

As may be expected, because of the heterogeneity of the methodology, outcomes of mCIMT are inconsistent. A meta-analysis by Shi et al. (2011) of 13 randomized controlled trials of mCIMT for adults post stroke found fairly strong evidence to suggest that mCIMT, compared with traditional therapy, results in improved motor ability. However, the results were inconsistent. For example, gains in kinematic variables (e.g., movement time) were limited post-mCIMT; this finding may be attributable to differences in dosage and to the heterogeneity of the inclusion criteria for participants in these studies (Nijland et al., 2010; Shi et al., 2011; Woodbury et al., 2009; Wu, Chen, et al., 2007).

A retrospective analysis of the EXCITE trial found that for a 6-hour session of signature CIMT, only about 3.95 hours of the session were typically used for task-specific training (Kaplon, Prettyman, Kushi, & Winstein, 2007). Perhaps a more distributed form of CIMT would provide an appropriate solution because participants would receive an equal duration of total treatment time in half the number of days as signature CIMT (Dettmers et al., 2005). To date, the most effective optimal dosage of mCIMT for producing meaningful and sustainable improvements in function is unclear. Furthermore,

alternative CIMT programs do not have defined protocols for home-based training by clients or caregivers; therefore, these programs cannot be replicated and studied.

SELF-TRAINING AND HOME-BASED TRAINING

Various protocols for self-training (Hosomi et al., 2011) and home-based training have been explored (Barzel et al., 2009; Richards et al., 2006; Tariah, Almalty, & Al-Oraibi, 2010) as ways to address the limitations in feasibility of the standard CIMT methodology. Intervention procedures for one self-training study included direct supervision by a practitioner for 40% of total training time, with the remainder designated for in-clinic self-training (Hosomi et al., 2011). The dosage was similar to that of signature CIMT, with 5 hours per day of therapy for 10 consecutive weekdays. Although direct comparisons need to be studied under controlled trial conditions, Hosomi et al. (2011) found a magnitude of improvements similar to that of signature CIMT.

Home-based therapy is another promising avenue to investigate; home-based therapy has been shown to be scientifically defensible and of at least short-term value (Tariah et al., 2010; Wolf, 2011). Clients subjectively reported a preference for practitioner-guided training, however, noting greater use and quality of movement of the affected limb compared with the home-based program independent protocol (Wolf, 2011). Furthermore, beyond the fact that home-training mCIMT protocols are not well defined, a residual perception and expectation that caregivers must rely on professionals to oversee or deliver the intervention remain.

In most countries, continuing constrictions in service delivery because of limited resources and trained staff will demand that family members of poststroke clients become more proactively engaged in the rehabilitation process irrespective of diagnosis or age. The extent to which family members should be trained and overseen and by whom are open-ended questions that have not received adequate attention. Professional oversight most logically should be relegated to occupational therapists, physical therapists, nurses, or physicians. The most appropriate person in a given locale might be a function of issues ranging from reimbursement criteria to cultural considerations. Moreover, alternatives for providing mCIMT protocols need to be clearly specified so that they can be replicated and used clinically.

REIMBURSEMENT OPTIONS

Progressively shortened hospital lengths of stay for adults post stroke are becoming a major concern in neurorehabilitation in both acute and rehabilitation facilities. The patient's physical, occupational, and vocational needs must be identified and met within a typical stay of 2 to 3 weeks, requiring prioritization of multiple, complex goals and treatment programs.

Emphasis is often placed on optimizing function and, for the UE, fostering compensatory behaviors regardless of the potential for use of the more impaired limb. This approach, although suboptimal, is often promoted because of the emerging time limits for therapy reimbursement and the goal of achieving favorable scores on the FIM™ (a trademark of the Uniform Data System for Medical Rehabilitation, a division of UB Foundation Activities, Inc.). This tool was originally designed to assess performance and improvement during rehabilitation and has evolved as a major outcome measurement that permits comparison across facilities (Granger, Markello, Graham, Deutsch, & Ottenbacher, 2009; Keith, Granger, Hamilton, & Sherwin, 1987). Unfortunately, clients can obtain a high score on the FIM by using only the less-affected UE in functional tasks. This focus on compensatory behaviors to gain functional independence may promote increased learned nonuse of the more-affected UE and give an inaccurate description of true neurological recovery.

Undoubtedly, shortened rehabilitation time frames have made the signature form of CIMT less practical and have fostered exploration of mCIMT programs and alternative environments for administration, such as home- or community-based (outpatient) settings. An emphasis on client-centered goals for improved functional gains can potentially be accomplished in the home environment if the specific program is elucidated and the appropriate personnel are trained and committed to successful oversight. This situation warrants careful review and underscores the need for further research on therapy delivery in non-clinic-based settings.

Currently, reimbursement of intense forms of CIMT occurs through fee-for-service or insurance plans that offer extensive coverage for rehabilitation services. Modified and intensive forms of CIMT may be billed similarly. The actual dosage, frequency, and duration of therapy sessions are based on the client's individual needs and insurance coverage.

Presently, no specific *Current Procedural Terminology™* (or *CPT™*) billing code (American Medical Association, 2013) has been designated for CIMT; consequently, the intensive exercise portion of the intervention may be billed in time units under the designation of neuromuscular reeducation, functional retraining, or therapeutic exercise. The behavioral component that addresses instruction in wearing the mitt and review of the home diary may be billed as patient or family education. Currently, actual billing and reimbursement practices across insurance policies, clinicians, and facilities nationwide have not been evaluated but warrant further assessment.

Options for delivery in a climate of cost containment include group-based CIMT programs or development of home-based delivery protocols with integration of more structured caregiver education. Efforts have been made to encourage insurance providers to accept CIMT by presenting the therapy as a mode of best practice that should be offered to those known to benefit most—that is, stroke survivors with mild to moderate impairment and great potential for further participation. The obstacle impeding this approach, however, is the belief that such an intervention might not be needed if individuals can already demonstrate adequate compensatory behavior with the less-impaired UE or can use the paretic limb in a reasonable assistive manner.

SUMMARY

Historically, neurorehabilitation approaches were based on the assumption that the CNS was "hardwired"—that is, incapable of change or repair. This assumption contributed to widespread clinical beliefs that functional improvement plateaued or ceased at a certain point post stroke (e.g., 6 months). The CIMT literature adds to a growing body of literature that challenges the idea of a plateau. CIMT studies clearly demonstrate that functional improvements can continue well into the chronic stage post stroke (>6 months) and can occur even in clients for whom recovery had previously plateaued. If traditional concepts of plateau represent a loss of hope, contemporary evidence, much of which has been generated by CIMT studies, represents renewed optimism in the potential for poststroke recovery. Applications of CIMT to the rehabilitation of adults with stroke have paved the way for contemporary applications of CIMT to the rehabilitation of children with hemiplegia. The following chapters explore the creative and thought-provoking ways in which CIMT has been translated into its pediatric applications.

Ultimately, the challenge to all neurorehabilitationists, regardless of the age of their clients, is to determine the optimal sequencing and dosing of interventions such as CIMT. This challenge can be met only if practitioners clearly define and measure client (adult or pediatric) performance at both the body function and activity and participation levels. In other words, the question is, How do we engage the pathological adult or pediatric nervous system so that we can optimize activity-dependent neuroplastic events that best enable progression toward maximal functional use of the impaired limb? Clearly, a great need exists for continued efforts to understand how a specific intervention, such as CIMT or other task-oriented intervention, drives functional improvements and facilitates the neuroplastic processes underlying these improvements in adult and pediatric populations.

REFERENCES

American Medical Association. (2013). *CPT 2013*. Chicago: Author.

Ausenda, C., & Carnovali, M. (2011). Transfer of motor skill learning from the healthy hand to the paretic hand in stroke patients: A randomized controlled trial. *European Journal of Physical and Rehabilitation Medicine, 47,* 417–425.

Barzel, A., Liepert, J., Haevernick, K., Eisele, M., Ketels, G., Rijntjes, M., & van den Bussche, H. (2009). Comparison of two types of constraint-induced movement therapy in chronic stroke patients: A pilot study. *Restorative Neurology and Neuroscience, 27,* 673–680.

Bobath, B., & Chartered Society of Physiotherapy (Great Britian). (1971). *Abnormal postural reflex activity caused by brain lesions* (2nd ed.). London: Heinemann Medical.

Bolognini, N., Vallar, G., Casati, C., Latif, L. A., El-Nazer, R., Williams, J., . . . Fregni, F. (2011). Neurophysiological and behavioral effects of tDCS combined with constraint-induced movement therapy in poststroke patients. *Neurorehabilitation and Neural Repair, 25,* 819–829.

Boyd, L., & Winstein, C. (2006). Explicit information interferes with implicit motor learning of both continuous and discrete movement tasks after stroke. *Journal of Neurologic Physical Therapy, 30,* 46–57.

Brunnstrom, S. (1956). Associated reactions of the upper extremity in adult patients with hemiplegia: An approach to training. *Physical Therapy Review, 36,* 225–236.

Caimmi, M., Carda, S., Giovanzana, C., Maini, E. S., Sabatini, A. M., Smania, N., & Moltini, F. (2008). Using kinematic analysis to evaluate constraint-induced movement therapy in chronic stroke patients. *Neurorehabilitation and Neural Repair, 22,* 31–39.

Carr, J. H., & Shepherd, R. B. (2000). *Movement science: Foundations for physical therapy in rehabilitation* (2nd ed.). Gaithersburg, MD: Aspen.

Celnik, P., Paik, N. J., Vandermeeren, Y., Dimyan, M., & Cohen, L. G. (2009). Effects of combined peripheral nerve stimulation and brain polarization on performance of a motor sequence task after chronic stroke. *Stroke, 40,* 1764–1771.

Chen, S., Wolf, S. L., Zhang, Q., Thompson, P. A., & Winstein, C. J. (2012). Minimal detectable change of the Actual Amount of Use Test and the Motor Activity Log: The EXCITE trial. *Neurorehabilitation and Neural Repair, 26,* 507–514. http://dx.doi.org/10.1177/15459683114225048

Cimolin, V., Beretta, E., Piccinini, L., Turconi, A. C., Locatelli, F., Galli, M., & Strazzer, S. (2012). Constraint-induced movement therapy for children with hemiplegia after traumatic brain injury: A quantitative study. *Journal of Head Trauma Rehabilitation, 27,* 177–187.

Cirstea, M. C., Ptito, A., & Levin, M. F. (2003). Arm reaching improvements with short-term practice depend on the severity of the motor deficit in stroke. *Experimental Brain Research, 152,* 476–188.

Cohen, L. G., Brasil-Neto, J. P., Pascual-Leone, A., & Hallett, M. (1993). Plasticity of cortical motor output organization following deafferentation, cerebral lesions, and skill acquisition. *Advances in Neurology, 63,* 187–200.

Combs, S. A., Finley, M. A., Henss, M., Himmler, S., Lapota, K., & Stillwell, D. (2012). Effects of a repetitive gaming intervention on upper extremity impairments and function in persons with chronic stroke: A preliminary study. *Disability Rehabilitation, 34,* 1291–1298.

Corbetta, D., Sirtori, V., Moja, L., & Gatti, R. (2010). Constraint-induced movement therapy in stroke patients: Systematic review and meta-analysis. *European Journal of Physical and Rehabilitation Medicine, 46,* 537–544.

Corti, M., McGuirk, T. E., Wu, S. S., & Patten, C. (2012). Differential effects of power training versus functional task practice on compensation and restoration of arm function after stroke. *Neurorehabilitation and Neural Repair, 26,* 842–854.

Daniel, L., Howard, W., Braun, D., & Page, S. J. (2012). Opinions of constraint-induced movement therapy among therapists in southwestern Ohio. *Topics in Stroke Rehabilitation, 19,* 268–275.

de Bode, S., Fritz, S. L., Weir-Haynes, K., & Mathern, G. W. (2009). Constraint-induced movement therapy for individuals after cerebral hemispherectomy: A case series. *Physical Therapy, 89,* 361–369. http://dx.doi.org/10.2522/ptj.20070240

DeLuca, S. C., Case-Smith, J., Stevenson, R., & Ramey, S. L. (2012). Constraint-induced movement therapy (CIMT) for young children with cerebral palsy: Effects of therapeutic dosage. *Journal of Pediatric Rehabilitation Medicine, 5,* 133–142. http://dx.doi.org/10.3238/prm-2012-0206

Dettmers, C., Teske, U., Hamzei, F., Uswatte, G., Taub, E., & Weiller, C. (2005). Distributed form of constraint-induced movement therapy improves functional outcome and quality of life after stroke. *Archives of Physical Medicine and Rehabilitation, 86,* 204–209.

Dromerick, A. W., Lang, C. E., Birkenmeier, R. L., Wagner, J. M., Miller, J. P., Videen, T. O., . . . Edwards, D. F. (2009). Very early constraint-induced movement during stroke rehabilitation (VECTORS): A single-center RCT. *Neurology, 73,* 195–201.

Duncan, P. (1997). Synthesis of intervention trials to improve motor recovery following stroke. *Topics in Stroke Rehabilitation, 3,* 1–20.

Ellis, M. D., Sukal-Moulton, T., & Dewald, J. P. (2009). Progressive shoulder abduction loading is a crucial element of arm rehabilitation in chronic stroke. *Neurorehabilitation and Neural Repair, 23,* 862–869.

Ertelt, D., Small, S., Solodkin, A., Dettmers, C., McNamara, A., Binkofski, F., & Buccino, G. (2007). Action observation has a positive impact on rehabilitation of motor deficits after stroke. *Neuroimage, 36*(Suppl. 2), T164–T173.

Franz, S. I., Scheetz, M. E., & Wilson, A. A. (1915). Hemiplegia. *JAMA, 65,* 2154–2155.

Fritz, S., Light, K., Clifford, S., Patterson, T., Behrman, A., & Davis, S. (2006). Descriptive predictors of outcomes following constraint-induced movement therapy for individuals with post-stroke hemiparesis. *Physical Therapy, 86,* 825–832.

Fritz, S. L., Light, K., Patterson, T., Behrman, A., & Davis, S. (2005). Active finger extension predicts outcomes after constraint-induced movement therapy for individuals with hemiparesis after stroke. *Stroke, 36,* 1172–1177. http://dx.doi.org/10.1161/01.sjr.0000165922.96430.d0

Fugl-Meyer, A. R., Jääskö, L., Leyman, I., Olsson, S., & Steglind, S. (1975). The post-stroke hemiplegic patient: A method for evaluation of physical performance. *Scandinavian Journal of Rehabilitation Medicine, 7,* 13–31.

Granger, C. V., Markello, S. J., Graham, J. E., Deutsch, A., & Ottenbacher, K. J. (2009). The uniform data system for medical rehabilitation: Report of patients with stroke discharged from comprehensive medical programs in 2000–2007. *American Journal of Physical Medicine and Rehabilitation, 88,* 961–972.

Guadagnoli, M. A., & Lee, T. D. (2004). Challenge point: A framework for conceptualizing the effects of various practice conditions in motor learning. *Journal of Motor Behavior, 36,* 212–224.

Harris-Love, M. L., Morton, S. M., Perez, M. A., & Cohen, L. G. (2011). Mechanisms of short-term training-induced reaching improvement in severely hemiparetic stroke patients: A TMS study. *Neurorehabilitation and Neural Repair, 25,* 398–411.

Hosomi, M., Koyama, T., Takebayashi, T., Terayama, S., Kodama, N., Matsumoto, K., & Domen, K. (2011). A modified method for constraint-induced movement therapy: A supervised self-training protocol. *Journal of Stroke and Cerebrovascular Disease, 21,* 767–775.

Jackson, J. H., Taylor, J., Holmes, G. M., & Walshe, F. M. R. (1931). *Selected writings of John Hughlings Jackson.* London: Hodder & Stoughton.

Jones, T. A., Kleim, J. A., & Greenough, W. T. (1996). Synaptogenesis and dendritic growth in the cortex opposite unilateral sensorimotor cortex damage in adult rats: A quantitative electron microscopic examination. *Brain Research, 733,* 142–148.

Kaplon, R. T., Prettyman, M. G., Kushi, C. L., & Winstein, C. J. (2007). Six hours in the laboratory: A quantification of practice time during constraint-induced therapy (CIT). *Clinical Rehabilitation, 21,* 950–958.

Keith, R. A., Granger, C. V., Hamilton, B. B., & Sherwin, F. S. (1987). The Functional Independence Measure: A new tool for rehabilitation. *Advances in Clinical Rehabilitation, 1,* 6–18.

Kleim, J. A., Barbay, S., & Nudo, R. J. (1998). Functional reorganization of the rat motor cortex following motor skill learning. *Journal of Neurophysiology, 80,* 3321–3325.

Kleim, J. A., Jones, T. A., & Schallert, T. (2003). Motor enrichment and the induction of plasticity before or after brain injury. *Neurochemical Research, 28,* 1757–1769.

Kleim, J. A., Swain, R. A., Czerlanis, C. M., Kelly, J. L., Pipitone, M. A., & Greenough, W. T. (1997). Learning-dependent dendritic hypertrophy of cerebellar stellate cells: Plasticity of local circuit neurons. *Neurobiology of Learning and Memory, 67,* 29–33.

Knapp, H., Taub, E., & Berman, A. (1963). Movements in monkeys with deafferented forearms. *Experimental Neurology, 7,* 305–315.

Kopp, B., Kunkel, A., Flor, H., Platz, T., Rose, U., Mauritz, K. H., … Taub, E. (1997). The Arm Motor Ability Test: Reliability, validity, and sensitivity to change of an instrument for assessing disabilities in activities of daily living. *Archives of Physical Medicine and Rehabilitation, 78,* 615–620.

Kunkel, A., Kopp, B., Muller, G., Villringer, K., Villringer, A., Taub, E., & Flor, H. (1999). Constraint-induced movement therapy for motor recovery in chronic stroke patients. *Archives of Physical Medicine and Rehabilitation, 80,* 624–628.

Lafleur, M. F., Jackson, P. L., Malouin, F., Richards, C. L., Evans, A. C., & Doyon, J. (2002). Motor learning produces parallel dynamic functional changes during the execution and imagination of sequential foot movements. *Neuroimage, 16,* 142–157.

Lang, C. E., MacDonald, J. R., & Gnip, C. (2007). Counting repetitions: An observational study of outpatient therapy for people with hemiparesis post-stroke. *Journal of Neurologic Physical Therapy, 31,* 3–10.

Laver, K., George, S., Thomas, S., Deutsch, J. E., & Crotty, M. (2012). Cochrane review: Virtual reality for stroke rehabilitation. *European Journal of Physical and Rehabilitation Medicine, 48,* 523–530.

Levin, M. F., & Panturin, E. (2011). Sensorimotor integration for functional recovery and the Bobath approach. *Motor Control, 15,* 285–301.

Liepert, J., Bauder, H., Miltner, W. H. R., Taub E., & Weiller, C. (2000). Treatment-induced cortical reorganization after stroke in humans. *Stroke, 31,* 1210–1216.

Liepert, J., Miltner, W. H. R., Bauder, H., Sommer, M., Dettmers, C., Taub, E., & Weiller, C. (1998). Motor cortex plasticity during constraint-induced movement therapy in stroke patients. *Neuroscience Letters, 250,* 5–8.

Liepert, J., Uhde, I., Graf, S., Leidner, O., & Weiller, C. (2001). Motor cortex plasticity during forced-use therapy in stroke patients: A preliminary study. *Journal of Neurology, 248,* 315–321.

Lin, K. C., Wu, C. Y., Wei, T. H., Lee, C. Y., & Liu, J. S. (2007). Effects of modified constraint-induced movement therapy on reach-to-grasp movements and functional performance after chronic stroke: A randomized controlled study. *Clinical Rehabilitation, 21,* 1075–1086.

Lo, A. C., Guarino, P., Krebs, H. I., Volpe, B. T., Bever, C. T., Duncan, P. W., . . . Paduzzi, P. (2009). Multicenter randomized trial of robot-assisted rehabilitation for chronic stroke: Methods and entry characteristics for VA ROBOTICS. *Neurorehabilitation and Neural Repair, 23,* 775–783.

Lotze, M., Braun, C., Birbaumer, N., Anders, S., & Cohen, L. G. (2003). Motor learning elicited by voluntary drive. *Brain, 126*(Pt. 4), 866–872.

Lyle, R. C. (1981). A performance test for assessment of upper limb function in physical rehabilitation treatment and research. *International Journal of Rehabilitation Research, 4,* 483–492.

Massie, C., Malcolm, M. P., Greene, D., & Thaut, M. (2009). The effects of constraint-induced therapy on kinematic outcomes and compensatory movement patterns: An exploratory study. *Archives of Physical Medicine and Rehabilitation, 90,* 571–579.

Mehrholz, J., Hadrich, A., Platz, T., Kugler, J., & Pohl, M. (2012). Electromechanical and robot-assisted arm training for improving generic activities of daily living, arm function, and arm muscle strength after stroke. *Cochrane Database of Systematic Reviews, 6,* CD006876.

Miltner, W., Bauder, H., Sommer, M., Dettmers, C., & Taub, E. (1999). Effects of constraint-induced movement therapy on patients with chronic motor deficits after stroke: A replication. *Stroke, 30,* 586–592.

Morris, D., Crago, J., DeLuca, S., Pidikiti, R., & Taub, E. (1997). Constraint-induced (CI) movement therapy for motor recovery after stroke. *Neurorehabilitation, 9,* 29–43.

Morris, D. M., Uswatte, G., Crago, J. E., Cook, E. W., & Taub, E. (2001). The reliability of the Wolf Motor Function Test for assessing upper extremity function after stroke. *Archives of Physical Medicine and Rehabilitation, 82,* 750–755.

Nijland, R., van Wegen, E., Verbunt, J., van Wijk, R., van Kordelaar, J., & Kwakkel, G. A. (2010). Comparison of two validated tests for upper limb function after stroke: The Wolf Motor Function Test and the Action Research Arm Test. *Journal of Rehabilitation Medicine, 42,* 694–696.

Nudo, R. J., Milliken, G. W., Jenkins, W. M., & Merzenich, M. M. (1996). Use-dependent alterations of movement representations in primary motor cortex of adult squirrel monkeys. *Journal of Neuroscience, 16,* 785–807.

Nudo, R. J., Plautz, E. J., & Frost, S. B. (2001). Role of adaptive plasticity in recovery of function after damage to motor cortex. *Muscle and Nerve, 24,* 1000–1019.

Ogden, R., & Franz, S. I. (1917). On cerebral motor control: The recovery from experimentally produced hemiplegia. *Psychobiology, 1,* 33–47.

Ostendorf, C. G., & Wolf, S. L. (1981). Effect of forced use of the upper extremity of a hemiplegic patient on changes in function: A single-case design. *Physical Therapy, 61,* 1022–1028.

Page, S. J., Boe, S., & Levine, P. (2013). What are the "ingredients" of modified constraint-induced therapy? An evidence-based review, recipe, and recommendations. *Restorative Neurology and Neuroscience, 31,* 299–309.

Page, S. J., & Levine, P. (2007). Modified constraint-induced therapy in patients with chronic stroke exhibiting minimal movement ability in the affected arm. *Physical Therapy, 87,* 872–878.

Page, S., Sisto, S., Levine, P., Johnston, M., & Hughes, M. (2001). Modified constraint-induced therapy: A randomized feasibility and efficacy study. *Journal of Rehabilitation Research and Development, 38,* 583–590.

Page, S. J., Sisto, S., Levine, P., & McGrath, R. E. (2004). Efficacy of modified constraint-induced movement therapy in chronic stroke: A single-blinded randomized controlled trial. *Archives of Physical Medicine and Rehabilitation, 85,* 14–18.

Page, S. J., Szaflarski, J. P., Eliassen, J. C., Pan, H., & Cramer, S. C. (2009). Cortical plasticity following motor skill learning during mental practice in stroke. *Neurorehabilitation and Neural Repair, 23,* 382–388.

Pang, M. Y., Harris, J. E., & Eng, J. J. (2006). A community-based upper-extremity group exercise program improves motor function and performance of functional activities in chronic stroke: A randomized controlled trial. *Archives of Physical Medicine and Rehabilitation, 87,* 1–9.

Platz, T. (2004). Impairment-oriented training (IOT)—Scientific concept and evidence-based treatment strategies. *Restorative Neurology and Neuroscience, 22,* 301–315.

Platz, T., van Kaick, S., Mehrholz, J., Leidner, O., Eickhof, C., & Pohl, M. (2009). Best conventional therapy versus modular impairment-oriented training for arm paresis after stroke: A single-blind, multicenter randomized controlled trial. *Neurorehabilitation and Neural Repair, 23,* 706–716.

Plautz, E. J., Milliken, G. W., & Nudo, R. J. (2000). Effects of repetitive motor training on movement representations in adult squirrel monkeys: Role of use versus learning. *Neurobiology of Learning and Memory, 74,* 27–55.

Ramachandran, V. S., & Altschuler, E. L. (2009). The use of visual feedback, in particular mirror visual feedback, in restoring brain function. *Brain, 132*(Pt. 7), 1693–1710.

Reiss, A. P., Wolf, S. L., Hammel, E. A., McLeod, E. L., & Williams, E. A. (2012). Constraint-induced movement therapy (CIMT): Current perspectives and future directions. *Stroke Research and Treatment, 2012,* 159–391. http://dx.doi.org/10.1155/2012/159391

Renner, C. I., Woldag, H., Atanasova, R., & Hummelsheim, H. (2005). Change of facilitation during voluntary bilateral hand activation after stroke. *Journal of the Neurological Sciences, 239,* 25–30.

Richards, L., Gonzalez Rothi, L. J., Davis, S., Wu, S. S., & Nadeau, S. E. (2006). Limited dose response to constraint-induced movement therapy in patients with chronic stroke. *Clinical Rehabilitation, 20,* 1066–1077.

Russo, S. (1995). Hemiplegic upper extremity rehabilitation: A review of the forced-use paradigm. *Neurology Report, 19,* 17–21.

Sawaki, L., Butler, A. J., Leng, X., Wassenaar, P. A., Mohammad, Y. M., Blanton, S., . . . Wittenberg, G. F. (2008). Constraint-induced movement therapy results in increased motor map area in subjects 3 to 9 months after stroke. *Neurorehabilitation and Neural Repair, 22,* 505–513. http://dx.doi.org/10.1177/1545968308317531

Schaumburg, S., Pierce, S., Gaffney, K., & Gershkoff, A. (1999, October). *Constraint induced therapy: Moving research into practice.* Paper presented at the meeting of the American Congress of Rehabilitation Medicine, Orlando, FL.

Schmidt, R. A., & Lee, T. D. (1999). *Motor control and learning: A behavioral emphasis* (3rd ed.). Champaign, IL: Human Kinetics.

Shi, Y. X., Tian, J. H., Yang, K. H., & Zhao, Y. (2011). Modified constraint-induced movement therapy versus traditional rehabilitation in patients with upper-extremity dysfunction after stroke: A systematic review and meta-analysis. *Archives of Physical Medicine and Rehabilitation, 92,* 972–982.

Shumway-Cook, A., & Woollacott, M. H. (2011). *Motor control: Translating research into clinical practice* (4th ed.). Philadelphia: Lippincott Williams & Wilkins.

Sirtori, V., Corbetta, D., Moja, L., & Gatti, R. (2010). Constraint-induced movement therapy for upper extremities in patients with stroke. *Stroke, 41,* e57–e58.

Smania, N., Gandolfi, M., Paolucci, S., Iosa, M., Ianes, P., Recchia, S., . . . Farina, S. (2012). Reduced-intensity modified constraint-induced movement therapy versus conventional therapy for upper extremity rehabilitation after stroke: A multicenter trial. *Neurorehabilitation and Neural Repair, 26,* 1035–1045.

Sterr, A., Elbert, T., Berthold, I., Kolbel, S., Rockstroh, B., & Taub, E. (2002). Longer versus shorter daily constraint-induced movement therapy of chronic hemiparesis: An exploratory study. *Archives of Physical Medicine and Rehabilitation, 83,* 1374–1377.

Stinear, J. W., & Byblow, W. D. (2004). Rhythmic bilateral movement training modulates corticomotor excitability and enhances upper limb motricity poststroke: A pilot study. *Journal of Clinical Neurophysiology, 21,* 124–131.

Stoykov, M. E., & Corcos, D. M. (2009). A review of bilateral training for upper extremity hemiparesis. *Occupational Therapy International, 16,* 190–203.

Takeuchi, N., Tada, T., Toshima, M., Chuma, T., Matsuo, Y., & Ikoma, K. (2008). Inhibition of the unaffected motor cortex by 1 Hz repetitive transcranial magnetic stimulation enhances motor performance and training effect of the paretic hand in patients with chronic stroke. *Journal of Rehabilitation Medicine, 40,* 298–303.

Takeuchi, N., Tada, T., Toshima, M., Matsuo, Y., & Ikoma, K. (2009). Repetitive transcranial magnetic stimulation over bilateral hemispheres enhances motor function and training effect of paretic hand in patients after stroke. *Journal of Rehabilitation Medicine, 41,* 1049–1054.

Tariah, H., Almalty, A. Z. S., & Al-Oraibi, S. (2010). Constraint-induced movement therapy for stroke survivors in Jordan: A home-based model. *International Journal of Therapy and Rehabilitation, 17,* 638–646.

Taub, E., Crago, J. E., Burgio, L. D., Groomes, T. E., Cook, E. W., III, DeLuca S. C., & Miller, N. E. (1994). An operant approach to rehabilitation medicine: Overcoming learned nonuse by shaping. *Journal of the Experimental Analysis of Behavior, 61,* 281–293.

Taub, E., Crago, J., & Uswatte, G. (1998). Constraint-induced movement therapy: A new approach to treatment in physical rehabilitation. *Rehabilitation Psychology, 43,* 152–170.

Taub, E., Lum, P. S., Hardin, P., Mark, V. W., & Uswatte, G. (2005). AutoCITE: Automated delivery of CI therapy with reduced effort by therapists. *Stroke, 36,* 1301–1304.

Taub, E., Miller, N. E., Novack, T. A., Cook, E. W., Fleming, W. C., Nepomuceno, C. S., . . . Crago, J. E. (1993). Technique to improve chronic motor deficit after stroke. *Archives of Physical Medicine and Rehabilitation, 74,* 347–354.

Taub, E., & Morris, D. M. (2001). Constraint-induced movement therapy to enhance recovery after stroke. *Current Atherosclerosis Reports, 3,* 279–286.

Taub, E., Uswatte, G., & Pidikiti, R. (1999). Constraint-induced movement therapy: A new family of techniques with broad application to physical rehabilitation: A clinical review. *Journal of Rehabilitation Research and Development, 36,* 237–251.

Thieme, H., Mehrholz, J., Pohl, M., Behrens, J., & Dohle, C. (2012). Mirror therapy for improving motor function after stroke. *Cochrane Database of Systematic Reviews, 3,* CD008449.

Timmermans, A. A., Spooren, A. I., Kingma, H., & Seelen, H. A. (2010). Influence of task-oriented training content on skilled arm–hand performance in stroke: A systematic review. *Neurorehabilitation and Neural Repair, 24,* 858–870.

Whitall, J., Waller, S. M., Sorkin, J. D., Forrester, L. W., Macko, R. F., Hanley, D. F., . . . Luft, A. (2011). Bilateral and unilateral arm training improve motor function through differing neuroplastic mechanisms: A single-blinded randomized controlled trial. *Neurorehabilitation and Neural Repair, 25,* 118–129.

Whyte, J. (2009). Defining the active ingredients of rehabilitation. *Health Policy Newsletter, 22*(4), 13.

Winstein, C. J., Miller, J. P., Blanton, S., Taub, E., Uswatte, G., Morris, D., . . . Wolf, S. (2003). Methods for a multisite randomized trial to investigate the effect of constraint-induced movement therapy in improving upper extremity function among adults recovering from a cerebrovascular stroke. *Neurorehabilitation and Neural Repair, 17,* 137–152. http://dx.doi.org/10.1177/0888439003255511

Winstein, C. J., Rose, D. K., Tan, S. M., Lewthwaite, R., Chui, H. C., & Azen, S. P. (2004). A randomized controlled comparison of upper-extremity rehabilitation strategies in acute stroke: A pilot study of immediate and long-term outcomes. *Archives of Physical Medicine and Rehabilitation, 85,* 620–628.

Winstein, C. J., & Wolf, S. L. (2009). Task-oriented training to promote upper extremity recovery. In J. Stein, R. L. Harvey, R. F. Macko, C. J. Winstein, & R. D. Zorowitz (Eds.), *Stroke recovery and rehabilitation* (pp. 267–290). New York: Demos Medical.

Winstein, C. J., Wolf, S. L., Dromerick, A. W., Lane, C. J., Nelsen, M. A., Lewthwaite, R., . . . ICARE Investigative Team. (2013). Interdisciplinary Comprehensive Arm Rehabilitation Evaluation (ICARE): A randomized controlled trial protocol. *BioMedCentral Neurology, 13,* 5. http://dx.doi.org/10.1186/1471-2377-13-5

Wittenberg, G. F., Chen, R., Ishii, K., Bushara, K. O., Taub, E., Gerber, L. H., . . . Cohen, L. G. (2003). Constraint-induced movement therapy: Magnetic-stimulation motor maps and cerebral activation. *Neurorehabilitation and Neural Repair, 17,* 48–57.

Wittenberg, G. F., & Schaechter, J. D. (2009). The neural basis of constraint-induced movement therapy. *Current Opinion in Neurology, 22,* 582–588. http://dx.doi.org/10.1097/WCO.06013e323320229

Wolf, S. L. (2007). Revisiting constraint-induced movement therapy: Are we too smitten with the mitten? Is all nonuse "learned"? and other quandaries. *Physical Therapy, 87,* 1212–1223.

Wolf, S. L. (2011). Correspondence: Home based therapy can be of, at least, short term value. *International Journal of Therapy and Rehabilitation, 18,* 116–117.

Wolf, S. L., & Binder-MacLeod, S. A. (1983). Electromyographic biofeedback applications to the hemiplegic patient: Changes in upper extremity neuromuscular and functional status. *Physical Therapy, 63,* 1393–1403.

Wolf, S. L., Blanton, S., Baer, H., Breshears, J., & Butler, A. J. (2002). Repetitive task practice: A critical review of constraint-induced movement therapy in stroke.

Neurology, 8, 325–338. http://dx.doi.org/10.1097/01.nrl.0000031014.85777.76

Wolf, S. L., Lecraw, D. E., Barton, L. A., & Jann, B. B. (1989). Forced use of hemiplegic upper extremities to reverse the effect of learned nonuse among chronic stroke and head-injured patients. *Experimental Neurology, 104,* 125–132.

Wolf, S. L., Newton, H., Maddy, D., Blanton, S., Zhang, Q., Winstein, C. J., . . . Light, K. (2007). The EXCITE trial: Relationship of intensity of constraint induced movement therapy to improvement in the Wolf Motor Function Test. *Restorative Neurology and Neuroscience, 25,* 549–562.

Wolf, S. L., Thompson, P. A., Estes, E., Lonergan, T., Merchant, R., & Richardson, N. (2011). The EXCITE trial: Analysis of "noncompleted" Wolf Motor Function Test items. *Neurorehabilitation and Neural Repair, 26,* 178–187. http://dx.doi.org/10.1177/1545968311426437

Wolf, S. L., Thompson, P. A., Winstein, C. J., Miller, J. P., Blanton, S. R., Nichols-Larsen D. S., . . . Sawaki, L. (2010). The EXCITE stroke trial: Comparing early and delayed constraint-induced movement therapy. *Stroke, 41,* 2309–2315. http://dx.doi.org/10.1161/STROKEAHA.110.588723

Wolf, S. L., Winstein, C. J., Miller, J. P., Taub, E., Uswatte, G., Morris, D., . . . EXCITE Investigators. (2006). Effect of constraint-induced movement therapy on upper extremity function 3 to 9 months after stroke: The EXCITE randomized clinical trial. *JAMA, 296,* 2095–2104. http://dx.doi.org/10.1001/jama.296.17.2095

Woodbury, M. L., Howland, D. R., McGuirk, T. E., Davis, S. B., Senesac, C. R., Kautz, S., & Richards, L. G. (2009). Effects of trunk restraint combined with intensive task practice on poststroke upper extremity reach and function: A pilot study. *Neurorehabilitation and Neural Repair, 23,* 78–91. http://dx.doi.org/10.1177/1545968308318836

World Health Organization. (2001). *International classification of functioning, disability and health.* Geneva: Author.

Wu, C. Y., Chen, Y. A., Lin, K. C., Chao, C. P., & Chen, Y. T. (2012). Constraint-induced therapy with trunk restraint for improving functional outcomes and trunk–arm control after stroke: A randomized controlled trial. *Physical Therapy, 92,* 483–492.

Wu, C. Y., Chen, C. L., Tang, S. F., Lin, K. C., & Huang, Y. Y. (2007). Kinematic and clinical analyses of upper-extremity movements after constraint-induced movement therapy in patients with stroke: A randomized controlled trial. *Archives of Physical Medicine and Rehabilitation, 88,* 964–970.

Wu, C. Y., Lin, K. C., Chen, H. C., Chen, I. H., & Hong, W. H. (2007). Effects of modified constraint-induced movement therapy on movement kinematics and daily function in patients with stroke: A kinematic study of motor control mechanisms. *Neurorehabilitation and Neural Repair, 21,* 460–466.

SHARON LANDESMAN RAMEY, PhD, and STEPHANIE C. DeLUCA, PhD

2

Pediatric CIMT: History and Definition

CHAPTER HIGHLIGHTS

- Terminology and concepts
- Early case studies of pediatric constraint-induced movement therapy (P–CIMT)
- Accumulating evidence from clinical trials of P–CIMT
- Recent research focused on answering questions relevant to precision practice
- Neuroplasticity and P–CIMT.

I n this chapter, we strive to bring together the two worlds of clinical experience and published scientific studies to provide a broad history of constraint-induced movement therapy (CIMT) as applied to children. This history is one in which there has been worldwide interest in adapting the fundamentals of CIMT into a wide array of treatment strategies for use with children from infancy through adolescence and young adulthood. **Pediatric CIMT (P–CIMT)** represents a class of therapeutic interventions, rather than a single, manualized protocol, that has—at minimum—three distinguishing characteristics:

1. Some form of constraint to the unimpaired or less-impaired arm, hand, or both;
2. Systematic efforts to shape new skills in the impaired (nonconstrained) upper extremity (UE) and provide opportunity for repetitive practice of these skills; and
3. Relatively high levels (dosage or intensity) of therapy for the hemiparetic UE.

KEY TERMS

Activation and reward thresholds
Activity-induced neuroplasticity
Anticipatory motor activity
Brain reorganization
Developmental disregard
Forced use
Functional neuroimaging
Interhemispheric inhibition
Learned nonuse
Learning
Massed practice
Modified P–CIMT
Pediatric application treatment
Pediatric CIMT
Shaping techniques
Visualization

P–CIMT is thus a concentrated, multicomponent form of pediatric therapy focused on promoting increased voluntary control and functional competence of the hemiparetic UE.

TERMINOLOGY AND CONCEPTS

In the published literature, there has been no consistent naming of the therapies that qualify as belonging to the class of P–CIMT. The terms used include *pediatric constraint-induced movement therapy, constraint-induced (CI) therapy, CI movement therapy, modified CI therapy,* and *forced use.* Often, the terms are not specifically defined; other times, they are defined in contradictory ways—such as the term *forced use,* which some define as the use of constraint alone (which does not qualify as P–CIMT because it does not include the use of systematic shaping and a relatively high dosage of therapy for the more-impaired UE).

When reading the original articles, as well as the clinical and scientific review articles, one must carefully attend to the precise therapy procedures and definitions; considerable misunderstanding could occur if readers relied primarily on the major conclusions in the abstract or the authors' summary. This text advocates adopting standard terminology and reporting requirements for P–CIMT with the goal of accelerating the acquisition of empirical evidence of the effects of alternative forms of P–CIMT—alone and in combination with other treatments and activities—on children's outcomes at the clinical, behavioral, subjective, and neurobiological levels.

We propose that the general term *P–CIMT* be applied to treatment strategies that meet these five conditions:

1. Constraint of the less-impaired or unimpaired UE to induce changes in the child's attention to movement of the other, more-impaired, unconstrained UE;
2. Specific use of systematic techniques to help shape, refine, and practice movements and functional use of the unconstrained UE;
3. Relatively high intensity of systematic training;
4. Delivered in naturalistic settings; and
5. Includes a plan to help transfer learned skills and activities to a posttherapy period designed to generalize these skills and activities to the child's daily life.

Appendix 2.A includes terms and definitions often used in P–CIMT.

PEDIATRIC APPLICATION

Pediatric application treatment is prescribed or approved by a clinician with relevant pediatric expertise for a child from infancy through young adulthood with the goal of improving UE functioning of a child with hemiparesis or asymmetrical impairment. Designating P–CIMT as distinct from adult CIMT is intentional, because P–CIMT takes into account multiple aspects of development itself that are not critical to the treatment protocol of adult CIMT for patients with stroke and because the adults did not previously have neuromotor impairment of their UEs. P–CIMT is thus a developmental therapy that considers the natural progression of UE development, both gross and fine motor skills, that shows rapid and important changes during the first decade of life. P–CIMT also incorporates other treatment elements relevant to children (but not essential for adults with stroke) such as motivation, attention span, generalization to everyday functional activities, and use of individualized reinforcers.

Particularly in the first few years of life, daily use of UEs has direct consequences for many other aspects of development, including posture, mobility, protective reflexes, arm and hand gestures for communication, and social engagement. Almost all published articles about P–CIMT include thoughtful elements that reflect understanding of how a child's age, interests, and prior experiences influence the setting of treatment goals, activities selected to include in the P–CIMT protocol, appropriate ways to measure progress, and how to prevent and then monitor for potential adverse events (which fortunately have been extremely rare; e.g., Charles, Wolf, Schneider, & Gordon, 2006; DeLuca, Echols, & Ramey, 2007; Eliasson, Krumlinde-Sundholm, Shaw, & Wang, 2005; Taub, Ramey, DeLuca, & Echols, 2004). In addition, the *P* in P–CIMT indicates that the treatment is designed with an explicit recognition that children learn best when they are engaged in the occupations of play and everyday activities that are personally rewarding, challenging, and meaningful to them and their families (Case-Smith & O'Brien, 2010; Gordon, Charles, & Wolf, 2006; Humphry, 2002).

CONSTRAINT OF ONE UE TO INDUCE CHANGES IN THE CHILD'S ATTENTION TO MOVEMENT OF THE OTHER (UNCONSTRAINED) UE

Children who receive P–CIMT usually have a clinical presentation of hemiplegia or hemiparesis, sometimes labeled *unilateral cerebral palsy* (cf. "Definition and Classification of Cerebral Palsy," 2007), although children with a diagnosis of quadriplegia—but with at least some functional skills greater on one side than the other—have also benefited greatly from receiving P–CIMT (DeLuca et al., 2007; DeLuca, Echols, Ramey, & Taub, 2003). The theoretical and practical intention of applying constraint to the unimpaired or less-impaired UE is to create an environmental press that "induces" the child to use the impaired arm and hand to accomplish tasks.

Many of the clinical case studies and trials using full-time constraint of the less-impaired UE have reported that infants, toddlers, and preschool-age children often show new levels of awareness of their impaired UE (e.g., DeLuca, Echols, Law, & Ramey, 2006; DeLuca et al., 2003). Whether this attentional shift is directly due to the reduction in the functional use of the less-affected UE, the novelty of wearing a constraint, the reduction of competing sensory and motor input from the more functional UE while it is constrained, the encouragement of the therapist or parent, or the child's own motivation to participate in P–CIMT is an intriguing and as-yet-unresolved question. The constraint must, at a minimum, be applied for the majority of the time the child receives active therapy; at a maximum, the constraint is worn throughout the day and night during the entire course of treatment. A frequently used intermediate-level protocol is having the child wear the constraint during the majority of waking hours during a multiweek course of P–CIMT.

Similarly, the actual methods for constraint have varied considerably. They include casting a long-arm or full-arm constraint extending to the end of the child's fingertips (this form of constraint almost always uses lightweight, semirigid, and permeable materials that are much more child friendly than old-fashioned, heavy plaster casts), constructing a variety of individualized splints that range from short (e.g., hand only or hand and wrist) to long (e.g., covering hand to beyond elbow), using generic cloth slings, and applying hand mitts or puppets.

Although verbal constraint or self-directed and voluntary constraint could technically qualify as a method of constraint, and could perhaps be highly effective with some children, we propose that this form of mental or social constraint differs sufficiently that it would not qualify for the class of P–CIMT treatments currently developed and studied. Verbal and self-applied forms of constraint are also particularly challenging to monitor and document and may represent a safety risk. (See Chapter 16, "Research Priorities: Understanding and Transcending the Limits of Current Knowledge to Inform Best Practices in Pediatric CIMT," for a detailed discussion of the importance of testing and understanding the different forms of constraint as an integral component of P–CIMT.)

SPECIFICALLY USE SYSTEMATIC TECHNIQUES TO HELP SHAPE, REFINE, AND PRACTICE MOVEMENTS AND FUNCTIONAL USE OF THE UNCONSTRAINED UE

The term *movement therapy* does not denote a highly specific or widely agreed-on set of therapy activities. Rather, the inclusion of movement therapy as part of the designation of P–CIMT reflects that it combines use of constraint with intentional therapy to promote improved movement and voluntary control of the unconstrained UE. That is, if a child is wearing a constraint and is merely encouraged by an adult to play and

try to use the unrestrained arm and hand, it would not qualify as P–CIMT. Of course, encouragement and play activities are valuable as adjuncts and are almost always included as part of an overall treatment plan, but P–CIMT requires systematic efforts that involve individualized application of techniques to promote effective use of the child's unrestrained arm and hand.

Formal shaping techniques, described in detail in many other chapters in this handbook, particularly Chapter 7, "Operationalizing Pediatric CIMT: Guidelines for Transforming Basic Principles and Scientific Evidence Into Clinical Practice for Individual Children," and Chapter 8, "ACQUIREc Protocol: What We Have Learned From a Decade of Delivering a Signature Form of Pediatric CIMT," involve providing well-timed, accurate, and informative feedback to the child as he or she moves and engages in activities.

Shaping techniques are a systematic set of activities in which the practitioner provides immediate feedback (e.g., performance-based, response-contingent reinforcement) to the child about voluntary behavior, then encourages the child to repeat the behavior and continues to provide immediate, informative feedback to the child until the child demonstrates a high level of performance of that movement (which is often considered achieving 80% success). As the child achieves higher levels of success, the practitioner gradually increases the expectations to perform the behavior at a more mature or higher level. This increased expectation is expressed by providing reinforcement only when the child achieves the higher level of performance.

Thus, shaping involves pacing the therapy activities in such a way as to maximize success (e.g., Skinner, 1968). Depending on the particular UE behavior being shaped, the parameters that define higher levels will vary. Examples include having the child reach a farther distance, increasing the speed of a movement, increasing precision in touching an object, increasing the strength of a grasp, or adding a new dimension to the behavior (e.g., grasping an object and then moving the object, scooping food with a spoon and then lifting the spoon to one's mouth, picking up and then rapidly releasing an object). The practitioner often includes verbal instructions or physical demonstrations or offers strategic physical prompts to assist a child in understanding the next level of performance.

Shaping activities, although highly structured, can also be gamelike and engaging, particularly when the behavior and reinforcers are selected to be motivating and engaging for the child. (For children who have experience with computer-based games or videogames, the practitioner can sometimes mention that the therapy shaping process is similar to going to a higher level of a game.) Sometimes, shaping involves a focus on acquiring and improving individual small components that can then later be chained together to create a more complex activity with observable functional outcomes. Other times, shaping activities concentrate on improving a feature of a particular movement or becoming faster, stronger, and more accurate in completing a movement or executing a functional task. For an overview of the history and terms related to operant conditioning, including the process of shaping by successive approximations and chaining, see Bijou and Baer (1961), Catania (2007), and Iversen and Lattal (1991).

With children who initially have minimal voluntary control to enact certain movements, the practitioner can notice even their small, partial, or incomplete movements and immediately reward them with feedback. Eventually, these very preliminary efforts can be practiced until the child shows better control and the behavior becomes more automatic. When a child achieves a specified level of performance for a given behavior, the practitioner then promotes moving to a higher level of performance through a combination of techniques such as demonstration, prompting, verbal description, and use of toys and devices that have inherent feedback built into them. For most children, shaping multiple basic behaviors such as reaching, grasping, pushing, pulling, picking up, and manipulating objects can easily be incorporated into playful, gamelike activities. These basic behaviors can also be repetitively practiced and extended in the course of many everyday self-help tasks and negotiating the environment at home, at school, and in community settings. Adult CIMT as a therapy package is also notably distinguished by the skillful application of systematic shaping procedures and repetitive practice.

RELATIVELY HIGH INTENSITY OF TRAINING

The most widely recognized feature of the original CIMT protocol for both adults with stroke and children with unilateral spastic cerebral palsy (CP) is its high intensity. The first successful CIMT applications with adults involved 6 hours of supervised practice for 10 of 14 days while wearing constraint during at least 90% of waking hours (Morris, Crago, DeLuca, Pidikiti, & Taub, 1997; Taub et al., 1994; see also Chapter 1). Similarly, the first studies with children involved 6 hours of systematic shaping and **massed practice** (i.e., high-density repetition of a newly learned or improved skill with the goal of having the new behavior become more automatic, skillful, and integrated into everyday behavior) daily under the guidance of a trained practitioner for 21 consecutive days while continuously wearing a semirigid, full-arm constraint (cf. Taub et al., 2007). These high therapy dosage levels were in dramatic contrast to the typical therapy dosages these patient populations had been receiving, often about 1 to 2 hours per week (e.g., DeLuca et al., 2006)

Determining therapy dosage

Exactly what does *relatively high intensity* mean? One of the most pressing topics in P–CIMT revolves around determining

the correct therapy dosage. Wide consensus exists among practitioners about the potential value of providing therapy at substantially higher levels than usual and customary care, although somewhat surprisingly, it has not yet become widely practiced. Moreover, a small increase in therapy dosage and the addition of a family support worker are insufficient to produce measurable neuromotor benefits (Weindling, Cunningham, Glenn, Edwards, & Reeves, 2007). In contrast, high-intensity therapy, including bimanual therapy as well as P–CIMT, has repeatedly produced significant benefits (e.g., Gordon et al., 2011). (See Chapter 9, "Alternative Pediatric CIMT: Understanding the How and Why of Clinical Variations in Pediatric CIMT," for more details about other high-intensity therapies, Chapter 13, "Intensive Bimanual Training Approaches to Upper-Extremity Rehabilitation in Children With Cerebral Palsy," for intensive bimanual therapy protocols for this clinical population, and Chapter 16, "Research Priorities: Understanding and Transcending the Limits of Current Knowledge to Inform Best Practices in Pediatric CIMT," for delineation of future research focused on dosage intensity.)

For decades, an ongoing debate concerning adult CIMT has concerned the extent to which benefits result from the high dosage itself rather than from the full package of treatment elements (Reiss, Wolf, Hammel, Mcleod, & Williams, 2012). In our judgment, this debate overlooks the tremendous originality in CIMT, which was the first treatment to include such high-intensity therapy as a critical feature. Understandably, many practitioners, parents, and insurance companies are concerned about what makes a dosage sufficiently intensive.

What we find noteworthy, however, is that most studies have addressed modified forms of P–CIMT rather than the traditional, or signature, form of P–CIMT. One of the major features that differentiates **modified P–CIMT** is its decreased intensity, usually resulting in sessions of shorter duration and fewer total hours of individualized shaping and practice. At this stage, no one can state with certainty what the minimal threshold is to produce significant effects, nor have ideal maximal thresholds been identified.

As described later in this chapter, many systematic research reviews have been completed, each launched with the goal of better delineating the dosage or intensity parameter (as well as other critical features of P–CIMT), but none have succeeded in answering the critical threshold question, because of inherent limitations (that cannot be retrospectively overcome) in how the early clinical trials were conducted, reported, and analyzed.

In the absence of definitive data, what guidelines can anchor the term *relatively high intensity*? Our review of the published studies supports the observation that most forms of P–CIMT that produce significant benefits to objective outcomes and gains that endure for at least 3 months provide therapy for at least 1.5 to 3.0 hours per day for a minimum of 10 days, with a lower density level of three sessions per week.

Many forms of modified P–CIMT combine two types of sessions: (1) those led by trained therapists and (2) those conducted by parents (after receiving special training and guidance), usually in the home setting. Thus, as a preliminary guideline for qualifying a treatment as a form of P–CIMT— including modified P–CIMT—we recommend the lowest threshold be at least 3 sessions per week with a minimum session time of 1.5 hours and probably for at least 2 weeks (although modified P–CIMT is being offered for much longer periods of time, such as the multisite trial in Italy that offered modified P–CIMT for 3 hours per day for 7 days per week for 10 weeks, combining both the practitioner-delivered and the parent-provided sessions; Facchin et al., 2011).

We are optimistic that leading professional and scientific organizations, including the American Occupational Therapy Association, the American Academy for Cerebral Palsy and Developmental Medicine, the American Physical Therapy Association, and the American Academy of Physical Medicine and Rehabilitation, will be interested in working collaboratively to develop a standardized way to quantify and report the dosage of all rehabilitation therapies (in treatment units per session, sessions per week, and number of consecutive weeks or total duration), thus yielding objective measures of total dosage and the density of the treatment schedule. Chapter 7, "Operationalizing Pediatric CIMT: Guidelines for Transforming Basic Principles and Scientific Evidence Into Clinical Practice for Individual Children," proposes using precise terms when reporting dosage, including intended and implemented (actually delivered) dosage, so that systematic comparisons can be made across clinical reports and research studies. Briefly, we suggest keeping reports that include documentation of the dosage per session; the total number of sessions; the spacing, or density, of sessions; the total duration of treatment; and the total amount of therapy (length of each session × number of sessions).

The central hypothesis guiding the recommendation for high-dosage rehabilitation is straightforward: To acquire and refine neuromotor skills necessitates large amounts of time (in both shaping new skills and refining them through repetitive practice with specific feedback). In typical development, children spend literally hundreds and perhaps thousands of hours using one or both of their UEs in a mix of activities that include trial-and-error learning, imitation, repetitive practice, explicit instruction, and naturalistic shaping opportunities that occur as an infant progresses from reflexive and minimal skill levels to far more differentiated, skillful gross and fine motor movements. By the time of diagnosis, children with hemiplegia often do not use their impaired side much or at all; when they do try to use the hemiparetic arm and hand, they must exert high levels of concentration and effort, and they frequently experience failure, fatigue, and frustration (cf. "The Definition and Classification of Cerebral Palsy," 2007).

Taub and colleagues (e.g., Taub et al., 1994) labeled this phenomenon **learned nonuse** in adults with chronic stroke to describe what occurs post injury when a person has repeated unsuccessful efforts with voluntary movement—thus leading to the CIMT goal of overcoming learned nonuse. Note that learned nonuse is not the same as the psychological construct of learned helplessness. In a review article, Taub, Uswatte, Mark, and Morris (2006) defined *learned nonuse* as follows:

> The general principle is that a certain portion of the motor deficit resulting from damage to the nervous system is the result not of the damage per se but of a learning phenomenon stemming from the damage, but whose core is the learned suppression of movement. (p. 242)

Central to the idea of learned nonuse is that the experience of repeated failures to complete a voluntary (intended) movement causes the suppression of future similar efforts. In contrast, *learned helplessness* is a psychological construct describing the condition in which a person behaves helplessly even when opportunities exist for help or to resolve a problem, but the person perseveres with a belief that he or she has no power to improve the situation (cf. Peterson, Maier, & Seligman, 1995). This learned helplessness is often accompanied by signs of depression, anxiety, or other symptoms of psychological distress. The presumed mechanisms for learned nonuse are physiological in nature and are thus likely not conscious or associated with a generalized form of perceived helplessness.

Developmental disregard

A related construct for pediatric populations is that of developmental disregard (DeLuca et al., 2006; Taub et al., 2004). **Developmental disregard** is the observable pattern of a child neglecting to attend to part of his or her body, which is often seen in children with hemiparesis, as they behave as though the impaired UE is "not there" or available to use. Developmental disregard represents the cumulative effect of unsuccessful experiences in using the hemiparetic arm and hand, and it occurs among children who have a stroke or other acquired brain injury very early in development. Developmental disregard in its severe manifestation is expressed when a child behaves as though the impaired arm and hand do not exist. Clinically, it is often observed to include differential sensory and motor activity, with many children showing a strong tendency to avoid voluntary use and sensory experiences with the impaired UE. Figure 2.1 illustrates developmental disregard and its multiple consequences for the child's developmental progression.

Figure 2.1   ORIGINS AND SEQUELAE OF DEVELOPMENTAL DISREGARD.

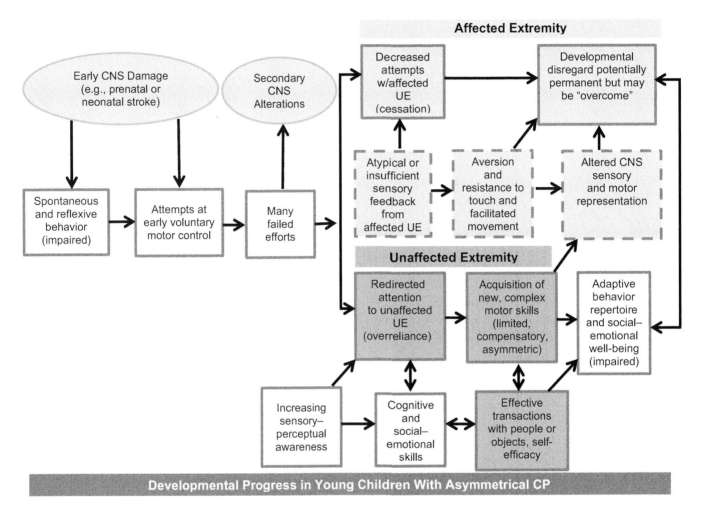

Note. Taub, Ramey, DeLuca, & Echols (2004); DeLuca, Echols, & Ramey (2007). CNS = central nervous system; CP = cerebral palsy; UE = upper extremity.

As shown in Figure 2.1, central nervous system (CNS) organization occurs through the establishment of functional sensory–motor systems that are intimately intertwined. In this model, sensations, perceptions, learning, and functions exert interdependent effects on developmental outcomes. Experience is a driving force that shapes the CNS and influences behavior in everyday settings. Seemingly random, uncoordinated, and reflexive early motor movements start in utero. These motor movements then experientially support the development of more coordinated and voluntary motor movements, likely associated with natural physiological rewards versus punishments that constitute feedback information to the CNS. Early movements and consequential experiences create thresholds that may stimulate (vs. inhibit or impair) levels of neuronal connectivity and shaping the brain's architecture (e.g., Als et al., 2004; Gillick & Zirpel, 2012). The feedback information is multimodal. **Learning** includes receiving and reacting to stimuli and progresses through a combination of many trial-and-error efforts that provide immediate, useful, and highly specific information for developing neuromotor competence.

Much of infant motor learning progresses from predominately reflexive, disorganized, and exploratory movements to increasingly intentional and successful voluntary movements that can be characterized by increased ease, speed, accuracy, smoothness, and integration into a complex, multimodal behavioral repertoire. In addition, postnatal motor learning clearly builds on remembered activities and consequences, sensations, anticipatory and visualized behavior, and observation and imitation of the behavior of others (Case-Smith & O'Brien, 2010).

What remains uncertain are the critical CNS threshold levels of activation that either are needed to support normal development or lead to **brain reorganization** (i.e., developing new connections and increased representation in key areas of the brain associated with voluntary control of motor behavior).

Theoretically, P–CIMT leads to overcoming developmental disregard as well as acquiring new skills and frequently displaying them in everyday activities. The child's improved control of the hemiparetic side is hypothesized to create a cascade of events, including development of new synapses and neural connections, strengthening and diversifying existing connections, and ultimately building new and intertwined neuronal tracts to support increased voluntary control of the impaired side and coordination of the two sides of the body (e.g., Sterling et al., 2013).

The longevity and future maturation of these new neuronal connections are then likely to be dependent on post rehabilitation activity and input. Effective rehabilitation will likely also include measurable gains for the unimpaired or less impaired side because of previous deprivation of typical bilateral sensory–motor experiences. In other words, the functional competency of each UE includes a combination of unilateral skills and movements that can be completed without the use of the other side and a large repertoire of behaviors that engage both UEs, sometimes in parallel, coordinated activity and sometimes with one side assisting or supporting the other side.

For children with very early damage to the CNS, notably infants diagnosed with spastic hemiparetic CP caused by presumed prenatal stroke, developmental disregard represents the cumulative consequences of both structural and functional disruption to the CNS before the establishment of more mature neuronal tracks (e.g., motor, premotor, sensory–motor) for a specific movement or set of movements (DeLuca et al., 2007). In these cases, the initial damage usually contributes to a multimodal loss or disruption of sensory–motor input and subsequent prevention of the establishment of age-typical synaptic connections and neuronal tracks.

Children with hemiparesis have major differences in the experience-driven connectivity between the two sides of their body, affecting both the early acquisition of their unilateral and bilateral skills and their degree of voluntary control. Multimodal sensory and motor inputs influence the organization of the brain, leading to distinctly atypical neuronal representation between the two sides of the body. When input is markedly reduced, and the child's attempts at voluntary movement of the hemiparetic side require high effort yet result in low (or no) success, a situation is created that reduces the child's willingness to use the hemiparetic side. Eventually, as the child adapts to the situation, he or she increasingly relies on the side that requires less effort and produces positive outcomes.

We hypothesize that young children rapidly learn that it is functionally efficient to ignore the impaired side, particularly if the impairment is severe. At one level, this functional accommodation represents the developmental principle of adaptation to achieve optimal practical and immediate outcomes, but it creates a situation in which overcoming the disregard of the impaired side may necessitate major intervention. We hypothesize that the phenomenon of developmental disregard is represented at both the structural and the functional levels of the brain with accompanying psychological and behavioral resistance to engaging in nonrewarding behavior.

Although prospective longitudinal studies of developmental disregard, especially those of overcoming developmental disregard, are lacking, changing a child's successful daily use of the hemiparetic side should theoretically result in marked reorganization of the brain and support future continued neuromotor control and behavioral progress (Taub et al., 2011). What remains unknown is whether therapy-induced neuroplasticity and overcoming developmental disregard will produce effects that extend beyond the specific neuromotor and sensory–motor domains. An intriguing but unanswered question is whether improved voluntary control of the hemiplegic UE will increase neuroplasticity throughout the brain and result in accelerated improvements in other domains, such as language, executive function (prefrontal cortex), and emotional self-regulation. In addition, Figure 2.1 shows that deviations and delays in motor development can result in social and emotional consequences for children, altering how others interact with them, the opportunities they have for participating in age-typical activities in their communities, and their own self-appraisal.

EARLY CASE STUDIES OF P–CIMT

The application of CIMT to children has a direct lineage from both the theoretical and the clinical literature on treatment for adults with chronic stroke. In fact, many practitioners have shared with us how they experimented on their own with variations of adult constraint-induced therapy. The two most salient features that pediatric practitioners have used are restraint of the unimpaired UE, thus creating a condition that forces the child to use the impaired arm and hand, and a high dosage of therapy, often in the form of multiple hours of systematic shaping and repetitive task practice on a daily basis.

Lois Wolf, a physical therapist, may have been the first to pioneer the principle of behavioral "forced use" with an infant from 1982 to 1984 (see our recollections and clinical notes about this case history in Exhibit 2.1). She did this shortly after early adult stroke case studies reported positive benefits in adult patients who were deemed to have reached a clinical plateau after their stroke and receipt of traditional therapy (e.g., Ostendorf & Wolf, 1981).

A few rehabilitation clinics had started to use CIMT for adults with stroke, yet at that time no randomized controlled

Exhibit 2.1   RECOLLECTIONS OF CASE HISTORY

We learned from Steve Wolf at Emory University, one of the pioneers in CIMT therapy for adults, about a very early application that his wife, Lois Wolf, a physical therapist, tried with an infant in the early 1980s. We interviewed Lois Wolf about this experience, which she supported by reviewing her original clinical records and having recent phone conversations with the patient (now in his early 30s) and his mother.

In the 1980s, a few therapists had begun exploring the idea of forced use with adults, which involved both restraining the nonimpaired UE and requiring the patient to engage in concentrated periods of using the impaired (hemiparetic) side to accomplish certain tasks. When Lois Wolf was asked by a colleague to assume responsibility for treating an infant (pediatrics was not her specialty or usual professional practice), she decided to adapt this new therapy approach for use in 3 2-hour sessions per week (weekly dosage = 6 hours). The patient was a 10-month-old infant diagnosed at age 4 months with a ministroke, resulting in right hemiparesis. The first period of outpatient treatment involved 8 months of thrice-weekly 2-hour sessions (total dosage = approximately 192 hours). The second period involved therapy for 2 2-hour sessions for the next 2 years until the child turned 4, yielding an additional dosage of about 200 or more hours per year. (The child's mother remembered that her young son also joined in weekly basketball play sessions with Steve Wolf and his sons during this time.)

One of Lois's first recollections was that there were times when this 10-month-old became very frustrated ("He had some screaming fits") when she insisted he use only his impaired side. This frustration was very difficult for the mother to observe. The mother now recollects this situation as a "battle of wills" and said her son always was and still is a strong-willed person. Moreover, the child's fits during therapy were not new; the mother remembered clearly that what led them to see their pediatrician and then a pediatric neurologist was that during tantrums, the child flailed his arm and leg on only one side, but not the other.

In retrospect, the therapist and mother suspect that these fits reflected frustration largely associated with the child's hemiparesis. Almost all of the therapy time, however, was described as being embedded in very active play. Lois Wolf told us she needed at least 2 hours for each therapy session, so there would be enough time to play, to communicate with the mother, and to be able to have the child really make some progress from his repeated efforts. The activities in this forced-use protocol closely followed the natural progress of UE and lower-extremity development, from proximal to distal, and with increasingly complex sequences. In addition, these sessions did not use a physical constraint.

In today's terminology, the therapy included a strong emphasis on acquiring and refining unilateral UE skills but also blended these skills into a variety of bilateral activities, such as crawling and ball play. Lois Wolf made several home visits and also met with the child's teachers to be sure that the other adults would consistently focus on use of the hemiparetic side and would have the skills to support generalization of the child's progress seen in therapy sessions. Three decades later, the mother credits her son's fabulous ability to interact and communicate with others to his early childhood experiences with so many caring adults who focused a lot of attention on him.

This young man has his own vivid memories of therapy. He remembers and expresses deep gratitude for his therapy and believes it helped him become very capable. As an adult, he earned an advanced college degree, is working, and engages in a full range of sports and recreational activities, such as doing daily push-ups, playing pool, and driving with both hands. He does not, however, use the impaired hand in typing (his one-handed typing is apparently rather amazing).

Lois also credits his highly dedicated mother, who took a full year of leave from work to learn how to help maximize her young child's prospects. The mother also enrolled her 4-year-old in gymnastics, soccer, and other sports activities in the community. Recently, the young man acknowledged that his peers have repeatedly celebrated him for overcoming obstacles, and although he has both reflected on and spoken publicly about it, he is also ready to move on and perhaps drop this self-labeling as being someone with a disability. Originally, the neurologist had given the parents a prognosis that he would show impairments in both speech and cognitive development.

Whether the child's intensive and successful therapy and participation in age-typical (rather than disability-focused) activities contributed directly to his many successes can never be known with certainty. Rather, we think this case history stands as a valuable lesson that a child's course of development is never entirely determined by damage early in life, thus the idea of making prognoses about an infant's future achievement levels is likely inadequately informed and perhaps somewhat misguided.

In concluding her reflections, Lois Wolf remarked that "this type of therapy demands incredible stamina and energy—not just on the part of the child, but for the therapist!" At the same time, we had no doubt that the therapist, the mother, and the now-adult child all had vivid and fond memories of having a lot of fun and seeing remarkable advances.

—**Sharon Landesman Ramey, PhD,** based on interviews and e-mail exchanges with Lois Wolf

---

trials (RCTs) had been conducted to provide strong efficacy data. Indeed, even before generating positive results from the first multisite RCT of adult CI therapy (known as the EXCITE trial, described in Chapter 1, "History and Development of CIMT"), Taub and Crago (1995a, 1995b) proposed that CIMT might be particularly beneficial for children with unilateral hemiparesis on the basis of the hypothesis of increased neuroplasticity in young children. Wolf's experience as a clinician demonstrated that applying the principles of actively redirecting a child's attention to the hemiparetic UE (forcing the child to use the impaired arm and hand), combined with administering a relatively high dosage of therapy and specifically working to ensure that the child received extensive environmental supports to promote repetitive practice and everyday usage, was highly effective.

Between 2001 and 2003, the first three peer-reviewed articles reporting the outcomes from individual case histories were published (Charles, Lavinder, & Gordon, 2001; DeLuca et al., 2003; Karman, Maryles, Baker, Simpser, & Berger-Gross, 2003). All used forms of intervention that met the previously discussed criteria for P–CIMT. In addition, embedded in a letter to the editor, Eliasson, Bonnier, and Krumlinde-Sundholm (2003) nominated a novel group approach and provided empirical data from a camp-based model of P–CIMT offered to older adolescents in Sweden.

The authors of all four of these reports (Charles et al., 2001; DeLuca et al., 2003; Eliasson et al., 2003; Karman et al., 2003) strongly credited adult clinical and laboratory experimental work as a foundation for the approaches they developed and tested. Interestingly, as a collection, these articles, although based on a small number of children—a total of 20 children ranging in age from 15 months to 18 years—foreshadowed almost all of the key issues (i.e., determining the optimal dosage, how a child responds to constraint, engaging parents to extend newly acquired skills and functions, embedding high-intensity therapy into the child's natural environment or daily functions), findings, and central questions about P–CIMT that have surfaced since then. Accordingly, we review the clinical descriptions of the children's responses to P–CIMT and describe the results from some of earliest variations in P–CIMT protocols that were implemented.

Charles et al. (2001) developed a form of P–CIMT that was delivered in the homes of three boys—aged 9, 11, and 13 years old—for 6 hours per day for 14 consecutive days (total dosage = 84 hours). During the 6 hours of daily treatment, each child wore a cotton sling fastened around the neck, secured to his waist, and covering the entire arm and hand. The sessions included a combination of many different play activities, inside and outside, including video-based games, and functional activities, such as dressing, eating and drinking, writing, and carrying objects. Although the child could request to be out of the sling during the session, no child had more than 20 minutes without the sling during a given session. These three children differed considerably in their baseline skill levels and their engagement in age-typical activities. Not unexpectedly, the types of changes observed and documented varied for each child and displayed different posttreatment time courses. Both the children and the families anecdotally reported seeing changes in everyday use, and these changes are described in detail in the article. Objective measures included discrete aspects of manual dexterity, sensory discrimination, and coordination of fingertip forces.

For some outcomes, two of the children showed improvement; for others, all three children did. Moreover, fluctuations in precise measurements over the next 6 months varied across the children. Charles et al. (2001) wrote,

> These changes may suggest that the time at which changes occur post intervention for each child, as well as which parameters change, may vary from child to child and this may depend on factors such as the degree of impairment or the location and extent of the CNS lesion. Furthermore, because some parameters returned to baseline level at the

four-week or six-month posttests, a home practice program may be warranted. (p. 75)

In their final concluding statement, these authors proposed that other measures such as range of motion and more detailed analyses of reaching and grasping behaviors and functional use might need to be included.

This first published clinical description identified several themes that remain salient today in the field of P–CIMT (Charles et al., 2001): (1) the importance of large individual differences in baseline competencies and differential types of impairments in children; (2) the difficulty in fully capturing the changes that occur by relying on only a small set of standardized measures (because these measures may be more or less sensitive to the treatment goals for certain children); and (3) the fact that posttreatment planning and engagement of parents to help maintain and extend improvements would need to become part of what P–CIMT embraces as a multicomponent therapeutic approach.

In 2003, DeLuca et al. published data from a single case history in which a toddler with a diagnosis of quadriparetic CP received P–CIMT in 5 weekly 6-hour sessions for 3 consecutive weeks when she was 15 months old and then had a second course of PCIMT when she was 21 months old. The second course of treatment involved 6 hours of P–CIMT per day for 21 consecutive treatment days.

As with the Charles et al. (2001) protocol, this treatment was implemented in the child's home (DeLuca et al., 2003). Before treatment, the child did not use her right UE for any unilateral or bilateral activities. By 15 months of age, she lagged approximately 3 to 7 months behind same-age peers on items on the Denver II (Frankenberg, Dodds, Archer, Shapiro, & Bresnick, 1992). Two interesting differences in the P–CIMT protocol for this toddler, compared with that for the 3 older boys in Charles et al. (2001), concerned constraint. First, her less-impaired UE was constrained using a lightweight, fiberglass cast (at 90° of elbow flexion and with wrist and fingers in a neutral position) rather than a soft and removable sling. Second, she wore the constraint continuously (i.e., 24 hours per day) for 3 consecutive weeks. Weekly checks on the casted arm involved removing the bivalved cast for about 15 minutes to assess her range of motion, skin integrity, and functional use of the constrained UE.

The rationale behind trying this casting approach, highly novel at that time, was that a very young child with almost no experience using one side of the body would need to become highly motivated to overcome learned use and developmental disregard (DeLuca et al., 2003). A cast constraining the more functional side clearly imposed high motivation for a child to try to move the impaired side to achieve desired goals (e.g., eating a favorite food, playing with a toy, waving to get attention). What was unknown then was how readily and happily a child would adapt to wearing a full-arm, full-time cast while receiving such a high daily dose of therapy in a compact (dense) period of 5 days per week over 3 weeks.

The DeLuca et al. (2003) case history provided interesting clinical documentation of the child's daily progress, showing that new behaviors emerged even on the 1st day of the intervention (e.g., placing an object in her mouth) followed by additional new behaviors daily. Self-feeding and voluntary reach, never previously observed, occurred on the 2nd and 3rd days, for example. By Day 13, she demonstrated weight bearing on all extremities when placed in a quadruped position (with cast removed) and showed bilateral coordination and independent sitting by Day 15.

During nontherapy hours, the child showed frequent spontaneous use of the affected UE. The mother's comments emphasized how much the child now seemed to notice the entire affected side of her body, which occurred even without parent reminders. DeLuca et al.'s (2003) report did mention, however, that the child was often more reluctant to practice new skills for the parents than for the therapist.

The child's fine motor skills quotient on the Peabody Developmental Motor Scales (Folio & Fewell, 1983) went from 43 to 62 within 3 weeks (DeLuca et al., 2003). Denver II scores also increased for all four subscales—fine motor/adaptive, gross motor, personal–social, and language. The increases in the latter two areas were somewhat surprising, because they were not designated therapy goals for the P–CIMT activities. Finally, DeLuca et al. (2003) developed a pediatric version of the adult scale known as the Motor Activity Log (Taub et al., 1993), a self-report tool concerning both the frequency of use and the skill level (quality of movement) of the hemiparetic UE in everyday activities. The Pediatric Motor Activity Log was a new tool (Taub et al., 2004) that had not yet been standardized, but DeLuca et al. considered it important to try to monitor the child's behavior outside the therapy context. The parent reports showed large gains in the child's engagement in the 17 daily activities judged appropriate for young children for both frequency and quality of use.

DeLuca et al.'s (2003) case history was the first reported involving a second treatment episode. The parents were eager to participate, based on their child's continued progress and the possibility that she could advance to even more mature hand–finger coordination and self-help skills as she became older and more independent. Interestingly, the child was very cooperative during the second casting and did not show resistance or stress related to wearing the full-arm constraint. Similar to the first treatment protocol of P–CIMT, the child (now age 21 months) showed daily progress during treatment and pretreatment–posttreatment gains in her use of the more impaired UE, confirmed by scoring videotaped standardized assessment sessions and supported by parent ratings using the Pediatric

Motor Activity Log. Maturation, of course, was identified as a factor that could have contributed to overall levels of improvement, although it was unlikely to fully account for the rapid and large changes during the 3-week epochs of P–CIMT.

A single case history is inherently limited, but it can identify clinical issues that might arise for others and can provide much-needed data related to the safety and feasibility of a therapeutic approach. DeLuca et al. (2003) acknowledged the need to conduct a larger RCT (which they had already begun and later reported in Taub et al., 2004, and DeLuca et al., 2006), while nominating the following as central topics for future study:

- Applicability of P–CIMT to children with diagnoses other than CP
- Relation of functional changes to cortical reorganization
- Consideration of the value of multiple interventions or repeated episodes of P–CIMT
- The urgent need for cost–benefit analysis, which is essential to the eventual adoption of a new treatment as a recommended standard of care.

Karman et al. (2003) provided the third clinical portrayal of individual children receiving P–CIMT. The P–CIMT protocol they developed and administered differed in several ways from the preceding reports. First, all children were treated in an inpatient rehabilitation hospital rather than in their homes. Second, the therapy included at least 4 hours per day delivered by professional therapy staff, although important additional portions were provided by teachers, teaching and nursing assistants, recreation staff, and parents, all of whom received instruction in the task and reinforcement techniques. Also, the constraint was a mitt applied only to the hand (rather than to the full arm and hand). The 7 children ranged in age from 7.7 to 17.1 years, and 3 were described as having "reached a plateau after long periods of standard therapies aimed at improving upper extremity function" (Karman et al., 2003, p. 261). The results showed that all the children showed gains in the amount and quality of use that Karman et al. described as "clinically and psychometrically 'large,'" (p. 265), yet they also reported that 2 children had gains that were not significant. They noted that neither of these children had a parent able to provide shaping instruction; moreover, one of the parents interfered with the treatment to "protect" the child from the "difficult work."

The Karman et al. (2003) study of inpatient P–CIMT reaffirmed the reality of individual differences, the likely importance of parental support and engagement, and how neuroimaging could be used to advance understanding of cortical reorganization. Two new issues Karman et al. introduced were the consideration that nonprofessionals could be trained to provide substantial portions of the intervention and the need to develop a complete manual to increase the procedural control over P–CIMT. They realized that such a manual would systematize the treatment for research purposes and provide clearer guidelines to clinicians who each use the tasks in their own idiosyncratic ways. A manualized protocol for a treatment that provides observable results in a short time frame would mobilize families, friends and community-based pediatric providers to pitch in to help provide treatment. (p. 266)

The same year, Eliasson et al. (2003) presented the results from a 2-week summer camp based on principles of CIMT they designed for youths aged 13 to 19 years who volunteered to participate in camp with the stated goal of improving use of their hemiplegic hand. The camp was 7 hours a day, 5 days a week for 2 consecutive weeks. Constraint was a glovelike splint of the well-functioning hand, and

> the activities included Frisbee golf, basketball, boules, baseball, volleyball, canoeing, water games, and various fine motor skills games, including board, dice, and card games. The participants were also engaged in the preparation of meals as well as washing up and all food intake was performed with the hemiplegic hand. In addition, manipulative exercises were performed every morning. (Eliasson et al., 2003, p. 357)

On the basis of pre- and postcamp experiences, all of which were performed in a group, the hemiparetic hand skills of almost all the youths improved, as measured by the Jebsen–Taylor Hand Function Test (Bovend'Eerdt, Dawes, Johansen-Berg, & Wade, 2004) and the Bruininks–Oseretsky Test of Motor Proficiency (Bruininks & Bruininks, 2005), and, to a lesser extent, improvements occurred in common daily activities. The youths maintained almost all of these improvements 5 months later. Eliasson et al. (2003) observed,

> by restraining the dominant hand, the participants were forced to use their hemiplegic hand more frequently and in a different manner than they would usually have done. . . . *Interestingly, this is at an age where the hand dysfunction may be considered to be in a persistent condition and it is, therefore, common practice to diminish frequency of treatment. Given this, it was surprising that such a short intervention period resulted in sustained improvement of several measured parameters.* (pp. 357–358, italics added)

Spontaneous comments by camp participants at follow-up indicated that they enjoyed the camp and felt more secure and more competent in using their hand, even though 8 of the 9 students had only mild degrees of impairment.

Collectively, these early teams of clinicians and scientists recognized what would become the major issues in the field of P–CIMT. Specifically, these issues included challenges related to addressing each child's individual differences so that the P–CIMT treatment protocol could be adjusted to promote "next levels" of skills, functional outcomes, and participation in everyday activities. A closely related issue was that there was and still is not one best set of assessment tools to use for all children. The tools available are not appropriate for use with children of all ages; some tools require the child to show certain minimal levels of functioning to administer them; and many tools do not sufficiently address treatment goals set by parents, children, and therapists. (See Chapter 6, "Assessment Tools to Measure Upper-Limb Function and Impact of Therapy," for more discussion about multiple dimensions to consider in selecting assessment methods and measures.)

These early clinical studies affirmed that including parents and addressing motivational issues are important to consider and that development of manualized protocols for training therapists and others may be of great value in ensuring that the treatment components are well understood and implemented with high fidelity to the treatment model. In addition, after children make rapid progress in a relatively short period of time, variation in maintenance of these gains is likely to occur, in part attributable to environmental supports, follow-up therapy, and motivational factors. Thus, a transfer package or posttreatment planning is now considered by many to be a strongly recommended component of the P–CIMT protocol. Finally, the huge variation in the early CIMT protocols for children and the wide range in ages and ability levels pointed to what has become well appreciated—that is, a variety of formats for P–CIMT can produce clinically and personally meaningful benefits to a heterogeneous group of children.

ACCUMULATING EVIDENCE FROM CLINICAL TRIALS OF P–CIMT

At the time of publication, we had identified more than 55 published studies that presented clinical outcome data on the effects of P–CIMT, including case reports, single-group clinical studies, quasi-experimental comparisons, and RCTs. In these studies, the type of constraint varied considerably (mitt, splint, sling, cast), as did where the constraint was applied (hand only, hand and forearm, forearm only, full arm) and the amount of time per day the child wore the constraint (from a low of 2 hours per day to many mid-levels of 6 to 10 hours per day to full-time, or 24 hours per day). The dosage of therapy and practice also ranged widely, from levels that would not be considered intensive, such as only 1 or 1.5 hours per day for a few days per week, to much higher levels of 4 and 6 hours per day, 5 to 7 days per week, for 2 or more weeks. The total treatment period for P–CIMT and modified P–CIMT ranged from just 1 week to as much as 10 weeks.

Replications of the same total treatment package have been few, and when they have occurred, they usually have been led by or affiliated with the same team of clinical investigators. Moreover, the vast majority of the articles concern modified P–CIMT. Interestingly, from early on, multiple, thoughtful efforts have been made to provide integrative and insightful reviews. Indeed, at times it has almost seemed as though more reviews and commentaries about P–CIMT were published than original studies reporting new findings.

Among the most influential reviews are two Cochrane systematic reviews, one by Hoare, Imms, Carey, and Wasiak (2007) and another by Sakzewski, Ziviani, and Boyd (2009). Each review identified only 3 RCTs that met their inclusion criteria for rigor, and even these trials had some methodological limits. Both reviews affirmed the need to conduct studies with larger sample sizes (i.e., with adequate power to test the study's primary hypotheses); increase the use of valid and reliable assessment tools, because many relied on study-specific measures and subjective ratings; and increase the rigor in monitoring the fidelity of treatment implementation. The RCTs that met the high-rigor criteria for different review articles varied considerably, as did the case histories reported earlier, in terms of their study participants' characteristics, the protocol used for the P–CIMT, and outcome measures selected.

Similarly, a review by Brady and Garcia (2009) recognized these same methodological limits and further identified the following topics as important for future research: determining whether an optimal age for intervention exists; providing guidelines on how to match child characteristics to specific treatment protocol parameters; and including measures of collateral benefits associated with clinical observations, such as improved balance and ambulation and decreased sensory aversion in children who received P–CIMT.

In the same year, Huang, Fetters, Hale, and McBride (2009) also reviewed the same body of research; they too lamented the wide variation in type and rigor of study design. They provided a useful summary of the types of constraint and dosage reported in 21 separate publications and classified these studies by their rigor. Their final conclusions reflect what has become a virtual consensus in the field of P–CIMT. Accordingly, we present their major conclusions in full:

> Studies varied widely in type and rigor of design; subject, constraint, and intervention characteristics; and ICF [*International Classification of Functioning, Disability, and Health;* World Health Organization, 2001] level for outcome measures. One measure at the body functions and structure level and 4

outcome measures at the activity level had large and significant treatment effects (d > or = .80), and these findings were from the most rigorous studies. Evidence from more-rigorous studies demonstrated an increased frequency of use of the [UE] following CIMT for children with hemiplegic [CP]. *The critical threshold for intensity that constitutes an adequate dose cannot be determined from the available research. Further research should include a priori power calculations, more-rigorous designs and comparisons of different components of CIMT in relation to specific children, and measures of potential impacts on the developing brain.* (p. 1126, italics added)

We strongly endorse the compatible conclusions of the previously discussed reviews. The limitations in the first decade of P–CIMT research cannot be overcome by more detailed analyses, nor can formal meta-analyses be conducted. Until very recently, virtually no true replication studies or multisite clinical trials were done. Moreover, some of the psychometrically solid assessment tools and strategies now available to measure pediatric treatment outcomes were not even available when the early P–CIMT trials began. To this day, major concerns still exist about the adequacy, range, and sensitivity of instruments that assess actual UE performance, whether for adults or for children (cf. Lemmens, Timmermans, Janssen-Potten, Smeets, & Seelen, 2012). For example, comparing the magnitude of changes for toddlers and preschool-age children with that for older children and adolescents is a thorny issue that will remain problematic to resolve.

Other problems in the early research that prevent useful cross-study comparisons are the large differences in the enrollment criteria. For example, some studies included children who had almost no functional use of or measurable skills with their hemiparetic UE (DeLuca et al., 2003), and many studies set a minimum threshold that required children to have considerable baseline skills in reaching, grasping, or releasing (Gordon, Charles, & Wolf, 2005). Thus, we look forward to the second generation of P–CIMT research that will increasingly meet the standards for greater rigor in design, implementation, and detailed reporting so that the empirical foundations for greater "precision practice" as envisioned in the introduction to this handbook will be established.

RECENT RESEARCH FOCUSED ON ANSWERING QUESTIONS RELEVANT TO PRECISION PRACTICE

In the past few years, several studies not included in the major research reviews previously cited have been published and provide relevant new findings. Increasingly, studies are focused on systematically varying some aspect of the treatment while controlling for the types of children enrolled, using the same pre- and posttreatment measures, and carefully documenting the treatment protocols as actually delivered. One study addressed the topic of therapy setting, comparing the same P–CIMT protocol delivered in the home versus in a clinic setting. Another systematically compared dosage levels, from the original 6 hours per day for 21 days to a half-dosage of the same type of P–CIMT. A larger scale multisite study compared outcomes for P–CIMT (using constraint and a primary focus on unilateral skill development) and bimanual training of comparable intensity. In this section, we discuss some of these studies because they help illustrate the next era of P–CIMT scientific inquiry and they provide findings that are intriguing and worthy of replication.

Rostami and Malamiri (2012) recently reported results from a study in Iran about the possible effects of the treatment setting in which children receive P–CIMT. They enrolled 14 children, aged 4 to 8 years, with spastic hemiplegic CP, who were randomly assigned to receive an identical form of modified CIMT in either their home or a clinic setting. The protocol involved 15 hours of individualized CIMT for 3 1.5-hour sessions per week for a total of 10 sessions (resulting in a relatively low total dosage of 15 hours). Constraint in both groups involved splinting the more functional arm with a thermoplastic material; the child was to wear the splint during most of the waking hours for the 3 or more weeks of therapy. In addition, children in both treatment groups received 1 hour of daily practice in their home (provided by parents), and the types of activities they practiced were the same regardless of the treatment environment.

On the basis of parent ratings, children in both the clinic and the home settings improved their use of the hemiparetic arm significantly, although the magnitude was significantly greater for children in the home setting. At the follow-up session 3 months later, however, only the children in the home treatment group continued to show significant improvements in both amount and quality of movement.

At the end of treatment, both groups showed significant gains on Subtest 8 (Manual Dexterity) of the Bruininks–Oseretsky test, but not on Subtest 5 (Upper-Limb Coordination). At the 3-month follow-up, however, children in the home group showed significant gains on scores of upper-limb coordination and speed and dexterity, whereas those in the clinic group did not. Despite the limits of the small sample size, this study provides a model for the type of systematic comparative research needed to better delineate the effective components of CIMT protocols for children. The reason treatment setting is important is that many theories of children's learning emphasize that learning in an everyday setting promotes both generalization and maintenance of new learning.

Another example of the next generation of P–CIMT research is the multisite trial by DeLuca, Case-Smith, Stevenson, and Ramey (2012) that randomly assigned children from ages 3 to 7 years to receive either 3 hours per day or 6 hours per day of the same form of CIMT. The P–CIMT protocol adhered to the manualized protocol known as ACQUIREc (DeLuca et al., 2007) that had previously been assessed in clinical trials and in use with more than 300 children in a research clinical setting.

The ACQUIREc protocol called for application of a lightweight, full-arm cast that the child wore continuously for the first 18 days of treatment when receiving therapy (6 hours per day for 21 days within a 4-week period), which involved systematic shaping and repetitive practice in unilateral activities in a home or homelike setting. The cast was then removed, and the child received another 3 days of shaping and practice focused on integrating new unilateral activities into bilateral, everyday use. The results immediately after treatment, 1 month later, and then 6 months later showed that both dosage levels produced significant benefits on multiple outcomes, but DeLuca et al. (2012) found no evidence that statistically larger benefits were obtained from the more intensive treatment.

DeLuca et al. (2012) noted the sample size was relatively small (only 9 children at each dosage level) and, despite random assignment, the groups were not equivalent at baseline. Controlling for baseline differences, the effect size for the objective outcome measures—the Assisting Hand Assessment (Krumlinde-Sundholm, Holmefur, Kottorp, & Eliasson, 2007) and the Quality of Upper Extremity Skills Test (QUEST; DeMatteo et al., 1992) Dissociated Movements subscale (which involves arm movements that are carried out without using the trunk to assist)—were large, .78 and .76, respectively. DeLuca et al. interpreted the findings in two ways: (1) The 3 hours of intensive therapy for 21 days may have sufficed to produce significant benefits that lasted for 6 months and (2) the inclusion of parents, who were required to be present for at least one treatment session per week as part of the protocol, may have led to children in both groups receiving almost comparable amounts of daily practice and encouragement over the month of therapy. Again, this study did not try to address the issue of whether the constraint per se contributed an independent effect on the observed outcomes, but DeLuca et al. noted the children and parents readily adapted to the constraint condition, and no negative side effects occurred from the casting of the less-impaired UE.

Facchin et al. (2011) conducted a multisite, cluster-randomized controlled clinical trial in Italy that enrolled 105 children with hemiplegic CP, 2 to 8 years old, whose motor impairment ranged from mild to severe at time of enrollment.

They compared the effects of three alternative treatments: (1) modified CIMT (n = 39 children), (2) equally intensive bimanual training (n = 33), and (3) a standard treatment group (n = 33). The modified CIMT involved a glove with a plastic splint on the child's dominant hand worn for 3 hours a day, every day for 10 weeks, with accompanying therapeutic training, provided at a rehabilitation center, focused on a diverse set of unilateral activities. The center-based treatment occurred 3 days a week in 3-hour sessions over a 10-week period. In each therapy session, the trained therapist delivered the first half of the session, followed by the parent delivering activities in the second half. Parents received instruction in how to interact with their child to promote unilateral skills. On the other 4 days each week, the parent was to spend 3 hours a day engaged in similar activities while the child wore the constraint at home.

The bimanual program followed a schedule identical to that of modified CIMT and included active parent training and engagement as well. The difference was that constraint was not used and bilateral activities were the focus of the treatment. In the traditional treatment group, infants received two 1-hour therapy sessions per week, and older children received occupational therapy once a week for 40 to 60 minutes. Facchin et al. (2011) identified as primary outcomes global scores on the QUEST and Besta Scale (Facchin et al., 2011). Both P–CIMT and bimanual training produced significant gains on the global scores, and the standard treatment did not. Looking at the subscales, an interesting note is that bimanual spontaneous use improved regardless of which intensive treatment the children received—the unilateral CIMT or the bimanual training.

For grasp, however, only the CIMT showed significant gains (on both the QUEST and Besta Scale) and dissociated movements and protective extension improved significantly only in the CIMT group (Facchin et al., 2011). Activities of daily living (ADLs) significantly improved in both of the intensive treatment groups for the 2- to 6-year-olds but not for the 7- to 8-year-olds, with a slight decline in the older children who received CIMT. This multisite trial demonstrated the short-term value of both forms of intensive training and some early differential effects. Facchin et al., however, cautioned that the more useful conclusions would be available when they analyzed the outcomes at 3, 6, and 12 months post treatment. Moreover, they collected valuable data related to secondary outcome measurements, including parental ratings, cognitive and behavioral changes, and parental treatment satisfaction and compliance, that have not yet been published.

Thus, the Facchin et al. (2011) study is an excellent example of the next-generation clinical trials that can provide more precise information about particular protocols and their contribution to children's progress. The study cannot answer the question about whether even higher levels of either CIMT or bimanual training would have produced different results, nor did it address the unresolved topic of whether the type of constraint used (i.e., hand only, 3 hours per day) led to different responses than would occur with a different type of constraint used for more hours per day or continuously.

There are many other important and interesting next-generation topics. Beyond the topics of optimal constraint, dosage, and location, among the pressing ones are the longitudinal course of development for children who receive P–CIMT and the impact of repeated epochs of P–CIMT at strategic times or stages in a child's development. Conducting this research will necessitate obtaining sufficient sample sizes, procuring the resources to maintain contact with study participants, and developing ways to obtain prospective data about posttreatment engagement and therapies the children receive (e.g., when and what types and amounts of engagement children have in particular sports, music, and art activities; other forms of neurorehabilitation; surgery; and pharmacologic treatment) that are sufficiently detailed and valid. Fortunately, efforts are being made in many university and clinical settings throughout the world that seek to enrich the knowledge base on a larger scale.

NEUROPLASTICITY AND P–CIMT

The field of P–CIMT has been fundamentally guided by the scientific principle of **activity-induced neuroplasticity,** which refers to the induction of changes in the CNS—primarily in the brain—by a person's actual activity or behavior. Such changes are in contrast to changes in the CNS resulting from biological maturation or from disease- or illness-related changes in the nervous system. A few published studies (cited in the following paragraphs) have reported results from neuroimaging of children before and after receiving P–CIMT—almost always the versions labeled as modified CIMT. In addition, many presentations at professional meetings (with results not yet published) have identified both opportunities and ongoing methodological and theoretical challenges to documenting neuroplasticity. In this section, we advocate more systematic investigations of structural and functional reorganization of the nervous system, primarily at the level of the brain, with a strong additional interest in changes in the peripheral nervous system and at the level of specific neuromuscular sites.

Carey and Seitz (2007) provided a critical overview of the limits as well as the promise of **functional neuroimaging,** which is an array of scientific methods used to record dimensions of brain activity while a person is engaged in tasks, in contrast to structural neuroimaging that detects anatomical features of the brain but not its direct functional activity, to explore mechanisms of recovery and neurorehabilitation from stroke. Although their review concentrates on adults with stroke, their conclusions apply to pediatric neurorehabilitation as well. Specifically, they advanced five hypotheses to help inform the design, analysis, and interpretation of neuroimaging data collected before and after specific interventions are applied. These interrelated hypotheses, succinctly presented in the reviewers' own words, are that

1. Adaptation occurs at the level of functional brain systems;
2. The brain–behavior relationship varies with recovery and over time;
3. Functional neuroimaging can improve our ability to predict recovery and select individuals for rehabilitation;
4. Mechanisms of recovery reflect different pathophysiological phases; and
5. Brain adaptation may be modulated by experience and specific rehabilitation. (p. 245)

In their review, Carey and Seitz (2007) provided examples of how a particular class of therapy interventions is linked to both theories of learning and features of neuroplasticity. They strongly argued for hypothesis-based approaches to neurorehabilitation that incorporate multiple methods of investigation capable of yielding crucial data about mechanisms of change and how changes occur over time.

Similarly, Gillick and Zirpel (2012) prepared a broad, integrative review titled "Neuroplasticity: Synapse to System," in which they detailed how brain lesions of the kind that affect children who present with hemiparesis or asymmetrical UE functioning can, in theory, result in alternative types of brain reorganization. In other words, lesions do not lead to only one pattern of reorganization. It is worth observing that among children who experience early prenatal stroke, stroke may result in differential brain development rather than reorganization of the kind that occurs in a more mature brain that once displayed normal organization. In theory, the age at which the lesion occurred as well as the location and extent of the lesion could influence the baseline or pretreatment functioning of a given child. Similarly, different specified types of intervention, such as those that include versus exclude constraint of the nonparetic or less-impaired UE, may lead to distinctive outcomes concerning interhemispheric activity. Other therapy parameters, such as specific activities and motor learning goals, as well as intensity (dosage) of rehabilitation, can also be conceptualized in terms of the brain regions that will be involved and, more particularly, the functional brain systems and neural networks likely to be affected.

Not all neuroplasticity results in desirable outcomes; that is, some neural reorganization could increase loss of function or compete with other natural patterns of developmental progression. Accordingly, models of the imbalance of **interhemispheric inhibition** in hemiplegia (i.e., how a region of one hemisphere of the brain limits or precludes engagement of the similar region in the other hemisphere), the role of **anticipatory motor activity** (i.e., mental planning of subsequent or sequential motor movements) and **visualization** (i.e., internal representation of what a motor behavior looks like, which can presumably facilitate skill in enacting the behavior), **activation and reward thresholds** (i.e., the levels needed to trigger brain activity in certain regions of interest or between regions of interest or the amount needed to produce sensations of pleasure associated with effective reward), and repetitive practice of movements that shift from initial high levels of effort to near automaticity are important in guiding decisions about the protocols and methods for neuroimaging.

An example of the thinking about neural mechanisms that Gillick and Zirpel (2012) provided relates to use of constraint in P–CIMT. They hypothesized that a transient depression in activity in the undamaged hemisphere could lead to increased neuronal activity in the damaged hemisphere, thus improving recovery:

> CIMT may inhibit overuse of the contralesional hemisphere, entreating the ipsilesional hemisphere to become more actively involved in the use of the affected limb. The effect produced by CIMT may be the result of decreased influence of GABA-mediated inhibition from the non-lesioned hemisphere and overall reduction of exaggerated interhemispheric inhibition. Emergent activity in the affected limb may contribute to increased synaptic efficacy and synaptogenesis. Understanding neuroplasticity, and the potential benefit of interventions can indeed now be studied at a translational, clinical level and can strengthen our appreciation of the ability of the nervous system to change and our practice in rehabilitation. (p. 1853)

Concerning neural reorganization in adults with stroke, CIMT is the first specified motor rehabilitation protocol that has identified changes in both brain structure and function (Mark, Taub, & Morris, 2006; Wittenberg & Schaechter, 2009). There is no reason to think that changes do not occur in children as well. In fact, structural and functional MRI (fMRI) and transcranial magnetic stimulation have documented changes, although the findings have diverged concerning the degree of changes in the lesioned and the unlesioned hemispheres. Similarly, the direct pathways or causal mechanisms responsible for these detected changes remain elusive. Concerning children, 6 articles (from 5 separate studies) have now been published that focus on the topic of cortical reorganization after receiving modified P–CIMT (Boyd et al., 2010; Cope et al., 2010; Sterling et al., 2013;

Sutcliffe, Gaetz, Logan, Cheyne, & Fehlings, 2007; Sutcliffe, Logan, & Fehlings, 2009; Szaflarski et al., 2006). These articles represent pioneering efforts rather than firm evidence and provide some useful information about feasibility and methodological issues as well.

Sutcliffe and colleagues (2007) in Canada first presented a single case history for an 8-year-old who was constrained full time with a cast while receiving only 1 hour of regular occupational therapy per week. In our judgment, the treatment does not qualify as P–CIMT but is rather an example of using constraint alone, or what is often termed *forced use.* After 3 weeks of this constraint protocol, Sutcliffe et al. detected evidence of cortical reorganization associated with some improvement on clinical measures, and these improvements persisted 6 months post constraint. Sutcliffe et al. complemented the *f*MRI data with use of magnetoencephalography to provide temporal data about cortical activation before and after movement onset, thus distinguishing between motor and somatosensory cortex activity.

After constraint therapy, Sutcliffe et al. (2007) found that increased contralateral movement evoked field activity at the level of the somatosensory cortex while increasing ipsilateral motor field activation in the motor cortex. They stated that

> Poor sensory input of an extremity is felt to lead to a condition of neglect, decreased use, and ultimately, poor motor function. . . . Improved hand function [may result from] a mechanism that enhances sensory input by way of the somatosensory cortex. (p. 1286)

The investigators recognized many limits to the single case study, but by itself, it supported the idea that constraint per se, rather than intensive therapy, can produce some detectable and enduring changes.

In 2009, Sutcliffe et al. expanded this neuroimaging assessment to include 4 additional children who received the same continuous casting for 3 weeks with 1 hour of therapy per week. One child did not adapt to the scanner, so data for that child were not available. Baseline data for the 4 children showed 2 with contralateral activation, 1 with ipsilateral activation, and 1 with no significant lateralization. After constraint therapy (i.e., used with the intention to force use of the more impaired, nonconstrained side), all children showed contralateral activation for the affected hand. Children who showed higher indices of developmental disregard before therapy were the ones who showed greater changes in brain lateralization indices.

Cope et al. (2010) used *f*MRI as one of the measures of the impact of a modified form of P–CIMT used with 10 children

aged 7 to 14 years. The modified P–CIMT involved constraint with a short arm cast 90% of waking hours for 2 weeks, during which children received 4 hours of therapy 5 days per week from a therapist and an additional 2 hours of planned practice. The therapy was described as neurodevelopmental therapy and, unlike other P–CIMT, did not explicitly provide immediate feedback to the child about his or her use of the hemiparetic UE (i.e., shaping techniques were not used). Instead, the therapist offered summary feedback later in the session. This therapy approach is markedly different from that used in adult and other P–CIMT protocols. In fact, only 7 of 10 children showed some improvement, with a modest effect size (.26) that was primarily due to 4 children.

Concerning *f*MRI changes, Cope et al. (2010) used a continuous tapping task but encountered substantial movement artifacts. Relying on a region-of-interest approach using data from 7 children, Cope et al. found that only 2 of the children had increases in signal change. Interestingly, these children were among those who showed the greatest clinical improvement. This study illustrates the need for greater refinement in the neuroimaging protocol to yield higher-quality data; the importance of considering whether the form of P–CIMT is sufficient to produce clinically meaningful changes (Cope et al. believed that the treatment may have been too short but overlooked the content of the therapeutic approach); and the need for much larger sample sizes.

For the next generation of P–CIMT research, innovation in neuroimaging protocols and activities studies during scanning, close alignment of data-analytic strategies to hypothesized changes induced by the key features of P–CIMT, and inclusion of much larger study samples will be central to understanding the interplay between therapy-induced behavioral changes and alterations in CNS structure and function.

SUMMARY

In the past two decades, CIMT has rapidly appeared as an innovative and highly promising therapy approach. P–CIMT has been adapted in many ways for implementation with children who have hemiparesis or other forms of asymmetrical CP. Well over 50 studies have reported significant positive changes from pretreatment to post treatment. Almost all studies that considered maintenance of benefits found they endured for at least 3 to 6 months, with a few exceptions.

This chapter provided a summary of the early case reports that identified many of the pressing topics that are important for clinicians and families to consider when recommending, designing, implementing, and documenting a course of P–CIMT. Next-generation research needs to focus on more rigorous comparisons of different P–CIMT protocols and on identifying more precise guidelines for determining when and for whom these diverse treatment protocols are well suited.

Collectively, this impressive group of studies has produced great benefits. However, for the studies that produced only small-magnitude benefits or reported some children did not benefit, careful consideration of the factors that likely contributed to these lower levels of benefits is worthwhile.

REFERENCES

Als, H., Duffy, F. H., McAnulty, G. B., Rivkin, M. J., Vajapeyam, S., Mulkern, R. V., & Eichenwald, E. C. (2004). Early experience alters brain function and structure. *Pediatrics, 113,* 846–857.

Bijou, S. W., & Baer, D. M. (1961). *Child development: A systematic and empirical therapy* (Vol. 1). New York: Appleton-Century-Crofts.

Bovend'Eerdt, T. J. H., Dawes, H., Johansen-Berg, H., & Wade, D. T. (2004). Evaluation of the Modified Jebsen Test of Hand Function and the University of Maryland Arm Questionnaire for Stroke. *Clinical Rehabilitation, 18,* 195–202.

Boyd, R, Sakzewski, L., Ziviani, J., Abbott, D. F., Badawy, R., Gilmore, R., . . . Jackson, G. D. (2010). INCITE: A randomized trial company contraint-induced movement therapy and bimanual training in children with congenital hemiplegia. *BMC Neurology, 12,* 4. http://dx.doi.org/10.1183/1471-2377-10-4

Brady, K., & Garcia, T. (2009). Constraint-induced movement therapy (CIMT): Pediatric applications. *Developmental Disabilities Research Reviews, 15,* 102–111. http://dx.doi.org/10.1002/ddrr.59

Bruininks, R. H., & Bruininks, B. D. (2005). *Bruinicks–Oseretsky Test of Motor Proficiency, 2nd Edition (BOT–2).* San Antonio, TX: Psychological Corp.

Carey, L. M., & Seitz, R. J. (2007). Functional neuroimaging in stroke recovery and neurorehabilitation: Conceptual issues and perspectives. *International Journal of Stroke, 2,* 245–264. http://dx.doi.org/10.1111/j.1747-4949.2007.00164.x

Case-Smith, J., & O'Brien, J. (Eds.). (2010). *Occupational therapy for children* (6th ed.). St. Louis: Mosby.

Catania, A. C. (2007). *Learning* (4th ed.). Cornwall-on-Hudson, NY: Sloan.

Charles, J., Lavinder, G., & Gordon, A. M. (2001). Effects of constraint-induced therapy on hand function in children with hemiplegic cerebral palsy. *Pediatric Physical Therapy, 13,* 68–76.

Charles, J. R., Wolf, S. L., Schneider, J. A., & Gordon, A. M. (2006). Efficacy of a child-friendly form of constraint-induced movement therapy in hemiplegic cerebral palsy: A randomized control trial. *Developmental Medicine and Child Neurology, 48,* 635–642. http://dx.doi.org/10.1111/j.1469-8749.2006.tb01332.x

Cope, S. M., Liu, X. C., Verber, M. D., Cayo, C., Rao, S., & Tassone, J. C. (2010). Upper-limb function and brain reorganization after constraint-induced movement therapy in children with hemiplegia. *Developmental Neurorehabilitation, 13,* 19–30. http://dx.doi.org/10.3109/17518420903236247

The definition and classification of cerebral palsy. (2007). *Developmental Medicine and Child Neurology, 49*(Suppl. 109), 1–44. http://dx.doi.org/10.1111/j.1469-8749.2007.00001.x

DeLuca, S. C., Case-Smith, J., Stevenson, R., & Ramey, S. L. (2012). Constraint-induced movement therapy (CIMT) for young children with cerebral palsy: Effects of therapeutic dosage. *Journal of Pediatric Rehabilitation Medicine, 5,* 133–142. http://dx.doi.org/10.3233/PRM-2012-0206

Deluca, S. C., Echols, K., Law, C. R., & Ramey, S. L. (2006). Intensive pediatric constraint-induced therapy for children with cerebral palsy: Randomized, controlled, crossover trial. *Journal of Child Neurology, 21,* 931–938. http://dx.doi.org/10.23107/7010.2006.00201

DeLuca, S. C., Echols, K., & Ramey, S. L. (2007). *ACQUIREc therapy: A training manual for effective application of pediatric constraint-induced movement therapy.* Hillsborough, NC: Mindnurture.

DeLuca, S. C., Echols, K., Ramey, S. L., & Taub, E. (2003). Pediatric constraint-induced movement therapy for a young child with cerebral palsy: Two episodes of care. *Physical Therapy, 83,* 1003–1013. PMID: 14577827

DeMatteo, C., Law, M., Russell, D., Pollock, N., Rosenbaum, P., & Walter, S. (1992). *QUEST: Quality of Upper Extremity Skills Test manual.* Hamilton, Ontario: Neurodevelopmental Research Unit, Chedoke Campus, Chedokee-McMasters Hospital.

Eliasson, A. C., Bonnier, B., & Krumlinde-Sundholm, L. (2003). Clinical experience of constraint induced movement therapy in adolescents with hemiplegic cerebral palsy—A day camp model. *Developmental Medicine and Child Neurology, 45,* 357–359. http://dx.doi.org/10.1111/j.1469-8749.2003tb00409.x

Eliasson, A. C., Krumlinde-Sundholm, L., Shaw, K., & Wang, C. (2005). Effects of constraint-induced movement therapy in young children with hemiplegic cerebral palsy: An adapted model. *Developmental Medicine and Child Neurology, 47,* 266-275. http://dx.doi.org/10.1111/j.1469-8749.2005tb01132.x

Facchin, P., Rosa-Rizzotto, M., Visonà Dalla Pozza, L., Turconi, A. C., Pagliano, E., Signorini, S., . . . Fedrizzi, E.; GIPCI Study Group. (2011). Multisite trial comparing the efficacy of constraint-induced movement therapy with that of bimanual intensive training in children with hemiplegic cerebral palsy: Postintervention results. *American Journal of Physical Medicine and Rehabilitation, 90,* 539–553. http://dx.doi.org/10.1097/PHM.0b013e3182247076

Folio, R., & Fewell, R. (1983). *Peabody Developmental Motor Scales and Activity Cards.* Hingham, MA: DLM Teaching Resources.

Frankenburg, W. K., Dodds, J., Archer, P., Shapiro, H., & Bresnick, B. (1992). The Denver II: A major revision and restandardization of the Denver Developmental Screening Test. *Pediatrics, 89,* 91–97.

Gillick, B. T., & Zirpel, L. (2012). Neuroplasticity: Synapse to system. *Archives of Physical Medicine and Rehabilitation, 93,* 1846–1855. http://dx.doi.org/10.1016/j.apmr.2012.04.026

Gordon A. M., Charles J., & Wolf S. L. (2005). Methods of constraint-induced movement therapy for children with hemiplegic cerebral palsy: Development of a child-friendly intervention for improving upper-extremity function. *Archives of Physical Medicine and Rehabilitation, 86,* 837–844. http://dx.doi.org/10.1016j.apmr.2004.10.0008

Gordon A. M., Charles J., & Wolf, S. L. (2006). Efficacy of constraint-induced movement therapy on involved-upper extremity use in children with hemiplegic cerebral palsy is not age-dependent. *Pediatrics, 117,* 363–373. http://dx.doi.org/10.1542/peds.2005-1009

Gordon, A. M., Hung, Y. C., Brandao, M., Ferre, C. L., Kuo, H.-C., Friel, K., . . . Charles, J. R. (2011). Bimanual training and constraint-induced movement therapy in children with hemiplegic cerebral palsy: A randomized trial. *Neurorehabilitation and Neural Repair, 25,* 692–702.

Hoare, B. J., Imms, C., Carey, L., & Wasiak, J. (2007). Constraint-induced movement therapy in the treatment of the upper limb in children with hemiplegic cerebral palsy: A Cochrane systematic review. *Clinical Rehabilitation, 21,* 675–685.

Huang, H. H., Fetters, L., Hale, J., & McBride, A. (2009). Bound for success: A systematic review of constraint-induced movement therapy in children with cerebral palsy supports improved arm and hand use. *Physical Therapy, 89,* 1126–1141. http://dx.doi.org/10.2522/ptj.20080111

Humphry, R. (2002). Young children's occupations: Explicating the dynamics of developmental processes. *American Journal of Occupational Therapy, 56,* 171–179. http://dx.doi.org/10.5014/ajot.56.2.171

Iversen, I. H., & Lattal, K. A. (1991). *Experimental analysis of behavior, part 1: Techniques in the behavioral and neural sciences.* Oxford, England: Elsevier Science & Technology.

Karman, N., Maryles, J., Baker, R. W., Simpser, E., & Berger-Gross, P. (2003). Constraint-induced movement therapy for hemiplegic children with acquired brain injuries. *Journal of Head Trauma Rehabilitation, 18,* 259–267.

Krumlinde-Sundholm, L., Holmefur, M., Kottorp, A., & Eliasson, A. (2007). The Assisting Hand Assessment: Current evidence of validity, reliability, and responsiveness to change. *Developmental Medicine and Child Neurology, 49,* 259–264.

Lemmens, R. J. M., Timmermans, A. A. A., Janssen-Potten, Y. J., Smeets, R. J. E. M., & Seelen, H. A. M. (2012). Valid and reliable instruments for arm-hand assessment at ICF activity level in persons with hemiplegia: A systematic review. *BMC Neurology, 12,* 21. http://dx.doi.org/10.1186/1471-2377-12-21

Mark, V., Taub, E., & Morris, D. (2006). Neuroplasticity and constraint-induced movement therapy. *Europa Medicophysica, 42,* 269–284.

Morris, D., Crago, J., DeLuca, S., Pidikiti, R., & Taub, E. (1997). Constraint-induced (CI) movement therapy for motor recovery after stroke. *Neurorehabilitation, 9,* 29–43.

Ostendorf, C. G., & Wolf, S. L. (1981). Effect of forced use of the upper extremity of a hemiplegic patient on changes in function: A single-case design. *Physical Therapy, 61,* 1022–1028.

Peterson, C., Maier, S. F., & Seligman, M. E. P. (1995). *Learned helplessness: A theory for the age of personal control.* New York: Oxford University Press.

Reiss, A. P., Wolfe, S. L., Hammel, E. A., McLeod, E. L, & Williams, E. A. (2012). Constraint-induced movement therapy (CIMT): Current perspectives and future directions. *Stroke Research and Treatment.* http://dx.doi.org/10.1155/2012/159391

Rostami, H. R., & Malamiri, R. A. (2012). Effects of treatment environment on modified constraint-induced movement therapy results in children with spastic hemiplegic cerebral palsy: A randomized controlled trial. *Disability and Rehabilitation, 34,* 40–44. http://dx.doi.org/10.3109/09638288.2011.585214

Sakzewski, L., Ziviani, J., & Boyd, R. (2009). Systematic review and meta-analysis of therapeutic management of upper-limb dysfunction in children with congenital hemiplegia. *Pediatrics, 123,* e1111–e1122. http://dx.doi.org/10.1542/peds.2008-3335

Skinner, B. F. (1968). *The technology of teaching.* East Norwalk, CT: Appleton-Century-Crofts.

Sterling, C., Taub, E., Davis, D., Rickards, T., Gauthier, L.V., Griffin, A., & Uswatte, G. (2013). Structural neuroplasticity change after constraint-induced movement therapy in children with cerebral palsy. *Pediatrics, 4,* e1664–e1669. http://dx.doi.org/10.1542/peds.2012-2051

Sutcliffe, T. L., Gaetz, W. C., Logan, W. J., Cheyne, D. O., & Fehlings, D. L. (2007). Cortical reorganization after modified constraint-induced movement therapy in pediatric hemiplegic cerebral palsy. *Journal of Child Neurology, 22,* 1281–1287.

Sutcliffe, T. L., Logan, W. J., & Fehlings, D. L. (2009). Pediatric constraint-induced movement therapy is associated with increased contralateral cortical activity on functional magnetic resonance imaging. *Journal of Child Neurology, 24,* 1230–1235.

Szaflarski, J. P., Page, S. J., Kissela, B. M., Lee, J. H., Levine, P., & Strakowski, S. M. (2006). Cortical reorganization following modified constraint-induced movement therapy: A study of four patients with chronic stroke. *Archives of Physical Medicine and Rehabilitation, 87,* 1052–1058. PMID: 16876549

Taub, E., & Crago, J. E. (1995a). Behavioral plasticity following central nervous system damage in monkeys and man. In B. Julesz & I. Kovacs (Eds.), *Maturational windows and adult cortical plasticity* (Vol. 23, pp. 201–215). Redwood City, CA: Addison-Wesley.

Taub, E., & Crago, J. E. (1995b). Overcoming learned nonuse: A new behavioral approach to physical medicine. In T. Kikuchi, H. Sakuma, I. Saito, & K. Tsuboi (Eds.), *Biobehavioral self-regulation: Eastern and Western perspectives* (pp. 2–9). Tokyo: Springer-Verlag.

Taub, E., Crago, J. E., Burgio, L. D., Groomes, T. E., Cook, E. W., III, DeLuca, S. C., & Miller, N. E. (1994). An operant approach to rehabilitation medicine: Overcoming learned nonuse by shaping. *Journal of the Experimental Analysis of Behavior, 61,* 281–293. http://dx.doi.org/10.1901/jeab.1994.61-281

Taub, E., Griffin, A., Nick, J., Gammons, K., Uswatte, G., & Law, C. R. (2007). Pediatric CI therapy for stroke-induced hemiparesis in young children. *Developmental Neurobiology, 10,* 3–18.

Taub, E., Griffin, A., Uswatte, G., Gammons, K., Nick, J., & Law, C. R. (2011). Treatment of congenital hemiparesis with pediatric constraint-induced movement therapy. *Journal of Child Neurology, 26,* 1163–1173. http://dx.doi.org/10.1177/0883073811408423

Taub, E. Miller, N. E., Novack, T. A., Cook, E. W., Fleming, W. C., Nepomuceno, C. S., . . . Crago, J. E. (1993). Technique to improve chronic motor deficit after stroke. *Archives of Physical Medicine and Rehabilitation, 74*(4), 347–354.

Taub, E., Ramey, S. L., DeLuca, S. C., & Echols, K. (2004). Efficacy of constraint-induced movement therapy for children with cerebral palsy with asymmetric motor impairment. *Pediatrics, 113,* 305–312. PMID: 14754942

Taub, E., Uswatte, G., Mark, V. W., & Morris, D. M. (2006). The learned use phenomenon: Implications for rehabilitation. *Eura Metaphysica, 42*(3), 241–255.

Weindling, A. M., Cunningham, C. C., Glenn, S. M., Edwards, R. T., & Reeves, D. J. (2007). Additional therapy for young children with spastic cerebral palsy: A randomised controlled trial. *Health Technology Assessment, 11*(16), iii–iv, ix–x, 1–71.

Wittenberg, G. F., & Schaechter, J. D. (2009). The neural basis of constraint-induced movement therapy. *Current Opinion in Neurology, 22,* 582–588. http://dx.doi.org/10.1097/WCO.0b013e323320229

World Health Organization. (2001) *International classification of functioning, disability and health.* Geneva: Author.

APPENDIX 2.A. DEFINITIONS OF P–CIMT TERMS

Upper-extremity (UE) constraint: *UE constraint* refers to any method that impedes or limits the natural or typical use of one UE. The constraint may be applied to the entire UE, from the shoulder to the end of the fingertips, resulting in almost total restraint of the use of the UE. Alternatively, the constraint may be applied to only some parts of the UE, such as from the elbow to the hand or just to the wrist and hand or the hand and fingers. Constraint as an essential component of pediatric constraint-induced movement therapy (P–CIMT) is always applied to the side that is either less severely impaired or not impaired.

Constraint should be described in terms of the following four dimensions. The first is the location of the constraint—that is, the parts of the UE that are restrained. The second is the method of constraint—rigid or semirigid casting, splint, sling, mitt, or direct physical constraint (e.g., the therapist holds part or almost all of the UE to prevent its use). The constraint methods reported as part of P–CIMT have almost always been flexible whole-arm casting, individual partial arm splints, soft slings, and hand mitts. Third is the amount of time per day the constraint is used; some forms of P–CIMT have used constraint throughout the night and day for the duration of the therapy (such as 3 or 4 weeks), although most have used constraint for either the majority of waking hours (6 to 10 hours per day) or just during the periods when active therapy (e.g., shaping and massed or repetitive practice) occurs. When constraint is not used continuously, it is important to describe both its intended time for use and its actual period of implementation. The last dimension is the total time period or duration for constraint, or the time from the start to the completion of the course of P–CIMT.

Active therapy to promote UE movement and skills: In P–CIMT, the term *active therapy* refers to a planned program of activities and strategies to increase competence in self-initiated movements and functional task performance in the UE targeted for therapy. In other words, a child's efforts to use the affected UE while wearing constraint do not comprise active therapy, although they are undoubtedly valuable and important to progress. Rather, the prescribed form of P–CIMT must specify how the specific features of the therapy will be implemented. Historically and theoretically, the driving elements of CIMT—for both adults and children—have been the application of systematic shaping procedures (defined earlier) followed by opportunities for repetitive practice with feedback to the person about progress and attainment of successive and sequential therapy goals. In the field of P–CIMT, active therapy has been further distinguished by high

intensity—that is, relatively long therapy sessions (often many hours per day) that are closely spaced (often daily for 5 or more days per week) over a specified time course (usually at least 2 weeks and frequently 4 or 8 weeks). At a minimum, all active therapy should be specified in terms of the following three dimensions:

1. *Who provides the active therapy:* What type of professional or trained person is delivering the P–CIMT? Sometimes the P–CIMT can be delivered by two or more people, such as a licensed and certified occupational therapist delivering some of the daily active therapy and a parent, teacher, or therapy assistant providing the remainder.

2. *The specified features of the active therapy:* P–CIMT was originally grounded in the active features of shaping, varied reinforcement, massed practice, and modeling techniques. Other examples of P–CIMT have engaged group and individual play activities, such as drama, sports, hand puppets, and computer-driven exercises and activities supervised by therapists and trained staff who provide individualized feedback during these activities. Ideally, a given form of P–CIMT should be sufficiently specified so that the fidelity of implementation or adherence to the treatment protocol can be measured. One example is the published manual about a high-intensity form of P–CIMT known as ACQUIREc that was originally tested in a randomized controlled trial with very young children and then later refined for use in a manualized format with a wider age range of children and young adults (DeLuca et al., 2007). In Chapter 7, "Operationalizing Pediatric CIMT: Guidelines for Transforming Basic Principles and Scientific Evidence Into Clinical Practice for Individual Children," we propose five components that should be included in all P–CIMT treatment protocols. All need to be documented when delivering P–CIMT. The five components include the (1) type of constraint used, (2) dosage prescribed of the P–CIMT protocol (described more thoroughly next), (3) use of systematic shaping principles, (4) delivery of the protocol in natural environments, and (5) inclusion of a transfer package to help children use any potential gains made in their daily lives.

3. *The dosage of P–CIMT:* Therapy dosage refers to the following parameters: time per treatment session, total number of treatment sessions, spacing of treatment sessions (i.e., density) over the course of treatment, total duration of treatment (i.e., calendar time from start to completion), and total dosage (time per treatment session × total number of treatment sessions).

Just as with the use of constraint, we recommend specifying both the intended or planned dosage and the actual dosage delivered for each child. Ideally, if a child receives less (or more) than the originally recommended dosage, the therapist would provide written documentation in the child's records that details reasons for this deviation and, if possible, an estimation of its impact.

Other relevant terms related to P–CIMT protocols: The terms most frequently encountered in the published articles reporting on P–CIMT include the adjectives *child friendly, family friendly, high intensity,* and *modified.* The nouns most often encountered include *natural environments, natural settings, functional outcomes, quality of life,* and *individualized goals.*

First, descriptive terms such as *child friendly, home version,* and *family friendly* carry a positive connotation that the P–CIMT is intentionally designed to be enjoyable, accessible, and accommodating of the different needs, interests, and life situations of children and families. We strongly endorse these

as features that, in an ideal world, would become universal with almost every form of treatment. At the same time, these terms have often carried with them the connotation that some other forms of P–CIMT are not friendly. With little doubt, both constraint and high intensity were initially thought to be possibly onerous or stress inducing because they clearly deviated from what had become the norm for relatively brief and infrequent therapy sessions that involved little or no constraint. Second, extensive published literature and many clinical discussions as well as online parent blogs and exchange groups indicate the majority of children and families have positive experiences with P–CIMT, and many have even suggested that it may be less stressful than traditional therapy models because the family and child see clear and rapid progress linked to therapy sessions.

JANE CASE-SMITH, EdD, OTR/L, BCP, FAOTA

3

Applying Occupation and Motor Learning Principles in Pediatric CIMT: Theoretical Foundations and Conceptual Framework

CHAPTER HIGHLIGHTS

- Foundational theories
- Transformational theories of CIMT
- Principles supporting transfer and generalization of learning.

Constraint-induced movement therapy (CIMT) has evolved since its original application with adults post stroke in the 1980s (e.g., Ostendorf & Wolf, 1981) into a comprehensive, theory-based intervention for children. Through this evolution, CIMT for children has transformed from a treatment with a singular focus on "forced use" of the affected upper extremity (UE) to an intensive and dynamic, multicomponent intervention. This chapter describes the current understanding of the pediatric form of CIMT (P–CIMT) and the theories and principles that guide the occupational therapy practitioner's critical thinking when planning and implementing a P–CIMT program.

The theories embedded in P–CIMT include foundational theories related to child development and learning, transformational theories that explain how P–CIMT promotes improved functional performance and why the techniques are effective, and principles that promote the child's skill transfer and generalization. Figure 3.1 presents a model showing how these theories and principles are linked. P–CIMT theories and principles primarily reflect those developed in the fields of psychology, education, occupational therapy, and physical therapy.

KEY TERMS

Achievement level of play
ACQUIREc therapy
Applied behavior analysis
Associative stage of learning
Autonomous stage of learning
Cognitive stage of learning
Competency level of play
Context therapy
Cortical reorganization
Developmental disregard
Dynamical systems theory
Exploratory level of play
Just-right challenge
Motor learning
MR3
Operant conditioning
Person–Environment–Occupation Model
Play
Play occupations
Positive behavior support
Scaffolding
Shaping
Upper-extremity constraint
Zone of proximal development

41

Figure 3.1   MODEL FOR THEORIES THAT UNDERLIE CIMT PRINCIPLES.

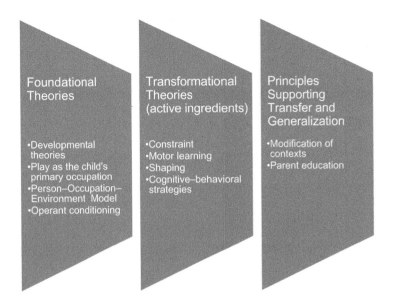

This chapter defines the primary tenets for the underlying theories of CIMT, applies these tenets to principles and strategies, and builds a conceptual framework for P–CIMT.

FOUNDATIONAL THEORIES

As in all neurorehabilitation interventions for children, practitioners must understand how children develop and learn from their environment. This critical foundational knowledge includes the stages of child development across performance domains and the theories that explain how children develop and learn. Foundational theories widely considered in pediatric rehabilitation include developmental theories, play as the child's primary occupation, the Person–Environment–Occupation (PEO) Model, and operant conditioning.

DEVELOPMENTAL THEORIES

Knowledge of how and when skills develop in typical children is essential to the practitioner's selection of individualized intervention goals and activities. The practitioner considers the child's developmental level when deciding which words (i.e., guiding language) to use in interactions with the child, what type of play activity will engage the child, and what task demands are likely to elicit the child's highest level of performance. By selecting activities that are developmentally appropriate across domains (e.g., social–emotional, language, cognitive, motor), the practitioner effectively engages the

child, sustains the child's participation, and appropriately supports the child's performance.

The original theories of psychologists Jean Piaget and Lev Vygotsky are foundational to understanding how children learn new skills through play and social interaction. Piaget posited that children adapt to their environment by assimilating new information or knowledge and then accommodating to new experiences (Flavell, 1985). He believed that children are active learners who continually adapt to their environment. Piaget documented children's intellectual development through observations of children's play and believed that a child's cognitive ability is best understood by observing his or her play (Piaget, 1971). His studies led to an understanding that children assimilate new knowledge into existing brain structures or adapt existing structures to accommodate new information. Therefore, by presenting new experiences to children, they accommodate to those experiences by modifying not only their play skills but also the brain structures that direct their play (Piaget, 1952, 1971).

Vygotsky (1978), another developmental theorist, expanded the work of Piaget to further explain how children learn. He emphasized the importance of social interaction to the child's development. Three aspects of his theory are foundational to P–CIMT principles: (1) learning with the assistance of another person, (2) the child's zone of proximal development, and (3) selecting activities that offer the "just-right" challenge.

First, a child initially learns a new skill with the assistance of another person, often an adult. Learning is therefore a social process before it is internalized by the child. **Scaffolding** is the process by which adults, including occupational therapy practitioners and caregivers, support or guide a child's actions to improve his or her competence (Case-Smith, Law, Missiuna, Pollock, & Stewart, 2010; Rowland, 1987). Examples of scaffolding include the practitioner modeling for the child, providing physical assistance, and prompting with verbal cues. The practitioner's scaffolding should be the just-right amount of support that enables the child to perform independently at a higher level. When using scaffolding to facilitate the child's learning, the adult gradually decreases or "fades" the amount of support provided so that the child can perform more independently (Tharp & Gallimore, 1998; Wood, Bruner, & Ross, 1976).

Second, the practitioner considers the child's zone of proximal development when designing the activity and determining the child's goals. Vygotsky's construct of **zone of proximal development** is defined as the distance between the child's level of independent performance and the level of potential performance when guided by an adult or supported by more capable peers (Vygotsky, 1978). The zone of proximal development helps the practitioner identify the next skill level that the child can achieve with adult support (Tharp & Gallimore, 1998).

A third component of Vygotsky's theory is the concept of selecting activities that offer the child a **just-right challenge:** The practitioner selects an activity for the child to perform that is slightly higher and more challenging than the child's current developmental performance level. The activity is just right because it is within the zone of proximal development and therefore is one that the child will likely succeed in mastering. The just-right challenge is also an activity that motivates the child to perform because it is novel but seems possible (i.e., within his or her zone of proximal development).

Occupational and physical therapy practitioners implementing P–CIMT must have a thorough understanding of child development, including the sequential steps of increasing competence across social–emotional, language, cognitive, and motor domains. Knowledge of child development and theories of developmental change allows the practitioner to identify activities in which the child can easily engage and the next steps that the child can accomplish.

In addition to understanding the developmental sequence, occupational therapy practitioners must understand how social–emotional, language, cognitive, and motor domains interact and progress to influence the child's performance. Although P–CIMT goals address the domain of motor development, the practitioner selects intervention activities that make demands appropriate to the child's cognitive and social developmental levels and that promote increased function (i.e., age-appropriate occupational activities). In addition, research has shown that P–CIMT outcomes include outcomes in developmental domains other than motor, such as social and cognitive (e.g., Aarts, Jongerius, Geerdink, van Limbeek, & Geurts, 2010; DeLuca, Echols, Law, & Ramey, 2006; Hsin et al., 2012; Sakzewski et al., 2011). Theories of human development are foundational to the active ingredients identified as key mediators in P–CIMT, presented later in this chapter.

PLAY AS THE CHILD'S PRIMARY OCCUPATION

Play is a primary occupation in which people engage and is an essential occupation of children. **Play** has been defined as "any spontaneous or organized activity that provides enjoyment, entertainment, amusement, or diversion" (Parham & Fazio, 2008, p. 448) and is a natural context for skill development. Most P–CIMT activities are embedded in play or playlike activities and are presented so that the child perceives the activity to be playful (DeLuca, Echols, & Ramey, 2007). Developmental scholars have suggested that a child's play is a highly effective vehicle by which children explore and then master their environment (Piaget, 1952, 1971; Reilly, 1969; Vygotsky, 1978), achieve important life skills, and learn to adapt to social demands (e.g., Parham, 2008). Reilly (1969), for example, posited that play prepares children for work by allowing them to practice and master skills that will prepare them to later function in work contexts. Although some describe play activities as those that allow children to expend physical energy and meet their arousal needs (e.g., quiet play can be calming, physical play can increase arousal), play activities primarily allow the child to practice and enhance cognitive, social, and motor performance.

Reilly (1974) defined three developmental levels of play through which the child learns to master his or her environment: (1) exploratory, (2) competency, and (3) achievement. These levels are similar to those of motor skill development described later in this chapter. All three levels of play can be used in P–CIMT sessions.

The **exploratory level of play** consists primarily of sensory experiences in which the goal is to explore and experience sensory input. Exploratory activities are the typical play of infants and toddlers and become less common in older children (Parham, 2008; Reilly, 1969). Infants are intrinsically motivated to explore the sensory attributes of toys and objects. P–CIMT play activities at this level may involve use of arms and hands in play activities (e.g., toys that make sounds or music, sand or bean buckets) with the goal of increasing the child's awareness of his or her arm and hand.

At the **competency level of play,** children's activities enable them to practice their emerging skills. Children seek opportunities to attempt new motor skills and to practice

Table 3.1. Developmental Stages of Play

STAGE	AGE (YEARS)	DESCRIPTION
Sensorimotor	0–2	Explores the sensory qualities of objects and activities Engages in first sensory–motor activities (e.g., mouthing) Enjoys moving to produce a sensory effect
Functional	1–2	Manipulates and acts on objects according to their functional use Understands appropriate use of objects (e.g., drinks from a cup, uses spoon to eat) but does not yet demonstrate true pretend play
Relational	1–2	Places two objects together Relates two or more objects by putting a block in a cup, a doll in a bed, or a pellet in a bottle
Pretend with self	2–3	Engages in pretend play with self (e.g., feeds self, drinks from a pretend bottle, pretend sleeps)
Pretend with others, symbolic play	2–4	Demonstrates symbolic play Begins make-believe and pretend play (e.g., washes a doll's face, drives a toy truck to the sandbox to be filled with sand)
Multistep pretend sequence	3–6	Engages in pretend play that involves several steps (e.g., feeds doll, rocks doll, puts doll to bed, covers doll with blanket)
Substitution or imaginative play	3–6	Uses an object for something different than its functional use (e.g., feeds the doll a cookie that is really a block)
Dramatic play, complex play	4–7	Pretends to be a dramatic character such as a princess, a superhero, a dentist, or a teacher Creates a role-play with different steps and parts, almost always in a social context with peers
Games with rules	7–12	Plays a game with rules and structure Plays with peers and follows accepted rules Engages in cooperative or competitive play

Sources. Belsky and Most (1981); Daunhauer, Coster, Tickle-Degnen, and Cermak (2007); Nicolich (1977); Parham (2008); Takata (1974).

them until they achieve mastery (Piaget, 1952, 1971). This intrinsic drive to achieve competency can be observed as a child attempts to stack blocks, complete a puzzle, fill a bucket with sand, balance on a curb, or ride a tricycle. P–CIMT activities often emphasize practice and precision of movements at a level that increases the child's sense of competence.

Children school age and older often seek activities in which they can demonstrate achievement. The **achievement level of play** often involves social activities, and children may seek external reinforcement for their performance (Reilly, 1969; Takata, 1974). Children become motivated to play games that have rules and to conform to social rules. For older children, P–CIMT activities can include games with rules; social activities such as those at a camp; and multistep activities with tangible outcomes, such as cooking muffins or making a stick ornament. The practitioner needs to consider these increasingly sophisticated levels of play to motivate

children, maintain their engagement to sustain performance, and build their confidence and sense of mastery.

When designing intervention activities, the practitioner should consider the child's initial level of play development. When play activities are developmentally appropriate, the child is more likely to fully participate and incorporate those activities into his or her other play opportunities. Table 3.1 lists stages of play with estimated ages at which each stage develops. A child attempts new play levels as he or she consolidates an easier type of play into his or her skill repertoire.

For example, functional play, in which children purposefully manipulate a toy or object for use and enjoyment in a manner that is consistent with the item's designed use, can easily become pretend play (a cognitively more mature form), in which children use make-believe or symbolic play, such as turning a marker into a pretend airplane that flies (with the child moving the marker in flight patterns). Likewise, single-step pretend activities can become multistep activities, such as lining up toy cars to create a car parade or a car race and then moving the cars in ways that follow the parade or race "rules." Using play stages to move from one level to another and increasing or decreasing the challenge according to the child's performance help maintain the child's engagement and effort in using his or her more impaired UE.

The practitioner uses play occupations within a P–CIMT session to accomplish four important aspects of the intervention:

1. Because play activities are meaningful and goal directed, the child is more likely to sustain his or her efforts in the activity until progress has been realized or the activity is completed.
2. Because the play activity reflects the child's preferred interests, the child is motivated to engage in and complete the activity.
3. Because the play activity is within the child's developmental play stage, he or she is optimally challenged, is interested in practicing the task, and is likely to be successful in achieving the play goal.
4. Because the play activity is fun, it generates positive affect, motivation, and sustained effort.

Practitioners ideally use play activities during P–CIMT sessions to achieve goals critical to intervention success. **Play occupations** are whole tasks with multiple steps that are meaningful to the child (Parham, 2008). Play activities should reflect the child's preferred interests, when possible should be selected by the child, and should be perceived to be fun. A well-designed play activity easily captures the child's attention and interest and sustains his or her engagement for a period of time sufficient for skill building. When children demonstrate new skills in the meaningful context of play, they are more likely to remember and learn those skills, later generalizing them to other self-initiated play activities (Munier, Myers, & Pierce, 2008).

PERSON–ENVIRONMENT–OCCUPATION MODEL

According to the **Person–Environment–Occupation Model** (Law et al., 1996), learning and performing are the result of the interaction of person, environment, and occupation. A child's performance cannot be separated from the context in which it is performed (Dunn, Brown, & McGuigan, 1994). The child's performance is highly influenced by the environment and the activity; further, the environment, particularly the social and cultural environment, is affected by the child's performance. This bidirectional and transactional nature of a child's behavior and the environment has been a well-established principle in the field of child development for the past 40 years (Sameroff, 2009).

In the PEO Model, the *environment* includes external cultural, socioeconomic, institutional, physical, and social factors that affect the child's experience and performance, and *occupation* is "any self-directed, functional task or activity in which a person engages" (Law et al., 1996, p. 16). In the PEO Model, the child's performance is the result of the dynamic, transactive relationships of person, environment, and occupation (Law et al., 1996). By appreciating the interrelatedness of person, environment, and occupation, an occupational therapy practitioner gains a comprehensive understanding of the variables that affect the child's performance and thus can plan intervention activities that are likely to work well in the context of P–CIMT. This model is the backdrop for the transformational theories described later in this chapter.

OPERANT CONDITIONING

Behavioral principles of how children learn have evolved from the learning theories developed in the early to mid-20th century (e.g., Ayllon & Michael, 1959; Bijou & Baer, 1961; Harris, Johnston, Kelley, & Wolf, 1964; Skinner, 1953). Behavioral learning theories are foundational to many interventions used with children, including applied behavior analysis techniques and positive behavior support (Cooper, Heron, & Heward, 2007; Dunlap, Carr, Horner, Zarcone, & Schwartz, 2008; Lutzker & Whitaker, 2005). These interventions use reinforcement to modify behavior and are based on the understanding that behavior is strengthened and maintained when it is rewarded with positive consequences (Skinner, 1953).

In **applied behavior analysis,** the practitioner applies his or her understanding of why and when behaviors occur to develop strategies that modify a targeted behavior. The practitioner analyzes what is prompting the child's behavior and then develops a consequence (e.g., reward, reinforcement) for that behavior to modify it (Mullick, 2006). **Positive behavior support** is an empirically validated, function-based approach to eliminate challenging behaviors and replace them with prosocial skills. The practitioner uses functional behavioral assessment to determine the antecedents and reinforcers of behavior. From this behavioral analysis, antecedents are eliminated and reinforcement of positive behavior is instituted. As a result, challenging behaviors are reduced and replaced with more positive behaviors (Carr et al., 1999).

Learning theories also form the basis for the highly specified shaping techniques that are used in P–CIMT to promote a child's higher level of performance. Skinner (1953), among others, observed a phenomenon in which a behavior that was reinforced was likely to be repeated and thus became "learned"; he termed this phenomenon *operant conditioning,* or *operant learning* (Harris et al., 1964; Skinner, 1953), essentially a type of instrumental learning. The expression *operant conditioning* originates from the fact that a person's voluntary behavior involves operating on the environment, and it is the consequences of these operations that result in learning. In other words, reward increases behavior, whereas neglect or punishment often extinguishes it.

The natural environment shapes behavior through behavioral consequences and contingencies: When given a stimulus, the child makes a behavioral response that is followed by an environmental consequence. Therefore, the child learns to associate certain behaviors with certain contingent responses (Skinner, 1953). When positive reinforcement follows the child's action, new behaviors are formed and existing behaviors are strengthened. To strengthen a behavior, it is important that the reinforcement be associated with the specific behavior, often in a very timely and obvious manner. The younger the child, the greater the need for a very short stimulus–consequence interval (e.g., Ramey & Ramey, 1999).

If reinforcement is absent or not given, a behavior is far less likely to be repeated or may be extinguished. Note that infants and preschool-age children enact certain behaviors that have their own inherent rewards or reinforcement (e.g., they produce interesting visual or auditory consequences that feel good). Thus, external reinforcement from others is not the only form of effective reward. In addition, if a behavior is punished or followed by aversive stimuli, it is not as likely to be repeated (e.g., Lutzker & Whitaker, 2005; Smith, 1994).

In P–CIMT, the practitioner actively uses operant learning principles by giving immediate verbal praise or tangible rewards to reinforce a target therapy behavior or by designing a therapy activity so that the child succeeds in achieving a goal, thereby providing a natural or intrinsic reinforcement (O'Brien & Williams, 2010). In these cases, the child's action is immediately reinforced, or the child makes a direct association between his or her voluntary action and reinforcement. This foundational theory has evolved into highly specific techniques used to modify behavior and is the basis for shaping techniques that are described in this book. (For a more detailed discussion of the concepts behind shaping and successive approximations, see Chapter 2, "Pediatric CIMT: History and Definition," and for operationalization of these concepts into practices within the framework of P–CIMT, see Chapter 7, "Operationalizing Pediatric CIMT: Guidelines for Transforming Basic Principles and Scientific Evidence into Clinical Practice for Individual Children.")

TRANSFORMATIONAL THEORIES OF P–CIMT

With an understanding of how children develop, play, and learn through interactions with the environment, P–CIMT

practitioners use four active ingredients to develop new skills and higher level performance in children with unilateral CP:
1. Constraint
2. Motor learning
3. Shaping
4. Cognitive and behavioral strategies.

Each concept and related principle has evolved from the theories defined earlier in this chapter or was developed through basic science research, and each has been validated, in part, through P–CIMT research.

CONSTRAINT

One active ingredient and important mediator of CIMT is the use of **upper-extremity constraint,** in which the less-affected or unaffected arm is constrained by applying a cast, mitt, or splint that prevents movement and functional use of this arm. (For a history of UE constraint, see Chapter 1, "History and Development of CIMT for Adults With Stroke.") Some researchers have speculated as to why constraint of the less-affected or unaffected UE affords new skill development and improved quality of movement in the affected UE of people with unilateral weakness (Gordon, 2011). As discussed in other chapters, the rationale or theory behind the effectiveness of constraint involves three considerations:
1. Developmental disregard
2. Repeated and extensive practice of the affected arm
3. Degree constraint is sustained.

Developmental disregard

Children with unilateral CP experience **developmental disregard** (DeLuca et al., 2006), that is, they ignore their affected arm or hand because it is less functional and reliable or provides limited sensory feedback when manipulating objects. Ignoring the affected arm is a natural consequence of congenital hemiparesis, and this neglect compounds the weakness because the child uses the arm and hand less over time. Limited use of the weaker arm results in a "contraction of cortical representation of the affected extremity" (DeLuca, Echols, Ramey, & Taub, 2003, p. 1004). Developmental disregard can remain throughout the lifespan unless specific intervention is provided to help the child establish motor skills and corresponding central nervous system pathways for sensory–motor function in the affected arm.

When the less-involved limb is constrained, the child becomes more aware of his or her affected limb, and of necessity it becomes the primary arm and hand used to achieve his or her functional goals (while the constraint is worn). Therefore, constraint effectively prevents or improves aspects of developmental disregard.

Repeated and extensive practice

Constraint of the less-affected arm provides the context for repeated, extensive practice with the more affected arm. The child is "forced" (or stimulated) to use his or her affected arm exclusively or primarily in play or functional activities that are designed to encourage specific repetitive movements. In therapy sessions in which the constraint of a cast or splint on the affected arm is not used, the practitioner would need to contrive an unnatural situation or hold the less involved arm to "force" the child to practice using the affected arm. With constraint established through use of a cast or splint, the practitioner can implement a more natural flow of playful activities to elicit the desired movement.

Degree constraint is sustained

In theory and through preliminary findings with functional magnetic resonance imaging (fMRI; Huang, Fetters, Hale, & McBride, 2009; Juenger et al., 2007; Sutcliffe, Gaetz, Logan, Cheyne, & Fehlings, 2007), sustained constraint, whether by casting maintained for 18 days or a splint applied up to 6 hours a day, allows for **cortical reorganization,** or reorganization of the brain structures that activate during UE movement. In particular, the constraint prevents or limits sensory–motor input to the arm, greatly limiting the flow of sensory information to the associated brain hemisphere. This slowing of neural activity in the unaffected hemisphere may facilitate activation in the impaired hemisphere. Although this slowing or limited neural input is temporary, it may still allow the development of new pathways (see Chapters 1 and 2) within the impaired hemisphere.

In summary, constraint of the less-affected arm or hand, which is one of the active ingredients of CIMT, is grounded in basic science (Taub et al., 2007) and has been supported by neuroimaging data (Juenger et al., 2007; Sutcliffe et al., 2007). Constraint, particularly a constant constraint, theoretically facilitates active and repetitive use of the affected arm and hand and may promote critical reorganization of neural pathways, with increased cortical representation of sensory–motor pathways for the affected arm and hand.

Neuroscience theories and research evidence for the effects of constraint on cortical reorganization show that the complementary active ingredients for P–CIMT, which are intensive exercise and intervention session activities, are grounded in learning and behavioral models. Both motor-learning principles and shaping techniques form the basis for P–CIMT intervention activities.

MOTOR LEARNING

In teaching a child a new movement pattern, the practitioner must consider how motor learning differs from learning other types of skills. **Motor learning** involves skill development through practice; skills are developed through motor learning at all levels, from acquiring a completely novel task or activity to refining a skill through practice. Motor performance is part of the dynamical systems that control human action. Motor performance depends on neuromusculoskeletal, sensory, perceptual, cognitive, and social–emotional systems, all of which permit the child to interact with the environment. For a child learning new movements, these systems play critical roles in the child's perception of feedback and reinforcement of movement patterns (Jongbloed-Pereboom, Janssen, Steenbergen, & Nijhuis-van der Sanden, 2012; Shumway-Cook & Woollacott, 2007).

Occupational therapy practitioners must consider the sensory and perceptual aspects of the task and ensure that the sensory feedback reinforces the child's learning (Sullivan, Kantak, & Burtner, 2008). Both frequent practice and consistent feedback about performance are important to children learning new motor skills. Sensory feedback can be augmented or reinforced by, for example, designing an activity in which the child moves against gravity, adding texture or weight to the objects he or she is manipulating, or performing the activity in a weight-bearing position. Auditory or visual feedback can also provide valuable reinforcement to enhance a child's motor activities and movements. Table 3.2 identifies the primary principles in motor learning.

Fitts and Posner (1967) described three stages of motor learning: (1) cognitive, (2) associative, and (3) autonomous. In the first stage, the **cognitive stage of learning,** the child attends to the activity to understand how to approach it or what the task demands. During this stage, the child uses trial-and-error movements that may or may not be successful. Movements are quite variable while the child is learning a strategy for performing the task. Cognitive skills can be important during this phase.

The second stage of learning a new motor skill is the **associative stage of learning.** In this phase, movements are less variable while the child is learning to refine his or her skill. In the third stage, the **autonomous stage of learning,** less attention and cognitive focus are required because the child is practicing the skill and demonstrating high consistency. During this stage, the skill becomes functional in that the child can demonstrate it in different activities under different conditions and can begin to incorporate that skill into play and other (e.g., self-help, school-related) occupations (O'Brien & Williams, 2010).

Four P–CIMT principles emerge from our understanding of **dynamical systems theory,** which suggests that performance

Table 3.2. Application of Motor Learning Principles

PRINCIPLE	APPLICATION
Specificity of learning	Practice experiences should resemble entire tasks that would naturally occur (e.g., put on pants and shoes).
Implicit learning	The child can learn from participating in a task without explicit reinforcement.
Maximized opportunities for practice	Repetition is essential for acquisition of motor skills.
Blocked and random practice	Blocked practice is repeated practice of the same action many times. Random practice is a practice sequence in which the related tasks are performed in no particular order.
Distribution of practice	Learning increases when practice is distributed across time (e.g., the child is given rest periods).
Extrinsic feedback	The practitioner provides extrinsic feedback in the form of information about the child's performance. More frequent feedback is helpful in early learning, and intermittent feedback is better in later learning.
Transfer of learning	The child must practice new learning in his or her natural routines and environments.

Sources. Case-Smith et al. (2010); Sheppard (2008).

is based on the interaction of systems in the context of activities and environments (O'Brien & Williams, 2010):

1. Learning a whole motor task is more effective and motivating than learning part of a movement.
2. Frequent, repetitive practice with consistent and immediate feedback is important for skill acquisition.
3. Variability in intervention activities allows the child to learn to adapt new motor skills to the variable demands of real-life contexts.
4. Intervention activities must be meaningful to the child.

These principles also reflect the PEO framework and the importance of learning in the context of meaningful occupation.

First, learning a whole motor task is more effective and motivating than learning a part of the movement (O'Brien & Williams, 2010). Children are motivated by and learn most

when engaged in play, social, or self-care occupations (Law et al., 1996). A whole activity (e.g., play activity, dressing, eating) engages the child more completely and for a longer period of time than does practice of a single movement or act. Using *f*MRI, Klingberg, Forssberg, and Westerberg (2002) found that when children were engaged in meaningful whole tasks rather than parts of tasks, more areas of the brain were activated. Therefore, engaging in a whole task, such as a game, an art activity, or a self-care activity, requires children to use multiple systems, building resilient mechanisms and multiple pathways for performance.

The second principle is that frequent, repetitive practice with consistent and immediate feedback is important for skill acquisition. Children who engage in frequent practice of a new motor skill and receive consistent feedback (e.g., every trial) demonstrate better retention and higher level performance than do those who engage in repetitive practice and receive reduced feedback (Sullivan et al., 2008). Practice is important for both adults and children; however, compared with adults, children benefit more from feedback (i.e., are more reliant on adult support of their learning), and their performance deteriorates when feedback is reduced (Sullivan et al., 2008). During P–CIMT, feedback to the child on performance is immediate and frequent.

The third principle is that by presenting variability in intervention activities, the child learns to adapt new motor skills to the variable demands of real-life contexts (Case-Smith et al., 2010; Shumway-Cook & Woollacott, 2007). Variability and adaptability are natural characteristics of play occupations and functional movement. In all natural contexts, variability can be expected. By presenting tasks with planned variations, the child's adaptability is reinforced; therefore, intervention activities should provide natural variability that can be achieved by practicing the same or similar movements while changing environments, materials, or task demands. By using planned variability when selecting activities rather than requiring the child to practice a consistent action, the practitioner helps the child develop more adaptable skills that can be more easily transferred to other contexts.

The fourth principle that emerges from dynamical systems theory is also core to engagement in play, school, or self-care occupations; intervention activities must be meaningful to the child (O'Brien & Williams, 2010). When engaged in an activity that he or she values or prefers and is of high interest, the child demonstrates higher level, sustained performance. Selecting a preferred object or activity engages the child more quickly and completely than does using a nonpreferred activity. Research has shown that when children view an activity as meaningful, they perform more repetitions and demonstrate higher quality movement (Gordon, Schneider, Chinnan, & Charles, 2007). Use of meaningful activities appears to promote engagement and quality of performance and is also hypothesized to promote retention (Fisher, 1998). To engage the child and promote sustained practice, occupational therapy practitioners select preferred play or social activities that match specific CIMT objectives. Using the child's preferred or motivating play occupations increases the likelihood of high effort and sustained practice. In addition, caregivers can replicate or adapt motivating play activities to support the child in generalizing new skills.

SHAPING

Shaping is a behavioral approach that uses operant conditioning techniques in a sequential manner to promote the child's development of a new skill or refinement of an existing skill. P–CIMT practitioners use shaping procedures to help the child develop a higher level of performance by breaking down a complex behavior into components and reinforcing each behavior individually and systematically until it approximates the desired behavior (DeLuca et al., 2006). Shaping is a systematic process of progressive acquisition of a new behavior through performance of successive acts that collectively represent a more advanced skill. To implement shaping techniques, the practitioner

- Identifies the target behavior,
- Determines small steps toward achieving that behavior (or, if the behavior is not composed of small steps, identifies the critical features of the movement, such as accuracy, speed, or efficiency, that can become more developmentally mature),
- Prompts and cues the child to demonstrate the movement at higher levels or higher quality, and
- Rewards each successive approximation of the skills (DeLuca et al., 2003, 2006; Taub et al., 2007).

Shaping is appropriate for multicomponent skills that can be divided into steps or levels of performance (e.g., using more controlled force when stirring, turning a knob, or playing a musical instrument) and for which a developmental progression in performance can be elicited.

Shaping is carried out in the context of explicit play and social interaction in which the practitioner and child interact one-on-one with high levels of reciprocity. Shaping tasks are selected by considering the family's and child's goals, intrinsically motivating aspects of the activity, the child's developmental level, and the potential for the activity to elicit targeted movements (Taub et al., 2007). The practitioner provides immediate feedback that is primarily social reinforcement, such as a smile, a high five, a positive tone of voice, and verbal praise. The practitioner's reinforcement may not be needed if the activity is intrinsically rewarding and the child appears to be highly engaged.

Shaping, in contrast to motor learning, involves breaking down activities into small steps that lead to a targeted goal or level of performance (e.g., moving an object higher, holding more pennies in a hand). When small steps are modeled, cued, and reinforced, often in multiple ways, it is important that the child perceive how his or her action reaches a play goal or meaningful outcome. When the activities used for shaping complex and multistep motor skills are carefully selected to be intrinsically motivating, the child will be more likely to perform those activities independently in other environments at times outside of the P–CIMT session (DeLuca et al., 2007). Occupational therapy practitioners often ask parents and children to identify favorite activities, reinforcers, and personal goals to help determine session activities. (See Chapter 7, "Operationalizing Pediatric CIMT: Guidelines for Transforming Basic Principles and Scientific Evidence Into Clinical Practice for Individual Children," for an in-depth explanation and examples of formal shaping processes.)

DeLuca et al. (2007) further defined the shaping techniques used in **ACQUIREc therapy,** a P–CIMT protocol that uses continuous casting and intensive therapy for a 21-day period. They defined an ongoing cycle within therapy sessions of shaping the child's performance in incremental steps leading toward a goal. In this cycle, termed *MR3* (movement, reinforcement, repetition, and refinement), the practitioner cues movement that is reinforced, repeated, and refined. When the child performs a new movement, it is reinforced, repeated, and refined into a higher level skill that is then reinforced, repeated, and refined. The concept of a cycle suggests a continual flow of P–CIMT session activities and a natural progression of skill development that characterizes the intervention episode. (Chapter 8, "ACQUIREc Protocol: What We Have Learned From a Decade of Delivering a Signature Form of Pediatric CIMT," describes ACQUIREc therapy in greater detail with clinical examples.)

COGNITIVE AND BEHAVIORAL STRATEGIES

When school-age children and adolescents participate in a P–CIMT program, it becomes increasingly important to use cognitive and behavioral theories and strategies to engage the child as a full participant. In older children, self-determination is an important motivational trait. Therefore, to encourage participation, the practitioner needs to allow the child to make decisions about goals and activities and to respect the child's decisions while maintaining the integrity of the intervention protocol.

In a conceptual model for children with CP proposed by Bartlett and Palisano (2002), motivation was the primary child characteristic, other than health condition, that was a determinant of change in motor abilities. The child's personal beliefs about how well he or she will be able to perform an activity and how much he or she values the activity are closely linked to whether the child will engage in the activity (Majnemer, Shevell, Law, Poulin, & Rosenbaum, 2010). Therefore, the practitioner encourages the child's participation by selecting activities the child values or prefers, selecting and grading each activity so that it matches the child's abilities, and supporting performance so that the child is successful.

Cognitive strategies to increase the child's motivation and willingness to attempt new skills in other environments include collaborating with the child to establish goals, allowing the child to select activities that align with those goals, and encouraging the child to self-evaluate how well he or she performs. The occupational therapy practitioner provides support in selecting goals that align with what he or she believes can be accomplished in a P–CIMT program. Although it is important to support the child's self-determination and decision making, it is equally important that the child succeed or master the activity; therefore, the practitioner guides the child and collaborates in decision making so that the goals and activities are both challenging and realistic.

Using the transformational theories and principles that are the active ingredients of P–CIMT, the occupational therapy practitioner selects intervention strategies and activities. These theories link directly to the increased likelihood of improved performance. To optimize the effects of P–CIMT, the practitioner also uses strategies to support the child's ability to generalize his or her learning from the intervention sessions to his or her everyday routines.

PRINCIPLES SUPPORTING TRANSFER AND GENERALIZATION OF LEARNING

P–CIMT includes methods to support the child's ability to transfer his or her learning to multiple contexts outside the therapy sessions and to adapt new skills to his or her everyday routine. Across different P–CIMT models, researchers and occupational therapy practitioners agree that successful intervention outcomes rely on the child's and family's ability to generalize learning to their daily routines and natural environments. Theories that support these aspects of P–CIMT have evolved from studies of neurorehabilitation with children. Two key elements to assist the child in generalizing new skills include

1. Modification of the context to accommodate new skills and
2. Parent education.

These elements of P–CIMT are part of therapy throughout the course of the P–CIMT protocol, but they are often emphasized during the final sessions and are essential to supporting transfer

of newly learned skills to the child's functional performance in his or her everyday routine.

MODIFICATION OF THE CONTEXT

Consistent with the PEO model, a primary concern of the occupational therapy practitioner is that the child's environment supports continued practice of new skills and transfer of new skills to his or her everyday routine. In the theoretical model of P–CIMT, the practitioner promotes the child's occupational participation by modifying the environment (e.g., by changing the task, activities, or materials) so that the child can accomplish the task or participate in the activity. Sometimes the environment needs to be modified to make the task demands sufficiently easy or sufficiently challenging for the child to be willing to try the activity. The goals for modifying the environment are to support the child's performance for successful and optimal participation and to ensure sustained engagement in targeted activities.

To facilitate skill transfer from P–CIMT therapy sessions to the child's daily routine, the occupational therapy practitioner recommends that parents or caregivers modify selected home activities, tasks, or environments. The first step in making recommendations is to ask the parents and child about their routine and daily activities (Case-Smith et al., 2010). Through these exchanges, the practitioner identifies activities the child participates in but could practice new skills for; activities the child does not participate in but could, leading to skill building; and activities the child partially participates in and could participate in more. The practitioner also identifies times during the day when the parents can implement therapeutic activities with the child and times when family activities are stressful or important or otherwise are not conducive to or appropriate for therapeutic activities.

Simple modifications of the home context can facilitate the child's functional gains when the associated activity occurs often in the child's daily routine or is highly motivating because it occurs in the context of family activity. For infants and toddlers, examples of modifications include crawling on the carpet like a caterpillar to get to the bedroom, opening containers to help mother make dinner, or helping father set the table; for older children, examples include doing homework that involves fine motor skills, helping with household chores, or participating in sports activities in the yard. When the child's context can be modified to support his or her performance of new and emerging skills, the probability that the skills will become consolidated into the child's routines and will become a daily habit greatly increases.

Darrah et al. (2011) described a context therapy approach in which practitioners focus on changing the characteristics of the task and the environment in an effort to change the child's performance. **Context therapy** uses the tenets of dynamical systems theory, positing "that motor behaviors are organized around functional tasks or goals and that the specific motor solution is influenced by the spontaneous interaction of variables from three sources: (1) child characteristics, (2) task demands, and (3) environmental influences" (Darrah et al., 2011, p. 617). With its emphasis on changing the task environment rather than the child, context therapy aligns with the PEO Model. In a randomized controlled trial, Law et al. (2011) compared context therapy to child-focused therapy with young children who had CP and found these interventions to be equally effective.

In P–CIMT, the emphasis on context is only part of the therapeutic program. Unlike the shaping techniques described earlier, which are used within the therapy session, practitioners using context therapy do not target a specific movement pattern but rather the child's ability to participate in a functional task toward a self- or family-identified goal (Law et al., 2011). Therefore, this conceptual model guides the practitioner's development of a home program. This emphasis on context may occur most appropriately at the end of a P–CIMT program when the practitioner and family make decisions about how best to continue the child's progress through activities in his or her natural environment.

PARENT EDUCATION

Parent education can be a critical element of P–CIMT and needs to be approached using a conceptual framework that leads to effective implementation. To motivate parents to partner and to contribute to P–CIMT, practitioners must consider critical tenets for caregiver coaching and education. Specific supports may be needed to help parents follow a home program or modify the home environment to reinforce or sustain the child's gains. Concepts designed to support successful parent education have been developed by educators, nurses, and psychotherapists as well as by occupational therapy practitioners (Caretto, Topolski, Linkous, Lowman, & Murphy, 2000; Dinnebeil, 1999; Schultz, Schmidt, & Stichter, 2011).

Before recommending a home program, the occupational therapy practitioner should develop a positive rapport with the parents and express interest by soliciting information about their priorities. Specifically, the practitioner asks the family about their daily routines and preferred interests, which might include participating in sports, church, or games or spending time with relatives. By understanding the family's priorities and interests, the practitioner can help parents identify how to fit practice opportunities for the child's new skills into their daily life. This understanding provides a context for naturally occurring activities that the practitioner

asks the parents to perform with the child (e.g., activities that can be folded into a bedtime routine, opportunities such as recreational swimming that can also be used for therapeutic benefit). Recommendations for at-home intervention activities should emphasize skill development that matches the family's priorities with performance areas that have the greatest meaning for both the child and family.

The practitioner should also consider the learning styles and needs of the parent and adapt his or her teaching to those individual needs. The parent's motivation, confidence, and skills highly influence how well he or she follows through with a home program or implements recommendations. Motivation to initiate a new activity in the daily routine or to change a daily routine is based on the parent's understanding of its importance and belief that he or she has the power to make a difference. Through a qualitative study of early intervention services, Fleming, Sawyer, and Campbell (2011) found that parent motivation and openness to try new activities were critical to their follow-through with a home program. Variables correlated with parent motivation were the parent's expectation of the child's progress, understanding of the therapy approach or techniques, and commitment to and investment in the child's therapy.

Many practitioners have defined strategies to motivate parents to participate in their child's intervention. A first step is to build a positive relationship with the family through open and honest communication (Jaffe, Humphry, & Case-Smith, 2010). Parents appreciate and respond to specific, objective information; flexibility in service delivery; sensitivity and responsiveness to their concerns; and positive, optimistic attitudes (McWilliam, Tocci, & Harbin, 1998; Jaffe et al., 2010). Although P–CIMT is a highly structured approach, practitioners can demonstrate sensitivity to parents' time demands and concerns. A practitioner's positive attitude, including optimism about child outcomes, also helps motivate parents and increase their participation.

In addition to motivation, parents also need to feel confidence that they have the skills to implement the activities and exercise program. When parents lack confidence, they often do not attempt a home program; therefore, it is important that parents not only understand the home activities but also feel sufficiently confident to implement them. Adult learning principles should be used to teach parents how to implement the activities (McWilliam, 2010). The occupational therapy practitioner should ask parents what learning style they prefer and should be flexible in presenting the home program information. Examples of adult learning principles include adapting information to parents' preferred learning style, presenting information to parents in writing and reviewing it verbally, modeling an activity for parents, and coaching parents through the steps as they perform an activity with the child. For certain activities, the practitioner might videotape himself or herself performing an activity with the child to provide the parent with a visual reminder of how to implement the procedure.

Parents are likely to require strong levels of instructional support in performing P–CIMT activities to enable them to extend formal shaping procedures in natural contexts and promote specific UE skills and newly acquired movement patterns. The practitioner should be flexible and thorough when setting up home programs, recognizing that parents have a wide range of learning styles and needs.

SUMMARY

P–CIMT is an effective and potentially broad-reaching intervention that is based on well-researched theories, although much remains to be empirically verified about key features of these theories. This chapter provides an overview of the foundational and transformative theories that form the conceptual framework for P–CIMT. With a solid understanding of the theories and conceptual framework underlying P–CIMT, occupational therapy practitioners have a useful approach for making informed clinical decisions and implementing a P–CIMT protocol with deep insight and high fidelity.

Foundational theories on child development, play, and learning in the context of rehabilitation afford a common understanding of principles that promote all children's performance and participation. More recently developed theories explain how and why the active ingredients of P–CIMT—namely, constraint, motor learning, shaping, and cognitive and behavioral strategies—are associated with meaningful gains in children's performance. An understanding of the research-based theories embedded in P–CIMT provides guidance for occupational therapy practitioners who implement the program and explains how gains from P–CIMT can result in long-term improvements in functional performance and quality of life for children with cerebral palsy.

REFERENCES

Aarts, P. B., Jongerius, P. H., Geerdink, Y. A., van Limbeek, J., & Geurts, A. C. (2010). Effectiveness of modified constraint-induced movement therapy in children with unilateral spastic cerebral palsy: A randomized controlled trial. *Neurorehabilitation and Neural Repair, 24,* 509–518.

Ayllon, T., & Michael, J. (1959). The psychiatric nurse as a behavioral engineer. *Journal of the Experimental Analysis of Behavior, 2,* 323–334.

Bartlett, D. J., & Palisano, R. J. (2002). Physical therapists' perceptions of factors influencing the acquisition of motor abilities of children with cerebral palsy: Implications for clinical reasoning. *Physical Therapy, 2,* 237–248.

Belsky, J., & Most, R. K. (1981). From exploration to play: A cross-sectional study of infant free play behavior. *Developmental Psychology, 17,* 630–639.

Bijou, S. W., & Baer, D. M. (1961). *Child development: A systematic and empirical theory* (Vol. 1). Englewood Cliffs, NJ: Prentice Hall.

Caretto, V., Topolski, K. F., Linkous, C. M., Lowman, D. K., & Murphy, S. M. (2000). Current parent education on infant feeding in the neonatal intensive care unit: The role of the occupational therapist. *American Journal of Occupational Therapy, 54,* 59–64. http://dx.doi.org/10.5014/ajot.54.1.59

Carr, E. G., Horner, R. H., Turnbull, A. P., Marquis, J. G., McLaughlin, D. M., McAtee, M. L., . . . Braddock, D. (1999). *Positive behavior support for people with developmental disabilities: A research synthesis.* Washington, DC: American Association on Mental Retardation.

Case-Smith, J., Law, M., Missiuna, C., Pollock, N., & Stewart, D. (2010). Foundations for occupational therapy practice with children. In J. Case-Smith & J. O'Brien (Eds.), *Occupational therapy for children* (6th ed., pp. 22–56). St. Louis: Mosby/Elsevier.

Cooper, J. O., Heron, T. E., & Heward, W. L. (2007). *Applied behavior analysis.* Upper Saddle River, NJ: Pearson/Merrill Hall.

Darrah, J., Law, M. C., Pollock, N., Wilson, B., Russell, D. J., Walter, S. D., . . . Galuppi, B. (2011). Context therapy: A new intervention approach for children with cerebral palsy. *Developmental Medicine and Child Neurology, 53,* 615–620.

Daunhauer, L. A., Coster, W. J., Tickle-Degnen, L., & Cermak, S. A. (2007). Effects of caregiver–child interactions on play occupations among young children institutionalized in Eastern Europe. *American Journal of Occupational Therapy, 61,* 429–440. http://dx.doi.org/10.5014/ajot.61.4.429

DeLuca, S. C., Echols, K., Law, C. R., & Ramey, S. L. (2006). Intensive pediatric constraint-induced therapy for children with cerebral palsy: Randomized, controlled, crossover trial. *Journal of Child Neurology, 21,* 931–938. http://dx.doi.org/10.23107/7010.2006.00201

DeLuca, S. C., Echols, K., & Ramey, S. L. (2007). *ACQUIREc therapy: A training manual for effective application of pediatric constraint-induced movement therapy.* Hillsborough, NC: MindNurture.

DeLuca, S. C., Echols, K., Ramey, S. L., & Taub, E. (2003). Pediatric constraint-induced movement therapy for a young child with cerebral palsy: Two episodes of care. *Journal of the American Physical Therapy Association, 83,* 1003–1013. PMID: 14577827

Dinnebeil, L. A. (1999). Defining parent education in early intervention. *Topics in Early Childhood Special Education, 19,* 161–165.

Dunlap, G., Carr, E. G., Horner, R. H., Zarcone, J. R., & Schwartz, I. (2008). Positive behavior support and applied behavior analysis: A familial alliance. *Behavior Modification, 32,* 682–698.

Dunn, W., Brown, C., & McGuigan, A. (1994). The ecology of human performance: A framework for considering the effect of context. *American Journal of Occupational Therapy, 48,* 595–607. http://dx.doi.org/10.5014/ajot.48.7.595

Fisher, A. G. (1998). Uniting practice and theory in an occupational framework (Eleanor Clarke Slagle Lecture). *American Journal of Occupational Therapy, 52,* 509–521. http://dx.doi.org/10.5014/ajot.52.7.509

Fitts, P. M., & Posner, M. I. (1967). *Human performance.* Belmont, CA: Brooks/Cole.

Flavell, J. (1985). *Cognitive development.* Englewood Cliffs, NJ: Prentice Hall.

Fleming, J. L., Sawyer, B., & Campbell, P. H. (2011). Early intervention providers' perspectives about implementing participation-based practices. *Topics in Early Childhood Special Education, 30,* 233–244.

Gordon, A. M. (2011). To constrain or not to constrain, and other stories of intensive upper extremity training for children with unilateral cerebral palsy. *Developmental Medicine and Child Neurology, 53*(Suppl. 4), 56–61.

Gordon, A. M., Schneider, J. A., Chinnan, A., & Charles, J. R. (2007). Efficacy of a hand–arm bimanual intensive therapy (HABIT) in children with hemiplegic cerebral palsy: A randomized control trial. *Developmental Medicine and Child Neurology, 49,* 830–838.

Harris, F. R., Johnston, M. K., Kelley, C. S., & Wolf, M. M. (1964). Effects of positive social reinforcement on regressed crawling of a nursery school child. *Journal of Educational Psychology, 55,* 34–41.

Hsin, Y.-J., Chen, F.-C., Lin, K.-C., Kang, L.-J., Chen, C.-I., & Chen, C.-Y. (2012). Efficacy of constraint-induced therapy on functional performance and health-related quality of life for children with cerebral palsy: A randomized controlled trial. *Journal of Child Neurology, 27,* 992–999.

Huang, H., Fetters, L., Hale, J., & McBride, A. (2009). Bound for success: A systematic review of constraint-induced movement therapy in children with cerebral palsy supports improved arm and hand use. *Physical Therapy, 89,* 1126–1141. http://dx.doi.org/10.2522/ptj.20080111

Jaffe, L., Humphry, R., & Case-Smith, J. (2010). Working with families. In J. Case-Smith & J. O'Brien (Eds.), *Occupational therapy for children* (6th ed., pp. 108–140). St. Louis: Mosby/Elsevier.

Jongbloed-Pereboom, M., Janssen, A. J. W. M., Steenbergen, B., & Nijhuis-van der Sanden, M. W. (2012). Motor learning and working memory in children born preterm: A systematic review. *Neuroscience and Biobehavioral Reviews, 36,* 1314–1330.

Juenger, H., Linder-Lucht, M., Walther, M., Berweck, S., Mall, V., & Staudt, M. (2007). Cortical neuromodulation by constraint-induced movement therapy in congenital hemiparesis: An *f*MRI study. *Neuropediatrics, 38,* 130–136.

Klingberg, T., Forssberg, H., & Westerberg, H. (2002). Increased brain activity in frontal and parietal cortex underlies the development of visuospatial working memory capacity during childhood. *Journal of Cognitive Neuroscience, 14,* 1–10.

Law, M., Cooper, B., Strong, S., Stewart, D., Rigby, P., & Letts, L. (1996). The Person–Environment–Occupation Model: A transactive approach to occupational performance. *Canadian Journal of Occupational Therapy, 63,* 9–23.

Law, M. C., Darrah, J., Pollock, N., Wilson, B., Russell, D. J., Walter, S. D., . . . Galuppi, B. (2011). Focus on function: A cluster, randomized controlled trial comparing child-versus context-focused intervention for young children with cerebral palsy. *Developmental Medicine and Child Neurology, 53,* 621–629.

Lutzker, J. R., & Whitaker, D. J. (2005). The expanding role of behavior analysis and support: Current status and future directions. *Behavior Modification, 29,* 575–594.

Majnemer, A., Shevell, M., Law, M., Poulin, C., & Rosenbaum, P. (2010). Level of motivation in mastering challenging tasks in children with cerebral palsy. *Developmental Medicine and Child Neurology, 52,* 1120–1126.

McWilliam, R. A. (2010). *Routines-based early intervention: Supporting young children and their families.* Baltimore: Paul H. Brookes.

McWilliam, R. A., Tocci, L., & Harbin, G. L. (1998). Family-centered services: Service providers' discourse and behavior. *Topics in Early Childhood Special Education, 18,* 206–221.

Mullick, J. A. (2006). Positive behavior support and applied behavior analysis. *Behavior Analyst, 29,* 51–74.

Munier, V., Myers, C., & Pierce, D. (2008). Power of object play for infants and toddlers. In L. D. Parham & L. Fazio (Eds.), *Play in occupational therapy for children* (2nd ed., pp. 219–250). St. Louis: Mosby/Elsevier.

Nicolich, L. M. (1977). Beyond sensorimotor intelligence: Assessment of symbolic maturity through analysis of pretend play. *Merrill-Palmer Quarterly, 2,* 90–99.

O'Brien, J., & Williams, H. (2010). Application of motor control/motor learning to practice. In J. Case-Smith & J. O'Brien (Eds.), *Occupational therapy for children* (6th ed., pp. 245–274). St. Louis: Mosby/Elsevier.

Ostendorf, C. G., & Wolf, S. L. (1981). Effect of forced use of the upper extremity of a hemiplegic patient on changes in function. *Physical Therapy, 61,* 1022–1028.

Parham, L. D. (2008). Play and occupational therapy. In L. D. Parham & L. Fazio (Eds.), *Play in occupational therapy for children* (2nd ed., pp. 3–42). St. Louis: Mosby/Elsevier.

Parham, L. D., & Fazio, L. (Eds.). (2008). *Play in occupational therapy for children* (2nd ed.). St. Louis: Mosby/Elsevier.

Piaget, J. (1952). *The origins of intelligence in children.* New York: International Universities.

Piaget, J. (1971). *Psychology and epistemology: Towards a theory of knowledge.* New York: Viking.

Ramey, C. T., & Ramey, S. L. (1999). *Right from birth: Building a child's foundation for life.* New York: Goddard Press.

Reilly, M. (1969). The educational process. *American Journal of Occupational Therapy, 23,* 299–307.

Reilly, M. (Ed.). (1974). *Play as exploratory learning.* Beverly Hills, CA: Sage.

Rowland, S. (1987). An interpretive model of teaching and learning. In A. Pollard (Ed.), *Children and their primary schools* (pp. 128–132). London: Falmer Press.

Sakzewski, L., Ziviani, J., Abbott, D. F., Macdonell, R. A., Jackson, G. D., & Boyd, R. N. (2011). Randomized trial of constraint-induced movement therapy and bimanual training on activity outcomes for children with congenital hemiplegia. *Developmental Medicine and Child Neurology, 53,* 313–320.

Sameroff, A. (2009). *The transactional model of development: How children and context shape each other.* Washington, DC: American Psychological Association.

Schultz, T. R., Schmidt, C. T., & Stichter, J. P. (2011). A review of parent education programs for parents of children with autism spectrum disorders. *Focus on Autism and Other Developmental Disabilities, 26,* 96–104.

Sheppard, J. J. (2008). Using motor learning approaches for treating swallowing and feeding disorders: A review. *Language, Speech, and Hearing Services in Schools, 39,* 227–236.

Shumway-Cook, A., & Woollacott, M. H. (2007). *Motor control: Translating research into clinical practice* (3rd ed.). Philadelphia: Lippincott Williams & Wilkins.

Skinner, B. F. (1953). *Science and human behavior.* New York: Free Press.

Smith, T. L. (1994). *Behavior and its causes: Philosophical foundations of operant psychology.* Boston: Kluwer Academic.

Sullivan, K. J., Kantak, S. S., & Burtner, P. A. (2008). Motor learning in children: Feedback effects on skill acquisition. *Physical Therapy, 88,* 720–732.

Sutcliffe, T. L., Gaetz, W. C., Logan, W. J., Cheyne, D. O., & Fehlings, D. L. (2007). Cortical reorganization after modified constraint-induced movement therapy in pediatric hemiplegic cerebral palsy. *Journal of Child Neurology, 22,* 1281–1287.

Takata, N. (1974). Play as prescription. In M. Reilly (Ed.), *Play as exploratory learning* (pp. 209–246). Beverly Hills, CA: Sage.

Taub, E., Griffin, A., Nick, J., Gammons, K., Uswatte, G., & Law, C. R. (2007). Pediatric CI therapy for stroke-induced hemiparesis in young children. *Developmental Neurorehabilitation, 10,* 3–18.

Tharp, R., & Gallimore, R. (1998). A theory of learning as assisted performance. In D. Faulkner, K. Littleton, & M. Woodhead (Eds.), *Learning relationships in the classroom* (pp. 93–110). London: Routledge.

Vygotsky, L. (1978). *Mind in society: The development of higher psychological processes.* Cambridge, MA: Harvard University Press.

Wood, D. J., Bruner, J., & Ross, G. (1976). The role of tutoring in problem solving. *Journal of Child Psychiatry, 17,* 89–100.

VALENTINA INTAGLIATA, MD, and RICHARD D. STEVENSON, MD

4

Motor Development and Physical Growth in Children With Cerebral Palsy

CHAPTER HIGHLIGHTS

- Definition and classification of cerebral palsy
- Prevalence of cerebral palsy
- Motor development of children with cerebral palsy
- Physical growth of children with cerebral palsy.

KEY TERMS

Cerebral palsy
Diplegia
Hemiplegia
Mechanostat
Quadriplegia
Skeletal maturation

Cerebral palsy (CP) is a well-recognized neuro-developmental condition that begins early in childhood and persists throughout the lifespan. The term is used to describe a group of heterogeneous disorders characterized primarily by motor impairment. Additionally, more than half of children with CP have associated conditions, such as epilepsy and intellectual disability (Himmelmann, Beckung, Hagberg, & Uvebrant, 2006). Many children with CP experience severe disability because of motor impairment affecting activities of daily living (ADLs) and participation in the community (Calley et al., 2012; McManus, Corcoran, & Perry, 2008; Morris, Kurinczuk, Fitzpatrick, & Rosenbaum, 2006). The associated comorbidities also can play a large role in overall disability (Bartlett & Palisano, 2000; Himmelmann et al., 2006; Kennes et al., 2002).

CP is the most common cause of motor impairment in children worldwide, with an estimated prevalence rate of between 2 and 3 per 1,000 live births. This rate increases to 40 to 100 per 1,000 live births among babies born very premature or with very low birth weight (VLBW; prevalence and characteristics of children with CP in Europe in 2002; Yeargin-Allsopp et al., 2008).

Over the past several decades, major medical advances in the care of children with CP have led to improved quality of life and increased survival. Currently, nearly half of children with severe impairment live into adulthood (Blair, 2010). Unfortunately, efforts to understand the etiologies of CP and implement preventive strategies have progressed slowly.

This chapter discusses the current definition and classification of CP and their importance for studying CP among populations across the world. Prevalence studies of large populations are discussed and statistics about children at increased risk for CP provided. The latter part of the chapter focuses on the motor development and physical growth of children with CP over time and the relationship between the two.

DEFINITION AND CLASSIFICATION OF CEREBRAL PALSY

Origins of the definition and classification of CP in the medical literature can be traced to the early 19th century and the influential work of the English orthopedist William Little (Morris, 2007). Little understood that the cause of "cerebral paresis" was damage to the brain during infancy. He described 47 cases and classified people with CP as *hemiplegic, paraplegic,* or *generalized* (Little, 1966). In 1957, a group called the "Little Club" convened in the United Kingdom to attempt to better define CP (Morris, 2007). Their initial description was later refined by Bax in 1964 as "a disorder of posture and movement due to a defect or lesion of the immature brain" excluding cases "which are of short duration, due to progressive disease or due solely to mental deficiency" (p. 295). This simple and brief description was deliberately broad so that services would not be limited for people with CP and Bax (1964) hoped that it would be readily translated for widespread approval (Rosenbaum, Paneth, Leviton, & Goldstein, 2007).

In an effort to produce an updated, practical, and universally accepted definition and classification scheme for CP, an international, multidisciplinary group met in Bethesda, Maryland, in 2004 for a workshop on the definition and classification of CP (Morris, 2007). The mission of this committee stemmed from changes in the delivery of care to children with disabilities and growing advancements in brain-imaging technology, neurobiology, and understanding of the etiologies of motor impairment (e.g., genetic factors). Rosenbaum and colleagues (2007) set forth a modified version of Bax's definition (Bax, 1964; Morris, 2007). The new definition was distinguished by the addition of a descriptor regarding the comorbid neurodevelopmental disorders that often accompany motor impairment in CP, such as cognitive impairment, sensory disturbances, and seizure disorder (Morris, 2007).

Because of the broad phenotypic definition of CP, it is valuable to further classify affected persons into categories or subgroups (Table 4.1). Subgroup classification provides

- A description of greater detail that more clearly explains the degree of a problem,
- Information to facilitate prediction of current and future services,
- Appropriate means for comparing people with the same problem in different places, and
- Sufficient information to evaluate change within a person at different points in time (Rosenbaum et al., 2007).

The information available for classification may differ depending on age, geographic region, and chosen characteristics. For a classification system to be useful, however, it must be reliable, provide specific definitions of characteristics, and enable consistent and reproducible classification of the same person when given identical information.

In the past, the anatomical distribution of impairment has been the primary emphasis for classification of CP. **Hemiplegia** is paralysis or paresis of the arm, trunk, and leg on the same side of the body; **diplegia** is paralysis of symmetrical parts of the body, characteristically the legs; and **quadriplegia** is paralysis that involves all four extremities. In addition to anatomical distribution, a second descriptor is used to describe the predominant type of tone or movement abnormality. The classification scheme for CP proposed by the committee includes multiple aspects of CP in four major dimensions:

1. Motor abnormalities,
2. Accompanying impairments,
3. Anatomical and neuroimaging findings, and
4. Causation and timing (Rosenbaum et al., 2007).

The motor abnormalities dimension contains a subcategory for the nature and type of movement disorder and a subcategory for functional impairment classification (Rosenbaum et al., 2007). Several measurement tools have been developed to describe specific areas of functioning, including the Manual Abilities Classification Scale (MACS; Eliasson, Krumlinde-Sundholm, et al., 2006; Morris et al., 2006) for upper-extremity (UE) and fine motor functioning and the Gross Motor Function Classification System (GMFCS; Bodkin, Robinson, & Perales, 2003; Palisano et al., 1997; Wood & Rosenbaum, 2000) for ambulation. Both the MACS and the GMFCS have been shown to be reliable and valid tools (Bodkin et al., 2003; Eliasson, Krumlinde-Sundholm, et al., 2006; Morris et al., 2006; Palisano et al., 1997; Wood & Rosenbaum, 2000). The GMFCS is widely used and classifies children on the basis of ability for self-initiated movement: Children at Level I walk without limitations, those at Level II walk with limitations, those at Level III walk using a handheld mobility device, those at Level IV engage in

Table 4.1   Cerebral Palsy Classification

MAIN DIMENSION	SUBCATEGORY	OTHER
Motor abnormalities	Nature and typology of the motor disorder Functional motor abilities	Type of hypertonia or movement abnormality (e.g., spasticity, ataxia, dystonia, athetosis) Extent to which individual is limited in motor function (e.g., GMFCS, MACS)
Accompanying impairments and secondary conditions	—	Musculoskeletal problems that develop later (e.g., contractures, scoliosis) Neurodevelopmental comorbidities (e.g., seizures, intellectual disability)
Anatomical and neuroimaging findings	Anatomical distribution Neuroimaging findings	Part of the body affected by motor impairment (e.g., limbs, trunk, bulbar) Neuroanatomical findings on CT or MRI (e.g., white matter loss, brain anomaly)
Causation and timing	—	Cause (if known) and associated timing of injury (if known; e.g., hypoxic ischemic encephalopathy at birth, schizencephaly during 2nd trimester)

Note. — = not applicable; CT = computed tomography; GMFCS = Gross Motor Function Classification System; MACS = Manual Abilities Classification Scale; MRI = magnetic resonance imaging.
Source. Rosenbaum, Paneth, Leviton, Goldstein, & Bax (2007).

self-mobility with limitations and may use powered mobility, and those at Level V require transportation in a manual wheelchair (Palisano et al., 1997; Palisano, Rosenbaum, Bartlett, & Livingston, 2008). Other instruments such as the Communication Function Classification (Hidecker et al., 2011) have not been studied as rigorously, and measurement tools for neuromotor function and community participation remain in development (Reilly, Skuse, Mathisen, & Wolke, 1995; Rosenbaum et al., 2007).

The category of accompanying impairments designates which associated conditions or secondary musculoskeletal complications are present. These should be listed as present or absent and described with a standardized instrument when possible (e.g., visual acuity measurement for vision impairment). At times, these associated conditions may cause more disability than the motor impairment, so it is valuable to include them.

The third dimension is intended to better describe anatomical and neuroimaging findings. Rosenbaum and colleagues (2007) advocated avoiding imprecise terminology such as *diplegia* and *quadriplegia* to describe impaired parts of the body. Rather, they favored use of the terms *bilateral* and *unilateral*, which have been shown to have better reliability. A practice parameter published by the American Academy of Neurology proposed that all children with CP undergo

neuroimaging (Ashwal et al., 2004). Although no universal classification scheme for neuroimaging exists currently, several experts support grouping findings into white matter lesions, grey matter lesions, brain malformations, and miscellaneous (Bax, Tydeman, & Flodmark, 2006; Krägeloh-Mann & Horber, 2007).

The causation and timing dimension provides an opportunity to indicate the etiology of the brain anomaly or damage, if it is known (e.g., brain malformation in the early second trimester). At this time, it is not possible to classify children solely on the basis of etiology, but advancements in radiological techniques are likely to make this possible in the future (Rosenbaum et al., 2007).

Rosenbaum and collegaues (2007) provided a greatly improved framework for describing CP and addressing the multiple dimensions of CP while focusing on motor impairment and allowing for individualization. However, some critics remain skeptical about the impact of these dimensions and have found no real improvement in the accuracy of diagnosis compared with previous definitions (Armstrong, 2007; Badawi et al., 2006; Carr, Reddy, Stevens, Blair, & Love, 2005). They argue that the new definition lacks clarification of the full range of disorders to include or exclude, the age limit for "immature brain," and the severity level for activity limitation. In addition to the need for further refinement, education and dissemination of this new system in the everyday clinical practice and education of health care professionals will be a challenge (Carr et al., 2005).

DIAGNOSIS AND DIFFERENTIAL DIAGNOSES

Despite continued changes in the conceptualization of CP, it remains a broad clinical diagnosis. Determining whether a person has CP relies on the clinical manifestations of motor impairment. Delayed motor milestones are often the initial cause for concern and bring the child to the attention of the clinician. Examination draws attention to abnormalities in muscle tone, spinal reflexes, and movement patterns. Diagnosis of young children—particularly infants and toddlers—can be challenging. The neurological exam of a neonate, for example, serves to demonstrate current status but is poorly predictive of subsequent neurodevelopmental disability (Nickel & Petersen, 2008). Also, infants and toddlers may require serial examinations as they age for accurate diagnosis. One study demonstrated that only 118 of 229 children with a diagnosis of CP at age 1 year still had the diagnosis at age 7 years (Nelson & Ellenberg, 1982). Assessment of movement patterns, including primitive and automatic reflexes and generalized movements, may improve the identification of CP in young children (Groen, de Blécourt, Postema, & Hadders-Algra, 2005; Hadders-Algra, 2004).

Medical history of risk factors and neuroimaging findings support the clinical suspicion of CP but are not essential for diagnosis. In fact, one study determined that only 63% of children with CP have a history of high-risk factors (Nelson & Ellenberg, 1986), and another study showed that approximately one-third of full-term infants later diagnosed with CP had normal brain imaging (Wu, Croen, Shah, Newman, & Najjar, 2006). Diagnosis is based on whether the definition criteria are met. Importantly, the motor impairment cannot be attributable solely to intellectual disability or a progressive neurological disorder. Observation over time may be necessary because some degenerative disorders cause slow deterioration and may not be obvious at initial presentation.

Several conditions may be confused with CP; these can be grouped into three categories: (1) static or idiopathic, (2) progressive, and (3) other treatable conditions (Nickel & Petersen, 2008). An example of an idiopathic condition is the habitual toe walker. This diagnosis is one of exclusion and is evident when no weakness or tone abnormalities are detected, although Achilles tendon contracture may occur (Sala, Shulman, Kennedy, Grant, & Chu, 1999). Sometimes family history can be useful, such as in the case of hereditary spastic paraplegia. This progressive disorder worsens into adulthood and is inherited through multiple mechanisms (autosomal dominant, autosomal recessive, X-linked; Gordon, 1993).

Ataxia and dystonia are less common subtypes of CP, but they are also present in several other neurological disorders. It is suggested that any child with pure dystonia undergo trial treatment with L-dopa or carbidopa because dopa-responsive dystonia is a treatable condition that often is misdiagnosed initially as CP (Jan, 2004).

In summary, several neurodevelopmental conditions have clinical presentations that may overlap with the presentation of CP. Thus, a careful history and physical examination are crucial, and other assessments may be indicated to exclude other conditions and corroborate clinical findings.

PREVALENCE OF CEREBRAL PALSY

To accurately monitor prevalence rates, it is essential to study large populations in a systematic manner. Various difficulties exist in monitoring CP rates over time and comparing them among different countries, including issues with definition changes, observer reliability, case ascertainment, and inclusion bias. Thus, determining whether a discrepant, or changing, prevalence rate is real can be a complex undertaking.

OVERALL PREVALENCE AND ASSOCIATED COMORBIDITIES

In 1998, the Surveillance of Cerebral Palsy in Europe (SCPE) was established as a network of 14 CP surveys and registers in 8 European countries to provide a framework for collaborative research on a large population of patients ("Prevalence and Characteristics," 2002). The task of the SCPE was to determine an overall prevalence rate, incorporating data from all 14 centers. More than 6,000 children born from 1976 to 1990, who were at least 5 years old at the time of registration, were included. Those with postnatal CP diagnosed with brain damage occurring after 28 days of life were included in the database but omitted from the analysis. This group of children with postnatally acquired CP accounted for 7.8% of the population.

The overall CP prevalence rate was 2.08 per 1,000 live births (95% confidence interval [CI] 2.02–2.14). The male-to-female ratio was 1.33:1, with all centers reporting more boys. Thirty-one percent of children were found to have severe intellectual disability, 21% had active seizures, and 11% had severe visual impairment. In general, about 1 in 5 children had severe CP, defined as having major cognitive deficit and nonambulatory status ("Prevalence and Characteristics," 2002).

Yeargin-Alsopp and colleagues (2008) conducted a multisite cross-sectional study in the United States using surveillance records from the Autism and Developmental Disabilities Monitoring Network. A retrospective review was performed on 415 8-year-olds with CP living in metropolitan Atlanta, northern Alabama, and southeastern Wisconsin in 2002. The average overall prevalence rate of CP was 3.6 per 1,000 live births, with similar rates among the three sites. Although the overall prevalence is notably higher in this study, many aspects of case definition and ascertainment can affect the calculated rate. For instance, this database did not systematically collect data on etiology of CP; thus, children with postnatal CP likely were included. Also, this study used the number of children in the population as the denominator, which can result in an increased rate compared with a calculation that instead uses live births (Yeargin-Allsopp et al., 2008).

Several registries in Australia have yielded prevalence rates for CP and have stratified prevalence based on factors such as severity level and birth weight. Combined data for all Australian territories yielded an overall prevalence rate of 1.9 per 1,000 live births between 1993 and 2003. In terms of severity level, this study classified children using the GMFCS with the following results: GMFCS Level I, 30.4%; GMFCS II, 19.8%; GMFCS III, 9.8%; GMFCS IV, 11.6%; GMFCS V, 13.8%; and unknown, 14.6% (Tables 4.2 and 4.3; Australian Cerebral Palsy Register Group, 2009).

The SPCE data indicate a statistically significant upward trend in the overall prevalence rate of CP, from less than 2 per 1,000 live births in 1976 to more than 2 per 1,000 in 1990. Additionally, the severity of CP gradually increased over time. These increases, however, occurred early on and were followed by a plateau in the 1980s ("Prevalence and Characteristics," 2002). Similarly, the United States had an 18% rise in the prevalence of CP from 1975 to 1991 as indicated by data from a surveillance program conducted by the Centers for Disease Control and Prevention and the Georgia Department of Health (Winter, Autry, Boyle, & Yeargin-Allsopp, 2002). This pattern of increase has been reported in several other studies, and the general consensus is that a peak in CP rates occurred in the late 1980s (Pharoah, Platt, & Cooke, 1996; Robertson, Watt, & Yasui, 2007; Vincer et al., 2006).

Data conflict on whether the reported increase is the result of the increased survival of preterm and low-birth-weight infants (Pharoah et al., 1996; Vincer et al., 2006; Winter et al., 2002). Controversy (and inadequate data) also exists about whether the prevalence rate since the 1980s has continued to increase, remains unchanged, or has decreased (Hagberg, Hagberg, Beckung, & Uvebrant, 2001; O'Shea, Preisser,

Table 4.2 Prevalence of Cerebral Palsy, by Country

COUNTRY OR REGION	OVERALL PREVALENCE	BOY:GIRL RATIO	ASSOCIATED IMPAIRMENTS
Europe (SPCE)	2.1 per 1,000 live births	1.3:1	Severe intellectual disability (31%) Active seizures (21%) Severe visual impairment (11%)
United States	3.6 per 1,000 children ages 8 years	1.4:1	Epilepsy (35%) Autism (8%)
Australia	1.9 per 1,000 live births	1.3:1	Moderate to severe cognitive impairment (20%) Active epilepsy (26%) Functional blindness (4%) GMFCS Levels I (31%), II (20%), III (10%), IV (12%), IV (14%), unknown (15%)
China	1.6 per 1,000 children ages 3 months to 7 years	1.6:1	N/A
Iceland	2.2 per 1,000 children ages 4–10 years	0.9:1	IQ/DQ <70 (46%) Epilepsy (28%) Visual impairment (15%) Hearing impairment (16%) GMFCS Levels I and II (67%), III (9%), IV and V (25%)
Malta	2.4 per 1,000 children ages 3–13 years	N/A	N/A

Note. GMFCS = Gross Motor Function Classification System; IQ/DQ = intellectual quotient or developmental quotient; N/A = not available; SPCE = Surveillance of Cerebral Palsy in Europe.
Sources: Australian Cerebral Palsy Register Group (2009); Kirby et al. (2011); Liu, Li, Lin, & Li (1999); Sciberras & Spencer (1999); Sigurdardóttir, Thórkelsson, Halldórsdóttir, Thorarensen, & Vik (2009); Yeargin-Allsop et al. (2008).

Table 4.3   Subtypes of Cerebral Palsy in Prevalence Studies

COUNTRY OR REGION	CEREBRAL PALSY SUBTYPE	OVERALL MOST COMMON	UNILATERAL OR HEMIPLEGIC CEREBRAL PALSY
Europe (SPCE)	Spastic 86% Dyskinetic 6.5% Ataxic 4.3% Other 3.7%	Bilateral spastic 55%	29%
United States	Spastic 77% Dyskinetic 2.6% Ataxic 2.4% Hypotonic 2.6%	Bilateral spastic 53%	23%
Australia	Spastic 91% Dyskinetic 4.4% Ataxic 5.0%	Bilateral spastic 62%	39%
Iceland	Spastic 83% Dyskinetic 12% Ataxic 3.0% Other 2.5%	Bilateral spastic 55%	28%
Malta	N/A	Bilateral overall 69%	11%

Note. N/A = not available; SPCE = Surveillance of Cerebral Palsy in Europe.
Sources. Australian Cerebral Palsy Register Group (2009); Kirby et al. (2011); Liu, Li, Lin, & Li (1999); Sciberras & Spencer (1999); Sigurdardóttir, Thórkelsson, Halldórsdóttir, Thorarensen, & Vik (2009); Yeargin-Allsop et al. (2008).

Klinepeter, & Dillard, 1998; Platt et al., 2007; "Prevalence and Characteristics," 2002; Robertson et al., 2007; Vincer et al., 2006; Winter et al., 2002).

SUBTYPES OF CEREBRAL PALSY IN PREVALENCE STUDIES

Because CP is not a single entity but a group of disorders that results in impairment of movement and posture, it is probable that the varying clinical presentations are a consequence of distinctive etiologies and, perhaps, different early interventions provided. Therefore, it is imperative that a system for classifying CP is reliable and valid to accurately compare and contrast subtypes. It is common for more than one type of motor problem to coexist in a child with CP, especially as the child grows older, making it even more challenging to distinguish precise motor types (Reid, Carlin, & Reddihough, 2011).

When classifying CP by subtype, the SPCE database revealed that 85.7% (95% CI 84.8–86.7) of children were spastic, 6.5% (95% CI 5.8–7.2) were dyskinetic, 4.3% (95% CI 3.8–4.9) were ataxic, and the remaining 3.7% were unknown. Bilateral spastic CP was the most common subtype, affecting slightly more than half of all children with CP (54.9%; 95% CI 53.5–56.4). Almost one-third of children (29.2%; 95%

CI 2.9–30.4) had unilateral spastic CP ("Prevalence and Characteristics," 2002). Data from the United States indicated that spastic CP was most common, accounting for 76.9% of all cases (Yeargin-Allsopp et al., 2008). Bilateral spastic CP was more frequent than unilateral, constituting 53.1% of cases. The relatively few remaining children had the following distribution of subtypes: dyskinetic, 2.6%; ataxic, 2.4%; and hypotonic, 2.6% (Yeargin-Allsopp et al., 2008).

PRETERM AND LOW-BIRTH-WEIGHT INFANTS

It is well established that children born preterm (<37 weeks gestational age) and with VLBW (<1,000 g) are at higher risk for CP than infants born at term (Pharoah et al., 1996; Platt et al., 2007; Winter et al., 2002). With the development of neonatal intensive care units and advancing therapies designed to minimize complications of prematurity (primarily respiratory and other infections), survival of these vulnerable infants has increased greatly.

SPCE data from 1976 to 1990 show that the overall prevalence rate for surviving children weighing less than 1,500 g at birth was 72.6 per 1,000 neonatal survivors (95% CI 67.4–77.8). Among those with birth weights of 1,500 g to 2,499 g (i.e., the heavier low-birth-weight infants), the prevalence was

11.1 per 1,000 neonatal survivors (95% CI 10.4–11.8), and for those weighing more than 2,500 g (i.e., normal birth weight), the prevalence was 1.2 per 1,000 neonatal survivors (95% CI 1.13–1.24; "Prevalence and Characteristics," 2002).

Gestational age is another measure for determining the prevalence of children at risk for CP and eliminates the issue of infants born small because of multiparous pregnancy or intrauterine growth restriction. Prevalence rates are 19% to 22% for those born at 24 to 26 weeks gestational age, 8% to 11% for those 28 to 30 weeks gestational age, and 4% to 5% for those 32 weeks gestational age (Ancel et al., 2006). One of the lowest reported rates for infants 20 to 27 weeks gestational age was in Canada for the years 2001 to 2003, with a prevalence of 19 per 1,000 live births (Robertson et al., 2007), or 1.9%. Although prevalence rates for VLBW and premature infants differ, these children as a group are at higher risk than the general population and contribute to about half of the cases of CP (Hagberg et al., 2001; Pharoah et al., 1996).

IMPACT OF SOCIOECONOMIC STATUS AND RACE AND ETHNICITY

Some evidence has suggested that distinct prevalence rates of CP exist on the basis of race and socioeconomic factors (Dolk, Pattenden, & Johnson, 2001; Dowding & Barry, 1990; Sundrum, Logan, Wallace, & Spencer, 2005; Wu et al., 2006, 2011; Yeargin-Allsopp et al., 2008). For instance, Black non-Hispanic children living in low- and middle-income neighborhoods in the United States are at highest risk for CP. The prevalence rate for Black non-Hispanic children is 4.7 per 1,000 live births (95% CI 3.6–4.9), compared with Hispanic children, who are at lowest risk, with a rate of 2.4 per 1,000 (95% CI 1.6–3.7; Yeargin-Allsopp et al., 2008). Children from low- and middle-income communities experience a 70% increase in prevalence over children from high-income communities (Yeargin-Allsopp et al., 2008).

In the United Kingdom, Dolk and colleagues (2001) estimated that "up to 17% of CP cases might be 'preventable'… if the whole population had the rate of CP of the most affluent quintile" (p. 362). Their study showed that the prevalence of CP was 3.33 per 1,000 live births in the most-deprived quintile and 2.08 in the most-affluent quintile. Although a greater proportion of births in the more-deprived quintiles were of low or VLBW, the trend held even for infants with normal birth weight (Dolk et al., 2001). Note that race and socioeconomic factors also affect rates of prematurity and low birth weight, and whether the reasons for this fact are biological or environmental is unclear. Overall, an association appears to exist between race and socioeconomic factors and risk for developing CP, although the nature of this relationship is not well established.

MOTOR DEVELOPMENT OF CHILDREN WITH CEREBRAL PALSY

Although CP has long been known as a disorder of motor function, only recently has the natural history of motor development over time in affected children been fully realized. Even children with mild impairment in the first few years of life are likely to show greater degrees of impairment in fine and gross motor skills when assessed at later ages (i.e., when these skills display more mature forms). Aspects of motor development include the ability to complete discrete and multicomponent motor tasks and the quality and efficiency of movement. In addition to being a disorder of movement and posture, about half of children with CP also have associated impairments and secondary conditions that further affect their ability to perform ADLs and participate in the community (Bartlett & Palisano, 2000; Himmelmann et al., 2006; Kennes et al., 2002).

FINE MOTOR AND UE DEVELOPMENT

In typically developing children, fine motor skills develop rapidly during the early years, and these skills later become more sophisticated as they enter middle childhood and adolescence (Holmefur, Krumlinde-Sundholm, Bergström, & Eliasson, 2010). Children with CP affecting the hands and UEs follow an altered developmental pattern and are impaired because of a combination of factors, including issues with strength, tone, speed, coordination, and sensation (Hanna et al., 2003). Great variation also exists independently of age in fine motor abilities among children with hemiplegia and quadriplegia (Hanna et al., 2003; Holmefur et al., 2010). Furthermore, children with diplegia have asymmetrically decreased hand function that is unrelated to genetically determined hand dominance (Beckung & Hagberg, 2002).

Longitudinal data are necessary to illustrate the average pattern of change in developing children and the variation in progress for individual children (Hanna et al., 2003). Such prospective observations have been repeated over time for children with hemiplegic and quadriplegic CP (Law et al., 1997). Hanna and colleagues (2003) published developmental curves for hand and UE function of children ages 16 to 70 months. Using linear mixed-effects modeling, these researchers estimated average developmental curves and degree of individual differences in severity of impairment; they assessed motor skills using the Peabody Developmental Motor Scales (PDMS; Folio & Fewell, 1983) and the Quality of Upper Extremity Skills Test (QUEST; Dematteo et al., 1993). Results of the work by Hanna and colleagues (2003) indicated that the average rate of motor development slows as children age. Interestingly, the data suggest that the same population of children showed a slightly different developmental pattern depending on the measurement tool used. With the PDMS for fine motor skills, scores increased over time for younger children, with the rate of change declining with age. In contrast, average QUEST scores tended to peak around 4 years of age and then decline. This perceived difference may be related to the "types of tasks that dominate each test" (Hanna et al., 2003, p. 454). The skills tested using the PDMS are functional manual tasks (e.g., cutting, drawing) that are probably amenable to improvement with practice, whereas the items in the QUEST are essentially a measure of the degree of UE physical impairment, which is presumably less likely to benefit from practice (Hanna et al., 2003). Also, physical impairments may be more subject to deterioration because of contractures, which increase as children with CP age. In general, it is important to appreciate that these estimates of motor development are dependent on the selected measurement tool as well as the type of CP (Hanna et al., 2003).

Hanna and colleagues (2003) observed substantial individual variation in the pattern of development using both measurement tools. The PDMS results suggested an increasing scope of manual skills as children become older. Although variability also existed at 16 months using the QUEST, the rate at which UE function improves with age decelerates more similarly among children. CP distribution and impairment severity also were significant predictors of the children's pattern of development using both measurement tools. Children with hemiplegia had better initial scores at 16 months and less decline in developmental rate than those with quadriplegia. Compared with children with moderate and severe impairment, children with mild CP had better hand function and a faster increase in developmental skills (Hanna et al., 2003).

Although some studies indicate that children with CP experience progress in fine motor development in the early years and have limited potential for improvement as they age, Eliasson, Forssberg, Hung, and Gordon (2006) demonstrated that improvement can continue even after adolescence, regardless of the initial severity of hand function. Children with CP were observed at ages 6 to 8 years and then followed up at ages 19 to 21 years. Between these intervals, participants experienced a 45% reduction in time to perform the Jebsen–Taylor Hand Function Test (Patterson Medical, Bolingbrook, IL) and a 22% decrease in time to complete the grip-lift task, both clinically significant differences when compared with typically developing peers performing the same tasks. However, these improvements in hand function did not result in typical hand function. The study participants as adolescents also showed signs of improved development in

terms of planning fine motor tasks and trial-to-trial variation (Eliasson, Forssberg, et al., 2006).

Regarding hand and UE function, hemiplegic CP has been more widely studied than other types of CP. Children with hemiplegic CP present a unique circumstance because they generally have one well-functioning arm and one impaired arm. The greatest challenge for the majority of these children is performing bimanual tasks, which affects their ability to complete ADLs (Eliasson, Forssberg, et al., 2006; Fedrizzi, Pagliano, Andreucci, & Oleari, 2003; Holmefur et al., 2010).

Numerous studies have made it clear that these children have considerably impaired spontaneous use of the affected hand, although they often are able to perform various activities with it if required to do so (Eliasson, Forssberg, et al., 2006; Fedrizzi et al., 2003). In a prospective longitudinal study, Fedrizzi and colleagues (2003) demonstrated that use of the affected hand in bilateral manipulation did not change greatly in adolescence for the group as a whole when compared with use in early childhood. The developmental inclination is for these children to acquire increasingly greater skill with the unaffected hand while further neglecting the impaired hand (Fedrizzi et al., 2003). Several reasons contribute to the impairment of bilateral hand manipulation, but sensory disturbances seem to play an important role (Cooper, Majnemer, Rosenblatt, & Birnbaum, 1995; Hoon et al., 2009; Wilke & Staudt, 2009).

Holmefur and colleagues (2010) followed children with hemiplegic CP prospectively using the Assisting Hand Assessment (AHA) to understand how bimanual activities develop over time and to create developmental curves using a nonlinear statistical growth model. Children were assessed at age 18 months and stratified into a low- and high-AHA group. A significant difference in both the limit and rate of development was found between the two groups. As expected, children with low AHA scores (22 to 40 raw score; do not perform bimanual play task independently) at the baseline age of 18 months had a lower average AHA maximum ability score at follow-up than children with a high AHA score (>40 raw score; perform bimanual tasks, although with difficulty; Holmefur et al., 2010).

For the rate of development, Holmefur and colleagues (2010) used the term *age-90* to represent the age in years by which children are expected to reach 90% of their motor development. Children with a low AHA score at initial assessment at age 18 months reached 90% of their average limit by approximately age 7 years. In contrast, children with an initial high AHA score completed 90% of their average limit by approximately age 3 years (Holmefur et al., 2010). This pattern of development is the opposite seen for gross motor function, in which children with more severe impairment (GMFCS Levels III to V) reach their limit sooner than those at GMFCS Levels I and II (Rosenbaum et al., 2002). These findings indicate that gross motor and fine motor development do not follow the same time course. The developmental curves using the AHA model are useful for predicting future bilateral manual abilities for children with hemiplegic CP (Holmefur et al., 2010).

GROSS MOTOR DEVELOPMENT

In children, gross motor development is frequently described in terms of the achievement of milestones, including rolling, sitting, walking, and jumping. Children with CP generally lag behind in accomplishing these skills and demonstrate abnormalities in movement, posture, and reflexes. After learning the diagnosis, families often seek guidance about how their child will function in the future. The GMFCS and the Gross Motor Function Measure (GMFM–66; Russell, Rosenbaum, Avery, & Lane, 2002) are measurement tools that can be used individually and in combination to specifically describe and predict gross motor development in children with CP (Rosenbaum et al., 2002). Both have been widely used and have been demonstrated to have good psychometric properties (Bodkin et al., 2003; Brunton & Bartlett, 2011; Nordmark, Hägglund, & Jarnlo, 1997; Palisano et al., 1997; Russell et al., 2000; Wood & Rosenbaum, 2000).

Until the landmark work of Rosenbaum and colleagues (2002), only clinical observations and cross-sectional data were available as references for patterns of motor development in children with CP (Palisano et al., 1997, 2008; Rosenbaum et al., 2002). Prior studies had not consistently used a valid and reliable classification system for functional abilities. In the study by Rosenbaum and colleagues, a cohort of children with varying severities of CP was followed prospectively, and the longitudinal data were used to create motor developmental curves based on GMFCS level. The curves were generated using GMFM–66 assessments over time and a nonlinear statistical growth model. Not only did the growth curves outline the average pattern of development for each GMFCS level, but the analysis allowed for systematic variations in the patterns of development based on data on individual variation (Rosenbaum et al., 2002).

The results of the study demonstrated that children with CP plateau in their motor development by ages 6 to 7 years, depending on their GMFCS level (Rosenbaum et al., 2002). For rate of development, the term *age-90* was used. A general trend was faster progression to age-90 as severity of impairment increased. Children with GMFCS Levels III to V progressed much faster than children at Level I. However, children at Level II did not progress faster than children at Level I. Importantly, "an earlier age-90 does not imply 'better' developmental progress—only that a child is closer to his/her

limit" (Rosenbaum et al., 2002, p. 1360). Again, this pattern of development is contrary to that seen for fine motor UE skills. Concerning the maximum level of motor skills, this study demonstrated that the limit of development is inversely related to impairment severity. Additionally, each GMFCS level curve is significantly statistically different from the others in terms of this limit parameter. For instance, children at GMFCS Level III would be expected to achieve a mean of 54.3 points on the GMFM–66, whereas children at GMFCS Level V would be expected to reach a mean of 22.3 points (Rosenbaum et al., 2002).

In summary, these curves provide clinicians and families with a major advance in the ability to predict future motor function in children with CP at a given level of severity. Stratification of severity is particularly useful to more accurately predict future motor progression. The data also are valuable for assessing whether a child is deviating from a projected pattern of gross motor development and for planning interventions and monitoring their effects (Rosenbaum et al., 2002). Important to consider, however, is that prognosis is invariably linked to the types and amounts of effective treatments and environmental opportunities available to children. Even carefully collected longitudinal data should be interpreted in an ecological context to reflect the fact that the observed pattern of development occurred for children born during certain years and living in certain places, where they did or did not receive certain types of interventions. The prospect of emerging treatments such as pediatric constraint-induced movement therapy and other interventions may yield higher functioning for children with CP in the future.

Hanna, Bartlett, Rivard, and Russell (2008) took this research a step further and used the data from Rosenbaum and colleagues (2002) to form reference percentiles for GMFM–66 scores within GMFCS level, and they evaluated the stability of these reference percentiles over time. The utility of reference percentiles lies in their ability to aid assessment of an individual child's standing relative to peers and abilities as they change over time. Hanna et al. demonstrated that over an interval of time, a child with CP may experience considerable change in motor function abilities, but this variation may still fall within an expected range based on GMFCS level. For example, there is an 80% chance that a child at GMFCS Level III will have a change of +15.9 points from one assessment to the next. Notably, these are cross-sectional reference percentiles, although the data come from a prospective longitudinal study. Thus, determination of a child's relative standing compared with peers represents his or her actual motor development only at that point in time (Hanna et al., 2008). Further, single-session assessments of children with CP may be highly sensitive to factors such as fatigue, interest or motivation, and perceived stress or comfort level during the assessment, which would result in greater intersession variation than occurs with typically developing children.

Children with CP have a period of progression in motor development in early childhood, but some children then experience a decline in gross motor function as they become adolescents and young adults. Most children with CP, however, maintain their abilities for ambulation (Day, Wu, Strauss, Shavelle, & Reynolds, 2007). Those who walk without difficulty at ages 10 and 25 years have the highest likelihood of maintaining that ability throughout their lifetime. Children with difficulty ambulating at age 10 years are most likely to have no change in ambulation abilities but are equally as likely to improve or decline over the next 15 years. Conversely, at age 25 years, these same children have little chance of improving ambulation and are much more likely to lose abilities (Day, Wu, et al., 2007). Of note, these data focus on children with a milder spectrum of disability and are retrospective rather than prospective.

A prospective study by Rosenbaum and colleagues (2002) showed that children at GMFCS Levels III, IV, and V are at risk of losing motor function as they enter adolescence and young adulthood, with those at Level IV experiencing the greatest declines (Hanna et al., 2009). It is not clear why these children experience gross motor decline over time, although it is likely that a combination of factors is responsible, including physical growth (Bartlett, Hanna, Avery, Stevenson, & Galuppi, 2010; Bottos & Gericke, 2003), environmental changes (Bottos & Gericke, 2003), joint deterioration and pain (Bartlett et al., 2010; Murphy, Molnar, & Lankasky, 1995), and fatigue (Jahnsen, Villien, Stanghelle, & Holm, 2003), which often occur as children age (Hanna et al., 2009).

Beckung, Carlsson, Carlsdotter, and Uvebrant (2007) created motor developmental curves using prospective data and GMFCS levels but subdivided the children with spastic CP on the basis of distribution of dysfunction. The resultant study population included 49% with spastic diplegia, 33% with spastic hemiplegia, 12% with dyskinesia, 3% with spastic tetraplegia, and 3% with ataxia. The majority of children were at GMFCS Levels I and II, and within this group, most were categorized as having spastic hemiplegia and spastic diplegia. Gross motor development did not vary between these two subtypes within levels. No children with hemiplegia were at GMFCS Level IV or V, and all children with spastic tetraplegia were at GMFCS Level V. Although some children performed at higher levels, most with dyskinesia performed at GMFCS Level V. The few children with ataxia in the study were not notably different from children with other types of CP within GMFCS levels. The authors concluded that gross motor development in a specific child cannot be predicted solely on the basis of the subtype of CP (Beckung et al., 2007).

INFLUENCE OF OTHER FACTORS ON MOTOR DEVELOPMENT

Although motor developmental curves now exist to describe how groups of children with CP progress over time, several other factors may affect an individual child's ability to function and participate (Bartlett & Palisano, 2000; Himmelmann et al., 2006; Kennes et al., 2002; Rosenbaum et al., 2002). It remains unclear how associated impairments such as intellectual disability and visual impairment contribute to individual variation in motor development. Other important variables that likely play a role include personal motivation and family environment. As new beneficial therapies surface, these developmental curves may need to be adapted to accommodate the effects of such interventions (Rosenbaum et al., 2002).

PHYSICAL GROWTH OF CHILDREN WITH CEREBRAL PALSY

Growth is a fundamental marker of health and well-being in children. The pattern of growth in typically developing children has been well studied and is predictable (de Onis et al., 2007; Kuczmarski et al., 2000; Ogden et al., 2002). Growth reference curves based on population averages allow for assessment of growth by comparing an individual child with the norm. Considerable deviation from the predicted average pattern of growth may indicate nutritional issues or other underlying pathology. Thus, the use of growth curves has become standard practice for health professionals in monitoring the health of all children (Kuczmarski et al., 2000; Ogden et al., 2002), and families also may use them to better understand how children typically grow.

GROWTH PATTERNS

Many studies have demonstrated that children with CP are shorter and lighter than age-matched peers and grow differently than typically developing children (Henderson et al., 2002; Krick, Murphy-Miller, Zeger, & Wright, 1996; Shapiro, Green, Krick, Allen, & Capute, 1986; Stallings, Charney, Davies, & Cronk, 1993a; Stevenson, Hayes, Cater, & Blackman, 1994). Even children with hemiplegia and diplegia are at risk for poor growth (Roberts, Vogtle, & Stevenson, 1994; Stallings, Charney, Davies, & Cronk, 1993b; Stevenson, Roberts, & Vogtle, 1995). Furthermore, differences exist in body composition, including decreased bone density (Henderson et al., 2002), muscle mass, and fat stores (Stallings et al., 1993a).

Plotting children with CP on standard growth curves for typically developing children reveals substantial deviation

(Krick et al., 1996). These plots, however, do not convey how these children grow compared with children who have comparable neurological impairment. Thus, it is not practical or highly informative to use typical pediatric growth charts for children with CP. Reference charts specific to children with CP provide the opportunity for a uniform assessment of growth and nutritional status and offer a mechanism for comparing similar children (Krick et al., 1996).

Krick and colleagues (1996) were the first to develop growth curves specific to children with quadriplegic CP and compare these with standards from the National Center for Health Statistics (NCHS). For both girls and boys with quadriplegic CP up to age 10 years, the 50th percentile was below the 10th percentile NCHS standards for weight and length for age and was approximately equal to the 10th percentile NCHS standards for weight and length. In general, boys were further below the norm than girls for all parameters. Children with CP also had more variability in growth than typical peers (Krick et al., 1996).

The rate of growth for children with CP was slower than that of typical peers; children were 5% shorter at age 2 years and more than 10% shorter at age 8 years (Krick et al., 1996). Other studies also revealed differences in *growth velocity*, defined as change in growth over a period of time, in children with CP (Samson-Fang & Stevenson, 1998; Stevenson et al., 1994). In a longitudinal study, Samson-Fang and Stevenson observed that some children with CP have suboptimal growth velocity compared with matched norms. They identified risk factors associated with decreased growth velocity, including young age, male gender, malnutrition, cognitive impairment, and nonambulatory status; type of CP and microcephaly were not associated with poor growth velocity. As the authors pointed out, decreased growth velocity implies that short children with CP are experiencing growth failure, which is notably different from constitutional short stature.

Growth velocity has the advantage of portraying how growth occurs over a period of time and how different variables affect it. Cross-sectional data, in contrast, convey the growth of persons at only one point in time. As a consequence, factors that potentially influence individual growth trajectories over time cannot be identified as reliably and the possibility of true cohort differences (e.g., age groups that received different amounts or types of high-quality interventions, age groups with higher proportions of children with CP because of more active early screening programs) cannot be addressed in cross-sectional studies (Samson-Fang & Stevenson, 1998).

Growth curves for children with CP stratified by level of disability are potentially more useful for the comparison and prediction of growth because they correspond to a particular group within a population of children with CP. Stevenson and colleagues (2006) initially developed such curves using knee height measurements for children classified at GMFCS Levels III to V. Day, Strauss, and colleagues (2007) used data from the California Department of Developmental Services to create growth curves in which children were classified into five groups on the basis of motor and feeding abilities. These curves were an extension of the work performed by Krick and colleagues (1996) and increased the age range to include 10- to 20-year-olds.

Not surprisingly, Day, Strauss, and colleagues (2007) showed that children with less-severe disability were closer to the growth norms of typically developing children than were children with more severely disabilities. Girls with CP in Group 1 (walk well for 6 minutes and balance well) were only slightly below the general population weight centiles at all ages except age 20, when the 90th percentile was actually slightly higher. The highest functioning boys with CP were slightly below the general population for all ages. For both genders in Group 2 (ambulate unsteadily alone or with supportive devices), the weight percentiles were noticeably below those of Group 1, and the gap widened with increasing age. For the girls and boys in Group 3 (crawl, creep, or scoot but do not walk) and Group 4 (do not crawl, creep, scoot, or walk; do not feed self but do not use gastrostomy tube), the difference in weight percentiles for age progressively worsened as disability increased. Children in Group 5 (similar to Group 4 but use gastrostomy tube) demonstrated a similar growth pattern to Group 4, except that the weight percentiles were 2 to 5 kg higher with a gastrostomy tube present (Day, Strauss, et al., 2007).

In terms of height for age percentiles for children with CP, the overall pattern generally corresponded to those for weight for age based on level of disability. Importantly, height data recorded in the California Department of Developmental Services database were not obtained via a validated measurement (Day, Strauss, et al., 2007). However, Oeffinger and colleagues (2010) demonstrated that tibial length is a reliable method for tracking bone growth in children with CP. Using data on tibial lengths, Oeffinger et al. developed growth curves for ambulatory children (GMFCS Levels I to III) and showed results similar to those of Day, Strauss, and colleagues (2007)—that is, children with worse GMFCS levels were shorter. Groups 3 through 5 in Day, Strauss, et al.'s study revealed a different pattern in weight gain over time, in which children with CP did not have the pubertal growth spurt of typically developing peers. In other words, a typical population of children tends to have a logistic (S-shaped) curve, whereas children with CP of more severe disability showed a straight-line increase in weight (Day, Strauss, et al., 2007). This finding was corroborated by other studies (e.g., Stevenson et al., 2006).

Worley and colleagues (2002) found that the pattern of sexual maturation in children with moderate-to-severe CP also differs. Compared with a typical population, puberty in White children with CP begins earlier and ends later. Also, more advanced sexual maturation was associated with increased body fat in girls with CP but decreased body fat in boys (Worley et al., 2002).

Another important aspect of growth, **skeletal maturation** (also known as *bone age*), is the rate at which bones are developing, usually relative to age-normed expectations, often ascertained by clinical tests such as radiography. Delayed skeletal maturation occurs commonly in children with CP and in one study occurred in 68% of children (Kong, Tse, & Lee, 1999). Delayed bone age also has been shown to correlate with diminished linear bone growth, reduced lumbar spine bone density, and decreased body fat in children with moderate to severe CP (Henderson et al., 2005). Henderson and colleagues demonstrated that delays in bone age of more than 2 years were most prevalent in children at GMFCS Level V, although the more profoundly affected children were the group more likely to have advances in bone age of more than 2 years.

Altered bone maturation has been recognized in children with hemiplegia in which the affected arm experiences diminished maturation. This unique situation, in which the unaffected arm is the study control, emphasizes the point that delayed bone age in children with CP occurs independently of malnutrition or other controlled factors (Roberts et al., 1994). Using this premise, one can postulate that early and repeated pediatric constraint-induced movement therapy might lead to improved growth and different long-term outcomes if the bone immaturity of the affected UE is related to diminished use.

IMPORTANCE OF POOR GROWTH

Although it is useful to have growth curves specific to children with CP, especially curves that are stratified by disability level, these reference charts are descriptive in nature. They do not necessarily represent the ideal growth for children with CP because they reflect the pattern of how a population of children *has grown*. It would be preferable to have prescriptive growth charts that demonstrate how children *should* grow (Grummer-Strawn, Garza, & Johnson, 2002). However, as Day, Strauss, and colleagues (2007) noted, "what an ideal weight or height might be for a child or young adult with CP is a complex question in any event, especially those with severe CP" (p. 171). Alternatively, it is possible to study the relationship between growth patterns of children stratified by disability level and to compare disability level with health and quality-of-life outcomes. Stevenson and colleagues (2006) investigated this relationship specifically and demonstrated that children with moderate and severe CP who were "larger" had better health and social participation compared with similar "smaller" children.

Brooks, Day, Shavelle, and Strauss (2011) studied the importance of differing growth patterns for morbidity and mortality in children with CP based on varying degrees of disability. This study used the same California Department of Developmental Services database used by Day, Strauss, and colleagues (2007) to stratify children on the basis of GMFCS level and identified weights associated with negative health outcomes. This growth chart methodology is consistent with that of both the Centers for Disease Control and Prevention and the World Health Organization growth curves. Brooks and colleagues showed that major comorbidities increased with worsening GMFCS level and were more common for children with weights below the 20th percentile in GMFCS Levels I through IV and in Level V without feeding tubes. Interestingly, the presence of a feeding tube was a marker for chronic medical conditions; children at GMFCS Level V–T (with gastrostomy) as a group had on average twice as many major comorbidities as those at GMFCS Level V–NT (no gastrostomy). Yet, children at GMFCS Level V–T and weight below the 20th percentile had fewer major medical conditions than the middle 60% (Brooks et al., 2011).

Brooks et al. (2011) also found an increased risk of death for children of low weight. The hazard ratio was 1.5 for those at GMFCS Levels III, IV, and V below the 20th centile and 2.2 for those at GMFCS Levels I and II below the 5th centile (Brooks et al., 2011). The mortality rate for those below the 20th percentile increased steadily with worsening GMFCS level, from 0.3 per 100 person–years for GMFCS Level I up to 26.0 per 100 person–years for GMFCS Level V–T. Brooks et al. found no increased rates of morbidity or mortality in children of high weight, although this finding does not necessarily signify that overweight is not a major health risk factor in children with CP. In summary, growth curves specific for children with CP correlate poor growth with medical comorbidities and mortality and provide a practical tool that may prove useful for care management decisions (Brooks et al., 2011).

FACTORS INFLUENCING GROWTH

Many factors may contribute to the differences in growth seen among children with CP. Poor nutrition certainly contributes to poor growth of children with CP (Fung et al., 2002; Shapiro et al., 1986; Stallings et al., 1993a, 1993b; Stevenson et al., 1994) and has been estimated to explain approximately 10% to 15% of linear growth when adjusting for other variables (Stallings et al., 1993a). In a study by Fung and colleagues (2002), children with the most severe feeding difficulties who received nutrition primarily via a feeding tube weighed more and had more muscle and fat mass than peers with similar disability who took all food orally. Although nutritional factors previously were thought to play a large role, it is now evident that nutritional factors are not exclusively responsible for growth issues in children with CP (Shapiro et al., 1986; Stallings et al., 1993a; Stevenson et al., 1994). For example, some children continue to have poor linear growth despite correction of malnutrition with a gastrostomy tube (Shapiro et al., 1986). Also, Stevenson and colleagues (1995) demonstrated that children with hemiplegic CP have smaller length and girth on the affected limb compared with the unaffected side.

Potential nonnutritional factors affecting growth include neuroendocrine abnormalities (Hamza, Ismail, & Hamed, 2011; Kuperminc et al., 2009); psychosocial influences (Henderson et al., 2007); and lack of potentially growth-promoting activity, which is discussed in the next section (Chen et al., 2011; Henderson et al., 2005; Ward, Caulton, Adams, & Mughal, 2006; Wilmshurst, Ward, Adams, Langton, & Mughal, 1996). For instance, the work of Kuperminc and colleagues (2009) indicated that children with CP at GMFCS Levels III through V have diminished circulating concentrations of insulin-like growth factor 1 and growth hormone and suggested that this finding may explain growth failure seen in this population. Henderson and colleagues (2007) investigated the effects of environment on growth and demonstrated that residential center living has a significant positive correlation with growth and nutrition independent of age, severity, and tube feeding.

RELATIONSHIP OF GROWTH AND MOTOR DEVELOPMENT

Considerable abnormalities in growth and development are seen in children with CP, including decreased body weight and height for age (Day, Strauss, et al., 2007; Krick et al., 1996; Shapiro et al., 1986; Stallings et al., 1993a; Stevenson et al., 1994), reduced linear growth velocity (Samson-Fang & Stevenson, 1998), and altered pubertal growth (Worley et al., 2002). Studies have documented that the severity of disability is associated with worse growth outcomes in terms of length, weight, and bone maturation (Day, Strauss, et al., 2007; Stevenson et al., 2006). As mentioned previously, multiple influences likely contribute to poor growth in children with CP, including nonnutritional factors such as lack of growth-promoting activities, in particular mechanical loading, which is fundamental for skeletal development (Ward et al., 2006).

According to Frost's (2003) model of bone development, mechanical forces result in bone "strains," which are sensed by a regulatory feedback system called the **mechanostat**. The mechanostat responds by adapting bone structure to whether the strain was strong or weak, a response that involves changes in bone size, architecture, and density (Frost, 2003). In typically developing children, longitudinal growth of bones occurs in reaction to muscular loading. The absence of typical musculature and weight bearing as seen in children with CP

and other neuromuscular diseases leads to abnormal bone development (Ward et al., 2006) and probably altered growth. Children with more severe motor limitations are expected to suffer more from poor bone growth and maturation according to the mechanostat model, undoubtedly because children with worse GMFCS levels by definition have more impaired mobility (Palisano et al., 1997), attributable to a combination of factors (tone issues, joint contractures, motor control, and muscle weakness).

Conversely, disturbances in growth also may have an effect on motor development. Supplementation for undernourished children has been shown to improve psychomotor development compared with children who do not receive supplementation (Grantham-McGregor, Powell, Walker, & Himes, 1991; Husaini et al., 1991). Little research exists on the motor function of undernourished children with CP. Campanozzi and colleagues (2007), however, showed that treatment of malnutrition and gastrointestinal disorders may improve motor function in children with CP. Overweight and obesity also may affect motor function, although this area has not been well studied. The prevalence of overweight and obesity has been estimated at about 15% in children with CP (Kwon et al., 2011; Rogozinski et al., 2007), and less-impaired children (GMFCS Level II) have twice the odds of becoming obese than children with greater involvement (GMFCS Level III; Rogozinski et al., 2007).

SUMMARY

CP is a relatively common neurodevelopmental condition that profoundly affects the lives of children and adults. How CP is conceptualized is evolving as research and technology advance. CP represents a group of heterogeneous disorders bound by an underlying impairment of the motor system. Within this diverse group, each child with CP is clearly unique, yet there is a critical need for improved ways of classifying and comparing children. Furthermore, the motor development and physical growth of affected children differ greatly from those of typically developing children. Although we are beginning to better understand how children with CP grow and develop over time, each child's course may be influenced by various factors.

Substantial progress in medical and social fields allows children affected by CP to live longer and more enriched lives (Blair, 2010). It has enabled very preterm and VLBW infants to survive past the neonatal period. With this improvement in survival, more children are developing CP with unclear provoking factors. As advances in research and technology continue, a more complete understanding of the mechanisms causing CP will inform the design of interventions that minimize the impact of CP on health and well-being. In turn, children with CP who are better able to function and participate in their roles early on will grow into healthier adults.

REFERENCES

Ancel, P. Y., Livinec, F., Larroque, B., Marret, S., Arnaud, C., Pierrat, V., . . . Kaminski, M.; EPIPAGE Study Group. (2006). Cerebral palsy among very preterm children in relation to gestational age and neonatal ultrasound abnormalities: The EPIPAGE cohort study. *Pediatrics, 117*, 828–835.

Armstrong, R. W. (2007). Definition and classification of cerebral palsy. *Developmental Medicine and Child Neurology, 49*, 166.

Ashwal, S., Russman, B. S., Blasco, P. A., Miller, G., Sandler, A., Shevell, M., & Stevenson, R.; Quality Standards Subcommittee of the American Academy of Neurology; Practice Committee of the Child Neurology Society. (2004). Practice parameter: Diagnostic assessment of the child with cerebral palsy: Report of the Quality Standards Subcommittee of the American Academy of Neurology and the Practice Committee of the Child Neurology Society. *Neurology, 62*, 851–863.

Australian Cerebral Palsy Register Group. (2009). *Report of the Australian Cerebral Palsy Register, birth years 1993–2003.* Auckland, New Zealand: Australasian Academy of Cerebral Palsy and Developmental Medicine.

Badawi, N., Novak, I., McIntyre, S., Edwards, K., Raye, S., deLacy, M., . . . Watson, L. (2006). Proposed new definition of cerebral palsy does not solve any of the problems of existing definitions. *Developmental Medicine and Child Neurology, 48*, 78; author reply 79.

Bartlett, D. J., Hanna, S. E., Avery, L., Stevenson, R. D., & Galuppi, B. (2010). Correlates of decline in gross motor capacity in adolescents with cerebral palsy in Gross Motor Function Classification System Levels III to V: An exploratory study. *Developmental Medicine and Child Neurology, 52*, e155–e160.

Bartlett, D. J., & Palisano, R. J. (2000). A multivariate model of determinants of motor change for children with cerebral palsy. *Physical Therapy, 80*, 598–614.

Bax, M. C. (1964). Terminology and classification of cerebral palsy. *Developmental Medicine and Child Neurology, 6*, 295–297.

Bax, M., Tydeman, C., & Flodmark, O. (2006). Clinical and MRI correlates of cerebral palsy: The European Cerebral Palsy Study. *JAMA, 296*, 1602–1608.

Beckung, E., Carlsson, G., Carlsdotter, S., & Uvebrant, P. (2007). The natural history of gross motor development in children with cerebral palsy aged 1 to 15 years. *Developmental Medicine and Child Neurology, 49*, 751–756.

Beckung, E., & Hagberg, G. (2002). Neuroimpairments, activity limitations, and participation restrictions in children with cerebral palsy. *Developmental Medicine and Child Neurology, 44*, 309–316.

Blair, E. (2010). Epidemiology of the cerebral palsies. *Orthopedic Clinics of North America, 41*, 441–455.

Bodkin, A. W., Robinson, C., & Perales, F. P. (2003). Reliability and validity of the Gross Motor Function Classification System for cerebral palsy. *Pediatric Physical Therapy, 15*, 247–252.

Bottos, M., & Gericke, C. (2003). Ambulatory capacity in cerebral palsy: Prognostic criteria and consequences for intervention. *Developmental Medicine and Child Neurology, 45*, 786–790.

Brooks, J., Day, S., Shavelle, R., & Strauss, D. (2011). Low weight, morbidity, and mortality in children with cerebral palsy: New clinical growth charts. *Pediatrics, 128*, e299–e307.

Brunton, L. K., & Bartlett, D. J. (2011). Validity and reliability of two abbreviated versions of the Gross Motor Function Measure. *Physical Therapy, 91*, 577–588.

Calley, A., Williams, S., Reid, S., Blair, E., Valentine, J., Girdler, S., & Elliott, C. (2012). A comparison of activity, participation and quality of life in children with and without spastic diplegia cerebral palsy. *Disability and Rehabilitation, 34*, 1306–1310.

Campanozzi, A., Capano, G., Miele, E., Romano, A., Scuccimarra, G., Del Giudice, E., . . . Staiano, A. (2007). Impact of malnutrition on gastrointestinal disorders and gross motor abilities in children with cerebral palsy. *Brain and Development, 29*, 25–29.

Carr, L. J., Reddy, S. K., Stevens, S., Blair, E., & Love, S. (2005). Definition and classification of cerebral palsy. *Developmental Medicine and Child Neurology, 47*, 508–510.

Chen, C. L., Lin, K. C., Wu, C. Y., Ke, J. Y., Wang, C. J., & Chen, C. Y. (2011). Relationships of muscle strength and bone mineral density in ambulatory children with cerebral palsy. *Osteoporosis International, 23*, 715–721.

Cooper, J., Majnemer, A., Rosenblatt, B., & Birnbaum, R. (1995). The determination of sensory deficits in children with hemiplegic cerebral palsy. *Journal of Child Neurology, 10*, 300–309.

Day, S. M., Strauss, D. J., Vachon, P. J., Rosenbloom, L., Shavelle, R. M., & Wu, Y. W. (2007). Growth patterns in a population of children and adolescents with cerebral palsy. *Developmental Medicine and Child Neurology, 49*, 167–171.

Day, S. M., Wu, Y. W., Strauss, D. J., Shavelle, R. M., & Reynolds, R. J. (2007). Change in ambulatory ability of adolescents and young adults with cerebral palsy. *Developmental Medicine and Child Neurology, 49,* 647–653.

DeMatteo, C., Law, M. C., Russell, D. J., Pollock, N., Rosenbaum, P. L., & Walter, S. D. (1993). The reliability and validity of the Quality of Upper Extremity Skills Test. *Physical and Occupational Therapy in Pediatrics, 13*(2), 1–18.

de Onis, M., Onyango, A. W., Borghi, E., Siyam, A., Nishida, C., & Siekmann, J. (2007). Development of a WHO growth reference for school-aged children and adolescents. *Bulletin of the World Health Organization, 85,* 660–667.

Dolk, H., Pattenden, S., & Johnson, A. (2001). Cerebral palsy, low birthweight and socio-economic deprivation: Inequalities in a major cause of childhood disability. *Paediatric and Perinatal Epidemiology, 15,* 359–363.

Dowding, V. M., & Barry, C. (1990). Cerebral palsy: Social class differences in prevalence in relation to birthweight and severity of disability. *Journal of Epidemiology and Community Health, 44,* 191–195.

Eliasson, A. C., Forssberg, H., Hung, Y. C., & Gordon, A. M. (2006). Development of hand function and precision grip control in individuals with cerebral palsy: A 13-year follow-up study. *Pediatrics, 118,* e1226–e1236.

Eliasson, A. C., Krumlinde-Sundholm, L., Rösblad, B., Beckung, E., Arner, M., Ohrvall, A. M., & Rosenbaum, P. (2006). The Manual Ability Classification System (MACS) for children with cerebral palsy: Scale development and evidence of validity and reliability. *Developmental Medicine and Child Neurology, 48,* 549–554.

Fedrizzi, E., Pagliano, E., Andreucci, E., & Oleari, G. (2003). Hand function in children with hemiplegic cerebral palsy: Prospective follow-up and functional outcome in adolescence. *Developmental Medicine and Child Neurology, 45,* 85–91.

Folio, R. M., & Fewell, R. F. (1983). *Peabody Developmental Motor Scales.* Allen, TX: DLM Teaching Resources.

Frost, H. M. (2003). Bone's mechanostat: A 2003 update. *Anatomical Record: Part A, Discoveries in Molecular, Cellular, and Evolutionary Biology, 275,* 1081–1101.

Fung, E. B., Samson-Fang, L., Stallings, V. A., Conaway, M., Liptak, G., Henderson, R. C., . . . Stevenson, R. D. (2002). Feeding dysfunction is associated with poor growth and health status in children with cerebral palsy. *Journal of the American Dietetic Association, 102,* 361–373.

Gordon, N. (1993). Hereditary spastic paraplegia: A diagnostic reminder. *Developmental Medicine and Child Neurology, 35,* 452–455.

Grantham-McGregor, S. M., Powell, C. A., Walker, S. P., & Himes, J. H. (1991). Nutritional supplementation, psychosocial stimulation, and mental development of stunted children: The Jamaican Study. *Lancet, 338,* 1–5.

Groen, S. E., de Blécourt, A. C., Postema, K., & Hadders-Algra, M. (2005). General movements in early infancy predict neuromotor development at 9 to 12 years of age. *Developmental Medicine and Child Neurology, 47,* 731–738.

Grummer-Strawn, L. M., Garza, C., & Johnson, C. L. (2002). Childhood growth charts. *Pediatrics, 109,* 141–142.

Hadders-Algra, M. (2004). General movements: A window for early identification of children at high risk for developmental disorders. *Journal of Pediatrics, 145*(Suppl.), S12–S18.

Hagberg, B., Hagberg, G., Beckung, E., & Uvebrant, P. (2001). Changing panorama of cerebral palsy in Sweden: VIII. Prevalence and origin in the birth year period 1991–94. *Acta Paediatrica (Oslo, Norway: 1992), 90,* 271–277.

Hamza, R. T., Ismail, M. A., & Hamed, A. I. (2011). Growth hormone deficiency in children and adolescents with cerebral palsy: Relation to gross motor function and degree of spasticity. *Pakistan Journal of Biological Sciences, 14,* 433–440.

Hanna, S. E., Bartlett, D. J., Rivard, L. M., & Russell, D. J. (2008). Reference curves for the Gross Motor Function Measure: Percentiles for clinical description and tracking over time among children with cerebral palsy. *Physical Therapy, 88,* 596–607.

Hanna, S. E., Law, M. C., Rosenbaum, P. L., King, G. A., Walter, S. D., Pollock, N., & Russell, D. J. (2003). Development of hand function among children with cerebral palsy: Growth curve analysis for ages 16 to 70 months. *Developmental Medicine and Child Neurology, 45,* 448–455.

Hanna, S. E., Rosenbaum, P. L., Bartlett, D. J., Palisano, R. J., Walter, S. D., Avery, L., & Russell, D. J. (2009). Stability and decline in gross motor function among children and youth with cerebral palsy aged 2 to 21 years. *Developmental Medicine and Child Neurology, 51,* 295–302.

Henderson, R. C., Gilbert, S. R., Clement, M. E., Abbas, A., Worley, G., & Stevenson, R. D. (2005). Altered skeletal maturation in moderate to severe cerebral palsy. *Developmental Medicine and Child Neurology, 47,* 229–236.

Henderson, R. C., Grossberg, R. I., Matuszewski, J., Menon, N., Johnson, J., Kecskemethy, H. H., . . . Stevenson, R. D. (2007). Growth and nutritional status in residential center versus home-living children and adolescents with quadriplegic cerebral palsy. *Journal of Pediatrics, 151,* 161–166.

Henderson, R. C., Lark, R. K., Gurka, M. J., Worley, G., Fung, E. B., Conaway, M., . . . Stevenson, R. D. (2002). Bone density and metabolism in children and adolescents with moderate to severe cerebral palsy. *Pediatrics, 110,* e5.

Hidecker, M. J., Paneth, N., Rosenbaum, P. L., Kent, R. D., Lillie, J., Eulenberg, J. B., . . . Taylor, K. (2011). Developing and validating the communication function classification system for individuals with cerebral palsy. *Developmental Medicine and Child Neurology, 53,* 704–710.

Himmelmann, K., Beckung, E., Hagberg, G., & Uvebrant, P. (2006). Gross and fine motor function and accompanying impairments in cerebral palsy. *Developmental Medicine and Child Neurology, 48,* 417–423.

Holmefur, M., Krumlinde-Sundholm, L., Bergström, J., & Eliasson, A. C. (2010). Longitudinal development of hand function in children with unilateral cerebral palsy. *Developmental Medicine and Child Neurology, 52,* 352–357.

Hoon, A. H., Jr., Stashinko, E. E., Nagae, L. M., Lin, D. D., Keller, J., Bastian, A., . . . Johnston, M. V. (2009). Sensory and motor deficits in children with cerebral palsy born preterm correlate with diffusion tensor imaging abnormalities in thalamocortical pathways. *Developmental Medicine and Child Neurology, 51,* 697–704.

Husaini, M. A., Karyadi, L., Husaini, Y. K., Sandjaja, B., Karyadi, D., & Pollitt, E. (1991). Developmental effects of short-term supplementary feeding in nutritionally-at-risk Indonesian infants. *American Journal of Clinical Nutrition, 54,* 799–804.

Jahnsen, R., Villien, L., Stanghelle, J. K., & Holm, I. (2003). Fatigue in adults with cerebral palsy in Norway compared with the general population. *Developmental Medicine and Child Neurology, 45,* 296–303.

Jan, M. M. (2004). Misdiagnoses in children with dopa-responsive dystonia. *Pediatric Neurology, 31,* 298–303.

Kennes, J., Rosenbaum, P., Hanna, S. E., Walter, S., Russell, D., Raina, P., . . . Galuppi, B. (2002). Health status of school-aged children with cerebral palsy: Information from a population-based sample. *Developmental Medicine and Child Neurology, 44,* 240–247.

Kirby, R., Wingate, M., Van Naarden, B., Doerneberg, N., Arneson, C., Benedict, R., . . . Yeargin-Allsopp, M. (2011). Prevalence and functioning of children with CP in four areas of the US in 2006: A report from the Autism & Developmental Disabilities Monitoring Network. *Research in Developmental Disabilities, 32,* 462–469.

Kong, C. K., Tse, P. W., & Lee, W. Y. (1999). Bone age and linear skeletal growth of children with cerebral palsy. *Developmental Medicine and Child Neurology, 41,* 758–765.

Krägeloh-Mann, I., & Horber, V. (2007). The role of magnetic resonance imaging in furthering understanding of the pathogenesis of cerebral palsy. *Developmental Medicine and Child Neurology, 49,* 948.

Krick, J., Murphy-Miller, P., Zeger, S., & Wright, E. (1996). Pattern of growth in children with cerebral palsy. *Journal of the American Dietetic Association, 96,* 680–685.

Kuczmarski, R. J., Ogden, C. L., Grummer-Strawn, L. M., Flegal, K. M., Guo, S. S., Wei, R., . . . Johnson, C. L. (2000). CDC growth charts: United States. *Advance Data, 314,* 1–27.

Kuperminc, M. N., Gurka, M. J., Houlihan, C. M., Henderson, R. C., Roemmich, J. N., Rogol, A. D., & Stevenson, R. D. (2009). Puberty, statural growth, and growth hormone release in children with cerebral palsy. *Journal of Pediatric Rehabilitation Medicine, 2,* 131–141.

Kwon, D. G., Kang, S. C., Chung, C. Y., Lee, S. H., Lee, K. M., Choi, I. H., . . . Park, M. S. (2011). Prevalence of obesity in ambulatory patients with cerebral palsy in the Korean population: A single institution's experience. *Clinics in Orthopedic Surgery, 3,* 211–216.

Law, M., Russell, D., Pollock, N., Rosenbaum, P., Walter, S., & King, G. (1997). A comparison of intensive neurodevelopmental therapy plus casting and a regular occupational therapy program for children with cerebral palsy. *Developmental Medicine and Child Neurology, 39,* 664–670.

Little, W. J. (1966). On the influence of abnormal parturition, difficult labours, premature birth, and asphyxia neonatorum, on the mental and physical condition of the child, especially in relation to deformities. *Clinical Orthopaedics and Related Research, 46,* 7–22.

Liu, J. M., Li, S., Lin, Q., & Li, Z. (1999). Prevalence of cerebral palsy in China. *International Journal of Epidemiology, 28,* 949–954.

McManus, V., Corcoran, P., & Perry, I. J. (2008). Participation in everyday activities and quality of life in pre-teenage children living with cerebral palsy in South West Ireland. *BMC Pediatrics, 8,* 50.

Morris, C. (2007). Definition and classification of cerebral palsy: A historical perspective. *Developmental Medicine and Child Neurology, 109*(Suppl.), 3–7.

Morris, C., Kurinczuk, J. J., Fitzpatrick, R., & Rosenbaum, P. L. (2006). Reliability of the Manual Ability Classification System for children with cerebral palsy. *Developmental Medicine and Child Neurology, 48,* 950–953.

Murphy, K. P., Molnar, G. E., & Lankasky, K. (1995). Medical and functional status of adults with cerebral palsy. *Developmental Medicine and Child Neurology, 37,* 1075–1084.

Nelson, K. B., & Ellenberg, J. H. (1982). Children who "outgrew" cerebral palsy. *Pediatrics, 69,* 529–536.

Nelson, K. B., & Ellenberg, J. H. (1986). Antecedents of cerebral palsy: Multivariate analysis of risk. *New England Journal of Medicine, 315,* 81–86.

Nickel, R., & Petersen, M. (2008). Motor disabilities and multiple handicapping conditions. In M. L. Wolraich, D. D. Drotar, P. H. Dworkin, & E. C. Perrin (Eds.), *Developmental–behavioral pediatrics: Evidence and practice* (pp. 483–519). Philadelphia: Mosby/Elsevier.

Nordmark, E., Hägglund, G., & Jarnlo, G. B. (1997). Reliability of the Gross Motor Function Measure in cerebral palsy. *Scandinavian Journal of Rehabilitation Medicine, 29,* 25–28.

Oeffinger, D., Conaway, M., Stevenson, R., Hall, J., Shapiro, R., & Tylkowski, C. (2010). Tibial length growth curves for ambulatory children and adolescents with cerebral palsy. *Developmental Medicine and Child Neurology, 52,* e195–e201.

Ogden, C. L., Kuczmarski, R. J., Flegal, K. M., Mei, Z., Guo, S., Wei, R., . . . Johnson, C. L. (2002). Centers for Disease Control and Prevention 2000 growth charts for the United States: Improvements to the 1977 National Center for Health Statistics version. *Pediatrics, 109,* 45–60.

O'Shea, T. M., Preisser, J. S., Klinepeter, K. L., & Dillard, R. G. (1998). Trends in mortality and cerebral palsy in a geographically based cohort of very low birth weight neonates born between 1982 to 1994. *Pediatrics, 101,* 642–647.

Palisano, R. J., Rosenbaum, P., Bartlett, D., & Livingston, M. H. (2008). Content validity of the expanded and revised Gross Motor Function Classification System. *Developmental Medicine and Child Neurology, 50,* 744–750.

Palisano, R., Rosenbaum, P., Walter, S., Russell, D., Wood, E., & Galuppi, B. (1997). Development and reliability of a system to classify gross motor function in children with cerebral palsy. *Developmental Medicine and Child Neurology, 39,* 214–223.

Pharoah, P. O., Platt, M. J., & Cooke, T. (1996). The changing epidemiology of cerebral palsy. *Archives of Disease in Childhood. Fetal and Neonatal Edition, 75,* F169–F173.

Platt, M. J., Cans, C., Johnson, A., Surman, G., Topp, M., Torrioli, M. G., & Krageloh-Mann, I. (2007). Trends in cerebral palsy among infants of very low birthweight (<1500 g) or born prematurely (<32 weeks) in 16 European centres: A database study. *Lancet, 369,* 43–50.

Prevalence and characteristics of children with cerebral palsy in Europe. (2002). *Developmental Medicine and Child Neurology, 44,* 633–640.

Reid, S. M., Carlin, J. B., & Reddihough, D. S. (2011). Distribution of motor types in cerebral palsy: How do registry data compare? *Developmental Medicine and Child Neurology, 53,* 233–238.

Reilly, S., Skuse, D., Mathisen, B., & Wolke, D. (1995). The objective rating of oral–motor functions during feeding. *Dysphagia, 10,* 177–191.

Roberts, C. D., Vogtle, L., & Stevenson, R. D. (1994). Effect of hemiplegia on skeletal maturation. *Journal of Pediatrics, 125,* 824–828.

Robertson, C. M., Watt, M. J., & Yasui, Y. (2007). Changes in the prevalence of cerebral palsy for children born very prematurely within a population-based program over 30 years. *JAMA, 297,* 2733–2740.

Rogozinski, B. M., Davids, J. R., Davis, R. B., Christopher, L. M., Anderson, J. P., Jameson, G. G., & Blackhurst, D. W. (2007). Prevalence of obesity in ambulatory children with cerebral palsy. *Journal of Bone and Joint Surgery, 89,* 2421–2426.

Rosenbaum, P., Paneth, N., Leviton, A., & Goldstein, M. (2007). The definition and classification of cerebral palsy. *Developmental Medicine and Child Neurology, 49*(Suppl. 109), 1–44.

Rosenbaum, P. L., Walter, S. D., Hanna, S. E., Palisano, R. J., Russell, D. J., Raina, P., . . . Galuppi, B. E. (2002). Prognosis for gross motor function in cerebral palsy: Creation of motor development curves. *JAMA, 288,* 1357–1363.

Russell, D. J., Avery, L. M., Rosenbaum, P. L., Raina, P. S., Walter, S. D., & Palisano, R. J. (2000). Improved scaling of the Gross Motor Function Measure for children with cerebral palsy: Evidence of reliability and validity. *Physical Therapy, 80,* 873–885.

Russell, D. J., Rosenbaum, P. L., Avery, L. M., & Lane, M. (2002). *Gross Motor Function Measure (GMFM–66 and GMFM 88) user's manual.* London: Mac Keith Press.

Sala, D. A., Shulman, L. H., Kennedy, R. F., Grant, A. D., & Chu, M. L. (1999). Idiopathic toe-walking: A review. *Developmental Medicine and Child Neurology, 41,* 846–848.

Samson-Fang, L., & Stevenson, R. D. (1998). Linear growth velocity in children with cerebral palsy. *Developmental Medicine and Child Neurology, 40,* 689–692.

Sciberras, C., & Spencer, N. (1999). Cerebral palsy in Malta 1981 to 1990. *Developmental Medicine and Child Neurology, 41,* 508–511.

Shapiro, B. K., Green, P., Krick, J., Allen, D., & Capute, A. J. (1986). Growth of severely impaired children: Neurological versus nutritional factors. *Developmental Medicine and Child Neurology, 28,* 729–733.

Sigurdardóttir, S., Thórkelsson, T., Halldórsdóttir, M., Thorarensen, O., & Vik, T. (2009). Trends in prevalence and characteristics of cerebral palsy among Icelandic children born 1990 to 2003. *Developmental Medicine and Child Neurology, 51,* 356–363.

Stallings, V. A., Charney, E. B., Davies, J. C., & Cronk, C. E. (1993a). Nutrition-related growth failure of children with quadriplegic cerebral palsy. *Developmental Medicine and Child Neurology, 35,* 126–138.

Stallings, V. A., Charney, E. B., Davies, J. C., & Cronk, C. E. (1993b). Nutritional status and growth of children with diplegic or hemiplegic cerebral palsy. *Developmental Medicine and Child Neurology, 35,* 997–1006.

Stevenson, R. D., Conaway, M., Chumlea, W. C., Rosenbaum, P., Fung, E. B., Henderson, R. C., . . . Stallings, V. A.; North American Growth in Cerebral Palsy Study. (2006). Growth and health in children with moderate-to-severe cerebral palsy. *Pediatrics, 118,* 1010–1018. http://dx.doi.org/10.1542/peds.2006-0298

Stevenson, R. D., Hayes, R. P., Cater, L. V., & Blackman, J. A. (1994). Clinical correlates of linear growth in children with cerebral palsy. *Developmental Medicine and Child Neurology, 36,* 135–142. PMID: 8132124

Stevenson, R. D., Roberts, C. D., & Vogtle, L. (1995). The effects of non-nutritional factors on growth in cerebral palsy. *Developmental Medicine and Child Neurology, 37,* 124–130. PMID: 7851668

Sundrum, R., Logan, S., Wallace, A., & Spencer, N. (2005). Cerebral palsy and socioeconomic status: A retrospective cohort study. *Archives of Disease in Childhood, 90,* 15–18.

Vincer, M. J., Allen, A. C., Joseph, K. S., Stinson, D. A., Scott, H., & Wood, E. (2006). Increasing prevalence of cerebral palsy among very preterm infants: A population-based study. *Pediatrics, 118*(6), e1621–e1626.

Ward, K. A., Caulton, J. M., Adams, J. E., & Mughal, M. Z. (2006). Perspective: Cerebral palsy as a model of bone development in the absence of postnatal mechanical factors. *Journal of Musculoskeletal and Neuronal Interactions, 6,* 154–159.

Wilke, M., & Staudt, M. (2009). Does damage to somatosensory circuits underlie motor impairment in cerebral palsy? *Developmental Medicine and Child Neurology, 51,* 686–687.

Wilmshurst, S., Ward, K., Adams, J. E., Langton, C. M., & Mughal, M. Z. (1996). Mobility status and bone density in cerebral palsy. *Archives of Disease in Childhood, 75,* 164–165.

Winter, S., Autry, A., Boyle, C., & Yeargin-Allsopp, M. (2002). Trends in the prevalence of cerebral palsy in a population-based study. *Pediatrics, 110,* 1220–1225.

Wood, E., & Rosenbaum, P. (2000). The Gross Motor Function Classification System for cerebral palsy: A study of reliability and stability over time. *Developmental Medicine and Child Neurology, 42,* 292–296.

Worley, G., Houlihan, C. M., Herman-Giddens, M. E., O'Donnell, M. E., Conaway, M., Stallings, V. A., . . . Stevenson, R. D. (2002). Secondary sexual characteristics in children with cerebral palsy and moderate to severe motor impairment: A cross-sectional survey. *Pediatrics, 110,* 897–902.

Wu, Y. W., Croen, L. A., Shah, S. J., Newman, T. B., & Najjar, D. V. (2006). Cerebral palsy in a term population: Risk factors and neuroimaging findings. *Pediatrics, 118,* 690–697.

Wu, Y. W., Xing, G., Fuentes-Afflick, E., Danielson, B., Smith, L. H., & Gilbert, W. M. (2011). Racial, ethnic, and socioeconomic disparities in the prevalence of cerebral palsy. *Pediatrics, 127,* e674–e681.

Yeargin-Allsopp, M., Van Naarden Braun, K., Doernberg, N. S., Benedict, R. E., Kirby, R. S., & Durkin, M. S. (2008). Prevalence of cerebral palsy in 8-year-old children in three areas of the United States in 2002: A multisite collaboration. *Pediatrics, 121,* 547–554.

NOELLE MOREAU, PT, PhD

5

Muscle Structural Adaptation in Cerebral Palsy and Relationship to Function

CHAPTER HIGHLIGHTS

- Overview of spasticity and muscle weakness
- Muscle structure–function relationships
- Current evidence for muscle structural adaptation in cerebral palsy
- Relationship to activity and participation in muscle structural adaptation in cerebral palsy
- Muscle plasticity and application to pediatric CIMT.

This chapter reviews the basic mechanisms of development related to two major systems—the muscle structural system and the central nervous system (CNS). These systems often have been studied in relative isolation, but in fact they work together dynamically and likely exert mutual influences with measurable consequences for a child's level of functioning over time. A child's initial muscle architecture and degree of voluntary control over particular muscles used in everyday activities are hypothesized to influence both the course and the consequences of pediatric constraint-induced movement therapy (P–CIMT).

Frequently, occupational therapy practitioners engage in activities (e.g., application of splints, training in stretching exercises) designed to alter or minimize a child's spasticity and increase range of motion. Similarly, physicians may prescribe medications and sometimes use surgery to achieve similar goals. These relatively passive strategies often are considered to set the stage to facilitate a child's future progress

KEY TERMS

Anatomical cross-sectional area
Aponeurosis
Cerebral palsy
Contractures
Epimysium
Fascicle angle
Fascicle length
Fascicles
Hypertonia
Isometric contraction
Isometric strength
Medial gastrocnemius muscle
Muscle architecture
Muscle endurance
Muscle plasticity
Muscle structural adaptation
Muscle thickness
Musculotendinous unit length
Myofibrils
Myogenesis
Palsy
Passive stiffness
Pennation angle
Perimysium
Perinatal asphyxia
Physiological cross-sectional area
Prenatal hypoxic ischemia
Rate of force development
Sarcomeres
Spasticity
Stretch reflex
Tendon compliance
Tendon length
Upper motor neuron disorder
Vicious circle
Voluntary activation

and to help prevent secondary conditions that lead to further impairments and decline in functioning as the child becomes older. By themselves, however, many of these techniques are now considered to be relatively ineffective (e.g., passive stretching and use of splinting alone; Autti-Ramo, Suoranta, Anttilla, Malmivaara, & Makela, 2006; Morris, Bowers, Ross, Stevens, & Phillips, 2011), especially if they are not used with an evidence-based form of therapy (see Chapter 16, "Research Priorities: Understanding and Transcending the Limits of Current Knowledge to Inform Best Practices in Pediatric CIMT," for ideas about future research that targets combining therapies and medical interventions). Perhaps these techniques are ineffective because they do not teach the child how to increase CNS voluntary control so that movements can become increasingly refined and integrated into the child's everyday repertoire. One cardinal feature of signature P–CIMT (discussed in depth in Chapter 2, "Pediatric CIMT: History and Definition," and Chapter 7, "Operationalizing Pediatric CIMT: Guidelines for Transforming Basic Princples and Scientific Evidence Into Clinical Practice for Individual Children") is its use of high-intensity shaping procedures and massed practice, presumably at levels sufficient to produce measurable changes in both muscle and brain architecture that in turn support stronger, faster, more accurate, and more coordinated complex movements.

Both muscle architecture and developing brains are highly plastic and moldable. People who spend long periods traveling in space, where they do not have to compete with Earth's gravity forces, lose muscle mass, strength, and control. Just as impressively, vigorous training and exercise routines (instead of a highly sedentary existence) result in large and impressive growth of muscles in both appearance and performance. Children engaged in P–CIMT can seem like young athletes training for the Olympics; indeed, many young star athletes train for 4 to 6 hours per day, many days per week, often for months and even years.

The findings in this chapter suggest possibilities for longitudinal research to follow children who receive P–CIMT (often along with other interventions and supports over the years) to see whether promoting higher neuromotor functioning at earlier ages will lead to markedly better long-term outcomes as reflected in both the structure and function of the muscular system and the CNS.

OVERVIEW OF SPASTICITY AND MUSCLE WEAKNESS

Cerebral palsy (CP) has been defined as "a group of disorders of the development of movement and posture, causing activity limitation, that are attributed to non-progressive disturbances that occurred in the developing fetal or infant brain" (Bax et al.,

2005, p. 572; see Chapter 4, "Motor Development and Physical Growth in Children With Cerebral Palsy," for a more complete history of definitions and classification schemes). Even though CP is classified as a nonprogressive **upper motor neuron (UMN) disorder,** defined as a lesion of the neural pathway above the anterior horn cell of the spinal cord or motor nuclei of the cranial nerves, it is widely known that muscles are significantly affected in CP and that the secondary effects on the musculoskeletal system are indeed progressive (Graham & Selber, 2003). The pathophysiology underlying muscle adaptation remains elusive, however. To appropriately design, plan, and implement a therapeutic intervention aimed at addressing a musculoskeletal impairment, it is important to first understand muscle adaptation in CP. This chapter focuses primarily on whole-muscle structural adaptation (i.e., change in the structure of muscle) in CP, the effects on muscle function, the relationship to activity such as P–CIMT, and participation limitations.

Spasticity and muscle weakness are considered primary impairments in CP, that is, they occur as a direct result of the upper motor neuron lesion. **Spasticity** is a velocity-dependent resistance to passive stretch, whereas **palsy** refers to paresis or weakness (Lance, 1980). Altered or atypical movement patterns, delayed attainment of neurodevelopmental milestones, decreased activity levels, and even immobilization early in infancy may occur as a result of CP (Bax et al., 2005; Morgan & Aldag, 1996). As illustrated in Figure 5.1, it is believed that over time, these altered use patterns lead to maladaptive muscle structural adaptations. These structural adaptations may lead to decreased range of motion (ROM) and joint **contractures** (i.e., limitations in joint ROM), further limiting movement and appropriate sensory input.

Because the architecture of a muscle is a primary determinant of muscle function, maladaptive adaptations produce decrements in muscle performance that not only cause muscle weakness but also decreases in muscle power and rate of force development (RFD). Diminished muscle performance combined with ROM limitations results in further activity and participation limitations, creating the vicious circle illustrated in Figure 5.1. A **vicious circle** is a complex set of events in which the response to one difficulty creates a new problem that aggravates the original difficulty (Bax et al., 2005). The set of events contains feedback loops in which each iteration of the cycle reinforces the previous one and continues unless an external factor breaks the cycle. Such a complex interaction of neural and muscular factors underlies much of the loss of function in people with CP.

Although muscle adaptation is believed to occur over time as a secondary consequence of altered activity and use patterns, altered muscle growth and development are certainly possible and have been observed in rat models of **perinatal asphyxia** (i.e., oxygen deprivation to the newborn infant during the birth process) and **prenatal hypoxic ischemia** (i.e.,

Figure 5.1 THE VICIOUS CIRCLE OF NEUROMUSCULAR IMPAIRMENTS IN CP.

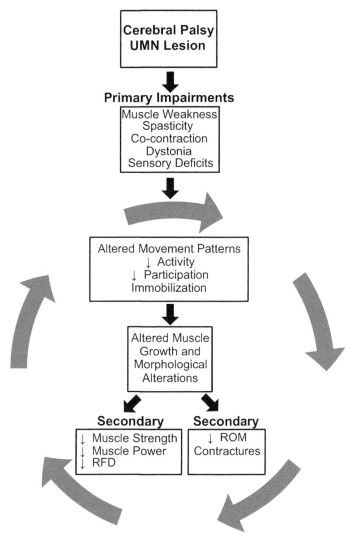

Note. CP = cerebral palsy; RFD = rate of force development; ROM = range of motion; UMN = upper motor neuron.

deprivation of the glucose and oxygen supply in utero, causing primary energy failure that leads to cell death and ultimately changes in brain metabolism), both of which are associated with CP (Coq et al., 2008; Delcour et al., 2011). In addition, the combined genetic, hormonal, nutritional, and inflammatory sequelae of perinatal brain injury provide some evidence for muscles being an initial impairment in CP (Ahmad et al., 2007; Girard, Kadhim, Beaudet, Sarret, & Sébire, 2009; Hay, Catz, Grave, & Yaffe, 1997; Hill, Threlkeld, & Fitch, 2011).

MUSCLE STRUCTURE–FUNCTION RELATIONSHIPS

Muscles appear to be inherently designed for specific functions. In particular, muscle architecture is considered to

be the primary determinant of muscle function (Lieber & Fridén, 2000). **Muscle architecture** refers to the arrangement of a muscle and the orientation of fibers, including **fascicles,** which are bundles of muscle fibers. Muscle architecture is characterized by **fascicle length,** which is the length of bundles of muscle fibers; **fascicle angle,** which is the angle at which the fascicles attach to the **aponeurosis** (i.e., layers of fascia that bind muscles together); and measures of muscle size such as **physiological cross-sectional area (PCSA),** or number of muscle fibers working together; **anatomical cross-sectional area (CSA),** or area of a section of muscle measured perpendicular to the long axis of a muscle; and **muscle thickness (MT),** or the distance between the superficial and deep aponeurosis. Other muscle structural parameters discussed in this chapter are musculotendinous unit length, muscle belly length, and tendon length and compliance.

A muscle's force-generating capacity is directly related to the PCSA (i.e., number of muscle fibers working in parallel). PCSA is equivalent to the sum of the CSA of all of the muscle fibers within a muscle and is estimated as the ratio of muscle volume to fascicle length multiplied by the cosine of the pennation angle (for pennate muscles; Lieber & Fridén, 2000). A pennate muscle has fascicles that attach obliquely to its tendon. **Pennation angle** is often estimated using the *fascicle angle;* the degree of pennation has both positive and negative consequences for force production. The amount of force transmitted directly to the tendon is reduced as a function of the cosine of the angle of pennation.

A unique design feature of a pennated muscle is that because of the arrangement of muscle fibers at an angle, it allows more muscle fibers and, thus, contractile material to be packed into a given space compared with a muscle in which the fibers run parallel to the axis of force generation (Kawakami, Abe, & Fukunaga, 1993). By allowing a greater PSCA, the force-generating capacity is increased far beyond the effect of the loss of transmitted force to the tendon. Given that most skeletal muscles have pennation angles of less than 30°, this effect is minimal (Ward, Eng, Smallwood, & Lieber, 2009). Other measures of muscle size, such as anatomical CSA and muscle thickness, also have been reported to be correlated with measures of force-generating capacity, such as muscle strength or peak torque production (Akagi, Kanehisa, Kawakami, & Fukunaga, 2008; Kanehisa, Ikegawa, & Fukunaga, 1994; Moreau, Simpson, Teefey, & Damiano, 2010).

Fiber length is indicative of the number of **sarcomeres** (i.e., long fibrous proteins) in series and is the primary determinant of muscle-shortening velocity and muscle excursion (Lieber & Fridén, 2000). Muscles with longer fibers have greater shortening velocities and a greater range over which they can produce force. In contrast, a muscle with a large PCSA is designed for high force production and smaller excursion.

Musculotendinous unit length refers to the combined length of the muscle belly and tendon, which are arranged in series with one another. Muscle belly length should not be confused with fascicle length, particularly in pennate muscle. Shortened muscle belly length has been associated with contractures; however, few studies have separated muscle belly from tendon length and thus report decreased overall musculotendinous unit length (Fry, Gough, & Shortland, 2004; Malaiya et al., 2007). Tendon length and compliance (discussed later in this chapter) also should be considered as important muscle structural parameters that can greatly affect the force velocity properties of muscle.

Figure 5.2 TWO-DIMENSIONAL B-MODE ULTRASOUND AXIAL IMAGE OF THE RECTUS FEMORIS.

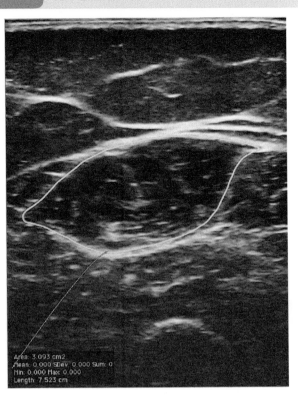

Note. The epimysium is traced in light blue and depicts the measurement of the cross-sectional area.

MUSCLE STRUCTURAL ADAPTATION IN CEREBRAL PALSY: CURRENT EVIDENCE

Numerous studies have identified alterations and differences in muscle architecture in children with CP compared with children who are developing typically (Cheatwood, 1995; Lieber & Fridén, 2002; Malaiya et al., 2007; Mohagheghi et al., 2008; Moreau, Teefey, & Damiano, 2009; Shortland, Harris, Gough, & Robinson, 2002). Reported measures of muscle size in people with CP include muscle volume, PCSA, CSA, and MT and were obtained with magnetic resonance imaging or with two- or three-dimensional B-mode ultrasonography. The **epimysium,** or connective tissue that surrounds the entire muscle belly, is highly reflective of ultrasound waves and produces hyperechoic (highly reflective) lines that can easily be seen in two-dimensional B-mode ultrasound imaging in both longitudinal and cross-sectional images (Figure 5.2). The connective tissue surrounding the fascicles, or **perimysium,** is also highly reflective and can be used to measure fascicle length and fascicle angle, as described in Figure 5.3 (Campbell & Wood, 2002).

Figure 5.3 TWO-DIMENSIONAL B-MODE ULTRASOUND LONGITUDINAL IMAGE OF THE VASTUS LATERALIS.

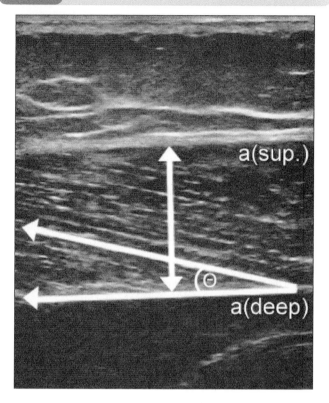

a(sup.)

(θ)

a(deep)

Note. Muscle thickness was calculated as the distance between superficial [a(sup.)] and deep aponeuroses [a(deep)] in the middle of the ultrasound image at a 90° angle from the deep aponeurosis as indicated by the vertical white arrow. Fascicle angle was the positive angle between the deep aponeurosis and the line of the fascicle as indicated by theta (θ) and corresponding arrows.

These studies of muscle architecture in CP are cross-sectional and involve older children (aged 5 to 19 years). Currently, no information is available in the literature regarding when such muscle architectural changes first occur and how these changes manifest in early motor development. However, Barber, Hastings-Ison, Baker, Barrett, and Lichtwark (2011) reported a 22% reduction in medial gastrocnemius muscle volume in children with CP aged 2 to 5 years, providing evidence that these changes may occur sooner than previously thought. Given the remarkable plasticity of muscle, it is not surprising that muscle adaptations may occur early in life. Future studies should investigate the time course of muscle development in children with CP to provide a better understanding of muscle growth and adaptation and of the development of secondary impairments such as contractures and muscle performance deficits.

The following sections discuss the evidence regarding **muscle structural adaptation** (i.e., change in the structure of the muscle) in CP in reference to three impairments of importance to clinicians—spasticity, muscle performance, and contractures. These sections emphasize the direct influence that muscle structural adaptations have on these impairments over time.

SPASTICITY

UMN lesions result in **hypertonia** (i.e., an increase in muscle tone) and an increased resistance to passive muscle lengthening (Stolov, 1966). Hypertonia is associated with an increased sensitivity of the **stretch reflex,** which is a muscle contraction in response to stretching within the muscle (reflex component), and with changes in muscle and connective tissue properties (nonreflexive component; Malouin, Bonneau, Pichard, & Corriveau, 1997). *Spasticity*, the reflexive component, is a velocity-dependent increased resistance to movement attributable to hyperexcitable stretch reflexes (Lance, 1980).

Unfortunately, the term *spasticity*, a component of hypertonia, is frequently and nonspecifically used to describe all aspects of hypertonia in addition to other UMN disorder signs and symptoms. For example, muscle structural adaptations in CP frequently have been referred to as changes secondary to spasticity or "spastic" muscle (Fridén & Lieber, 2003; Lieber & Fridén, 2002; Lieber, Steinman, Barash, & Chambers, 2004). An issue not addressed adequately in these studies of "spastic" muscle is the degree of spasticity present, if any, in the muscles sampled. Both clinically and experimentally, it is common to detect spasticity in certain muscle groups but not in others (Damiano et al., 2002; Damiano, Quinlivan, Owen, Shaffrey, & Abel, 2001; Katz, Rovai, Brait, & Rymer, 1992). Therefore, if spasticity is hypothesized to result in secondary myopathic changes, the presence and degree of spasticity should be documented for the muscles in question. Until they are documented and investigated experimentally, it cannot accurately be said that these findings are representative of "spastic" muscle. Rather, these findings are representative of muscles in children and adolescents with CP.

MUSCLE PERFORMANCE

Given that muscle architecture is the primary determinant of the force–velocity properties of muscle, identifying the muscle architectural adaptations that occur in CP provides a better understanding of why muscles perform the way they do. It has been reported consistently in the literature that lower-extremity (LE) muscle size is decreased when comparing youth with CP with age-matched typically developing children and when comparing the paretic with the nonparetic extremity in hemiplegia, even when corrected for body mass (Barber et al., 2011; Elder et al., 2003; Malaiya et al., 2007; Mohagheghi et al., 2007; Moreau et al., 2009).

Muscle volume has been widely reported across LE muscles, with deficits of 26% to 41% for the gastrocnemius (Elder et al., 2003; Malaiya et al., 2007), 18% to 50% for individual quadriceps muscles (Lampe, Grassl, Mitternacht, Gerdesmeyer, & Gradinger, 2006; Oberhofer, Stott, Mithraratne, & Anderson, 2010; Shortland, 2009), and 28% for the ankle dorsiflexors (Elder et al., 2003). Relatively similar deficits have been observed for PCSA, CSA, and MT in these same muscle groups when comparing youths with CP with typically developing youths, paretic with typically developing limbs, and paretic with nonparetic limbs in youths with hemiplegic CP (Bandholm, Magnusson, Jensen, & Sonne-Holm, 2009; Bland, Prosser, Bellini, Alter, & Damiano, 2011; Elder et al., 2003; Mohagheghi et al., 2007; Moreau et al., 2009).

Mechanisms responsible for the lack of muscle growth may include a reduced number of **myofibrils** (i.e., a muscle fiber's threads made up of sarcomeres, which are the contractile units of a myofibril) arranged in a series in parallel, decreased muscle fiber CSA, and altered expressions of genes involved in **myogenesis** (i.e., the formation of muscle tissue during embryonic development; Fridén & Lieber, 2003; Smith et al., 2009). Fridén and Lieber (2003) reported that the CSAs of single muscle fibers from the wrist flexors obtained from biopsies were one-third the size of those of a control group.

The clinical implications of decreased muscle size are noteworthy. Fewer sarcomeres working in parallel result in a decrease in force-generating capacity. Indeed, strength deficits ranging between 40% and 85% of normal have been reported for LE muscle groups (Eek & Beckung, 2008; Ross & Engsberg, 2002; Wiley & Damiano, 1998). Generally, the distal plantarflexors and dorsiflexors were reported to be the weakest.

Fewer published studies have reported quantitative measurements of strength deficits in the upper extremities of people with CP. Vaz, Cotta Mancini, Fonseca, Vieira, and de Melo Pertence (2006) reported that wrist flexor and extensor strength in children with hemiplegic CP was reduced by 50% and 70%, respectively, compared with typically developing children. Weakness is considered to be one of the primary impairments that contributes to functional limitations in children with CP. LE muscle strength has consistently been reported to be significantly correlated with the Gross Motor Function Measure (GMFM; Russell et al., 1989) and walking speed (Damiano et al., 2001; Eek & Beckung, 2008; Goh, Thompson, Huang, & Schafer, 2006; Ross & Engsberg, 2007). Furthermore, the ratio of wrist extensor strength to wrist flexor stiffness explained 46% of the variance in hand function (Vaz et al., 2006).

Muscle endurance, which is the ability of a muscle unit to sustain repeated contractions against resistance for an extended period of time, has been presumed to be limited in CP because of decreased cardiorespiratory fitness, muscle spasticity, and subjective complaints of generalized fatigue (Jahnsen, Villien, Stanghelle, & Holm, 2003; Lundberg, 1978). It is now known that muscles in people with CP are, in fact, highly durable; that is, the rate of decline in torque or force during both voluntary and electrically elicited repeated muscle contractions is slower compared with typically developing children (Moreau, Li, Geaghan, & Damiano, 2008; Stackhouse, Binder-Macleod, & Lee, 2005). Clinically, although muscles are more durable, the level of force that is able to be sustained may not be of sufficient magnitude to be functionally significant because of the amount of muscle weakness. Therefore, therapeutic programs targeting strength and power, rather than muscle endurance, are recommended to increase the overall force-generating capacity of the muscle and reduce relative effort of the task (Moreau, Li, et al., 2008).

Although muscle size does not fully explain the presence of weakness in people with CP, it does explain a significant portion. After controlling for age and Gross Motor Function Classification System (GMFCS; Palisano et al., 1997) level, vastus lateralis muscle thickness explains 82% of the variance in knee extensor **isometric strength** (i.e., maximal strength against resistance), whereas rectus femoris muscle thickness explains 32% of the variance after controlling for age (Moreau et al., 2010).

Other factors, such as voluntary activation, co-contraction of antagonist muscles, moment arm, fiber length, and intrinsic stiffness, also play a role in reduced voluntary force production. For example, **voluntary activation,** or the ability to activate available motor units within a muscle, was reported to be 33% and 50% lower in youths with CP compared with typically developing youths for the quadriceps and plantarflexors, respectively (Stackhouse et al., 2005). This concept is illustrated in Figure 5.4, which shows that an increase in vastus lateralis muscle thickness in a child with CP at any of the GMFCS levels yields a smaller increase in voluntary isometric peak torque compared with a typically developing child of the same age. Also note that isometric strength decreases as a function of GMFCS level, in that higher-functioning children (lower GMFCS levels) are stronger than lower-functioning children. Representative ultrasound images of rectus femoris muscle thickness in 12-year-old children with CP across GMFCS levels and in a typically developing child are illustrated in Figure 5.5. Rectus femoris muscle thickness decreases and subcutaneous fat increases with increasing GMFCS levels compared with a typically developing child of the same age.

Ongoing work suggests that rectus femoris muscle thickness is decreased across all GMFCS levels in children with CP compared with typically developing children after controlling for age and leg length (Moreau & Holthaus, 2011). In addition, independent ambulators (GMFCS Levels I and II) were shown to have larger quadriceps muscles than marginal

Figure 5.4 PREDICTION OF MAXIMUM ISOMETRIC KNEE EXTENSOR PEAK TORQUE FROM VARIOUS VL MUSCLE THICKNESS VALUES IN 12-YEAR-OLD CHILDREN WITH CP FOR GMFCS LEVELS I–IV AND FOR A 12-YEAR-OLD TYPICALLY DEVELOPING CHILD.

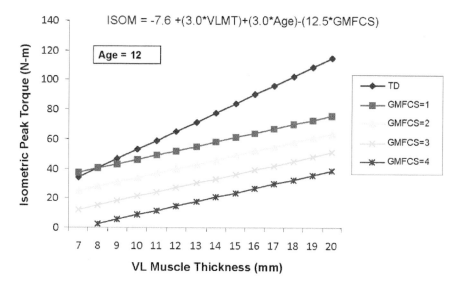

$$ISOM = -7.6 +(3.0*VLMT)+(3.0*Age)-(12.5*GMFCS)$$

Note. The equation is based on the VL muscle thickness predictive equations from Moreau, Simpson, Teefey, and Damiano (2010). CP = cerebral palsy; GMFCS = Gross Motor Function Classification System level; ISOM = isometric knee extensor peak torque (N-m); TD = typically developing; VL = vastus lateralis; VLMT = VL muscle thickness (mm).

Source. Reprinted from "Muscle Architecture Predicts Maximal Strength and Is Related to Activity Levels in Children with Cerebral Palsy," by N. G. Moreau, K. Simpson, S. Teefey, & D. L. Damiano, 2010, *Physical Therapy, 90,* Figure 3. Copyright © 2010 American Physical Therapy Association. Reprinted with permission.

ambulators (GMFCS IV) or nonambulators (GMFCS V). Furthermore, those who required assistance to ambulate (GMFCS III) were shown to have larger muscles than marginal ambulators (GMFCS IV) and nonambulators (GMFCS V; Moreau & Holthaus, 2011). Ohata, Tsuboyama, Ichihashi, and Minami (2006) also reported significant differences in quadriceps muscle thickness between GMFCS Levels III and V in adults with CP. Thickness of the triceps and the longissimus measured at the midthoracic level also varied by GMFCS level in adults with CP and were lowest in nonambulators. Collectively, these studies stress the importance of ambulation and weight-bearing activities on the maintenance of muscle mass not only in the lower extremities but also in the upper-extremity (UE) and trunk musculature.

Another parameter strongly influenced by muscle size is **RFD,** which is the rate of rise in force or torque from the onset of contraction. RFD is a measure of how quickly peak strength or torque can be reached. Although strength is important, it typically takes at least 300 milliseconds (ms) to reach peak torque in most human muscles. However, many everyday activities involve movements with faster contraction times between 50 ms and 200 ms (Aagaard, 2003). Therefore, if two people have the same peak strength for a given muscle group, the person with a higher RFD will be able to reach a higher level of torque earlier during an activity.

This concept does not apply only to athletic endeavors. A simple example is from the gait cycle. During normal walking, quadriceps torque must be generated within approximately 150 ms during early stance to achieve knee extension (Perry, 1992). Considering that it takes at least 300 ms to achieve peak torque, a higher RFD would allow a greater amount of torque to be generated within the initial 150 ms. Data show that knee extensor RFD calculated from a knee extension isometric task in youths with CP was reduced by 70% compared with a 50% decrement in strength (Moreau, Falvo, & Damiano, 2012). Muscle thickness of the vastus lateralis was shown to be the best predictor of RFD, explaining 32% of the variance in RFD. Furthermore, knee extensor RFD was a better predictor than strength of sports and physical functioning and the ability to perform transfers (Moreau et al., 2012). These data support the notion that time-dependent measures of force production, such as RFD, should be considered in addition to absolute strength to adequately characterize everyday performance of activities. Research is needed to explore the importance of RFD in gross motor activities of the UE, such as wheelchair propulsion.

Fascicle, or fiber length, is considered to be the single most important muscle architectural parameter (Lieber et al., 2004). Fascicle length represents the number of sarcomeres in series and therefore is the primary determinant of the

Figure 5.5 REPRESENTATIVE ULTRASOUND IMAGES OF RECTUS FEMORIS MUSCLE THICKNESS IN 12-YEAR-OLD CHILDREN WITH CP ACROSS GMFCS LEVELS AND IN A TYPICALLY DEVELOPING CHILD.

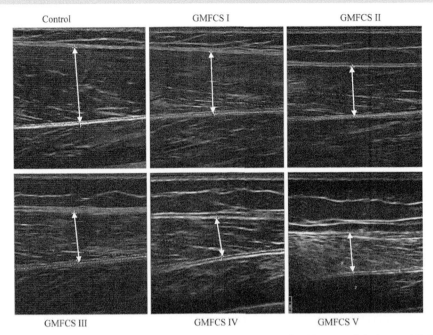

Note. Muscle thickness is the perpendicular distance between superficial and deep aponeuroses as indicated by the white arrows. Subcutaneous fat is located proximal to the superficial aponeurosis between the skin surface and the proximal arrowhead. CP = cerebral palsy; GMFCS = Gross Motor Function Clasification System.

shortening velocity and excursion of a muscle. Muscles with longer fibers have more sarcomeres in series and are capable of producing force through a larger ROM and at higher speeds than shorter fibers. The two-joint rectus femoris muscle crosses the hip and knee joints and has been implicated as a cause of stiff knee gait in people with CP, in whom knee joint excursion during walking is diminished. Rectus femoris fascicle length was found to be decreased by 27% in children with CP compared with typically developing children (Moreau et al., 2009).

The **medial gastrocnemius muscle,** which is the medial head of the gastrocnemius muscle located in the posterior lower leg, has been the muscle of interest in many architectural studies of children with CP because of the propensity of this muscle to be affected by spasticity and weakness. The results for the gastrocnemius, however, are equivocal. Although the original study by Shortland and colleagues (2002) reported no differences in fascicle length between children with CP (*n* = 7) and typically developing children (*n* = 5), this study had a small sample size with low statistical power to detect group differences. Since then, multiple reports of decreased fascicle lengths in the affected limbs of youths with hemiplegic and diplegic CP have provided evidence that fiber length may be decreased in the medial gastrocnemius muscle (Bland et al., 2011; Cheatwood, 1995; Gao, Zhao, Gaebler-Spira, & Zhang, 2011; Malaiya et al., 2007; Mohagheghi et al., 2007, 2008).

The combined effects of decreased muscle size and fascicle length have important functional implications. Muscle power, as the product of force and velocity, would be adversely affected by decreases in muscle size and fascicle length, respectively. In Figure 5.6, the maximum force that the two fibers can produce is equivalent because they have identical PCSAs. At any given contraction velocity, however, the muscle with the longer fibers is capable of producing higher levels of force and, thus, greater muscle power. In fact, average muscle power in youths with CP during a knee extension isokinetic test at 60° per second was shown to be only 18% of that of an age-matched comparison group of typically developing children (N. G. Moreau, unpublished data, 2012; Figure 5.7). Knee extensor strength during the same isokinetic test in these participants was 64% of that of the comparison group of typically developing participants. These data suggest that muscle power may be more affected than muscle strength in youths with CP.

The large decrement observed in muscle power is reflected in the fact that youths with CP have difficulty producing torque at higher speeds of movement, which is often required during daily activities. Particularly in the elderly population, muscle power is a more important muscle performance indicator than strength and a better predictor of physical function and mobility (Bassey et al., 1992; Skelton, Greig, Davies, & Young, 1994). Because of the similarities in muscle architecture and fiber type alterations between people with CP and elderly

| **Figure 5.6** | FORCE–VELOCITY RELATIONSHIPS OF TWO MUSCLES WITH DIFFERENT FIBER LENGTHS BUT IDENTICAL STRENGTH (I.E., IDENTICAL PHYSIOLOGICAL CROSS-SECTIONAL AREAS). |

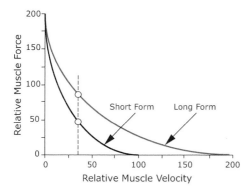

Note. The muscle with the longer fibers maintains a higher force at any given velocity (dashed vertical line). At an identical shortening velocity, the longer fibers have more sarcomeres in series, which allows each sarcomere to have a slower absolute contraction velocity compared to the shorter fibered muscle. This allows it to operate higher on the force–velocity curve. The difference between the muscles becomes smaller as shortening velocity decreases.

Reprinted from *Skeletal Muscle Structure, Function, and Plasticity: The Physiological Basis for Rehabilitation*, 3rd ed. (p. 148), by R. L. Lieber, 2010, Baltimore: Lippincott Williams & Wilkins. Copyright © 2010 Lippincott Williams & Wilkins. Reprinted with permission.

people (e.g., decreased fascicle length and muscle size, increase in Type I fibers), it is likely that muscle power may play an even greater role in functional limitations than previously believed.

| **Figure 5.7** | PEAK TORQUE, AS A MEASURE OF MUSCLE STRENGTH, AND MUSCLE POWER CALCULATED DURING AN ISOKINETIC KNEE EXTENSION TEST AT 60° PER SECOND IN CHILDREN WITH CP. $N = 11$; MEAN AGE = 10.6 ± 1.9 YR. |

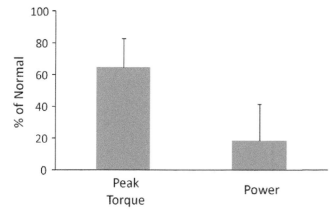

Note. Values are presented as a percentage of normal values obtained in a group of age-matched typically developing children ($N = 8$; mean age = 10.5 ± 2.5 yr; N. G. Moreau, unpublished data, 2012). CP = cerebral palsy.

| **Figure 5.8** | SCHEMATIC ILLUSTRATION OF THE EFFECTS OF FIBER LENGTH AND PENNATION ANGLE ON MUSCLE THICKNESS AND MUSCLE LENGTH. |

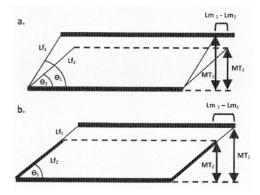

Note. In (a), the muscle has identical fiber lengths but different fascicle angles. A decrease in fascicle angle ($\Theta_2 < \Theta_1$) results in a corresponding decrease in muscle thickness ($MT_2 < MT_1$). In (b), the muscle has identical pennation angles but different fascicle lengths. A decrease in fascicle length ($Lf_2 < Lf_1$) results in a corresponding decrease in muscle thickness ($MT_2 < MT_1$). The overall effect is a decrease in muscle length ($Lm_2 < Lm_1$). Lf = fiber length; Lm = muscle length; MT = muscle thickness.

Fascicle angle differences between youths with CP and typically developing youths also are limited to the gastrocnemius and vastus lateralis and have produced equivocal results (Malaiya et al., 2007; Mohagheghi et al., 2008; Moreau et al., 2009; Shortland et al., 2002). Muscle atrophy can result in a decrease in fascicle angle, particularly in highly pennated muscles such as the vastus lateralis and gastrocnemius muscle, consistent with previously discussed reports of diminished muscle size in youth with CP (Barber et al., 2011; Elder et al., 2003; Malaiya et al., 2007; Mohagheghi et al., 2007; Moreau et al., 2009). Fascicle angle is also highly dependent on muscle thickness and fascicle length. Figure 5.8(a) illustrates a pennate muscle with identical fascicle lengths but different fascicle angles. Note that a decrease in fascicle angle ($\Theta_2 < \Theta_1$) results in a corresponding decrease in muscle thickness ($MT_2 < MT_1$). Furthermore, muscle hypertrophy has been associated with increases in pennation angle, which would allow more contractile material to be placed within a given volume, increasing the force production capability of the muscle (Blazevich, Gill, & Zhou, 2006; Kawakami et al., 1993).

CONTRACTURES

Contractures refers to the loss of joint ROM because of structural changes in muscle, tendon, or ligaments that contribute to an increase in passive stiffness. Contractures are common in CP, particularly in two-joint muscles such as the biceps brachii, wrist flexors, gastrocnemius, psoas, rectus femoris, and hamstrings (Panteliadis & Strassburg, 2004).

Figure 5.9 COMPARISON OF MUSCLE FORCE AND JOINT ANGLE IN TWO MUSCLES WITH DIFFERENT FIBER LENGTHS BUT IDENTICAL STRENGTH (I.E., IDENTICAL PHYSIOLOGICAL CROSS-SECTIONAL AREAS).

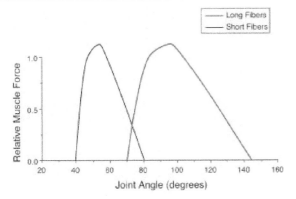

Note. The muscle with the longer fibers (red line) has a ROM of 75°, whereas the muscle with the short fibers (black line) has a ROM of only 40°. The reason for the difference is that the longer fibered muscle has a smaller change in sarcomere length per joint angle rotation.

Source. Reprinted from *Skeletal Muscle Structure, Function, and Plasticity: The Physiological Basis for Rehabilitation*, 3rd ed. (p. 139), by R. L. Lieber, 2010, Baltimore: Lippincott Williams & Wilkins. Copyright © 2010 Lippincott Williams & Wilkins. Reprinted with permission.

This section explores the muscle structural changes that are believed to cause contractures in CP.

Decreased muscle belly length is often implicated as a cause of contracture because of the limitations in joint ROM. However, internal architectural changes within the muscle also may contribute to contractures. Figure 5.9 illustrates two muscles with identical PSCAs but different fiber lengths. Note that the muscle with the longer fibers has a greater active ROM than the muscle with shorter fibers because there are more sarcomeres in series to take up the change in length. In this example, by increasing fiber length, active ROM increases from 40° to 75° (Lieber, 2010). Therefore, fiber length has a direct influence on active ROM.

The orientation of fibers within a muscle also must be considered when discussing the effect of fiber length on whole muscle length. In a parallel-fibered muscle, a decrease in fascicle length would have a direct effect on muscle length. An example of a parallel or fusiform muscle that is affected by contracture in CP is the biceps brachii. The biceps are composed of long fibers that run parallel to the long axis of the muscle. In this case, a decrease in fascicle length would have a reliable effect on muscle length. However, the relationship in pennate muscle is more complex. For example, Figure 5.8(b) illustrates a pennate muscle with identical fascicle angles but different fascicle lengths. A decrease in fascicle length ($Lf_2 < Lf_1$) results in a corresponding decrease in muscle thickness ($MT_2 < MT_1$) and a decrease in muscle length ($Lm_2 < Lm_1$).

However, the effect on muscle length in a pennate muscle is less than that on a parallel muscle.

Although several studies have reported decreased fascicle lengths in various LE muscles in children with CP (Bland et al., 2011; Cheatwood, 1995; Gao et al., 2011; Malaiya et al., 2007; Mohagheghi et al., 2007, 2008; Moreau et al., 2009), a limitation of ultrasound imaging is the inability to measure actual sarcomere length or to normalize fascicle length by sarcomere length. As such, fascicle length is not a direct measure of sarcomere number. However, using intraoperative techniques involving laser diffraction and muscle biopsies, researchers reported that shortened hamstring muscles in children with CP undergoing hamstring lengthenings were composed of fewer sarcomeres in series rather than shortened sarcomeres (Smith, Lee, Ward, Chambers, & Lieber, 2011). In fact, these authors determined that in vivo sarcomere length was actually longer than normal in the wrist flexors and hamstrings, two muscle groups commonly affected by contracture (Lieber & Fridén, 2002; Smith et al., 2011). In addition, these muscles experience higher stresses with increasing muscle length. What these findings describe is a maladaptive process in which the muscle's response to growth and stress is to increase sarcomere length rather than to add sarcomeres in series. Therefore, contracted or shortened muscles in CP may have fewer numbers of sarcomeres in series, but the sarcomeres may be overlengthened to compensate.

Shortland and colleagues (2002) proposed that contractures in the medial gastrocnemius muscle, a pennate muscle, are secondary to muscle atrophy and shortened aponeurosis rather than to a decrease in fiber length. Figure 5.10 illustrates this concept. This figure contains three muscles with identical numbers of fibers. The thickness or diameter of the muscle fibers in 5.10(b) is 20% larger than those in 5.10(a), resulting in an increase in muscle length. However, results from an increasing number of studies have reported decreases in fascicle length of the medial gastrocnemius (Cheatwood, 1995; Gao et al., 2011; Malaiya et al., 2007; Mohagheghi et al., 2007, 2008) and rectus femoris (Moreau et al., 2009) muscles in CP, indicating the possibility that a combination of decreased fiber length and muscle atrophy contributes to the development of contractures, as illustrated in Figure 5.10(c). The muscle in 5.10(c) has longer and thicker diameter fibers than the muscle in 5.10(a). As a result, the muscle itself in 5.10(c) is both longer and thicker.

Another proposed mechanism for contracture is an increase in **passive stiffness** (i.e., resistance to elongation or shortening) of muscle tissue. Lieber and colleagues investigated at the cellular level muscle fiber stiffness in CP and stiffness of fiber bundles, which contain muscle fibers and extracellular matrix material (Fridén & Lieber, 2003; Lieber, Runesson, Einarsson, & Fridén, 2003; Smith et al., 2011). Previous

Figure 5.10	SCHEMATIC ILLUSTRATION OF THREE MUSCLES WITH IDENTICAL NUMBERS OF FIBERS AND IDENTICAL PENNATION ANGLES.

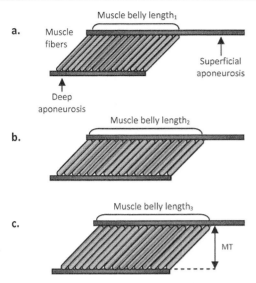

Note. The thickness or diameter of the muscle fibers in (b) is 20% greater than those in (a), resulting in an increase in muscle length. The muscle fibers in (c) are 20% thicker and 20% longer than those in (a), resulting in an increase in both muscle length and muscle thickness. MT = muscle thickness.

Figure 5.11	SCHEMATIC ILLUSTRATION OF THE EFFECTS OF TENDON PROPERTIES ON SARCOMERE LENGTH IN A MUSCLE WITH THREE SERIAL SARCOMERES.

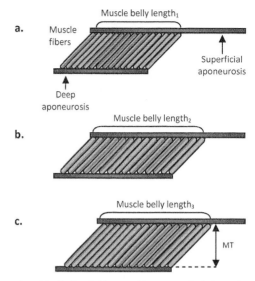

Note. (a) muscle and tendon length (L) at rest; (b) same muscle during an isometric contraction in which slack is taken up in the tendon (L1), allowing the sarcomeres to shorten; and (c) same muscle but with a more compliant tendon (L2) during an isometric contraction, allowing greater sarcomere shortening, placing the sarcomere in an unfavorable position for force production.

studies showed that muscle fibers themselves were stiffer across a variety of muscles and were attributed to the major load-bearing intracellular protein titin (Fridén & Lieber, 2003; Lieber et al., 2003). However, in a well-controlled study, Smith and colleagues (2011) reported an increase in stiffness of the fiber bundles in the hamstring muscles that was accompanied by an increase in collagen content. The authors concluded that the combination of increased passive stiffness of fiber bundles (rather than muscle fibers) and increased in vivo sarcomere lengths contribute to higher stresses and, ultimately, the development of contractures in CP. However, the mechanisms underlying these muscle property changes are unknown.

Up to this point, only muscle changes associated with contractures in CP have been discussed. **Tendon length,** which is the length of the tendon measured from the musculotendinous junction to the tendon insertion on the bone, and **tendon compliance,** which measures the ease with which the tendon yields to pressure or resistance without being deformed, are also important components of the overall musculotendinous unit. Tendons lengthen during muscle contraction to allow the sarcomeres to shorten during contraction and to absorb passive tension. Figure 5.11(a) represents a muscle at rest, whereas 5.11(b) represents a muscle during an **isometric contraction,** in which slack is taken up in the tendon, allowing the sarcomeres to shorten. In the presence of shortened muscles with stiffer fiber bundles

and overstretched sarcomeres, what happens to the tendons? As mentioned previously, partitioning muscle and tendon length from the musculotendinous unit complex during both morphological and biomechanical testing requires sophisticated techniques.

Some evidence exists in the literature of Achilles tendon elongation in youths with CP in response to muscle contracture (Gao et al., 2011; Wren et al., 2010). More specifically, Achilles tendon lengths in children with CP were reported to be longer than in typically developing children for those with and without ankle plantarflexion contractures, suggesting that tendon adaptation may occur before the development of contracture (Wren et al., 2010). Tendon elongation also may be an adaptation within the musculotendinous unit to compensate for stiffer fiber bundle properties and the inability to add sarcomeres in series in response to growth or stretch. Figure 5.11(c) illustrates an isometric muscle contraction with a longer, more compliant tendon than in 5.11(b). The negative consequence of increased tendon elongation is that the sarcomeres are allowed to shorten too much, allowing excessive actin and myosin overlap and placing them in an unfavorable position for force production.

Although there are fewer sarcomeres in series, the sarcomeres themselves may be overlengthened, at least as reported for the wrist flexors and hamstring muscles (Lieber et al., 2003; Smith et al., 2011). If sarcomeres are indeed overlengthened, then the additional shortening provided by the longer, more compliant tendon would have a positive contribution on force output because it would allow the sarcomere to operate at a more optimal length on the length–tension curve. Therefore, despite prevailing muscle weakness in youths with CP, tendon adaptation may play a role in preserving force output in the presence of overstretched sarcomeres.

MUSCLE STRUCTURAL ADAPTATION IN CP: RELATIONSHIP TO ACTIVITY AND PARTICIPATION

The investigation of muscle structural adaptations in CP is a relatively new field of investigation that has grown over the past 10 years. Therefore, the literature relating muscle structure to activity and participation is limited.

As described in Figure 5.1, inactivity and altered movement patterns are believed to lead to muscle structural adaptations, which influence muscle function. Altered muscle function affects activity levels, and ultimately participation in society, as part of a vicious circle. According to this theory, direct and indirect links should exist between muscle structure and activity and participation. A clinically meaningful relationship ($\rho = .49$; Moreau et al., 2010) has been observed between rectus femoris fascicle length and scores on the Sports and Physical Functioning scale of the Pediatric Outcomes Data Collection Instrument (PODCI; Daltroy, Liang, Fossel, & Goldberg, 1998). This scale includes higher level activities in addition to sports activity, and researchers have hypothesized that fascicle length is important for muscle-shortening velocity during these activities.

Another clinically meaningful relationship ($r = .50$; Moreau et al., 2010) was found between vastus lateralis fascicle angle and the Transfers and Basic Mobility scale of the PODCI ($r = .47$) and the Locomotion subdomain of the Activities Scale for Kids (ASK; Young, Yoshida, Williams, Bombardier, & Wright, 1995). Because the vastus lateralis was inherently designed for force production as a pennate muscle with a large PSCA, Moreau and colleagues (2010) hypothesized that the vastus lateralis is necessary for the movement against gravity necessary for gait, transfers, and moving from sit to stand. However, Moreau and colleagues (2010, 2012) observed that measures of muscle performance, such as strength and RFD, had stronger positive associations with activity and participation than muscle architecture. These findings are supported by Figure 5.1, which shows a direct relationship between muscle performance and activity and participation.

Ohata and colleagues (2008) tested 38 children and adolescents with CP and quantified the relationships among quadriceps thickness, consisting of combined rectus femoris and vastus intermedius thickness, and two measures of activity and participation: the GMFM shortened version (GMFM–66; Russell et al., 2000) and the Pediatric Evaluation of Disability Inventory (PEDI; Feldman, Haley, & Coryell, 1990). The GMFM–66 assesses a wide range of gross motor abilities and consists of items such as crawling, rolling, standing, walking, and jumping (Russell et al., 2000). Ohata and colleagues (2008) found that quadriceps muscle thickness was significantly correlated with the GMFM–66 aggregate score ($r = .52$), emphasizing that children with higher abilities have thicker quadriceps muscles. Quadriceps thickness also was significantly correlated with the PEDI Mobility and Self-Care domains ($r = .63$ and $.74$, respectively), which reflect self-reported daily activity in children with disabilities.

In walking, muscle thickness and fascicle length of the anterior tibialis were shown to be significantly correlated to fast walking speed (Bland et al., 2011). Fascicle lengths of the anterior tibialis and rectus femoris also have been reported to be positively correlated to step length during walking in children with CP (Bland et al., 2011; Moreau, Stanley, Teefey, & Damiano, 2008). Therefore, the excursion limitations of the rectus femoris about the hip and knee in children with CP that are secondary to decreased fascicle lengths may present during gait as shorter steps. Collectively, these data provide some support that altered muscle structure–function relationships are related to activity and participation limitations. However, more studies are needed that are adequately powered to answer these questions.

MUSCLE PLASTICITY AND APPLICATION TO PEDIATRIC CIMT

Muscle plasticity is the potential for muscle to adapt or change in response to stimuli. Because of the remarkable plasticity of muscle, muscle architecture also can readily adapt to positive stimuli, such as muscle loading from resistance training or weight-bearing activities. In fact, muscle adaptations, such as hypertrophy and other changes in internal muscle architecture, have been observed after resistance training activities in various populations such as elderly people, healthy adults, and even people with CP (Aagaard et al., 2001; McNee, Gough, Morrissey, & Shortland, 2009; Reeves, Narici, & Maganaris, 2004). The most important factor to consider to effect a change in muscle structure and function is the dosage (frequency, intensity, and duration) of the intervention—more specifically, matching dosage with the goal of the intervention.

For example, if a goal of P–CIMT for a particular child is to the improve coordination, timing, and accuracy of throwing a ball with the affected arm, then repetitive, massed practice of this activity would be an appropriate therapeutic activity. However, if triceps muscle weakness is the underlying factor limiting performance of this functional task, then muscle strengthening should be targeted. In this case, repetitive low-load activities will not provide an adequate stimulus for muscle strengthening. Rather, to sufficiently load the muscle, an activity should be designed that targets the triceps muscle group, with only 2 or 3 sets of 6 to 15 repetitions being performed at a given intensity or load. Strengthening should be performed 2 to 4 times per week on nonconsecutive days, and weight or intensity should be progressively increased when 15 repetitions can be performed with good form. If improving muscle power is the goal, 1 to 3 sets of 3 to 6 repetitions of an activity should be performed at a higher velocity of movement. These guidelines adhere to the American Academy of Pediatrics and National Strength and Conditioning Association position statement papers for youth resistance training, which provide more detailed information (Faigenbaum et al., 2009; McCambridge, Stricker, & American Academy of Pediatrics Council on Sports Medicine and Fitness, 2008).

When planning therapeutic interventions, dosage should be adjusted according to the underlying goal of therapy. Often, therapeutic interventions designed for children with disabilities are not intensive enough to induce permanent changes at the muscle level. Therefore, when impairments in muscle strength or power are a limiting factor affecting the performance of a functional task, these impairments should be specifically targeted through a carefully designed therapeutic intervention that adheres to pediatric and youth resistance training guidelines (Faigenbaum et al., 2009; McCambridge et al., 2008). As an adjunct to P–CIMT or other therapies, activities that target muscle power or strength in specific muscle groups could easily be incorporated into a P–CIMT program on nonconsecutive days of treatment.

SUMMARY

Although CP is the result of a CNS injury, the secondary effects on the musculoskeletal system are profound. The function of a muscle is strongly determined by its structural properties. In particular, the architecture of a muscle plays a critical role in the amount of force, shortening velocity, and ROM that can be produced. Because muscles are one of the most plastic tissues in the human body, they readily adapt to the level of use. Therefore, this chapter provided a summary of muscle structural adaptations that occur as a consequence of CP, with an emphasis on how these adaptations relate to common secondary impairments such as ROM deficits, contractures, and muscle weakness. Evidence was presented describing the relationship of muscle architecture to activity and participation.

A better understanding of the physiological basis for secondary impairments in CP should aid in the development of interventions aimed at exploiting the remarkable plasticity of muscle in a positive manner. When appropriate, therapy should be designed to effect change in muscle structure and function, ultimately improving mobility, activity, and participation in children with CP.

REFERENCES

Aagaard, P. (2003). Training-induced changes in neural function. *Exercise and Sport Sciences Reviews, 31,* 61–67.

Aagaard, P., Andersen, J. L., Dyhre-Poulsen, P., Leffers, A. M., Wagner, A., Magnusson, S. P., . . . Simonsen, E. B. (2001). A mechanism for increased contractile strength of human pennate muscle in response to strength training: Changes in muscle architecture. *Journal of Physiology, 534,* 613–623.

Ahmad, I., Zaldivar, F., Iwanaga, K., Koeppel, R., Grochow, D., Nemet, D., . . . Cooper, D. M. (2007). Inflammatory and growth mediators in growing preterm infants. *Journal of Pediatric Endocrinology and Metabolism, 20,* 387–396.

Akagi, R., Kanehisa, H., Kawakami, Y., & Fukunaga, T. (2008). Establishing a new index of muscle cross-sectional area and its relationship with isometric muscle strength. *Journal of Strength and Conditioning Research, 22,* 82–87.

Autti-Ramo, L., Suoranta, J., Anttilla, H., Malmivaara, A., & Makela, M. (2006). Effectiveness of upper and lower limb casting and orthoses in children with cerebral palsy: An overview of review articles. *American Journal of Physical Medicine and Rehabilitation, 85,* 89–103.

Bandholm, T., Magnusson, P., Jensen, B. R., & Sonne-Holm, S. (2009). Dorsiflexor muscle-group thickness in children with cerebral palsy: Relation to cross-sectional area. *NeuroRehabilitation, 24,* 299–306.

Barber, L., Hastings-Ison, T., Baker, R., Barrett, R., & Lichtwark, G. (2011). Medial gastrocnemius muscle volume and fascicle length in children aged 2 to 5 years with cerebral palsy. *Developmental Medicine and Child Neurology, 53,* 543–548.

Bassey, E. J., Fiatarone, M. A., O'Neill, E. F., Kelly, M., Evans, W. J., & Lipsitz, L. A. (1992). Leg extensor power and functional performance in very old men and women. *Clinical Science (London, England), 82,* 321–327.

Bax, M., Goldstein, M., Rosenbaum, P., Leviton, A., Paneth, N., Dan, B., . . . Damiano, D.; Executive Committee for the Definition of Cerebral Palsy. (2005). Proposed definition and classification of cerebral palsy, April 2005. *Developmental Medicine and Child Neurology, 47*, 571–576.

Bland, D. C., Prosser, L. A., Bellini, L. A., Alter, K. E., & Damiano, D. L. (2011). Tibialis anterior architecture, strength, and gait in individuals with cerebral palsy. *Muscle and Nerve, 44*, 509–517.

Blazevich, A. J., Gill, N. D., & Zhou, S. (2006). Intra- and intermuscular variation in human quadriceps femoris architecture assessed in vivo. *Journal of Anatomy, 209*, 289–310.

Campbell, R. S., & Wood, J. (2002). Ultrasound of muscle. *Imaging, 14*, 229–240.

Cheatwood, A. P. (1995). *Changes in medial gastrocnemius architecture with spasticity and contracture* (Unpublished doctoral dissertation). University of Southern California, Los Angeles.

Coq, J. O., Strata, F., Russier, M., Safadi, F. F., Merzenich, M. M., Byl, N. N., & Barbe, M. F. (2008). Impact of neonatal asphyxia and hind limb immobilization on musculoskeletal tissues and S1 map organization: Implications for cerebral palsy. *Experimental Neurology, 210*, 95–108.

Daltroy, L. H., Liang, M. H., Fossel, A. H., & Goldberg, M. J. (1998). The POSNA pediatric musculoskeletal functional health questionnaire: Report on reliability, validity, and sensitivity to change. Pediatric Outcomes Instrument Development Group. Pediatric Orthopaedic Society of North America. *Journal of Pediatric Orthopedics, 18*, 561–571.

Damiano, D. L., Quinlivan, J. M., Owen, B. F., Payne, P., Nelson, K. C., & Abel, M. F. (2002). What does the Ashworth scale really measure and are instrumented measures more valid and precise? *Developmental Medicine and Child Neurology, 44*, 112–118.

Damiano, D. L., Quinlivan, J., Owen, B. F., Shaffrey, M., & Abel, M. F. (2001). Spasticity versus strength in cerebral palsy: Relationships among involuntary resistance, voluntary torque, and motor function. *European Journal of Neurology, 8*(Suppl. 5), 40–49.

Delcour, M., Russier, M., Xin, D. L., Massicotte, V. S., Barbe, M. F., & Coq, J. O. (2011). Mild musculoskeletal and locomotor alterations in adult rats with white matter injury following prenatal ischemia. *International Journal of Developmental Neuroscience, 29*, 593–607.

Eek, M. N., & Beckung, E. (2008). Walking ability is related to muscle strength in children with cerebral palsy. *Gait and Posture, 28*, 366–371.

Elder, G. C., Kirk, J., Stewart, G., Cook, K., Weir, D., Marshall, A., & Leahey, L. (2003). Contributing factors to muscle weakness in children with cerebral palsy. *Developmental Medicine and Child Neurology, 45*, 542–550.

Faigenbaum, A. D., Kraemer, W. J., Blimkie, C. J., Jeffreys, I., Micheli, L. J., Nitka, M., & Rowland, T. W. (2009). Youth resistance training: Updated position statement paper from the National Strength and Conditioning Association. *Journal of Strength and Conditioning Research, 23*(Suppl.), S60–S79.

Feldman, A. B., Haley, S. M., & Coryell, J. (1990). Concurrent and construct validity of the Pediatric Evaluation of Disability Inventory. *Physical Therapy, 70*, 602–610.

Fridén, J., & Lieber, R. L. (2003). Spastic muscle cells are shorter and stiffer than normal cells. *Muscle and Nerve, 27*, 157–164.

Fry, N. R., Gough, M., & Shortland, A. P. (2004). Three-dimensional realisation of muscle morphology and architecture using ultrasound. *Gait and Posture, 20*, 177–182.

Gao, F., Zhao, H., Gaebler-Spira, D., & Zhang, L. Q. (2011). In vivo evaluations of morphologic changes of gastrocnemius muscle fascicles and Achilles tendon in children with cerebral palsy. *American Journal of Physical Medicine and Rehabilitation, 90*, 364–371.

Girard, S., Kadhim, H., Beaudet, N., Sarret, P., & Sébire, G. (2009). Developmental motor deficits induced by combined fetal exposure to lipopolysaccharide and early neonatal hypoxia/ischemia: A novel animal model for cerebral palsy in very premature infants. *Neuroscience, 158*, 673–682.

Goh, H. T., Thompson, M., Huang, W. B., & Schafer, S. (2006). Relationships among measures of knee musculoskeletal impairments, gross motor function, and walking efficiency in children with cerebral palsy. *Pediatric Physical Therapy, 18*, 253–261.

Graham, H. K., & Selber, P. (2003). Musculoskeletal aspects of cerebral palsy. *Journal of Bone and Joint Surgery, British Volume, 85*, 157–166.

Hay, W. W., Jr., Catz, C. S., Grave, G. D., & Yaffe, S. J. (1997). Workshop summary: Fetal growth: Its regulation and disorders. *Pediatrics, 99*, 585–591.

Hill, C. A., Threlkeld, S. W., & Fitch, R. H. (2011). Early testosterone modulated sex differences in behavioral outcome following neonatal hypoxia ischemia in rats. *International Journal of Developmental Neuroscience, 29*, 381–388.

Jahnsen, R., Villien, L., Stanghelle, J. K., & Holm, I. (2003). Fatigue in adults with cerebral palsy in Norway compared with the general population. *Developmental Medicine and Child Neurology, 45*, 296–303.

Kanehisa, H., Ikegawa, S., & Fukunaga, T. (1994). Comparison of muscle cross-sectional area and strength between untrained women and men. *European Journal of Applied Physiology and Occupational Physiology, 68,* 148–154.

Katz, R. T., Rovai, G. P., Brait, C., & Rymer, W. Z. (1992). Objective quantification of spastic hypertonia: Correlation with clinical findings. *Archives of Physical Medicine and Rehabilitation, 73,* 339–347.

Kawakami, Y., Abe, T., & Fukunaga, T. (1993). Muscle-fiber pennation angles are greater in hypertrophied than in normal muscles. *Journal of Applied Physiology, 74,* 2740–2744.

Lampe, R., Grassl, S., Mitternacht, J., Gerdesmeyer, L., & Gradinger, R. (2006). MRT-measurements of muscle volumes of the lower extremities of youths with spastic hemiplegia caused by cerebral palsy. *Brain and Development, 28,* 500–506.

Lance, J. W. (1980). Symposium synopsis. In R. G. Feldman, R. R. Young, & W. P. Koella (Eds.), *Spasticity: Disordered motor control* (pp. 485–500). Chicago: Yearbook Medical.

Lieber, R. L. (2010). *Skeletal muscle structure, function, and plasticity: The physiological basis for rehabilitation* (3rd ed.). Baltimore: Lippincott Williams & Wilkins.

Lieber, R. L., & Fridén, J. (2000). Functional and clinical significance of skeletal muscle architecture. *Muscle and Nerve, 23,* 1647–1666.

Lieber, R. L., & Fridén, J. (2002). Spasticity causes a fundamental rearrangement of muscle–joint interaction. *Muscle and Nerve, 25,* 265–270.

Lieber, R. L., Runesson, E., Einarsson, F., & Fridén, J. (2003). Inferior mechanical properties of spastic muscle bundles due to hypertrophic but compromised extracellular matrix material. *Muscle and Nerve, 28,* 464–471.

Lieber, R. L., Steinman, S., Barash, I. A., & Chambers, H. (2004). Structural and functional changes in spastic skeletal muscle. *Muscle and Nerve, 29,* 615–627.

Lundberg, A. (1978). Maximal aerobic capacity of young people with spastic cerebral palsy. *Developmental Medicine and Child Neurology, 20,* 205–210.

Malaiya, R., McNee, A. E., Fry, N. R., Eve, L. C., Gough, M., & Shortland, A. P. (2007). The morphology of the medial gastrocnemius in typically developing children and children with spastic hemiplegic cerebral palsy. *Journal of Electromyography and Kinesiology, 17,* 657–663.

Malouin, F., Bonneau, C., Pichard, L., & Corriveau, D. (1997). Non-reflex mediated changes in plantarflexor muscles early after stroke. *Scandinavian Journal of Rehabilitation Medicine, 29,* 147–153.

McCambridge, T. M., & Stricker, P. R.; American Academy of Pediatrics Council on Sports Medicine and Fitness. (2008). Strength training by children and adolescents. *Pediatrics, 121,* 835–840.

McNee, A. E., Gough, M., Morrissey, M. C., & Shortland, A. P. (2009). Increases in muscle volume after plantarflexor strength training in children with spastic cerebral palsy. *Developmental Medicine and Child Neurology, 51,* 429–435.

Mohagheghi, A. A., Khan, T., Meadows, T. H., Giannikas, K., Baltzopoulos, V., & Maganaris, C. N. (2007). Differences in gastrocnemius muscle architecture between the paretic and non-paretic legs in children with hemiplegic cerebral palsy. *Clinical Biomechanics, 22,* 718–724.

Mohagheghi, A. A., Khan, T., Meadows, T. H., Giannikas, K., Baltzopoulos, V., & Maganaris, C. N. (2008). In vivo gastrocnemius muscle fascicle length in children with and without diplegic cerebral palsy. *Developmental Medicine and Child Neurology, 50,* 44–50.

Moreau, N. G., Falvo, M. J., & Damiano, D. L. (2012). Rapid force generation is impaired in cerebral palsy and is related to decreased muscle size and functional mobility. *Gait and Posture, 35,* 154–158. http://dx.doi.org/10.1016/j.gaitpost.2011.08-027

Moreau, N. G., & Holthaus, K. (2011). Motor severity negatively affects muscle architecture in CP: A comparison between GMFCS levels, hemiplegia, and typically developing children. *Developmental Medicine and Child Neurology, 53,* 78.

Moreau, N. G., Li, L., Geaghan, J. P., & Damiano, D. L. (2008). Fatigue resistance during a voluntary performance task is associated with lower levels of mobility in cerebral palsy. *Archives of Physical Medicine and Rehabilitation, 89,* 2011–2016. http://dx.doi.org/10.1016/j.apmr.2008.03.012

Moreau, N. G., Simpson, K. N., Teefey, S. A., & Damiano, D. L. (2010). Muscle architecture predicts maximum strength and is related to activity levels in cerebral palsy. *Physical Therapy, 90,* 1619–1630. http://dx.doi.org/10.2522/ptj.20090377

Moreau, N. G., Stanley, C., Teefey, S. A., & Damiano, D. L. (2008, April). *Rectus femoris fascicle length is related to dynamic measures of knee excursion during gait in cerebral palsy.* Paper presented at the meeting of the Gait and Clinical Movement Analysis Society, Richmond, VA.

Moreau, N. G., Teefey, S. A., & Damiano, D. L. (2009). In vivo muscle architecture and size of the rectus femoris and vastus lateralis in children and adolescents with cerebral palsy. *Developmental Medicine and Child Neurology, 51,* 800–806. http://dx.doi.org/10.111/j.1469-8749.2009.03307

Morgan, A. M., & Aldag, J. C. (1996). Early identification of cerebral palsy using a profile of abnormal motor patterns. *Pediatrics, 98,* 692–697.

Morris, C., Bowers, R., Ross, K., Stevens, P., & Phillips, D. (2011). Orthotic management of cerebral palsy: Recommendations from a consensus panel. *NeuroRehabilitation, 28,* 37–46.

Oberhofer, K., Stott, N. S., Mithraratne, K., & Anderson, I. A. (2010). Subject-specific modelling of lower limb muscles in children with cerebral palsy. *Clinical Biomechanics, 25,* 88–94.

Ohata, K., Tsuboyama, T., Haruta, T., Ichihashi, N., Kato, T., & Nakamura, T. (2008). Relation between muscle thickness, spasticity, and activity limitations in children and adolescents with cerebral palsy. *Developmental Medicine and Child Neurology, 50,* 152–156.

Ohata, K., Tsuboyama, T., Ichihashi, N., & Minami, S. (2006). Measurement of muscle thickness as quantitative muscle evaluation for adults with severe cerebral palsy. *Physical Therapy, 86,* 1231–1239.

Panteliadis, C. P., & Strassburg, H. M. (2004). *Cerebral palsy: Principles and management.* New York: Thieme.

Perry, J. (1992). *Gait analysis: Normal and pathological function.* Thorofare, NJ: Slack.

Reeves, N. D., Narici, M. V., & Maganaris, C. N. (2004). In vivo human muscle structure and function: Adaptations to resistance training in old age. *Experimental Physiology, 89,* 675–689.

Ross, S. A., & Engsberg, J. R. (2002). Relation between spasticity and strength in individuals with spastic diplegic cerebral palsy. *Developmental Medicine and Child Neurology, 44,* 148–157.

Ross, S. A., & Engsberg, J. R. (2007). Relationships between spasticity, strength, gait, and the GMFM–66 in persons with spastic diplegia cerebral palsy. *Archives of Physical Medicine and Rehabilitation, 88,* 1114–1120.

Russell, D. J., Avery, L. M., Rosenbaum, P. L., Raina, P. S., Walter, S. D., & Palisano, R. J. (2000). Improved scaling of the Gross Motor Function Measure for children with cerebral palsy: Evidence of reliability and validity. *Physical Therapy, 80,* 873–885.

Russell, D. J., Rosenbaum, P. L., Cadman, D. T., Gowland, C., Hardy, S., & Jarvis, S. (1989). The Gross Motor Function Measure: A means to evaluate the effects of physical therapy. *Developmental Medicine and Child Neurology, 31,* 341–352.

Shortland, A. (2009). Muscle deficits in cerebral palsy and early loss of mobility: Can we learn something from our elders? *Developmental Medicine and Child Neurology, 51*(Suppl. 4), 59–63.

Shortland, A. P., Harris, C. A., Gough, M., & Robinson, R. O. (2002). Architecture of the medial gastrocnemius in children with spastic diplegia. *Developmental Medicine and Child Neurology, 44,* 158–163.

Skelton, D. A., Greig, C. A., Davies, J. M., & Young, A. (1994). Strength, power and related functional ability of healthy people aged 65–89 years. *Age and Ageing, 23,* 371–377.

Smith, L. R., Lee, K. S., Ward, S. R., Chambers, H. G., & Lieber, R. L. (2011). Hamstring contractures in children with spastic cerebral palsy result from a stiffer extracellular matrix and increased in vivo sarcomere length. *Journal of Physiology, 589,* 2625–2639.

Smith, L. R., Pontén, E., Hedström, Y., Ward, S. R., Chambers, H. G., Subramaniam, S., & Lieber, R. L. (2009). Novel transcriptional profile in wrist muscles from cerebral palsy patients. *BMC Medical Genomics, 2,* 44.

Stackhouse, S. K., Binder-Macleod, S. A., & Lee, S. C. (2005). Voluntary muscle activation, contractile properties, and fatigability in children with and without cerebral palsy. *Muscle and Nerve, 31,* 594–601.

Stolov, W. C. (1966). The concept of normal muscle tone, hypotonia and hypertonia. *Archives of Physical Medicine and Rehabilitation, 47,* 156–168.

Vaz, D. V., Cotta Mancini, M., Fonseca, S. T., Vieira, D. S., & de Melo Pertence, A. E. (2006). Muscle stiffness and strength and their relation to hand function in children with hemiplegic cerebral palsy. *Developmental Medicine and Child Neurology, 48,* 728–733.

Ward, S. R., Eng, C. M., Smallwood, L. H., & Lieber, R. L. (2009). Are current measurements of lower extremity muscle architecture accurate? *Clinical Orthopaedics and Related Research, 467,* 1074–1082.

Wiley, M. E., & Damiano, D. L. (1998). Lower-extremity strength profiles in spastic cerebral palsy. *Developmental Medicine and Child Neurology, 40,* 100–107.

Wren, T. A., Cheatwood, A. P., Rethlefsen, S. A., Hara, R., Perez, F. J., & Kay, R. M. (2010). Achilles tendon length and medial gastrocnemius architecture in children with cerebral palsy and equinus gait. *Journal of Pediatric Orthopedics, 30,* 479–484.

Young, N. L., Yoshida, K. K., Williams, J. I., Bombardier, C., & Wright, J. G. (1995). The role of children in reporting their physical disability. *Archives of Physical Medicine and Rehabilitation, 76,* 913–918.

ROSLYN N. BOYD, PhD, MSc, BSc, Pgrad, and
LEANNE SAKZEWSKI, PhD, BOccThy

6

Assessment Tools to Measure Upper-Limb Function and Impact of Therapy

CHAPTER HIGHLIGHTS

- Systematic reviews
- Measuring the goals of intervention from the child's perspective
- Activity outcomes
- Measuring unimanual capacity
- Measuring unimanual performance
- Measuring bimanual performance
- Assessment of executive function
- Assessment of mastery and motivation
- Participation outcomes
- Quality of life
- Monitoring feasibility and adverse events.

KEY TERMS

ABILHAND–Kids
Acceptability
Assessment of Life Habits
Assessment of Motor and Process Skills
Assisting Hand Assessment
Box and Block Test
Brief Rating Inventory of Executive Function
Canadian Occupational Performance Measure
Capacity
Children's Hand-Use Experience Questionnaire
Developmental disregard
Dimensions of Mastery Questionnaire
Feasibility
Goal Attainment Scaling
Interpretability
Jebsen–Taylor Hand Function Test
Melbourne Assessment of Unilateral Upper Limb Function
Participation
Pediatric Evaluation of Disability Inventory
Pediatric Motor Activity Log
Pediatric Volitional Questionnaire
Performance
Quality of Upper Extremity Skills Test
Reliability
Validity

he *International Classification of Functioning, Disability and Health (ICF)* provides a framework for measuring and documenting health outcomes at the body function and structure, activities, and participation levels (World Health Organization [WHO], 2001). It also considers the influence of contextual factors, including personal and environmental factors, on a child's health status (Majnemer & Mazer, 2004). Outcome measures therefore need to address the multidimensional nature of the *ICF* by focusing not only on body structure and function but also on activity and participation.

Increasingly, public bodies such as the U.S. Food and Drug Administration recommend the use of valid and reliable outcome measures capable of detecting clinically significant change (Cano & Hobart, 2008). Detecting change using an assessment tool that is not validated or proven reliable for the population, even if the tool has been used and reported in other clinical trials, does not give meaningful information about the outcome of an intervention. In measuring outcomes of intensive upper-limb training programs such as constraint-induced movement therapy (CIMT) and other adjunctive interventions (e.g., targeted use of intramuscular botulinum toxin A before implementing CIMT), it is important to use measures that are known to be reliable and valid for the population and that measure clinically important change.

The total time required for a CIMT program can be high, varying from <30 to 120 hours, consequently consuming a great amount of time and resources. It is therefore essential not only to use valid and reliable measures in domains on which the training is focused (e.g., activity limitations) but also to consider outcomes meaningful to the patients and families (e.g., goals, participation in activities, quality of life). From the health provider's perspective, important factors include additional risks, adverse events, and unintended effects possibly attributed to the treatment, as well as cost and consequences of the CIMT program compared with usual care.

This chapter describes measures considered useful in interpreting the outcomes of intensive models of upper-limb training in children with unilateral motor disability in both clinical and research settings. The selection of appropriate outcome measures from the broad group of measures reported in this chapter is contingent on the goals of the program, whether the program has a clinical or research focus, and the setting in which the program takes place.

SYSTEMATIC REVIEWS

Many relevant systematic reviews have evaluated the psychometric properties (validity, reliability, and responsiveness) and clinical utility of outcome measures in specific domains for use with children and adolescents with motor disability. The systematic reviews relevant to this chapter cover the domains of (1) upper-limb activity limitations (Gilmore, Sakzewski, & Boyd, 2010; Klingels et al., 2010), (2) participation restrictions (Sakzewski, Boyd, & Ziviani, 2007; Ziviani, Desha, Feeney, & Boyd, 2010), and (3) quality of life (Carlon et al., 2010).

In these systematic reviews, a modified version of the CanChild Outcome Measures Rating Form (Law, 2004a) was used to extract descriptive information and grade the psychometric properties and clinical utility of the assessment tools. The Outcome Measures Rating Form incorporates the ICF framework and was designed to rate the quality and clinical utility of outcome measures and therefore was deemed the most appropriate scale to evaluate the assessment tools. For each review, the CanChild rating form was tailored to measure the domain of the ICF relevant to the group of measures.

The characteristics (for both clinical and research settings) of the assessment tools extracted included target population, age range, purpose of tool, format, content, number of scales and items, time to administer, availability and cost of manual, and training required. An assessment was considered valid if it was found to measure what it is supposed to measure (Portney & Watkins, 2000). Information on **validity** included construct, criterion, and evaluative validity or responsiveness. *Evaluative validity* or *responsiveness* is the ability to detect minimal clinically important change over time (Guyatt, Walter, & Norman, 1987). **Reliability** measures the degree to which a test is stable, measuring a construct in a reproducible and consistent way (Law, 2004b). Internal consistency and interrater, intrarater, and test–retest reliability also were evaluated.

When interpreting the reliability coefficients, Portney and Watkins (2000) suggested considering values below .50 to represent poor reliability; .50 to .75, moderate reliability; and above .75, good reliability. They presented these values as a guideline only and emphasized that degree of acceptable reliability depends on how the results will be applied; for instance, they proposed using a value of at least .90 when interpreting results for an individual. These guidelines also can be applied to kappa statistics, which are appropriate for nominal data (Portney & Watkins, 2000). The CanChild Outcome Measures Rating Form guidelines for reliability coefficients are that above .80 are excellent; .60 to .79, adequate; and <.60, poor (Law, 2004b).

The clinical utility of outcome measures is rated according to **interpretability** (meaningfulness of scores), **feasibility** (ease of administration, scoring, and interpretation), and **acceptability** of the measure to assessors and respondents (utility vs. burden). Time of administration, availability of a manual and clarity of instructions, format of assessment, and requirement for further assessor training are reviewed. The availability of a test manual and normative data also is considered.

This chapter presents outcome measures considered useful for the measurement of intensive upper-limb training and summarizes information on their psychometric properties and clinical utility according to domains of the ICF. Recommendations regarding each measure's strengths and limitations in clinical and research settings also are provided.

MEASURING THE GOALS OF INTERVENTION FROM THE CHILD'S PERSPECTIVE

A family-centered approach underpins contemporary occupational therapy and physical therapy practice for children and youths with cerebral palsy (CP). Identification of meaningful goals of the child and family helps determine priorities for an individualized and family-focused intervention. Two goal-setting measures have been used in clinical settings and in a range of upper-limb rehabilitation trials for children with CP: the Canadian Occupational Performance Measure (COPM) and Goal Attainment Scaling (GAS).

CANADIAN OCCUPATIONAL PERFORMANCE MEASURE

The **Canadian Occupational Performance Measure (COPM)** is a standardized individualized, client-centered measure evaluating self-perception of occupational performance on identified goals over time (Law et al., 2005). It is the most commonly used individualized outcome measure in pediatric occupational therapy practice (Tam, Teachman, & Wright, 2008). The standardized administration procedure uses a semistructured interview of caregivers or children, or both, to identify areas of difficulty in self-care, productivity (school or preschool), and leisure. These difficulty areas are then rated on a scale of 1 to 10 for importance, enabling up to five areas of difficulty to be prioritized. Caregivers and children rate their perceived performance of and satisfaction with the prioritized areas of difficulty using a 10-point rating scale. Higher scores indicate higher perceived performance and greater satisfaction. Children aged 8 years or older can complete the COPM reliably (Law et al., 2005).

Benefits

The COPM has strong content, construct, and criterion validity and adequate test–retest reliability (intraclass correlation coefficient [ICC] = .76–.89). A change of 2 or more points on the COPM is considered clinically meaningful. Recent studies of pediatric CIMT (P–CIMT) have consistently demonstrated the COPM to be sensitive to change (Aarts, Jongerius, Geerdink, van Limbeek, & Geurts, 2010; Hoare, 2010; Sakzewski et al., 2011a; Wallen, O'Flaherty, & Waugh, 2007).

Limitations

It has been suggested that the process of engaging children and families in setting therapy goals and increasing their focus on those goal areas may in itself contribute to improved outcomes (Wallen & Ziviani, 2012). Accordingly, for benefits to be attributed to a particular form of therapy, the magnitude of change would need to be substantially larger to justify implementing the therapy.

GOAL ATTAINMENT SCALING

Goal Attainment Scaling (GAS) is a criterion-referenced individualized outcome measure of goal attainment (Kiresuk, Smith, & Cardillo, 1994). GAS can be used with all ages and disabilities and uses a semistructured interview to elicit client-identified goals. These individual goals are rated on a 5-point scale (from −2 = *less-than-expected outcome* to +2 = *greater-than-expected outcome*). Each goal is weighted according to

importance. A total *t* score can be calculated based on the weighted average of scores to provide a quantitative index of whether progress was equal to, greater than, or less than expected.

Benefits

GAS relies on prespecified criteria that can be objectively assessed as a measure of goal attainment, whereas the COPM provides a subjective rating (not anchored to behavioral criteria). GAS has been shown to identify some goal areas not addressed in standardized assessments (Steenbeek, Gorter, Ketelaar, Galama, & Lindeman, 2011). Changes in GAS goals following intervention, however, have been poorly correlated with changes on standardized assessments such as the Gross Motor Function Measure (GMFM–66; Steenbeck et al., 2011). One interpretation is that GAS is more responsive to capturing certain types of change in people. GAS has been used in several P–CIMT trials, demonstrating that it is responsive to clinical change (Gordon et al., 2011; Wallen et al., 2011).

Limitations

The accuracy of goal setting and rating relies on the clinical skills of the person setting the goals (Clark & Caudrey, 1983; Cytrynbaum, Ginath, Birdwell, & Brandt, 1979; Palisano, 1993). Some reports have indicated that scores can be biased because the practitioner is both the source of assessment and the person setting expected outcomes; for example, setting low levels for expected improvement could lead to higher levels of attainment after treatment (Palisano, 1993; Palisano, Haley, & Brown, 1992). Comparisons across studies also could be problematic with this tool because the magnitude of the goals and the criteria for measuring them could differ widely, even for children who show similar pretreatment to posttreatment changes. This concern has led to recommendations that goal setting and rating be performed by someone other than the treating clinician (Cytrynbaum et al., 1979). However, a recent study of interrater reliability among therapists of children with CP found that reliability was enhanced when the child's treating therapist set the goals (Steenbeek, Ketelaar, Lindeman, Galama, & Gorter, 2010).

ACTIVITY OUTCOMES

Children with hemiplegia usually have difficulty grasping, reaching, releasing, and manipulating objects with the impaired upper limb (Eliasson, Gordon, & Forssberg, 1991). Motor and sensory impairments can lead to the child learning to perform tasks mainly with his or her nonimpaired arm, which could contribute to what has been called **developmental disregard,** or learned nonuse of the involved upper limb (Charles & Gordon, 2005; Hoare, Imms, Carey, & Wasiak, 2007).

Intervention often is focused on improving both unimanual and bimanual function of the upper limbs during activity.

Assessments with excellent psychometric properties and clinical utility that specifically measure a child's impaired upper-limb use and bimanual use are necessary to ensure a broad and functionally useful measurement of outcomes in clinical trials of upper-limb training for children with congenital hemiplegia. Measurement of **capacity** of the impaired upper limb (i.e., what the child can do when asked) often can demonstrate skills and abilities that are not spontaneously used in bimanual tasks in real-life situations (i.e., **performance,** or what the child typically does in daily life). It is therefore important to capture aspects of both capacity and performance. Understanding the discrepancy between a child's capacity and performance also may assist with selection of the most appropriate model of upper-limb training (e.g., CIMT, bimanual training) at a given stage in the child's development.

This chapter reports on upper-limb activity assessments useful for measuring the outcomes of CIMT and modified CIMT (mCIMT). Aspects of unimanual capacity of the impaired upper limb include quality of movement (e.g., Melbourne Assessment of Unilateral Upper Limb Function [Melbourne

Assessment; Randall, Johnson, & Reddihough, 1999], Quality of Upper Extremity Skills Test [QUEST; DeMatteo et al., 1992]) and efficiency of movement (e.g., Jebsen–Taylor Hand Function Test [JTHFT; Taylor, Sand, & Jebsen, 1973]). Bimanual performance measures include the Assisting Hand Assessment (AHA; Krumlinde-Sundholm, Holmefur, Kottorp, & Eliasson, 2007), ABILHAND–Kids (Arnould, Penta, Renders, & Thonnard, 2004), and the recently developed Children's Hand-Use Experience Questionnaire (CHEQ; Sköld, Hermansson, Krumlinde-Sundholm, & Eliasson, 2011). The characteristics of these assessments are summarized in Table 6.1.

The ABILHAND–Kids, AHA, Melbourne Assessment, and CHEQ were designed specifically for assessment of children with CP or a unilateral disability. Published studies have reported data on all of these tools for children with congenital hemiplegia. In addition, the studies reporting data for the AHA incorporated children with unimanual impairment, including brachial plexus palsy and congenital hemiplegia. The validity and reliability of the Melbourne Assessment and the ABILHAND–Kids were investigated in children with various distribution and motor types of CP. Evidence for validity and evaluative validity for these assessments is reported in Table 6.2.

Table 6.1   Description of Major Pediatric Assessment Tools by Target Population, Activity, and Primary Use

MEASURE	TARGET POPULATION AND AGE	TYPE OF ACTIVITY MEASURED	PRIMARY PURPOSE[a]	PERFORMANCE OR CAPACITY[b]
Melbourne Assessment of Unilateral Upper Limb Function[c]	Children with CP or neurological impairment aged 30 months–15 years[c,d]	Unimanual	Discriminative Evaluative	Capacity
Quality of Upper Extremity Skills Test[e]	Children with CP or neurological impairment aged 18 months–8 years	Unimanual	Evaluative	Capacity
Jebsen–Taylor Hand Function Test[f]	Children with DD aged 5–18 years	Unimanual	Evaluative	Capacity
Pediatric Motor Activity Log–Revised[g]	Children with hemiplegic CP aged 6 months–8 years	Unimanual	Evaluative	Performance
Assisting Hand Assessment[h]	Children with a unilateral disability aged 18 months–12 years	Bimanual play	Discriminative Evaluative	Performance
ABILHAND–Kids[i]	Children with CP aged 6–15 years	Manual ability (bimanual and unimanual)	Discriminative	Performance
Children's Hand-Use Experience Questionnaire[j]	Children with unilateral upper-limb impairment aged 6–18 years	Bimanual	Evaluative	Performance
Box and Block Test[k]	Children aged 6–19 years and adults with unilateral upper-limb impairment	Unimanual	Discriminative	Capacity

Note. CP = cerebral palsy; DD = developmental disabilities.
[a]*Discriminative* assessments can discriminate between different client groups; *evaluative* assessments are better able to measure the magnitude of longitudinal changes for an individual or group (Kirschner & Guyatt, 1985). [b]*Performance* indicates what typically happens in daily life without prompting. *Capacity* indicates the best elicited response. [c]Randall, Johnson, & Reddihough, 1999. [d]Randall, Imms, & Carey, 2012. [e]DeMatteo et al., 1992. [f]Taylor, Sand, & Jebsen, 1973. [g]Wallen, Bundy, Pont, & Ziviani, 2009a. [h]Krumlinde-Sundholm & Eliasson, 2003. [i]Arnould, Penta, Renders, & Thonnard, 2004. [j]Sköld, Hermansson, Krumlinde-Sundholm, & Eliasson, 2011. [k]Mathiowetz, Volland, Kashman, & Weber, 1985; Desrosiers, Bravo, Hébert, Dutil, & Mercier, 1994.

Table 6.2   Content, Construct, Concurrent, and Evaluative Validity of Upper-Limb Activity Measures

ASSESSMENT	CONTENT VALIDITY	CONSTRUCT VALIDITY	CRITERION VALIDITY	EVALUATIVE VALIDITY
Melbourne Assessment of Unilateral Upper Limb Function (MUUL)[a]	Literature review, review of existing assessments, workshops with experienced occupational therapy practitioners[a]	Significant correlations with the PEDI on self-care (Spearman's ρ = .939), mobility (.783), and total functional skills (.718)[b]	Four experienced clinicians assessed according to usual methods ICC between clinicians = −.92 Average correlation between clinician score and MUUL = .87 (n = 11)[c]	SDD = 8.9% (5–8 years, n = 21)[d] SDD = 7.4% (5–16 years, n = 20)[e]
Quality of Upper Extremity Skills Test (QUEST)[f]	Literature review, discussion with clinicians and experts[f]	Correlation between therapists' judgment of child's hand function and QUEST scores for right and left hands (n = 71)[f] Significant correlation between MUUL and total QUEST (r = .84) for total score of QUEST and PDMS–FM (r = .83)[d] Rasch analysis: Not unidimensional, better fit of items in domains, posture items in grasp domain erratic[g]	NA	Smallest clinically significant difference in casting trial 4.89 units[h] SDD = 13.8% (total test score, 5–8 years, n = 21)[d]
Jebsen–Taylor Hand Function Test[i]	Initially developed for adults Lowest age limits established[j]	Significant negative correlation with SHUEE (r = −0.76)[k]	NA	NA
Pediatric Motor Activity Log–Revised[l]	Rasch analysis: Strong construct validity—How Often scale and How Well scale[l] Item analysis: Item correlation (r = .39–.78)[m]	NA	Fair concurrent validity with PMAL–QOM (WeeFIM, PDMS–G, PDMS–V)[n] Moderate convergent validity with PAFT limb preference scale (partial r = .36)[m]	Large differences on both scales between item difficulty and child ability estimates; insufficient items to discriminate between very low or very high functioning children[o] MDC = 0.67 for PMAL–AOU and 0.66 for PMAL–QOL[n] MCID change of 0.39–0.94 PMAL–AOU and 0.38–0.74 PMAL–QOL[n] SEM 3, MDC 8, SRM 4.4[m]
Assisting Hand Assessment (AHA)[p]	Developed by experts in the field[p] Rasch model (unidimensionality demonstrated for 91% of responses in a 22-item version)[q]	Discriminates between children with different levels of hand function (separation value = 6.16) and levels of impairment not related to age[p,q]	NA	Person-separation reliability estimate R = .97 Ability to separate and distribute person ability measures, which indicates sensitivity to change (18 months–12 years, n = 303, 409 assessments)[q] SDD was less than 4 raw score (n = 55, 18 months–12 years)[r]
ABILHAND–Kids[s]	Based on existing scales and expert advice[s] Rasch model	Significant relationship with type of school education, CP, and the GMFCS[s] Invariance verified across demographic and clinical subgroups of children with CP[t]	NA	Person separation reliability estimate R = .94 (n = 36)[s]

(Continued)

Table 6.2   Content, Construct, Concurrent, and Evaluative Validity of Upper-Limb Activity Measures *(Cont.)*

ASSESSMENT	CONTENT VALIDITY	CONSTRUCT VALIDITY	CRITERION VALIDITY	EVALUATIVE VALIDITY
Children's Hand-Use Experience Questionnaire[u]	Review of literature, previous assessments, interviews with children and adolescents and their parents, clinical experience Pilot testing with 18 families[u]	NA	NA	Person separation reliability estimate ranged from .90 to .94 for scales[u]
Box and Block Test	Developed with typical adults[v] and children[w]	Significant correlations with the AHA (Spearman's ρ = .88; $p < .01$) in children with unilateral CP[x]	NA	NA

Note. CP = cerebral palsy; GMFCS = Gross Motor Function Classification System; MCID = minimal clinically important difference; MDC = minimal detectible change; NA = no data available; PAFT = Pediatric Arm Function Test; PDMS–FM = Peabody Developmental Motor Scale–Fine Motor Scale; PDMS–G = Peabody Developmental Motor Scale–Grasping subtest; PDMS–V = Peabody Developmental Motor Scale–Visual–Motor Integration subtest; PEDI = Pediatric Evaluation of Disability Inventory; PMAL–AOU = Pediatric Motor Activity Log–Amount of Use; PMAL–QOL = Pediatric Motor Activity Log–Quality of Life; PMAL–QOM = Pediatric Motor Activity Log–Quality of Movement; SHUEE = Shriners Hospitals Upper Extremity Evaluation Tool; SDD = smallest detectable difference; SEM = standard error of measurement; SRM = standardized response mean; WeeFIM = Functional Independence Measure for children. [a]Randall, Johnson, & Reddihough, 1999. [b]Bourke-Taylor, 2003. [c]Johnson et al., 1994. [d]Klingels et al., 2008. [e]Sakzewski et al., 2011a. [f]DeMatteo et al., 1992. [g]Thorley, Lannin, Cusick, Novak, & Boyd, 2012a. [h]Law et al., 1991. [i]Taylor, Sand, & Jebsen, 1973. [j]Jebsen, Taylor, Trieschmann, Trotter, & Howard, 1969. [k]Davids et al., 2006. [l]Wallen, Bundy, Pont, & Ziviani, 2009a. [m]Uswatte et al., 2012. [n]Lin et al., 2012. [o]Wallen, Bundy, Pont, & Ziviani, 2009b. [p]Krumlinde-Sundholm & Eliasson, 2003. [q]Krumlinde-Sundholm, Holmefur, Kottorp, & Eliasson, 2007. [r]Holmefur, Aarts, Hoare, & Krumlinde-Sundholm, 2009. [s]Arnould, Penta, Renders, & Thonnard, 2004. [t]Arnould, 2006. [u]Sköld, Hermansson, Krumlinde-Sundholm, & Eliasson, 2011. [v]Mathiowetz, Volland, Kashman, & Weber, 1985. [w]Mathiowetz, Federman, & Wiemer, 1985. [x]Holmström et al., 2010.

Most of the assessments have adequate content and construct validity. Details on the reliability of assessments are reported in Table 6.3. Internal consistency was reported for the ABILHAND–Kids, the AHA, and the Melbourne Assessment. Strong inter- and intrarater reliability was reported for the AHA and Melbourne Assessment. Reported evidence for the test–retest reliability of the ABILHAND–Kids, however, provided only Pearson product–moment correlations (*r*); the ICC reflects both correlation and agreement and has therefore become the preferred statistic (Portney & Watkins, 2000). Excellent test–retest reliability has been reported for the Melbourne Assessment and AHA.

Evidence of the clinical utility of activity limitation assessments is summarized in Table 6.4. Administration time varies widely across the assessments, from 5 to 45 minutes. Assessor training is required for the AHA; for the other assessments, either training is not required or the need for training is not specified. The AHA method of administration includes practitioner observation of a child's performance in an upper-limb activity, whereas the Melbourne Assessment and JTHFT involve a practitioner systematically administering items. The ABILHAND–Kids is a parent-completed questionnaire. The Melbourne Assessment and AHA use videotaped assessments that are scored later by trained individuals.

MEASURING UNIMANUAL CAPACITY

MELBOURNE ASSESSMENT OF UNILATERAL UPPER LIMB FUNCTION

The **Melbourne Assessment of Unilateral Upper Limb Function** is a standardized measure of quality of movement of the impaired upper limb encompassing both impairment (body structure and function) and activity limitations (Hoare, 2010; Randall et al., 1999). It was specifically designed for children with CP aged 5 to 15 years. The test consists of 16 items examining aspects of reach, grasp, release, and manipulation and is videotaped for later scoring. Each item is scored according to specific criteria to rate quality of range of motion, accuracy, fluency, and dexterity, yielding a maximum possible raw score of 122. Raw scores can be converted to a percentage score.

Benefits

During test development, construct and content validity were established (Randall et al., 1999). Inter- and intrarater reliability was very high for total scores (ICC = .95 and .97, respectively) and moderate to high for individual items (ICC = .69–.91). The original version of the Melbourne Assessment has been extended to younger children, aged 2 to 4 years, with minor modification to scoring of two items (Randall, Pallant, Imms,

Table 6.3 Reliability of Upper-Limb Assessment Tools

ASSESSMENT	INTERNAL CONSISTENCY (CRONBACH'S α)	INTERRATER RELIABILITY (ICC)	INTRARATER RELIABILITY (ICC)	TEST–RETEST RELIABILITY
Melbourne Assessment of Unilateral Upper Limb Function[a]	.96 (n = 20, 5–16 years, variety of types of CP)[b] Trained and untrained raters = .99[c]	.95 (15 raters, total test scores, n = 20)[b] LOA = 14%[b] LOA with training = 5%[d] Original 12-item test: Kappa = .65 (1st scoring, 2 raters) and .72 (2nd scoring; n = 20, variety of types of CP)[e] .99 (12 trained raters) .98 (12 untrained raters) 5 years, 5 months–12 years[c] .87 (1st session, 5 raters, n = 10) .88 (2nd session, 5 raters, n = 10)[f] .96 total score (3 OTs, 34 videotapes; 6 years–14 years, 5 months)[g] .90 fluency items; .87 range items; .77 target accuracy; .68 quality of movement Individual items .37–.96[g]	.97 (20 raters, n = 20, total test scores, variety of types of CP)[b] LOA = 12%[b] LOA with training = 3.5%[d] Original 12-item test: Kappa = .82 for 1st therapist and .79 for 2nd therapist (n = 20, variety of types of CP)[e] .97–.99 (5 raters, 10 children aged 10–17 years)[f] .97 (2 raters, 21 children aged 5–8 years)[h]	CCC = .98 for 1st rater and .97 for 2nd rater[a]
Quality of Upper Extremity Skills Test[i]	.97 (n = 31 assessments, 2–12 years, variety of types of CP)[j]	.95 (two raters, total test scores, n = 16)[j] .96 (two raters, total test scores, n = 71)[j] .72–.90 (Spearman's ρ, used Wilcoxon signed rank test to confirm no systematic difference, 3 raters, total test scores, n = 21, 29% hemiplegia)[k] .96 (2 raters, total test scores, n = 21, 100% hemiplegia)[h] .91 (2 raters, total test scores, n = 26, 5 with hemiplegia)[j] .86 total score (2 raters, total test score)[j]	.69 Assessor 1 and .89 Assessor 2 (n = 26, 2–13 years) .95 Assessor 1 and .63 Assessor 2 (Spearman's ρ, n = 21, 2–4 years, 6 months) .96 (1 rater, total scores)[j]	.95 (ICC for total test score)[j] .85–.94 (Spearman's ρ)[k]
Jebsen–Taylor Hand Function Test[m]	NA	r = .99 (hemiplegia, n not known)[n]	r = .99 (hemiplegia, n not known)[n]	r = .97 dominant hand, r = .98 nondominant hand (children with stable hand disabilities)[m]
Pediatric Motor Activity Log–Revised[o]	.93 (n = 60, 2–8 years, CP)[p]	NA	NA	ICC = .94 How Often scale ICC = .93 How Well scale[q] ICC = .89[p]
Assisting Hand Assessment (AHA)[r]	.97 (person separation reliability estimate: 409 assessments, 18 months–12 years, 8 months, hemiplegic CP and OBPP)[s]	.98 (2 raters; 18 months–5 years, 11 months; 16 children with congenital hemiplegia and 2 with OBPP)[t] .97 (20 raters; 19 months–4 years, 2 months; 6 children with hemiplegia and 2 with OBPP)[t]	.99 (20 raters)[t]	Small Kids AHA ICC = .99 School Kids AHA ICC = .98 Alternate forms ICC = .99 between Small Kids and School Kids versions and .98 between board games[u]
ABILHAND–Kids[v]	.94 (person separation reliability estimate; n = 113, 6–15 years, variety of types of CP)[v]	NA	NA	r = .91 (n = 36)[v]

(Continued)

Table 6.3 Reliability of Upper-Limb Assessment Tools *(Cont.)*

ASSESSMENT	INTERNAL CONSISTENCY (CRONBACH'S α)	INTERRATER RELIABILITY (ICC)	INTRARATER RELIABILITY (ICC)	TEST–RETEST RELIABILITY
Children's Hand-Use Experience Questionnaire[w]	NA	NA	NA	NA
Box and Block Test	NA	Right hand r = 1.000, left hand r = .999[x]	NA	Rho coefficients of .976 and .937 for right and left hand[x]

Note. CCC = concordance correlation coefficient; CP = cerebral palsy; ICC = intraclass correlation coefficient; LOA = limits of agreement; NA = not available; OBPP = obstetric brachial plexus palsy; OT = occupational therapist; r = Pearson product–moment correlation.
[a]Randall, Johnson, & Reddihough, 1999. [b]Randall, Carlin, Chondros, & Reddihough, 2001. [c]Cusick, Vasquez, Knowles, & Wallen, 2005. [d]Corn et al., 2003. [e]Johnson et al., 1994. [f]Mackey et al., 2006. [g]Spirtos, O'Mahony, & Malone, 2011. [h]Klingels et al., 2008. [i]DeMatteo et al., 1992. [j]Thorley, Lannin, Cusick, Novak, & Boyd, 2012b. [k]Haga et al., 2007. [l]Sorsdahl, Moe-Nilssen, & Strand, 2008. [m]Taylor, Sand, & Jebsen, 1973. [n]Gordon, Charles, & Wolf, 2006. [o]Wallen, Bundy, Pont, & Ziviani, 2009b. [p]Uswatte et al., 2012. [q]Wallen, Bundy, Pont, & Ziviani, 2009b. [r]Krumlinde-Sundholm & Eliasson, 2003. [s]Krumlinde-Sundholm, Holmefur, Kottorp, & Eliasson, 2007. [t]Holmefur, Krumlinde-Sundholm, & Eliasson, 2007. [u]Holmefur, Aarts, Hoare, & Krumlinde-Sundholm, 2009. [v]Arnould, Penta, Renders, & Thonnard, 2004. [w]Sköld, Hermansson, Krumlinde-Sundholm, & Eliasson, 2011. [x]Mathiowetz, Volland, Kashman, & Weber, 1985.

& Carey, 2010). The assessment is quick to administer (10 to 30 minutes) and score (20 to 30 minutes). Assessor training is recommended but not required.

Limitations

Studies investigating reliability have suggested that the smallest detectable difference ranges from 7.4% (Sakzewski et al., 2011a) to 8.7% (Klingels et al., 2008). Several upper-limb rehabilitation studies for children with CP have called into question the sensitivity of the Melbourne Assessment to detect changes (Aarts et al., 2010; Sakzewski et al., 2011b; Wallen et al., 2007) because the small reported changes have not exceeded measurement error. This finding may reflect the fact that items on the Melbourne Assessment predominantly measure aspects of body function and structure (Hoare, Imms, Randall, & Carey, 2011), whereas the interventions being investigated (e.g., P–CIMT) were focused more on activity-based functions. The Melbourne Assessment recently underwent a Rasch analysis that found that items did not encompass a unidimensional scale but rather formed four distinct subscales (Randall, Pallant, et al., 2010). At this stage, however, it is unclear whether any of the subscales is better able to detect changes following intensive upper-limb training, including CIMT. The revised Melbourne Assessment 2 (Randall, Johnson, & Reddihough, 2010) is available but is costly.

QUALITY OF UPPER EXTREMITY SKILLS TEST

The **Quality of Upper Extremity Skills Test** is a criterion-referenced observational assessment comprising 34 items in four domains (dissociated movement, grasp, weight bearing, protective extension). Scores from each domain are summed and converted to a percentage score. According to the test manual, both the impaired and unimpaired upper limbs are assessed and included in the scoring.

Benefits

The QUEST has established content (DeMatteo et al., 1992) and construct validity (DeMatteo et al., 1992; Klingels et al., 2008). Evidence has been found of high interrater reliability for total scores and intrarater and test–retest reliability for children with CP aged 2 to 13 years (DeMatteo et al., 1992; Haga et al., 2007; Klingels et al., 2008; Thorley, Lannin, Cusick, Novak, & Boyd, 2012b).

Limitations

Items on the QUEST predominantly measure aspects of body structure and function (Gilmore et al., 2010; Hoare et al., 2011) and therefore may not adequately capture change following activity-based interventions such as CIMT. A recent Rasch analysis to investigate the construct validity of the QUEST indicated that total scores lacked unidimensionality but that domain scores had better construct validity, suggesting that total scores should not be reported. Posture items in the grasp domain were problematic, and it was recommended they be removed from the assessment (Thorley, Lannin, Cusick, Novak, & Boyd, 2012a).

Table 6.4 Clinical Utility of Upper-Limb Activity Measures

ASSESSMENT	FORMAT OF ADMINISTRATION	ADMINISTRATION TIME	ASSESSOR TRAINING	MANUAL AND EQUIPMENT	SCALES AND ITEMS	SCORING
Melbourne Assessment of Unilateral Upper Limb Function[a]	Practitioner administers items in a standardized procedure	10–30 minutes	Recommended but NR	Manual and kit must be purchased	16 upper-limb activity items rated on quality and task achievement	Raw scores converted to percentages
Quality of Upper Extremity Skills Test[b]	Practitioner administers items	30–45 minutes	NR, but recommended by others[c,d]	Free online	34 items, 4 domains: dissociated movements, grasp, protective extension, weight bearing; 3 subjective scales not scored	Raw scores converted to percentages
Jebsen–Taylor Hand Function Test[e]	Practitioner administers items and times	10–15 minutes	NR	Must be purchased	6 timed items (modified)	Each item is timed, maximum time allowable/item = 120 minutes; 6 items summed for total score
Pediatric Motor Activity Log–revised[f]	Caregiver-completed questionnaire	NS	NR	Must be purchased	2 scales: How Well, How Much	Revised scoring for both scales collapsed to 3 levels (0–2); Original scoring 6-step scale[g]
Assisting Hand Assessment[h]	Practitioner-led play session; Video recorded, scored later	10–15 minutes	Required	Manual received during training, kit must be purchased	22 items assess assisting hand general use, arm use, grasp–release, fine adjustment, coordination, and pace	Raw scores converted to percentage score; Calibrated in logits
ABILHAND-Kids[i]	Parent-completed questionnaire	NS	NR	Free online; No equipment	21 activity questions rated as impossible, difficult, or easy	Online analysis available; Calibrated in logits
Children's Hand-Use Experience Questionnaire[j]	Online parent- or child- (>13 years) completed questionnaire	NS	NR	Free online; No equipment	29 bimanual activities rated on 3 scales: perceived efficacy of grasp, time to perform, degree of feeling bothered	Online summary report generated; Conversion to logits by test developers (minimum of 20 assessments, cost unknown)
Box and Block Test	Practitioner administers items	3–5 minutes	NR	Published[k]	1 item, 1 scale	Number of blocks transferred in 1 min for total score

Note. NR = not required; NS = not specified.
[a]Randall, Johnson, & Reddihough, 1999. [b]DeMatteo et al., 1992. [c]Sorsdahl, Moe-Nilssen, & Strand, 2008. [d]Davies & Gavin, 1999. [e]Taylor, Sand, & Jebsen, 1973. [f]Wallen, Bundy, Pont, & Ziviani, 2009b. [g]Uswatte et al., 2012. [h]Krumlinde-Sundholm & Eliasson, 2003. [i]Arnould, Penta, Renders, & Thonnard, 2004. [j]Sköld, Hermansson, Krumlinde-Sundholm, & Eliasson, 2011. [k]Mathiowetz, Volland, Kashman, & Weber, 1985.

JEBSEN–TAYLOR HAND FUNCTION TEST

The **Jebsen–Taylor Hand Function Test** is used to evaluate speed and dexterity of the impaired upper limb on timed tasks (Taylor et al., 1973). The tasks are of varying complexity and use everyday items to assess grasp and release abilities. The original test was designed and validated in adults and typically developing children. Modification of the original test has been performed in several P–CIMT studies (Charles, Wolf, Schneider, & Gordon, 2006; Gordon et al., 2011; Sakzewski et al., 2011a). The writing task was omitted, and the maximum allowable time for each of the 6 remaining items was reduced to 2 minutes to both reduce frustration and allow comparison across studies.

Benefits

The JTHFT has been shown to be responsive to change after an intervention (Charles et al., 2006; Eliasson, Krumlinde-Sundholm, Shaw, & Wang, 2005; Eliasson, Shaw, Pontén, Boyd, & Krumlinde-Sundholm, 2009; Gordon, Schneider, Chinnan, & Charles, 2007). Test–retest reliability (Pearson $r = .87–.99$) was found to be excellent for children with stable hand conditions (including CP) across the 7 subtests for both the dominant and nondominant hands in a small sample (Taylor et al., 1973). The assessment is quick to administer and has the added advantage of measuring the capacity of the impaired and unimpaired limbs separately, essential for measuring improvements in the impaired limb and monitoring any impact of wearing a constraint on the unimpaired upper limb.

Limitations

Some evidence suggests difficulties with the stability of test–retest performance in the impaired limb (Eliasson et al., 2005). At present, the evidence for validity and reliability of the JTHFT is limited for children with congenital hemiplegia.

BOX AND BLOCK TEST

The **Box and Block Test** is used as a measure of speed and gross manual dexterity across various populations, including adults without disabilities (Mathiowetz, Volland, Kashman, & Weber, 1985), elderly persons (Desrosiers, Bravo, Hébert, Dutil, & Mercier, 1994), and typically developing children (Mathiowetz, Federman, & Wiemer, 1985). The test involves grasping and releasing as many blocks as possible, one at a time, from one compartment over a divider to another in 1 minute. The score for each hand is the number of blocks transferred, an objective measure enabling comparison of speed and dexterity between limbs and over time.

Benefits

The test is simple, quick, and easy to administer. Reliability, validity, and normative values have been established for children, adults, and elderly persons (Desrosiers et al., 1994; Mathiowetz, Federman, et al., 1985; Mathiowetz, Volland, et al., 1985). High interrater reliability was found for the right and left hand in 27 adults with two raters ($r = 1.000$ and .999, respectively). Test–retest reliability at 6-months intervals has been reported at .937 and .976 (left and right hand, respectively; Mathiowetz, Volland, et al., 1985). In children with CP, a high correlation was found between performance on the AHA and on the Box and Block Test (Spearman's $\rho = .88$; $p < .01$; Holmström et al., 2010).

Limitations

The Box and Block Test is purely a capacity measure of speed and dexterity and does not account for the effectiveness associated with different pinches and grips available to the hand (including hook, power grip, lateral pinch, and tip pinch). Thus, the ability of this test to determine changes in the quality of functional improvements is limited.

MEASURING UNIMANUAL PERFORMANCE

PEDIATRIC MOTOR ACTIVITY LOG

The **Pediatric Motor Activity Log (PMAL)** is a caregiver report questionnaire measuring real-world use of the impaired upper limb in common daily activities, capturing both perceived amount of use and quality of use. The PMAL was based on a validated adult assessment, the Motor Activity Scale, developed for adults after stroke (Taub et al., 1993). The PMAL was first reported by Taub, Ramey, DeLuca, and Echols (2004) to specifically measure change in real-world use of the impaired upper limb following CIMT in children aged 7 months to 8 years. At that time, no reliability or validity data were reported for the pediatric version.

Subsequently, three independent groups have looked at psychometric properties of the PMAL. Uswatte and colleagues (2012) examined the PMAL–Revised for ages 2 to 8 years and reported high internal consistency (Cronbach's $\alpha = .93$) and test–retest reliability ($r = .89$). The standard error of measurement was 0.15, and minimal detectable difference was 0.42 (Uswatte et al., 2012). They also reported moderate convergent validity based on ratings of videotaped play behavior (by masked or blinded observers) and parent PMAL ratings (Uswatte et al., 2012).

The PMAL underwent Rasch analysis and was found to have a disordered rating scale (Wallen, Bundy, Pont, & Ziviani,

2009a). A collapsed rating scale yielded strong evidence for both construct validity and reliability (one item—throw a ball or similar object—was deleted; Wallen et al., 2009a).

Finally, Lin and colleagues (2012) compared PMAL scores to scores on the Functional Independence Measure (WeeFIM; Ottenbacher et al., 2000) in children and the Peabody Developmental Motor Scales (Folio & Fewell, 2000). This team proposed that studies identify a "minimally clinically important change" on the PMAL. Using anchor-based and distributional-based approaches, they proposed that at least 0.67 points on the PMAL Amount of Use subscale and 0.66 points on the PMAL Quality of Movement subscale be considered a true change (i.e., above measurement error). They further concluded that both the Quality of Movement and Amount of Use subscales were responsive to treatment changes (Lin et al., 2012).

Benefits

As explained in the preceding section, strong evidence of validity and reliability has been reported from diverse sources and analyses. The assessment targets real-world use of the impaired upper limb, which reflects one of the primary benefits of CIMT, namely increased spontaneous use of the impaired upper limb. The original PMAL has been used in several studies of CIMT, suggesting sensitivity to change (Lin et al., 2011; Taub et al., 2011).

Limitations

Results of Rasch analysis have suggested that the PMAL may not be sensitive enough for children at the extremes of ability (i.e., very mild or very severe) because items that can discriminate among children at the extremes may be insufficient (Wallen et al., 2009a). Further, a PMAL tool is needed that has items better suited for older children with CP, which would necessitate further psychometric evaluation.

MEASURING BIMANUAL PERFORMANCE

ASSISTING HAND ASSESSMENT

The **Assisting Hand Assessment** is a Rasch-analyzed measure of the effectiveness with which a child with a unilateral impairment makes use of his or her impaired hand in bimanual tasks (Krumlinde-Sundholm & Eliasson, 2003). The AHA is a performance measure that assesses how children aged 18 months to 12 years typically or spontaneously use their impaired upper limb as an assisting hand in bimanual tasks. It consists of 22 items assessing general use, arm use, grasp–release, fine motor adjustment, coordination, and pace of the impaired upper limb. The test session is videotaped for later scoring.

Each item is scored on a 4-point scale, and possible raw scores range from 22 to 88. Raw scores can be transformed into scaled scores ranging from 25 to 100. The ordinal scores also can be transformed into equal interval logits as a result of the Rasch analysis. Interrater and intrarater reliability are excellent for summed scores (ICC = .98 and .99, respectively).

Two versions of the AHA are available, the Small Kids AHA for children aged 18 months to 5 years and the School Kids AHA for children aged 6 to 12 years. The Mini-AHA for children aged 6 to 18 months and the Ad-AHA for adolescents with hemiplegia and adults after a stroke are currently under development.

Benefits

Test–retest reliability is high for both the Small Kids and School Kids versions (ICC = .99 and .98, respectively), and there is high reliability between the two versions (ICC = .99). The AHA has been shown to be responsive to change in clinical trials (Aarts et al., 2010; Case-Smith, DeLuca, Stevenson, & Ramey, 2012; Eliasson et al., 2005; Gordon et al., 2011; Hoare, 2010; Sakzewski et al., 2011a). The smallest detectable difference is 3.89 for the Small Kids AHA and 3.65 for the School Kids AHA (raw scores).

Limitations

AHA raters must receive standardized training and formal certification by the test developers or a trained educator. Although this required certification can be seen as a benefit in ensuring a standardized administration and scoring of the assessment, it also can be seen as a limitation because of the cost (course fee, travel and lodging expenses), accessibility of training (offered once or twice a year), and time required for certification. Administration time is 10 to 15 minutes; however, scoring can take substantially longer (up to 60 minutes). Although the AHA has excellent interrater reliability, our experience in a large randomized controlled trial suggests that it is beneficial for one rater to complete both the pre- and posttest assessments for individual participants (Sakzewski et al., 2011b).

ABILHAND–KIDS

The **ABILHAND–Kids** is a parent- or caregiver-completed questionnaire that assesses manual abilities of children with impaired upper-limb function aged 6 to 15 years (Arnould et al., 2004). The scale consists of 21 items covering both unimanual and bimanual self-care activities. There are no age, gender, or handedness biases. Each item is rated as 0 = *impossible*, 1 = *difficult*, or 2 = *easy*, yielding a raw score range of 0 to 42.

Benefits

Good evidence has been found of content validity based on existing scales, expert advice, and Rasch measurement model. Evidence of construct validity has been established. Internal consistency (.94 person separation reliability estimate) and test–retest reliability ($r = .91$) are high. A manual is available, and analysis and conversion of scores to logits can be obtained online (www.rehab-scales.org/abilhand-kids.html). The ABILHAND–Kids was shown to be responsive to change in a randomized trial of P–CIMT (Aarts et al., 2010). It is a short questionnaire and provides information relevant to goal setting for occupational therapy.

Limitations

The sensitivity of the ABILHAND–Kids to change is as yet unclear because it has not been used frequently as an outcome measure in upper-limb intervention studies (Aarts et al., 2010).

CHILDREN'S HAND-USE EXPERIENCE QUESTIONNAIRE

The **Children's Hand-Use Experience Questionnaire** is a Rasch-analyzed questionnaire used to investigate the experiences of children and youths aged 6 to 18 years with unilateral hand dysfunction in using their impaired hand in bimanual activities (Sköld et al., 2011). The questionnaire assesses level of independence and whether one or two hands are used in completing 29 bimanual activities. In addition, respondents rate perceived efficacy of grasp, time taken to complete the activity, and degree of "being bothered" doing the activity for each of the bimanual activities. The CHEQ can be completed free online (www. cheq.se/questionnaire). The test developers recommend that caregivers assist children under age 13 years in completing the questionnaire. A summary report can be generated, but for research purposes, the test developers transform data into logit scores.

Benefits

Rasch analysis during test development on 86 children with unilateral impairment confirmed the internal scale validity and appropriateness of the rating scale (Sköld et al., 2011).

Limitations

No evidence is available regarding reliability. The CHEQ has not been used in clinical trials, and it remains unclear whether the CHEQ is sensitive to change.

PEDIATRIC EVALUATION OF DISABILITY INVENTORY

The **Pediatric Evaluation of Disability Inventory (PEDI)** was designed as a judgment-based assessment of key functional capabilities in children aged 6 months to 7.5 years with physical or combined physical and cognitive disabilities (Haley, Coster, Ludlow, Haltiwanger, & Andrellos, 1992). It also can be used to evaluate older children whose functional abilities are below those of a typically developing 7.5-year-old. Capability in and performance of functional activities are measured in 3 domains: (1) self-care, (2) mobility, and (3) social function. Capability is measured by the identification of skills in which the child has achieved mastery and is scored as 0 = *unable* or 1 = *capable*. Performance is measured by the level of caregiver assistance (0 = *total assistance* to 5 = *independent*) and modification required to accomplish functional activities (0 = *none* to 4 = *extensive modifications*). The PEDI evaluates 197 functional skill items and 20 caregiver assistance or modification items developed from existing assessments and reviewed by an expert panel.

Benefits

The PEDI has established strong content and construct validity (Haley et al., 1992). Concurrent validity is reported between the PEDI and the WeeFIM ($r = .80–.97$; Haley et al., 1992). Interinterviewer reliability is very high on the Caregiver Assistance scales (ICC = .96–.99) and adequate to high on the Modifications scales (ICC = .79–1.00; Haley et al., 1992; Ziviani et al., 2001). The PEDI is sensitive to change because of the wide range of items in each domain and has been identified as appropriate for use with children with CP (Debuse & Brace, 2011). PEDI Functional Skills and Caregiver Assistance scores in the self-care domain demonstrated a significant effect of CIMT compared with a control group ($d = 1.61$ and 1.37, respectively; de Brito Brandão, Mancini, Vaz, Pereira de Melo, & Fonseca, 2010).

Computer-adapted tests (PEDI–CAT) are being developed that meet precision requirements for research and clinical practice. The PEDI and PEDI–CAT have been found to effectively discriminate between children with and without disabilities. High test–retest reliability has been reported for the online PEDI–CAT in all 4 domains (ICC .96–.99; Dumas et al., 2012; Haley et al., 2011).

Limitations

Potential limitations of the PEDI are the restricted age range and the considerable time required to administer the assessment. Although practitioners can complete the PEDI independently, it is ideally administered through a structured parent interview that takes 30 minutes to 1 hour. The PEDI–CAT reduces the level of practitioner involvement and time required, taking only approximately 12 minutes to complete, and will be available for a wider age range.

ASSESSMENT OF EXECUTIVE FUNCTION

Planning of execution of tasks in everyday life can be considered in terms of the *ICF* domains of activity limitations and participation restrictions (WHO, 2001). Two measures, the Brief Rating Inventory of Executive Function (BRIEF; Chevignard et al., 2009) and the Assessment of Motor Processing Skills (AMPS; Fisher & Bray Jones, 2010), are useful for measuring motor planning capacity and performance in clinical trials of upper-limb training.

BRIEF RATING INVENTORY OF EXECUTIVE FUNCTION

The **Brief Rating Inventory of Executive Function** measures executive function in everyday life. Two index scores are obtained from the BRIEF: The Behavioral Regulation Index (BRI) is derived from the Inhibit, Shift, and Emotional Control subscales, and the Metacognition Index (MCI) is derived from the Initiate, Working Memory, Plan, Organization of Materials, and Monitor subscales. These 2 indexes combine to form an overall global executive composite score (GEC) and are useful in studies that relate cognitive measures of executive function to behavioral manifestation of executive function in everyday life.

Benefits

The BRIEF has been found to be an ecologically valid measure of executive functioning (Chevignard et al., 2009). It has been shown to have good internal consistency (Cronbach's α = .80–.98; Gioia, Isquith, Guy, & Kenworthy, 2000a, 2000b), and high test–retest reliability has been found for the parent form on the BRI (r = .92), MCI (r = .88), and GEC (r = .86; Gioia et al., 2000b). An overall measure of executive function like the BRIEF could be useful to classify global executive function across a sample.

Limitations

The BRIEF may be predictive of outcome in response to rehabilitation, but to date this possibility has not been tested. Comprehensive evaluation of executive function would require assessment of some domains the BRIEF does not cover (Anderson, 2002).

ASSESSMENT OF MOTOR AND PROCESS SKILLS

The **Assessment of Motor and Process Skills** is a standardized, observational assessment designed to be used by occupational and physical therapy practitioners to evaluate the quality of a

person's performance of activities of daily living (ADLs; Fisher & Bray Jones, 2010). It is appropriate for use with children aged 2 years or older with any functional limitation. Respondents select a minimum of 2 ADLs from 116 task options (e.g., putting on shoes, eating a meal, brushing teeth). Practitioners score the quality of performance in 16 ADL motor skills and 20 ADL processing skills on a 4-point, criterion-referenced rating scale: 1 = *unacceptable*, 2 = *ineffective*, 3 = *questionable*, and 4 = *competent*. Raw scores are entered into AMPS computer-scoring software and converted through many-faceted Rasch (MFR) analyses into linear ADL motor and ADL process ability measures expressed in logits, which adjust for differences in rater severity, task challenge, and skill item difficulty. Each ADL task performance takes approximately 10 to 15 minutes.

Benefits

The AMPS has been standardized on more than 148,000 respondents and 13,070 raters internationally (Fisher & Bray Jones, 2010). It has extensive evidence of validity across age groups and diagnoses and is free from bias related to cultural differences (Fisher & Bray Jones, 2010). Children and adolescents have demonstrated 95% goodness-of-fit on the AMPS process scale and 90% on the AMPS motor scale (Poulson, 1996). Acceptable goodness-of-fit has been shown in people with CP (Kottorp, Bernspång, & Fisher, 2003). Concurrent validity tests found that the ADL motor and process measures represent unique constructs that are not assessed by other ADL instruments and that cannot be equated to body functions (e.g., strength, memory). The AMPS has high test–retest reliability for the motor and process skill scales (r = .90 and .87, respectively) and high interrater and intrarater reliability, with 95% of raters in the standardization sample demonstrating acceptable goodness-of-fit to the MFR model (Fisher & Bray Jones, 2010). The AMPS can detect very small changes in quality of ADL task performance because it evaluates the smallest possible units of task performance, and responsiveness to change has been reported in clinical studies involving children with CP (Kang et al., 2008; Russo, Atkins, Haan, & Crotty, 2009; Van Zelst, Miller, Russo, Murchland, & Crotty, 2006). Changes of at least 0.5 logits on the AMPS motor scale and 0.4 logits on the process scale are considered statistically significant. Occupational therapy practitioners have reported high clinical utility of the AMPS in pediatric settings (Payne & Howell, 2005).

Limitations

Occupational and physical therapy practitioners must attend a 5-day training course and complete a further 10 assessments to become a certified AMPS rater. The AMPS can be administered in a clinic or home environment, although ideally the practitioner should evaluate the client's performance in the environment in which the client will be functioning (Park, Fisher, & Velozo, 1994), requiring additional time for a home visit in many circumstances. Although the AMPS was designed for use with children, adolescents, and adults, it was standardized primarily on adults. Caution should be used in interpreting AMPS motor scale scores in children younger than age 8 years because 10% of children score outside the range for their age (10% misfit on Rasch-analyzed scale). The scale can still administered to this age group, but in addition to caution in interpretation this use requires further validation.

ASSESSMENT OF MASTERY AND MOTIVATION

Motivation is considered a personal factor within the *ICF* model and is defined as "mental functions that produce the incentive to act; the conscious or unconscious driving force for action" (WHO, 2007, p. 51). School-age children with CP report lower levels of motivation, including cognitive-oriented persistence, gross motor persistence, social persistence with adults and peers, and mastery pleasure compared with their typically developing peers (Majnemer, Shevell, Law, Poulin, & Rosenbaum, 2010).

DIMENSIONS OF MASTERY QUESTIONNAIRE AND PEDIATRIC VOLITIONAL QUESTIONNAIRE

The **Dimensions of Mastery Questionnaire (DMQ)** is an assessment of adults' and children's perceptions of children's mastery-related behaviors and motivation (Morgan, Busch-Rossnagel, Barrett, & Wang, 2009). The DMQ has Infant and Toddler/Preschool versions for parents and teachers to complete and School Aged and Teen versions that are self-completed. It contains 45 items rated on a 5-point Likert scale grouped in five scales: (1) persistence at object/cognitive tasks, (2) gross motor persistence, (3) social mastery with adults, (4) social mastery with peers/children, and (5) expressive aspects—mastery pleasure and negative reactions to failures.

The **Pediatric Volitional Questionnaire (PVQ)** is an observational assessment questionnaire completed by practitioners (Basu, Kafkes, Schatz, Kiraly, & Kielhofner, 2008). The practitioner observes the child in different settings and in activities that enable social interaction and then rates the child on a 14-item scale across three areas of volitional development: (1) exploration (tries new things, tries to produce effect, shows preference, initiates actions, shows curiosity), (2) competency (pursues activity to completion, tries to solve problems, practices skill, expresses mastery pleasure, is task directed, stays engaged), and (3) achievement (uses imagination, organizes/modifies environment, seeks challenges).

Benefits

The DMQ and PVQ have some evidence of adequate content and construct validity (Basu et al., 2008; Morgan et al., 2009). The DMQ has preliminary evidence of test–retest reliability. Both measures have good clinical utility, with administration time of 10 to 30 minutes (Morgan et al., 2009).

Limitations

The DMQ can be self-completed; however, interviews are recommended for children under age 10 years. To date, no evidence is available of evaluative validity for either measure in children with CP or in terms of sensitivity to treatment effects.

PARTICIPATION OUTCOMES

Participation is defined by the WHO (2001) as "involvement in a life situation" (p. 14) and is multidimensional in nature, requiring broad consideration of the child, family, and environment. Practitioners choosing participation assessments to measure the impact of an activity-based intervention should consider using specific domains (e.g., personal care) rather than an entire measurement scale. In general, it seems unlikely that an intervention targeting training of upper-limb skills and functional independence (activity limitations) will have a broad-ranging impact on global participation scores because many other personal and environmental factors may influence the intensity and diversity of participation. Instead, practitioners should consider the specific domains of participation measures that require hand use and independence in daily life skills and reflect on the specific goals identified by children and their caregivers, because these factors are more likely to mirror the content of the intervention and may elucidate whether functional gains more broadly affect specific aspects of societal participation.

Table 6.5 briefly summarizes several measurement tools evaluating various aspects of participation. Clinical trials cannot possibly measure all potential areas of improvement; however, anecdotal reports suggest positive changes in areas not directly targeted as part of the intervention (e.g., social–emotional and language areas, increased self-confidence). The Assessment of Life Habits is discussed in more detail in the next section because some evidence suggests that specific domains such as personal self-care may be sensitive to change in response to modified CIMT (Sakzewski et al., 2011b).

ASSESSMENT OF LIFE HABITS

The **Assessment of Life Habits (LIFE–H)** is designed for children aged 5 to 13 years and measures life habits in the

Table 6.5 Examples of Participation Outcome Measures

OUTCOME	AGE	POPULATION	FORMAT	ITEMS AND DOMAINS
Activities Scale for Kids–Performance[a]	5–15 years	Musculoskeletal disorders	Self-report questionnaire	30 items, 7 domains: personal care, dressing, other skills, locomotion, play, standing skills, transfers
Assessment of Life Habits (LIFE–H)[b]	5–13 years	With disabilities	Self-report or interviewer questionnaire	197 items (long version), 64 items (short version); 12 domains: nutrition, personal care, fitness, mobility, communication, interpersonal, housing, responsibilities, recreation, education, employment, community
Assistance to Participate Scale[c]	5–18 years	With disabilities	Caregiver report questionnaire	Amount of assistance required to participate in 8 play and leisure activities
Children's Assessment of Participation and Enjoyment/Preferences for Activities of Children (CAPE/PAC)[d]	6–21 years	With or without disabilities	Self- or interviewer report Individual or group	2 domains (informal, formal); 5 dimensions assessed for each domain (diversity, intensity, with whom, where, enjoyment) 5 activity types (recreational, active physical, social, skill-based, self-improvement)
Children Helping Out: Responsibilities, Expectations and Supports (CHORES)[e]	6–11 years	With or without disabilities	Caregiver report questionnaire	33 items, 2 subscales (self-care, family) 2 items parent rated: importance, satisfaction
Children's Leisure Assessment Scale[f]	10–18 years	With or without disabilities	Self-report questionnaire	30 items, 4 domains (instrumental indoor, outdoor, self-enrichment, games and sports)
Children Participation Questionnaire[g]	4–6 years	With or without disabilities	Caregiver report questionnaire	44 items, 6 domains: ADLs, IADLs, play, leisure, social participation, education
Pediatric Activity Card Sort[h]	5–14 years	With or without disabilities	Child interview	75 items, 4 domains: personal care, school and productivity, hobbies and social activities, sports
Pediatric Interest Profile[i]	6–12 years	With or without disabilities	Self-report questionnaire	50-item kid version, 59-item preteen version; 8 domains: sports, outdoor, summer, winter, indoor, creative, lessons, socializing
Participation and Environment Measure for Children and Youth[j]	5–17 years	With or without disabilities	Caregiver report questionnaire (paper or online)	Participation evaluated in 3 areas: home (10 items), school (5 items), community (10 items) Frequency, level of involvement, desire to change evaluated Level of environmental support for community (16 items), school (17 items), and home (12 items)
Pediatric Community Participation Questionnaire[k]	8–20 years	Physical disabilities	Child or youth interview	19 items rated on a 6-point scale
Preschool Activity Card Sort[l]	3–6 years	With or without disabilities	Caregiver interview	85 items, 7 domains: self-care, community mobility, high-demand leisure, low-demand leisure, social interaction, domestic chores, education
School Function Assessment–Participation[m]	5–12 years	Physical or sensory impairment	Teacher interview	6 major school activity settings: classroom, playground and recess, transportation, bathroom and toileting, transitions, mealtime

Note. ADLs = activities of daily living; IADLs = instrumental activities of daily living.
[a]Bagley et al., 2011. [b]Noreau, Fougeyrollas, & Vincent, 2002. [c]Bourke-Taylor, Law, Howie, & Pallant, 2009. [d]King et al., 2004. [e]Dunn, 2004. [f]Rosenblum, Sachs, & Schreuer, 2010. [g]Rosenberg, Jarus, & Bart, 2010. [h]Mandich, Polatajko, Miller, & Baum, 2004. [i]Henry, 2000. [j]Coster et al., 2011. [k]Washington, Wilson, Engel, & Jensen, 2007. [l]Berg & LaVesser, 2006. [m]Coster, Deeney, Haltiwanger, & Haley, 1998.

home, school, and neighborhood environments (Fougeyrollas, Noreau, & Lepage, 2002; Noreau, Fougeyrollas, & Vincent, 2002). It is a questionnaire completed by the parent or caregiver about the child. The child form is based on an adult version (Noreau et al., 2002). The long form consists of 197 items divided into 12 categories and includes regular activities (e.g., eating meals, communication, mobility) and social roles. A weighted score ranging from 0 to 10 is generated for each category and for an overall total. A version of the LIFE–H is available for children aged 0 to 4 years (www.indcp.qc.ca/assessment-tools/introduction/life-h); however, no evidence of validity or reliability has been reported for this version.

Benefits

Evidence has been reported of construct validity (Fougeyrollas et al., 2002) and criterion validity for the version for children aged 5 to 13 years, as well as strong correlations between the LIFE–H and the PEDI and WeeFIM (Noreau et al., 2004). Adequate to excellent internal consistency (α = .73–.90 for categories, .97 for daily activities, and .90 for social roles), intrarater reliability (ICC = .83–.95 for daily activities), interrater reliability (ICC = .80–.91 for daily activities and .63–.90 for social roles), and test–retest reliability (ICC = .73 for total score) also have been established (Noreau et al., 2007). Some evidence exists that specific domains of the LIFE–H (e.g., personal care) may be sensitive to changes following mCIMT (Sakzewski et al., 2011b).

Limitations

The LIFE–H long form can be very time consuming to complete (192 questions); therefore, it is recommended that practitioners select specific domains related to the intervention that can be scored and reported by domain. Some evidence has been found of minor scoring difficulties, which may be remediated by using an interview method (Sakzewski et al., 2011b).

QUALITY OF LIFE

WHO (1997) defines **quality of life (QOL)** as "individuals' perception of their position in life in the context of the culture and value systems in which they live and in relation to their goals, expectations, standards and concerns" (p. 1). QOL also is defined as a person's feelings of well-being across many domains, including physical, social, emotional, and spiritual (Ziviani et al., 2010). Outcome measures that purport to evaluate QOL should take a broad approach to measuring well-being and not just measure outcomes on the functional domain (Carlon et al., 2010). It is therefore crucial that measures of QOL are consistent with the perspective of changes in well-being rather than merely assessing for an absence of ill-being (Waters et al., 2007).

QOL measures can be generic (i.e., measure the well-being of any child, developing typically or with a disability, e.g., the KIDSCREEN; KIDSCREEN Group Europe, 2006) or condition specific (i.e., focused specifically on a defined population and tailored to the issues that might affect the QOL of that population, e.g., Cerebral Palsy Quality of Life Questionnaire for Children [CPQOL–Child], Davis, Shelly, Waters, & Davern, 2010; Waters et al., 2007). Condition-specific measures of QOL have a role to play for children with CP because they include all domains that are highly salient to the clinical population, such as physical functioning and adaptive equipment as well as psychosocial domains (Ziviani et al., 2010).

When available, a condition-specific measure is preferable to a generic measure because it addresses aspects of life unique to a given population group. For children with unilateral CP undergoing a program of P–CIMT (original or mCIMT), it is therefore important to use condition-specific measures of QOL validated and reliable for the age range included. A comprehensive systematic review of the clinimetric properties of measures of QOL (Carlon et al., 2010) identified 2 condition-specific measures—the CPQOL–Child (Davis et al., 2010) and the Cerebral Palsy Quality of Life Questionnaire for Teens (CPQOL–Teen; Davis et al., 2012)—and 1 generic measure—the KIDSCREEN (KIDSCREEN Group Europe, 2006)—relevant to QOL in school-age children with unilateral CP. Although other condition-specific CP QOL measures are available, such as the Child Health Index of Life With Disabilities (Narayanan et al., 2006), the Pediatric Quality of Life Inventory CP Module (Varni et al., 2006), and the DISABKIDS CP Module (Baars et al., 2005), these instruments have some limitations. They have been criticized for focusing on measurement of function (e.g., what the child can do, limitations in specific activities) from the perspective of ill-being (e.g., "What are you having difficulties with . . .") rather than focusing on children's overall well-being (e.g., how children feel about their life, "What are your feelings about . . . ," "How happy you are about . . ."; Shelly et al., 2008). Presentation of QOL measure items from the context of ill-being is problematic because an absence of ill-being does not necessarily imply improvement in well-being (Davis et al., 2010).

The CPQOL–Child and CPQOL–Teen were developed using grounded theory and are based on topics and themes garnered from interviews with parents of children with CP and health care professionals. Importantly, the process for developing both the CPQOL–Child and CPQOL–Teen included discussion and consultation with children who have CP. These QOL measures were designed to be completed by parents but also have a child or teen self-report version for children aged 9 years and older (Davis et al., 2010, 2012). Results of a factor analysis demonstrated that the CPQOL–Child measures seven broad domains of quality of life: (1) social well-being and acceptance, (2) functioning, (3) participation and physical health, (4) emotional well-being, (5) access to services, (6) pain and impact of disability, and (7) family health.

The available data on the psychometric properties of the two measures are presented in Table 6.6. Both measures have evidence of construct validity using the Gross Motor Function Classification System (GMFCS; Davis et al., 2012; Waters et al., 2007). Both measures reported content (face) validity and concurrent validity. Data are reported on the internal reliability of the domains and test–retest reliability; however, evidence of interrater reliability, measurement error, and responsiveness to change is limited. Two recent studies of P–CIMT have shown the CPQOL–Child to be sensitive to domain-specific changes in QOL (Hsin et al., 2012; Sakzewski et al., 2012). Specifically, domains of "feelings about functioning" and "participation and physical health" demonstrated significant changes following both intensive P–CIMT and intensive bimanual training (Sakzewski et al., 2012). The CPQOL–Child and CPQOL–Teen are both quick to administer (15 to 20 minutes) and are freely available for all users (www.cpqol.org.au).

Correlation between parent-proxy and child reports are good on CPQOL–Child domains (ICC = .52–.77; Waters et al., 2007) and CPQOL–Teen domains (ICC = .40–.61; Davis et al., 2012). Reasons for parent–child discordance in domains of QOL for both typically developing children and those with CP have been variously and inconsistently reported. Factors associated with greater parent–child agreement are extremely diverse, including male gender of the child (Majnemer, Shevell, Law, Poulin, & Rosenbaum, 2008), female gender of the child (Gates, Otsuka, Sanders, & McGee-Brown, 2010), observable outcomes (e.g., function, comfort) compared with social–emotional domains (Daltroy, Liang, Fossel, & Goldberg, 1998), older age (Majnemer et al., 2008), greater social competency and functional independence (Majnemer et al., 2008), fewer emotional symptoms (Majnemer et al., 2008), reporting of less-extreme scores by children (Waters, Stewart-Brown, & Fitzpatrick, 2003), reporting of more-extreme scores by children (KIDSCREEN Group Europe, 2006), and basing responses on single events (KIDSCREEN Group Europe, 2006).

A further complicating factor is that children with unilateral CP have been shown to have significantly greater psychological problems than typically developing peers (Parkes, White-Koning, McCullough, & Colver, 2009), and this factor also may contribute to differing perspectives between parents and children on QOL. It is therefore recommended that, when possible, children and youths report their own QOL, while recognizing that the views of parents may provide an important alternative perspective.

MONITORING FEASIBILITY AND ADVERSE EVENTS

In a clinical and research setting, monitoring the feasibility of and compliance with a P–CIMT program and the fidelity of implementation on the part of the practitioner is essential. Ethically, this monitoring should be done by personnel who are not directly involved in delivering the intervention to ensure an unbiased approach. Use of a constraint (e.g., glove, cast, sling) in either a clinical or research setting requires supervision for safety (see Chapter 7, "Operationalizing Pediatric CIMT: Guidelines for Transforming Basic Principles and Scientific Evidence into Clinical Practice for Individual Children," and Chapter 16, "Research Priorities: Understanding and Transcending the Limits of Current Knowledge to Inform Best Practices in Pediatric CIMT," which list potential side effects to be monitored) and appropriate support to provide engaging activities to minimize frustration (Gilmore, Ziviani, Sakzewski, Shields, & Boyd, 2010). We do not advocate the use of constraint alone (often referred to as *forced use*) without also using motivating and engaging activities to maximize engagement, compliance, and motor learning.

In a research setting, the potential for adverse events related to the use of constraint in the P–CIMT program should be monitored by an investigator masked to group allocation so that both objective measures and open-ended questions can reveal any negative or unintended effects of the treatment protocol. This effort often requires careful thinking about a full range of consequences, including how each event should be graded or documented and how long study participants should be followed after treatment ends (National Cancer Institute, 2009). Adverse events also should be graded in terms of likely relationship to the intervention being studied (e.g., use of constraint, prior use of intramuscular injections of botulinum toxin A). This grading can be attributed on the basis of patient history, onset and duration, family history, consistency, and literature in terms of documented adverse events known to be temporally related to the treatment. The relationship of events to interventions should be classified as definite, probable, possible, or unlikely (Naranjo et al., 1981).

SUMMARY

In a research setting, the selection of appropriate outcome measures for a P–CIMT program should focus primarily on the domains that the intervention specifically addresses or targets for change, such as unimanual capacity, bimanual capacity, or functional and occupational outcomes in daily life. Researchers may also wish to measure indirect outcomes (e.g., participation, QOL) or to interpret the mechanisms associated with behavioral changes attributable to the therapy

Table 6.6 Selected Quality of Life Measures

OUTCOME MEASURE	AGE	DOMAINS AND ITEMS	CONTENT VALIDITY	CONCURRENT VALIDITY	CONSTRUCT (CONVERGENT AND DIVERGENT) VALIDITY	INTERNAL RELIABILITY	RETEST (ICC) RELIABILITY
CP QOL–Child[a]	4–12 years parent report; 9–12 years child report	Self-report 53 items, parent-proxy report 66 items, in 7 domains: Social well-being and acceptance Participation and physical health Functioning Emotional well-being Pain and impact of disability Access to services Family	Domains determined in consultation with children with CP and their parents (*n* = 28 families)	Domains moderately correlated with those of KIDSCREEN and CHQ	Global QOL *r* = .18–.62 Global Health *r* = .21–.56	α = .74–.92 (caregivers; *n* = 205) α = .80–.90 (child self-report; *n* = 53)	.76–.89
CP QOL–Teen[b]	Youth 12–18 years	72 items in 7 domains: Well-being and participation Communication and physical health School well-being Social well-being Access to services Family health Feelings about functioning	Domains determined in consultation with adolescents and caregivers	NA	Adolescent self-report: Moderate correlation with KIDSCREEN–10 (*r* = .63–.68), GMFCS for well-being and participation (*r* = .36), communication and physical health (*r* = .29), feelings about function (*r* = .40) Weak-to-moderate correlation with PedsQL generic domains and moderate correlation with condition-specific PedsQL domains Caregiver report: Moderate correlation with KIDSCREEN–10 (*r* = .43–.66), GMFCS for well-being and participation, communication and physical health, feelings about functioning Moderate correlation with generic and condition-specific PedsQL on some domains	α = .81–.96 (caregivers; *n* = 112) α = .78–.95 (adolescents; *n* = 87)	.57–.88 (adolescents) .29–.83 (caregivers)

Note. CPQOL = Cerebral Palsy Quality of Life; CP = cerebral palsy; CHQ = Child Health Questionnaire; GMFCS = Gross Motor Function Classification Scale; ICC = intraclass correlation coefficient; NA = not available; PedsQL = Pediatric Quality of Life Inventory; QOL = quality of life; *r* = Pearson product–moment correlation.
[a]Davis, Shelly, Waters, & Davern, 2010. [b]Davis et al., 2012.

or intervention (e.g., by including neuroscience or sensory function measures). In this chapter, we have described tools that are suitable for these primary and secondary aims and that have strong psychometric properties, including sensitivity to change, in a variety of age groups.

In a clinical setting, the selection of appropriate outcome measures used in a P–CIMT program should focus on measuring outcomes meaningful to the participating child and family (patient-reported outcomes) and applicable to the setting in which the program is conducted (e.g., real-world use). To achieve the best results, family-centered measures such as the COPM and GAS may help prioritize the focus and intended goals of the P–CIMT program, taking into account the perspective of the child or youth. The clinician must, however, recognize that the setting of goals (using the COPM or GAS) may contribute to expectations regarding the outcomes of the program. Many personal goal-related tasks involving the upper limb are inherently bimanual, so combining P–CIMT with specific goal-directed bimanual training may be required to achieve goals.

REFERENCES

Aarts, P. B., Jongerius, P. H., Geerdink, Y. A., van Limbeek, J., & Geurts, A. C. (2010). Effectiveness of modified constraint-induced movement therapy in children with unilateral spastic cerebral palsy: A randomized controlled trial. *Neurorehabilitation and Neural Repair, 24,* 509–518.

Anderson, P. (2002). Assessment and development of executive function (EF) during childhood. *Child Neuropsychology, 8,* 71–82.

Arnould, C. (2006). *Hand functioning in children with cerebral palsy.* Louvain-La-Neuve, Belgium: Université Catholique de Louvain.

Arnould, C., Penta, M., Renders, A., & Thonnard, J. L. (2004). ABILHAND–Kids: A measure of manual ability in children with cerebral palsy. *Neurology, 63,* 1045–1052.

Baars, R. M., Atherton, C. I., Koopman, H. M., Bullinger, M., & Power, M.; DISABKIDS Group. (2005). The European DISABKIDS project: Development of seven condition-specific modules to measure health related quality of life in children and adolescents. *Health and Quality of Life Outcomes, 3,* 70–79.

Bagley, A. M., Gorton, G. E., Bjornson, K., Bevans, K., Stout, J. L., Narayanan, U., & Tucker, C. A. (2011). Factor- and item-level analyses of the 38-item Activities Scale for Kids—Performance. *Developmental Medicine and Child Neurology, 53,* 161–166.

Basu, S., Kafkes, A., Schatz, R., Kiraly, A., & Kielhofner, G. (2008). *A user's manual for the Pediatric Volitional Questionnaire* (Version 2.1). Chicago: Model of Human Occupation Clearinghouse, Department of Occupational Therapy, University of Illinois at Chicago.

Berg, C., & LaVesser, P. (2006). The Preschool Activity Card Sort. *OTJR: Occupation, Participation and Health, 26,* 143–151.

Bourke-Taylor, H. (2003). Melbourne Assessment of Unilateral Upper Limb Function: Construct validity and correlation with the Pediatric Evaluation of Disability Inventory. *Developmental Medicine and Child Neurology, 45,* 92–96.

Bourke-Taylor, H., Law, M., Howie, L., & Pallant, J. F. (2009). Development of the Assistance to Participate Scale (APS) for children's play and leisure activities. *Child: Care, Health and Development, 35,* 738–745.

Cano, S. J., & Hobart, J. C. (2008). Watch out, watch out, the FDA are about. *Developmental Medicine and Child Neurology, 50,* 408–409.

Carlon, S., Shields, N., Yong, K., Gilmore, R., Sakzewski, L., & Boyd, R. (2010). A systematic review of the psychometric properties of quality of life measures for school aged children with cerebral palsy. *BMC Pediatrics, 10,* 81.

Case-Smith, J., DeLuca, S. C., Stevenson, R., & Ramey, S. L. (2012). Multicenter randomized controlled trial of pediatric constraint-induced movement therapy: 6-month follow-up. *American Journal of Occupational Therapy, 66,* 15–23. http://dx.doi.org/10.5014/ajot.2012.002386

Charles, J., & Gordon, A. M. (2005). A critical review of constraint-induced movement therapy and forced use in children with hemiplegia. *Neural Plasticity, 12,* 245–261; discussion 263–272.

Charles, J. R., Wolf, S. L., Schneider, J. A., & Gordon, A. M. (2006). Efficacy of a child-friendly form of constraint-induced movement therapy in hemiplegic cerebral palsy: A randomized control trial. *Developmental Medicine and Child Neurology, 48,* 635–642.

Chevignard, M. P., Servant, V., Mariller, A., Abada, G., Pradat-Diehl, P., & Laurent-Vannier, A. (2009). Assessment of executive functioning in children after TBI with a naturalistic open-ended task: A pilot study. *Developmental Neurorehabilitation, 12,* 76–91.

Clark, M. S., & Caudrey, D. J. (1983). Evaluation of rehabilitation services: The use of goal attainment scaling. *International Rehabilitation Medicine, 5,* 41–45.

Corn, K., Imms, C., Timewell, G., Carter, C., Collins, L., Dubbeld, S., … Froude, E. (2003). Impact of second skin lycra splinting on the quality of upper limb movement in children. *British Journal of Occupational Therapy, 66,* 464–472.

Coster, W., Bedell, G., Law, M., Khetani, M. A., Teplicky, R., Liljenquist, K., . . . Kao, Y. C. (2011). Psychometric evaluation of the Participation and Environment Measure for Children and Youth. *Developmental Medicine and Child Neurology, 53,* 1030–1037.

Coster, W., Deeney, T., Haltiwanger, J., & Haley, S. (1998). *School Function Assessment user's manual.* San Antonio, TX: Psychological Corporation/Therapy Skill Builders.

Cusick, A., Vasquez, M., Knowles, L., & Wallen, M. (2005). Effect of rater training on reliability of Melbourne Assessment of Unilateral Upper Limb Function scores. *Developmental Medicine and Child Neurology, 47,* 39–45.

Cytrynbaum, S., Ginath, Y., Birdwell, J., & Brandt, L. (1979). Goal Attainment Scaling: A critical review. *Evaluation Quarterly, 3,* 5–40.

Daltroy, L. H., Liang, M. H., Fossel, A. H., & Goldberg, M. J.; Pediatric Outcomes Instrument Development Group, Pediatric Orthopaedic Society of North America. (1998). The POSNA Pediatric Musculoskeletal Functional Health Questionnaire: Report on reliability, validity, and sensitivity to change. *Journal of Pediatric Orthopedics, 18,* 561–571.

Davids, J. R., Peace, L. C., Wagner, L. V., Gidewall, M. A., Blackhurst, D. W., & Roberson, W. M. (2006). Validation of the Shriners Hospital for Children Upper Extremity Evaluation (SHUEE) for children with hemiplegic cerebral palsy. *Journal of Bone and Joint Surgery: American Volume, 88,* 326–333.

Davies, P. L., & Gavin, W. J. (1999). Measurement issues in treatment effectiveness studies. *American Journal of Occupational Therapy, 53,* 363–372. http://dx.doi.org/10.5014/ajot.53.4.363

Davis, E., MacKinnon, A., Davern, M., Boyd, R., Bohanna, I., Waters, E., . . . Reddihough, D. (2012). Description and psychometric properties of the CP QOL–Teen: A quality of life questionnaire for adolescents with cerebral palsy. *Research in Developmental Disabilities, 34,* 344–352.

Davis, E., Shelly, A., Waters, E., & Davern, M. (2010). Measuring the quality of life of children with cerebral palsy: Comparing the conceptual differences and psychometric properties of three instruments. *Developmental Medicine and Child Neurology, 52,* 174–180.

de Brito Brandão, M., Mancini, M. C., Vaz, D. V., Pereira de Melo, A. P., & Fonseca, S. T. (2010). Adapted version of constraint-induced movement therapy promotes functioning in children with cerebral palsy: A randomized controlled trial. *Clinical Rehabilitation, 24,* 639–647.

Debuse, D., & Brace, H. (2011). Outcome measures of activity for children with cerebral palsy: A systematic review. *Pediatric Physical Therapy, 23,* 221–231.

DeMatteo, C., Law, M., Russell, D., Pollock, N., Rosenbaum, P., & Walter, S. (1992). *QUEST: Quality of Upper Extremity Skills Test manual.* Hamilton, ON: Neurodevelopmental Research Unit, Chedoke Campus, Chedoke-McMasters Hospital.

Desrosiers, J., Bravo, G., Hébert, R., Dutil, E., & Mercier, L. (1994). Validation of the Box and Block Test as a measure of dexterity of elderly people: Reliability, validity, and norms studies. *Archives of Physical Medicine and Rehabilitation, 75,* 751–755.

Dumas, H. M., Fragala-Pinkham, M. A., Haley, S. M., Ni, P. S., Coster, W., Kramer, J. M., . . . Ludlow, L. H. (2012). Computer adaptive test performance in children with and without disabilities: Prospective field study of the PEDI–CAT. *Disability and Rehabilitation, 34,* 393–401.

Dunn, L. (2004). Validation of the CHORES: A measure of school-aged children's participation in household tasks. *Scandinavian Journal of Occupational Therapy, 11,* 179–190.

Eliasson, A.-C., Gordon, A. M., & Forssberg, H. (1991). Basic co-ordination of manipulative forces of children with cerebral palsy. *Developmental Medicine and Child Neurology, 33,* 661–670.

Eliasson, A. C., Krumlinde-Sundholm, L., Shaw, K., & Wang, C. (2005). Effects of constraint-induced movement therapy in young children with hemiplegic cerebral palsy: An adapted model. *Developmental Medicine and Child Neurology, 47,* 266–275.

Eliasson, A. C., Shaw, K., Pontén, E., Boyd, R., & Krumlinde-Sundholm, L. (2009). Feasibility of a day-camp model of modified constraint-induced movement therapy with and without botulinum toxin A injection for children with hemiplegia. *Physical and Occupational Therapy in Pediatrics, 29,* 311–333.

Fisher, A., & Bray Jones, K. (2010). *Assessment of Motor and Process Skills: Vol. 1. Development, standardization, and administration manual* (7th ed.). Fort Collins, CO: Three Star Press.

Folio, M. R., & Fewell, R. R. (2000). *Peabody Developmental Motor Scales: Examiner's manual.* Chicago: Riverside.

Fougeyrollas, P., Noreau, L., & Lepage, C. (2002). *Assessment of Life Habits, Children–Long form.* Quebec: Réseau International sur le Processus de Production du Handicap/International Network on the Disability Creation Process.

Gates, P., Otsuka, N., Sanders, J., & McGee-Brown, J. (2010). Functioning and health-related quality of life of adolescents with cerebral palsy: Self versus parent perspectives. *Developmental Medicine and Child Neurology, 52,* 843–849.

Gilmore, R., Sakzewski, L., & Boyd, R. (2010). Upper limb activity measures for 5- to 16-year-old children with congenital hemiplegia: A systematic review. *Developmental Medicine and Child Neurology, 52,* 14–21.

Gilmore, R., Ziviani, J., Sakzewski, L., Shields, N., & Boyd, R. (2010). A balancing act: Children's experience of modified constraint-induced movement therapy. *Developmental Neurorehabilitation, 13,* 88–94.

Gioia, G., Isquith, P., Guy, S., & Kenworthy, L. (2000a). *Behavior Rating Inventory of Executive Function.* Odessa, FL: Psychological Assessment Resources.

Gioia, G. A., Isquith, P. K., Guy, S. C., & Kenworthy, L. (2000b). Behavior Rating Inventory of Executive Function. *Child Neuropsychology, 6*, 235–238.

Gordon, A. M., Charles, J., & Wolf, S. L. (2006). Efficacy of constraint-induced movement therapy on involved upper-extremity use in children with hemiplegic cerebral palsy is not age-dependent. *Pediatrics, 117*, e363–e373.

Gordon, A. M., Hung, Y. C., Brandao, M., Ferre, C. L., Kuo, H. C., Friel, K., . . . Charles, J. R. (2011). Bimanual training and constraint-induced movement therapy in children with hemiplegic cerebral palsy: A randomized trial. *Neurorehabilitation and Neural Repair, 25*, 692–702.

Gordon, A. M., Schneider, J. A., Chinnan, A., & Charles, J. R. (2007). Efficacy of a hand–arm bimanual intensive therapy (HABIT) in children with hemiplegic cerebral palsy: A randomized control trial. *Developmental Medicine and Child Neurology, 49*, 830–838.

Guyatt, G., Walter, S., & Norman, G. (1987). Measuring change over time: Assessing the usefulness of evaluative instruments. *Journal of Chronic Diseases, 40*, 171–178.

Haga, N., van der Heijden-Maessen, H. C., van Hoorn, J. F., Boonstra, A. M., & Hadders-Algra, M. (2007). Test–retest and inter- and intrareliability of the Quality of the Upper-Extremity Skills Test in preschool-age children with cerebral palsy. *Archives of Physical Medicine and Rehabilitation, 88*, 1686–1689.

Haley, S. M., Coster, W. J., Dumas, H. M., Fragala-Pinkham, M. A., Kramer, J., Ni, P. S., . . . Ludlow, L. H. (2011). Accuracy and precision of the Pediatric Evaluation of Disability Inventory Computer-Adaptive Tests (PEDI–CAT). *Developmental Medicine and Child Neurology, 53*, 1100–1106.

Haley, S. M., Coster, W. J., Ludlow, L. H., Haltiwanger, J. T., & Andrellos, P. J. (1992). *Pediatric Evaluation of Disability Inventory (PEDI): Development, standardization and administration manual.* Boston: New England Medical Center Hospitals, Inc., and PEDI Research Group.

Henry, A. (2000). *Pediatric Interest Profiles: Surveys of play for children and adolescents.* San Antonio, TX: Therapy Skill Builders.

Hoare, B. (2010). *Upper limb intervention following botulinum toxin-A in young children with hemiplegic cerebral palsy.* Melbourne, Australia: Latrobe University.

Hoare, B., Imms, C., Carey, L., & Wasiak, J. (2007). Constraint-induced movement therapy in the treatment of the upper limb in children with hemiplegic cerebral palsy: A Cochrane systematic review. *Clinical Rehabilitation, 21*, 675–685.

Hoare, B., Imms, C., Randall, M., & Carey, L. (2011). Linking cerebral palsy upper limb measures to the *International Classification of Functioning, Disability and Health. Journal of Rehabilitation Medicine, 43*, 987–996.

Holmefur, M., Aarts, P., Hoare, B., & Krumlinde-Sundholm, L. (2009). Test–retest and alternate forms reliability of the Assisting Hand Assessment. *Journal of Rehabilitation Medicine, 41*, 886–891.

Holmefur, M., Krumlinde-Sundholm, L., & Eliasson, A.-C. (2007). Interrater and intrarater reliability of the Assisting Hand Assessment. *American Journal of Occupational Therapy, 61*, 79–84. http://dx.doi.org/10.5014/ajot.61.1.79

Holmström, L., Vollmer, B., Tedroff, K., Islam, M., Persson, J. K., Kits, A., . . . Eliasson, A. C. (2010). Hand function in relation to brain lesions and corticomotor-projection pattern in children with unilateral cerebral palsy. *Developmental Medicine and Child Neurology, 52*, 145–152.

Hsin, Y. J., Chen, F. C., Lin, K. C., Kang, L. J., Chen, C. L., & Chen, C. Y. (2012). Efficacy of constraint-induced therapy on functional performance and health-related quality of life for children with cerebral palsy: A randomized controlled trial. *Journal of Child Neurology, 27*, 992–999.

Jebsen, R. H., Taylor, N., Trieschmann, R. B., Trotter, M. J., & Howard, L. A. (1969). An objective and standardized test of hand function. *Archives of Physical Medicine and Rehabilitation, 50*, 311–319.

Johnson, L. M., Randall, M. J., Reddihough, D. S., Oke, L. E., Byrt, T. A., & Bach, T. M. (1994). Development of a clinical assessment of quality of movement for unilateral upper-limb function. *Developmental Medicine and Child Neurology, 36*, 965–973.

Kang, D. H., Yoo, E. Y., Chung, B. I., Jung, M. Y., Chang, K. Y., & Jeon, H. S. (2008). The application of client-centred occupational therapy for Korean children with developmental disabilities. *Occupational Therapy International, 15*, 253–268.

KIDSCREEN Group Europe. (2006). *The KIDSCREEN Questionnaires: Quality of life questionnaires for children and adolescents handbook.* Lengerich, Germany: Pabst Science.

King, G., Law, M., King, S., Hurley, P., Rosenbaum, P., Hanna, S., . . . Young, N. (2004). *Children's Assessment of Participation and Enjoyment (CAPE) and Preferences for Activities of Children (PAC).* San Antonio, TX: Harcourt Assessment.

Kiresuk, T., Smith, A., & Cardillo, J. (1994). *Goal Attainment Scaling: Applications, theory, and measurement.* Hillsdale, NJ: Lawrence Erlbaum.

Kirschner, B., & Guyatt, G. (1985). A methodological framework for assessment health indices. *Journal of Chronic Disease, 38*, 27–36.

Klingels, K., De Cock, P., Desloovere, K., Huenaerts, C., Molenaers, G., Van Nuland, I., . . . Feys, H. (2008). Comparison of the Melbourne Assessment of Unilateral Upper Limb Function and the Quality of Upper Extremity Skills Test in hemiplegic CP. *Developmental Medicine and Child Neurology, 50*, 904–909.

Klingels, K., Jaspers, E., Van de Winckel, A., De Cock, P., Molenaers, G., & Feys, H. (2010). A systematic review of arm activity measures for children with hemiplegic cerebral palsy. *Clinical Rehabilitation, 24*, 887–900.

Kottorp, A., Bernspång, B., & Fisher, A. G. (2003). Validity of a performance assessment of activities of daily living for people with developmental disabilities. *Journal of Intellectual Disability Research, 47*, 597–605.

Krumlinde-Sundholm, L., & Eliasson, A. (2003). Development of the Assisting Hand Assessment: A Rasch-built measure intended for children with unilateral upper limb impairments. *Scandinavian Journal of Occupational Therapy, 10*, 16–26.

Krumlinde-Sundholm, L., Holmefur, M., Kottorp, A., & Eliasson, A. C. (2007). The Assisting Hand Assessment: Current evidence of validity, reliability, and responsiveness to change. *Developmental Medicine and Child Neurology, 49*, 259–264.

Law, M. (2004a). *Outcome measures rating form.* Hamilton, Ontario: CanChild Centre for Disability Research. Retrieved from www.canchild.ca/en/canchildresources/resources/measrate.pdf

Law, M. (2004b). *Outcome measures rating form guidelines.* Hamilton, Ontario: CanChild Centre for Disability Research. Retrieved from www.canchild.ca/en/canchildresources/resources/measguid.pdf

Law, M., Baptiste, S., Carswell, A., McColl, M., Polatajko, H., & Pollock, N. (2005). *Canadian Occupational Performance Measure* (3rd ed.). Ottawa: CAOT Publications ACE.

Law, M., Cadman, D., Rosenbaum, P., Walter, S., Russell, D., & DeMatteo, C. (1991). Neurodevelopmental therapy and upper-extremity inhibitive casting for children with cerebral palsy. *Developmental Medicine and Child Neurology, 33*, 379–387.

Lin, K. C., Chen, H. F., Chen, C. L., Wang, T. N., Wu, C. Y., Hsieh, Y. W., & Wu, L. L. (2012). Validity, responsiveness, minimal detectable change, and minimal clinically important change of the Pediatric Motor Activity Log in children with cerebral palsy. *Research in Developmental Disabilities, 33*, 570–577.

Lin, K. C., Wang, T. N., Wu, C. Y., Chen, C. L., Chang, K. C., Lin, Y. C., & Chen, Y. J. (2011). Effects of home-based constraint-induced therapy versus dose-matched control intervention on functional outcomes and caregiver well-being in children with cerebral palsy. *Research in Developmental Disabilities, 32*, 1483–1491.

Mackey, A. H., Miller, F., Kilgour, G., Gitner, A., Richman, E., Hamer, J., & Stott, S. (2006). Reliability of the Melbourne Assessment in children with hemiplegia. *Developmental Medicine and Child Neurology, 48*(Suppl. 106), 23–24.

Majnemer, A., & Mazer, B. (2004). New directions in the outcome evaluation of children with cerebral palsy. *Seminars in Pediatric Neurology, 11*, 11–17.

Majnemer, A., Shevell, M., Law, M., Poulin, C., & Rosenbaum, P. (2008). Reliability in the ratings of quality of life between parents and their children of school age with cerebral palsy. *Quality of Life Research, 17*, 1163–1171.

Majnemer, A., Shevell, M., Law, M., Poulin, C., & Rosenbaum, P. (2010). Level of motivation in mastering challenging tasks in children with cerebral palsy. *Developmental Medicine and Child Neurology, 52*, 1120–1126.

Mandich, A., Polatajko, H., Miller, L., & Baum, C. (2004). *Paediatric Activity Card Sort (PACS)*. Ottawa: CAOT Publications ACE.

Mathiowetz, V., Federman, S., & Wiemer, D. (1985). Box and Block Test of manual dexterity: Norms for 6–19 year olds. *Canadian Journal of Occupational Therapy, 52*, 241–245.

Mathiowetz, V., Volland, G., Kashman, N., & Weber, K. (1985). Adult norms for the Box and Block Test of manual dexterity. *American Journal of Occupational Therapy, 39*, 386–391. http://dx.doi.org/10.5014/ajot.39.6.386

Morgan, G., Busch-Rossnagel, N., Barrett, K., & Wang, J. (2009). *The Dimensions of Mastery Questionnaire (DMQ): A manual about its development, psychometrics, and use.* Fort Collins: Colorado State University.

Naranjo, C. A., Busto, U., Sellers, E. M., Sandor, P., Ruiz, I., Roberts, E. A., . . . Greenblatt, D. J. (1981). A method for estimating the probability of adverse drug reactions. *Clinical Pharmacology and Therapeutics, 30*, 239–245.

Narayanan, U. G., Fehlings, D., Weir, S., Knights, S., Kiran, S., & Campbell, K. (2006). Initial development and validation of the Caregiver Priorities and Child Health Index of Life with Disabilities (CPCHILD). *Developmental Medicine and Child Neurology, 48*, 804–812.

National Cancer Institute. (2009). *Common Terminology Criteria for Adverse Events (CTCAE) Version 4.0: NCI, NIH.* Washington, DC: U.S. Department of Health and Human Services.

Noreau, L., Fougeyrollas, P., & Vincent, C. (2002). The LIFE–H: Assessment of the quality of social participation. *Technology and Disability, 14*, 113–118.

Noreau, L., Lepage, C., Boissière, L., Picard, R., Fougeyrollas, P., Mathieu, J., . . . Nadeau, L. (2004). Social participation in children with cerebral palsy: Measurement issues and applications. *Developmental Medicine and Child Neurology, 45*, 43–44.

Noreau, L., Lepage, C., Boissière, L., Picard, R., Fougeyrollas, P., Mathieu, J., . . . Nadeau, L. (2007). Measuring participation in children with disabilities using the Assessment of Life Habits. *Developmental Medicine and Child Neurology, 49*, 666–671.

Ottenbacher, K. J., Msall, M. E., Lyon, N., Duffy, L. C., Ziviani, J., Granger, C. V., . . . Feidler, R. C. (2000). The WeeFIM instrument: Its utility in detecting change in children with developmental disabilities. *Archives of Physical Medicine and Rehabilitation, 81*, 1317–1326.

Palisano, R. J. (1993). Validity of Goal Attainment Scaling in infants with motor delays. *Physical Therapy, 73,* 651–658; discussion 658–660.

Palisano, R. J., Haley, S. M., & Brown, D. A. (1992). Goal Attainment Scaling as a measure of change in infants with motor delays. *Physical Therapy, 72,* 432–437.

Park, S., Fisher, A. G., & Velozo, C. A. (1994). Using the Assessment of Motor and Process Skills to compare occupational performance between clinic and home settings. *American Journal of Occupational Therapy, 48,* 697–709. http://dx.doi.org/10.5014/ajot.48.8.697

Parkes, J., White-Koning, M., McCullough, N., & Colver, A. (2009). Psychological problems in children with hemiplegia: A European multicentre survey. *Archives of Disease in Childhood, 94,* 429–433.

Payne, S., & Howell, C. (2005). An evaluation of the clinical use of the Assessment of Motor and Process Skills with children. *British Journal of Occupational Therapy, 68,* 277–280.

Portney, L. G., & Watkins, M. P. (2000). *Foundations of clinical research: Application to practice* (2nd ed.). Englewood Cliffs, NJ: Prentice Hall.

Poulson, T. L. (1996). *Validity of the AMPS for children and adolescents.* Fort Collins: Colorado State University.

Randall, M., Carlin, J. B., Chondros, P., & Reddihough, D. (2001). Reliability of the Melbourne Assessment of Unilateral Upper Limb Function. *Developmental Medicine and Child Neurology, 43,* 761–767.

Randall, M., Imms, C., & Carey, L. (2012). Further evidence of validity of the Modified Melbourne Assessment for neurologically impaired children aged 2 to 4 years. *Developmental Medicine and Child Neurology, 54,* 424–428.

Randall, M., Johnson, I., & Reddihough, D. (1999). *The Melbourne Assessment of Unilateral Upper Limb Function: Test administration manual.* Melbourne, Australia: Royal Children's Hospital.

Randall, M. J., Johnson, L. M., & Reddihough, D. S. (2010). *The Melbourne Assessment 2 of Unilateral Upper Limb Function: Test administration manual.* Melbourne, Australia: Royal Children's Hospital.

Randall, M., Pallant, J., Imms, C., & Carey, L. (2010). Psychometric properties of the "extended" Melbourne Assessment of Unilateral Upper Limb Function based on Rasch analysis. *Developmental Medicine and Child Neurology, 52,* 12.

Rosenberg, L., Jarus, T., & Bart, O. (2010). Development and initial validation of the Children Participation Questionnaire (CPQ). *Disability and Rehabilitation, 32,* 1633–1644.

Rosenblum, S., Sachs, D., & Schreuer, N. (2010). Reliability and validity of the Children's Leisure Assessment Scale. *American Journal of Occupational Therapy, 64,* 633–641. http://dx.doi.org/10.5014/ajot.2010.08173

Russo, R. N., Atkins, R., Haan, E., & Crotty, M. (2009). Upper limb orthoses and assistive technology utilization in children

with hemiplegic cerebral palsy recruited from a population register. *Developmental Neurorehabilitation, 12,* 92–99.

Sakzewski, L., Boyd, R., & Ziviani, J. (2007). Clinimetric properties of participation measures for 5- to 13-year-old children with cerebral palsy: A systematic review. *Developmental Medicine and Child Neurology, 49,* 232–240. PMID: 1735548

Sakzewski, L., Carlon, S., Shields, N., Ziviani, J., Ware, R. S., & Boyd, R. N. (2012). Impact of intensive upper limb rehabilitation on quality of life: A randomized trial in children with unilateral cerebral palsy. *Developmental Medicine and Child Neurology, 54,* 415–423. http://dx.doi.org/10.1111/j.1469-8749.2012.04272.x

Sakzewski, L., Ziviani, J., Abbott, D. F., Macdonell, R. A., Jackson, G. D., & Boyd, R. N. (2011a). Participation outcomes in a randomized trial of 2 models of upper-limb rehabilitation for children with congenital hemiplegia. *Archives of Physical Medicine and Rehabilitation, 92,* 531–539. http://dx.doi.org/10.1016/j.apar.2010.11.022

Sakzewski, L., Ziviani, J., Abbott, D. F., Macdonell, R. A. L., Jackson, G. D., & Boyd, R. N. (2011b). Randomized trial of constraint-induced movement therapy and bimanual training on activity outcomes for children with congenital hemiplegia. *Developmental Medicine and Child Neurology, 53,* 313–320. http://dx.doi.org/10.1111/j.1469-8749.2010.03859.x

Shelly, A., Davis, E., Waters, E., Mackinnon, A., Reddihough, D., Boyd, R., . . . Graham, H. K. (2008). The relationship between quality of life and functioning for children with cerebral palsy. *Developmental Medicine and Child Neurology, 50,* 199–203.

Sköld, A., Hermansson, L. N., Krumlinde-Sundholm, L., & Eliasson, A. C. (2011). Development and evidence of validity for the Children's Hand-Use Experience Questionnaire (CHEQ). *Developmental Medicine and Child Neurology, 53,* 436–442.

Sorsdahl, A. B., Moe-Nilssen, R., & Strand, L. I. (2008). Observer reliability of the Gross Motor Performance Measure and the Quality of Upper Extremity Skills Test, based on video recordings. *Developmental Medicine and Child Neurology, 50,* 146–151.

Spirtos, M., O'Mahony, P., & Malone, J. (2011). Interrater reliability of the Melbourne Assessment of Unilateral Upper Limb Function for children with hemiplegic cerebral palsy. *American Journal of Occupational Therapy, 65,* 378–383. http://dx.doi.org/10.5014/ajot.2011.001222

Steenbeek, D., Gorter, J. W., Ketelaar, M., Galama, K., & Lindeman, E. (2011). Responsiveness of Goal Attainment Scaling in comparison to two standardized measures in outcome evaluation of children with cerebral palsy. *Clinical Rehabilitation, 25,* 1128–1139.

Steenbeek, D., Ketelaar, M., Lindeman, E., Galama, K., & Gorter, J. W. (2010). Interrater reliability of Goal Attainment Scaling in rehabilitation of children with cerebral palsy. *Archives of Physical Medicine and Rehabilitation, 91,* 429–435.

Tam, C., Teachman, G., & Wright, V. (2008). Paediatric application of individualised client-centred outcome measures: A literature review. *British Journal of Occupational Therapy, 71,* 286–296.

Taub, E., Griffin, A., Uswatte, G., Gammons, K., Nick, J., & Law, C. R. (2011). Treatment of congenital hemiparesis with pediatric constraint-induced movement therapy. *Journal of Child Neurology, 26,* 1163–1173.

Taub, E., Miller, N. E., Novack, T. A., Cook, E. W., III, Fleming, W. C., Nepomuceno, C. S., ... Crago, J. E. (1993). Technique to improve chronic motor deficit after stroke. *Archives of Physical Medicine and Rehabilitation, 74,* 347–354.

Taub, E., Ramey, S. L., DeLuca, S., & Echols, K. (2004). Efficacy of constraint-induced movement therapy for children with cerebral palsy with asymmetric motor impairment. *Pediatrics, 113,* 305–312.

Taylor, N., Sand, P. L., & Jebsen, R. H. (1973). Evaluation of hand function in children. *Archives of Physical Medicine and Rehabilitation, 54,* 129–135.

Thorley, M., Lannin, N., Cusick, A., Novak, I., & Boyd, R. (2012a). Construct validity of the Quality of Upper Extremity Skills Test for children with cerebral palsy. *Developmental Medicine and Child Neurology, 54,* 1037–1043.

Thorley, M., Lannin, N., Cusick, A., Novak, I., & Boyd, R. (2012b). Reliability of the Quality of Upper Extremity Skills Test for children with cerebral palsy aged 2 to 12 years. *Physical and Occupational Therapy in Pediatrics, 32,* 4–21.

Uswatte, G., Taub, E., Griffin, A., Vogtle, L., Rowe, J., & Barman, J. (2012). The Pediatric Motor Activity Log–Revised: Assessing real-world arm use in children with cerebral palsy. *Rehabilitation Psychology, 57,* 149–158.

Van Zelst, B. R., Miller, M. D., Russo, R., Murchland, S., & Crotty, M. (2006). Activities of daily living in children with hemiplegic cerebral palsy: A cross-sectional evaluation using the Assessment of Motor and Process Skills. *Developmental Medicine and Child Neurology, 48,* 723–727.

Varni, J. W., Burwinkle, T. M., Berrin, S. J., Sherman, S. A., Artavia, K., Malcarne, V. L., & Chambers, H. G. (2006). The PedsQL in pediatric cerebral palsy: Reliability, validity, and sensitivity of the Generic Core Scales and Cerebral Palsy Module. *Developmental Medicine and Child Neurology, 48,* 442–449.

Wallen, M., Bundy, A., Pont, K., & Ziviani, J. (2009a). Psychometric properties of the Pediatric Motor Activity Log used for children with cerebral palsy. *Developmental Medicine and Child Neurology, 51,* 200–208.

Wallen, M., Bundy, A., Pont, K., & Ziviani, J. (2009b). The revised Pediatric Motor Activity Log to measure upper limb outcome in children with hemiplegic cerebral palsy. *Developmental Medicine and Child Neurology, 51,* 29.

Wallen, M., O'Flaherty, S. J., & Waugh, M. C. (2007). Functional outcomes of intramuscular botulinum toxin type A and occupational therapy in the upper limbs of children with cerebral palsy: A randomized controlled trial. *Archives of Physical Medicine and Rehabilitation, 88,* 1–10.

Wallen, M. A., & Ziviani, J. M. (2012). Canadian Occupational Performance Measure: Impact of blinded parent-proxy ratings on outcome. *Canadian Journal of Occupational Therapy, 79*(1), 7–14.

Wallen, M., Ziviani, J., Naylor, O., Evans, R., Novak, I., & Herbert, R. D. (2011). Modified constraint-induced therapy for children with hemiplegic cerebral palsy: A randomized trial. *Developmental Medicine and Child Neurology, 53,* 1091–1099.

Washington, L. A., Wilson, S., Engel, J. M., & Jensen, M. P. (2007). Development and preliminary evaluation of a pediatric measure of community integration: The Pediatric Community Participation Questionnaire (PCPQ). *Rehabilitation Psychology, 52,* 241–245.

Waters, E., Davis, E., Mackinnon, A., Boyd, R., Graham, H. K., Kai Lo, S., . . . Reddihough, D. (2007). Psychometric properties of the Quality of Life Questionnaire for children with CP. *Developmental Medicine and Child Neurology, 49,* 49–55.

Waters, E., Stewart-Brown, S., & Fitzpatrick, R. (2003). Agreement between adolescent self-report and parent reports of health and well-being: Results of an epidemiological study. *Child: Care, Health and Development, 29,* 501–509.

World Health Organization. (1997). *WHOQOL: Measuring quality of life.* Geneva: Author.

World Health Organization. (2001). *International classification of functioning, disability and health.* Geneva: Author.

World Health Organization. (2007). *International classification of functioning, disability and health–Children and youth version.* Geneva: Author.

Ziviani, J., Desha, L., Feeney, R., & Boyd, R. (2010). Measures of participation outcomes and environmental considerations for children with acquired brain injury: A systematic review. *Brain Impairment, 11,* 93–112.

Ziviani, J., Ottenbacher, K. J., Shephard, K., Foreman, S., Astbury, W., & Ireland, P. (2001). Concurrent validity of the Functional Independence Measure for Children (WeeFIM) and the Pediatric Evaluation of Disabilities Inventory in children with developmental disabilities and acquired brain injuries. *Physical and Occupational Therapy in Pediatrics, 21,* 91–101.

section II

Clinical Applications, Protocols, and Individualization

SHARON LANDESMAN RAMEY, PhD; STEPHANIE C. DeLUCA, PhD; and PATTY COKER-BOLT, PhD, OTR/L

7

Operationalizing Pediatric CIMT: Guidelines for Transforming Basic Principles and Scientific Evidence Into Clinical Practice for Individual Children

CHAPTER HIGHLIGHTS

- Clinical appraisal of children to assess appropriateness for pediatric constraint-induced movement therapy (CIMT)
- Making the clinical decision to recommend pediatric CIMT
- Operationalization: Linking critical features of pediatric CIMT to components of a treatment plan
- Supplemental components of pediatric CIMT
- Developing a fidelity measure of pediatric CIMT
- Becoming qualified to deliver evidence-based forms of pediatric CIMT
- Tension between the ideal and practical: Strategies for providing signature pediatric CIMT to children of different ages, temperaments, and functional levels
- How to keep a child engaged in high-intensity therapy.

KEY TERMS

ACQUIREc therapy
Applied behavioral analysis
Alternative pediatric CIMT
Cerebral palsy
Compensatory movements
Forced use
Hemiparesis
Massed repetitive practice
Modified pediatric CIMT
Neuroplasticity
Prompting techniques
Shaping techniques
Signature pediatric CIMT
Standardized treatment logs
Unilateral motor impairment
Varied repetitive practice

This chapter describes the history and diversity of research and clinical practice in the field of pediatric constraint-induced movement therapy (P–CIMT). Scientific evidence shows that this approach to rehabilitation for children with **hemiparesis,** a condition in which one side of the body is markedly impaired in terms of voluntary control, strength, coordination, speed, accuracy, and functional use compared with the other side, produces clinically meaningful improvement in use of the arm and hand in a relatively short period of time (Brady & Garcia, 2009; Hoare, Imms, Carey, & Wasiak 2007; Huang, Fetters, Hale, & McBride, 2009;

Sakzewski, Ziviani, & Boyd, 2009; Taub et al., 2007; see Chapter 2, "Pediatric CIMT: History and Definition," for the history and a summary of P–CIMT research findings).

However, many urgent questions remain unanswered regarding the optimal protocol for P–CIMT in terms of its intensity or dosage, the type and duration of constraint, and the specific therapeutic techniques used during the treatment sessions. (See Chapter 16, "Reasearch Priorities: Understanding and Transcending the Limits of Our Current Knowledge to Inform Best Practices in Pediatric CIMT," for a proposed future research agenda that addresses many important issues, including the effects of repeated treatment epochs, combined therapeutic approaches, use of technology, and individual differences in response to treatment interventions.) Practitioners worldwide have embraced the central ideas supporting the delivery of P–CIMT and begun to experiment in their own clinical practices with a wide range of modifications.

This chapter provides useful information to practitioners and families so they can understand and apply the central ideas of P–CIMT. Guidelines for clinical planning and practice to maximize clinical benefits and link measurement of progress to participation in therapy are included. To achieve high-quality systems of care that implement evidence-based treatments in a timely and equitable manner to all children who are eligible, practitioners and policymakers need to work closely to ensure that all key stakeholders are well-informed and prepared to implement treatments with high fidelity to the original protocols that produced benefits.

Michie, Fixsen, Grimshaw, and Eccles (2009) emphasized the importance of providing standardized descriptions and reporting about complex intervention behavior. Indeed, clarity about complex interventions is vital to the field of implementation science, which represents the translation of clinically efficacious treatments into routine, community-based clinical service. In other words, the goal of bringing the behavior of health care professionals in line with evidence-based practice can be realized only if the field produces "greater clarity about the functional components of those interventions. These should then be matched to population, setting, and other contextual characteristics" (Michie et al., 2009, p. 40). Thus, this chapter provides the functional components of P–CIMT and how they can be adjusted for different children, clinic settings, and functional or occupational outcomes.

CLINICAL APPRAISAL OF CHILDREN TO ASSESS APPROPRIATENESS FOR P–CIMT

Children with hemiparesis frequently face a long-term reality of everyday challenges as the result of injury to their nervous system, primarily at the central nervous system or brain level. The current understanding of the cause of **cerebral palsy (CP)** for most children diagnosed early in life (within the first 2 years) is that a prenatal stroke (i.e., damage to the brain during the fetal period that results in cell death and brain lesions caused by altered blood supply to specific regions of the brain; Govaert, Ramenghi, Taal, DeVries, & deVeber, 2009; Özduman et al., 2004) or, more likely, a series of prenatal strokes occurred, attributable to a variety of possible factors that result in damage to the developing brain.

For most children, stroke and CP are not inherently progressive conditions, that is, the primary brain lesion will not change over time. For children who develop hemiparesis after the age of 2 years, the acquired brain injury can be caused by many factors, including head trauma (most commonly from automobile injuries, sports injuries, and physical falls; Broman & Michel, 1995), infections, extended very high fever associated with diverse conditions, and other diseases that increase the risk of stroke (e.g., sickle cell disease. See Chapter 4, "Motor Development and Physical Growth in Children With Cerebral Palsy," for more details about biomedical considerations related to CP).

To date, P–CIMT appears to an effective treatment strategy for children with **unilateral motor impairment** (i.e., when one side of the body displays measurably lower functional competence or strength than the other side), regardless of the specific cause of their neuromotor impairment. Hopefully, future research findings will provide greater specification about the relationship among the etiology, timing of brain injury, and extent and location of brain injury and the variation in individual children's responses to P–CIMT. Thus far, most of the studies on individual differences in response to P–CIMT (post hoc) have not detected any consistent differences associated with the child's age, gender, or initial severity of functional impairment (e.g., DeLuca, Case-Smith, Stevenson, & Ramey, 2012; DeLuca, Echols, Law, & Ramey, 2006; Gordon, Charles, & Wolf, 2006). These studies, however, often had fairly small sample sizes that limited their power to detect such differences.

Although P–CIMT leads to improved upper-extremity (UE) functioning, it does not totally eliminate the condition of hemiparesis, nor is it expected to do so. Accordingly, P–CIMT is most accurately viewed as (1) an evidence-based therapy approach applicable to a diverse group of children with hemiparesis and (2) an effective rehabilitation strategy to be incorporated into a longer-term and broader, multiyear treatment plan for each child (rather than a singular, stand-alone treatment). P–CIMT needs to be considered part of a longer-term plan because the majority of children with hemiparesis also face challenges beyond just having reduced or altered function of their UE. Typically, a child with hemiparesis is likely to show measurable differences relative to his or her typically developing age-matched peers in multiple, age-appropriate activities. These other areas of altered development for many children with hemiparesis may include one or more of the following:

- Neuromotor impairments that affect the child's posture and postural control
- Reduced mobility (e.g., ambulation) skills with lower efficiency, more effortfulness, increased injury risk, and possible need for orthoses (e.g., ankle–foot orthotics, crutches, walkers, wheelchairs)
- Impaired or delayed speech and language development
- Decreased or atypical facial expressiveness
- Sensory and perceptual impairments (e.g., increased or decreased sensitivity to touch, pressure, pain, heat or cold, spatial–body awareness)
- Delayed or uneven neurocognitive functioning, as displayed in the prefrontal cortex executive function (EF) skills (key areas are sustained attention, planning, working memory, response inhibition, emotional self-regulation, behavioral flexibility, anticipating and valuing the future, and evaluating one's own behavior in relation to that of others) and overall tested intelligence
- Social–emotional challenges, likely attributable to a combination of basic brain changes associated with the original injury, limited or atypical environmental opportunities to acquire a full repertoire of social and emotional competencies, and additional demands and frustrations associated with the child's primary disability
- Additional medical problems and comorbidities (e.g., elevated rates of seizures that may further exacerbate other aspects of the child's overall pattern of development, autism spectrum disorders, behavior problems).

Many of the associated differences in the development of children with hemiparesis are likely to reflect conditions secondary to their primary diagnosis, such as limited social–emotional skills, behavioral problems, and growth disorders. (See Chapter 4, "Motor Development and Physical Growth in Children With Cerebral Palsy," for an overview of CP and development.) It also is true that many children with a primary diagnosis of CP are quite healthy and have few or no additional problems in their overall development in other domains.

MAKING THE CLINICAL DECISION TO RECOMMEND P–CIMT

The decision to recommend providing P–CIMT for a given child occurs within the context of the total appraisal of the child's clinical, social, and educational needs and the child's life situation. Almost all children with hemiparesis

are excellent candidates for P–CIMT, provided the therapy delivered adheres to the central components of P–CIMT as tested thus far (Table 7.1). As in all ethical and informed health care decisions, professionals should never base their recommendation to a client and family primarily on factors such as cost, convenience, and local availability. Instead, the recommendation should be guided by the reasonable expectation that a given treatment—in this case, P–CIMT—will result in improved health outcomes, increased functional use of the UE, prevention of secondary and atypical compensatory behaviors, and improved quality of life.

Although P–CIMT is no longer a new form of rehabilitation, it has not yet been formally adopted as a standard of care. Many practitioners seek additional information about when and for whom to recommend this treatment. The clinical decision-making process to consider P–CIMT is supported, in part, by extensive scientific evidence that the usual and customary forms of therapy for children with hemiparetic CP do not, in fact, produce significant benefits (see Barry, 2001; Butler & Darrah, 2001). These forms of usual and customary therapy, still widely prescribed and implemented, often involve low-dosage therapy sessions that last about 1 hour and occur either 1 or 2 times per week and continue for many months throughout the year, using general principles of neurodevelopmental therapy, along with an eclectic combination of rehabilitation practices (e.g., prompting, encouragement, undirected practice, modeling or imitation, direct facilitation, range-of-motion exercises, play or activities of daily living that require use of the impaired UE).

Unfortunately, these traditional pediatric therapy approaches used by both occupational therapists and physical therapists lack evidence that they produce measurable and long-lasting benefits. Recognizing that the usual and customary therapies children with CP receive do not meet standards for being evidence-based increases the need to search for and apply forms of therapy that have demonstrated positive effects and that offer greater likelihood of producing notable functional improvement. Thus, practitioners are advised to actively look for evidence from rigorous clinical trials, particularly those that are later replicated and those that show sustained gains for children similar to those they are treating, to support their clinical decision making and choice of therapy protocols to implement.

In the eagerness to increase the provision of evidence-based P–CIMT, it is vital that implementation adhere to the components of the therapy protocols that have produced results. If high fidelity to the treatment model is not maintained, P–CIMT is at risk for being considered a poorly defined therapy approach that is so weakly or incompletely delivered that practitioners and families alike may incorrectly conclude that it is not effective in producing change in clients.

Table 7.1   FIVE ESSENTIAL OR CORE COMPONENTS OF P–CIMT IN SIGNATURE AND MODIFIED PROTOCOLS

FIVE ESSENTIAL COMPONENTS OF P–CIMT	SIGNATURE OR TRADITIONAL P–CIMT	MODIFIED P–CIMT
1. Constraint of the less-impaired or unimpaired UE	Constraint of the less-impaired or unimpaired UE for the majority of waking hours and during active treatment	Constraint of the less-impaired or unimpaired UE at least during active treatment
2. High dosage (likely minimum threshold: 2-hr sessions per day for 5 days/week) for at least 2 weeks	High dosage of therapy in a concentrated period of time involving active treatment for a minimum of 3 hours per day for 5 days/week for at least 2 weeks	High dosage of therapy in a concentrated period of time with a minimum of 2 hours/day for 5 days/week for multiple weeks
3. Use of shaping techniques and repetitive practice with task variation	Use of shaping techniques to review, extend, practice, and refine skills that use formal operant learning techniques with immediate feedback and reinforcement in all treatment sessions	Use of shaping techniques to review, extend, practice, and refine skills as an active component of treatment
4. Learning functional skills in natural and diverse settings	Learning functional skills in natural and diverse settings (i.e., treatment is in these settings)	Treatment may occur in clinics, although emphasis is on functional skills for use in natural and diverse settings
5. Transition (posttherapy) planning for maintenance of gains	Posttherapy planning to promote functional bilateral and unilateral UE development and continued practice of new skills with more-impaired UE	Posttherapy planning to promote functional bilateral and unilateral UE development and continued practice of new skills with more-impaired UE

Note. P–CIMT = pediatric constraint-induced movement therapy; UE = upper extremity.

One great practical challenge in working in this field is that specialized training in the use and application of new techniques such as P–CIMT often is not readily available. Further, the training offered has not yet been consistently monitored for its quality, rigor, and adherence to the scientific evidence. Most clinics, as well as community-based or school-based therapy programs, face another barrier for treatment recommendation—namely, these programs are designed primarily to provide weekly, usually 1-hour, therapy sessions, often in the clinic or hospital setting or during school hours. Logistically, these providers would need to redesign their operations and reschedule their practitioners so that they could deliver the much higher dosage and higher density protocol of P–CIMT to children.

Another major obstacle for these traditional, clinic-based operations is how to deliver the therapy in natural home and community environments rather than in a clinical setting. The dominant model of clinic-based services supports the way customary therapy services are billed, approved, and reimbursed for a fixed number of therapy visits from third-party payers, usually with reauthorization for ongoing treatment sessions or those beyond routine care.

OPERATIONALIZATION: LINKING CRITICAL FEATURES OF P–CIMT TO COMPONENTS OF A TREATMENT PLAN

A review of scientific findings and clinical reports reveals that many practitioners have conducted their own review of the published findings and tried to determine how to provide at least some of the features of P–CIMT to the children being served. It is a concern that in many places children are receiving therapy labeled as "constraint-induced therapy" when, in fact, the therapy does not replicate or contain the key P–CIMT elements that produced significant and lasting benefits in rigorous clinical trials (e.g., see letter to the editor by Ramey, DeLuca, Case-Smith, & Stevenson, 2012). Administering only some (rather than all) of the essential elements of P–CIMT and creating convenience-based adaptations that are not sufficiently supported by rigorous scientific evidence may waste time and money, fail to realize full benefits for individual children, and, in some cases, possibly cause unintended harm.

Therapy modifications that do not sufficiently adhere to a specified treatment protocol that has demonstrated significant benefits may fail to produce intended benefits and place a child in a situation that could lead to unexpected negative (iatrogenic) side effects.

The most widespread examples of inappropriate and ineffective forms of "alternative" CIMT include the following:

- Children receiving only 1 or 2 relatively brief sessions (usually less than 2 hours) per week that involve placing constraint on at the start and then taking it off at the end of each session. These very low dosage therapy sessions with only brief intervals of applying constraint seldom produce clinically significant benefits for the child. Repeated application of the constraint also can be frustrating for both the practitioner and the child.
- Use of constraint only without the intensive shaping therapy component (other than having parents and teachers encourage the child to use his or her arm) has been problematic and ineffective.
- Improper casting or splinting techniques have caused constriction of fingers and thumb or created undue physical stress on other parts of the arm and elbow.

Research and experience show that very low therapy dosages with limited, improper, or no-constraint approaches should never be labeled as P–CIMT.

Five central features or essential therapeutic components of P–CIMT qualify a multicomponent treatment program as being a form of evidence-based P–CIMT (also see Table 7.1):

1. Constraint of the less-impaired or unimpaired UE in a systematic way during the course of active treatment;
2. High dosage of therapy in a relatively concentrated period;
3. Primary reliance on **shaping techniques** (i.e., systematic procedures in which behavior is progressively modified through a sequence of activities by applying reinforcement for increasingly higher levels of performance) that include structured opportunities for repetitive practice that focus on increasing ease, speed, accuracy, and control of movements as well as extending new skills into the child's everyday behavioral repertoire;
4. Learning functional skills in natural and diverse settings; and
5. Transition to or planning for posttherapy activities.

Together, the five central features of P–CIMT are a bundled package of rehabilitation techniques aimed at engaging a child in a treatment course of P–CIMT. Excluding any one of these features disqualifies the treatment from being considered P–CIMT. Adhering to this operationalized definition promotes identifying a specific protocol (amenable to measuring its fidelity of implementation) for each P–CIMT intervention while still providing latitude for adaptation, individualization, and accommodation over the course of therapy for a given child.

Forms of children's constraint-induced therapy are designated as one of three primary categories—(1) signature, or standard; (2) modified; and (3) alternative—following the recommendations recently proposed for classifying adult constraint-induced therapy forms (Blanton, Wilsey, & Wolf, 2008; Reiss, Wolf, Hammel, McLeod, & Williams, 2012). Both **signature P–CIMT** and **modified P–CIMT** interventions include all five core components; in contrast, forms of alternative P–CIMT contain only some of the five components. This chapter focuses on versions of signature and modified P–CMIT, because many have produced considerable and lasting (i.e., 6 months post treatment) benefits.

For "alternative" P–CIMT protocols, the practitioner must identify a rationale for their selection and the evidence that supports the variations selected. If the alternative P–CIMT protocol lacks empirical support, the practitioner needs to explain this fact to the parents and child and indicate why a modified or signature form of P–CIMT was not selected. This conversation increases clarity in communication between practitioners and families and may provide opportunities to explore other treatment options. When an alternative P–CIMT protocol is identified and subjected to rigorous evaluation, the specific components of the protocol can be evaluated as a package in terms of impact on the outcomes for the types of children for whom the alternative P–CIMT was developed.

The five essential P–CIMT components (constraint, high dosage, shaping and repetitive practice, natural environments, and transition planning) will be described next in operational detail.

CONSTRAINT

The first component of P–CIMT is constraint of the less-impaired or unimpaired UE in a systematic way during the course of active treatment. The theory is that this intervention will redirect the child's attention to use the more-impaired UE and perhaps reduce competing sensory–motor activity and reliance on well-established habit patterns that do not include active use of the more-impaired UE in play and daily activities.

HIGH DOSAGE

High dosage of therapy in a relatively concentrated period is defined as a minimum of 2-hour daily sessions for 5 to 7 days per week, usually over multiple weeks, yielding a minimum total dosage of 30 hours, although most of the efficacious dosages have had a total between 60 and more than 126 hours (Taub et al., 2007).

High dosage of therapy was a cardinal feature of the adult form of constraint-induced therapy (see Chapter 1, "History and Theory of CIMT for Adults With Stroke," for the history of adult CIMT), and independent studies support the conclusion that high-intensity therapy can be beneficial (e.g., Gordon et al., 2011). Acquisition of new behavioral skills requires considerable effort, particularly at first, for these new skills to become more proficient and eventually to be as automatic and natural as skills for the less-impaired UE. This high-dosage and concentrated therapy is hypothesized to be a critical feature of P–CIMT.

Similarly, theories of **neuroplasticity,** which is the ability of the nervous system, particularly the brain, to structurally and functionally change, postulate that reshaping the architecture and functional efficiency of the brain is closely linked to use; therefore, higher levels of use lead to new areas of activation and larger or more integrated areas of neuromotor representation and functional activity in multiple brain regions and functional brain networks (Gillick & Zirpel, 2012).

SHAPING AND REPETITIVE PRACTICE

Primary reliance on shaping techniques includes structured opportunities to review, extend, and repeatedly practice (massed and varied) new and refined skills. Shaping uses a combination of strategies to prompt, reinforce, and continuously refine and improve behavior. Shaping for a given type of UE movement or skill begins with a functional behavioral assessment of both the task and the child's initial level of performance. **Massed repetitive practice** refers to many repetitions of the same or highly similar behavior within a concentrated continuous time (i.e., high density of repetition with minimal rest intervals between repetitions). **Varied repetitive practice** refers to implementing the behavior with intentional differences, such as pushing an object to one side, then pushing to the other side, then pushing forward, or lifting different size blocks and placing them in different places when returning them. Massed practice can improve the automaticity, ease, and confidence, with which the child can complete a specified motor act or movement. Variation in practice helps the child understand the diverse ways in which a particular behavior can be displayed and adapted, helping increase the realization that many motor behaviors can increase in their functional value through these variations in how they are used.

Formal shaping procedures belong to a large class of techniques used in the field known as **applied behavior analysis,** which is an area of study that involves the systematic and intentional application of scientific principles of learning and reinforcement with the goal of improving behavioral outcomes. (*Note:* This field is a specialty area in psychology and education in which professionals can earn formal certification. For an excellent book on applied behavior anlaysis, see Cooper, Heron, & Heward, 2007).

Most UE functional activities involve multiple components that eventually chain together. **Prompting techniques** represent a class of widely used therapeutic techniques in which a stimulus is applied to promote or induce movement or a particular neuromotor behavior. Prompting techniques are often incorporated into shaping procedures. Examples of prompting include verbal guidance and instructions, visual displays (e.g., photos, videos), positional prompts (e.g., placing a child in a sitting position that facilitates easier movement from the shoulder or elbow), and touching or stimulating a body part (e.g., a tap to the elbow to help the forearm move forward, a gentle push from below a finger to elicit an upward movement of that finger). Practitioners also frequently model (demonstrate or show) the behavior in a way that is easy for the child to observe and then try to imitate.

Once a child shows an effort to initiate a behavior in the direction of the intended function, the practitioner provides reinforcement immediately. The practitioner and parents individualize the reinforcement for each child on the basis of the child's likes, interests, motivators, and dislikes. Varied reinforcement over the course of the session, rather than overly rigid or mechanical actions, provides stronger and more enduring results. For young children, reinforcers should include a mix of verbal praise, smiles, clapping, offering small rewards that can accumulate (e.g., stickers, small healthy snacks), or doing something silly (e.g., making a funny sound, a gentle tickle that the child enjoys). For older children, immediate verbal reinforcements help the child identify more (vs. less) successful efforts. Older children often enjoy setting up rewards that include engaging in a favorite activity after achieving an identified goal for a particular portion of the therapy session.

As a child shows progress in measurable ways, such as the behavior becoming more predictable, more accurate, faster, better coordinated, or stronger, the practitioner increases the expectations for subsequent performance in gradual increments. This can involve describing the higher expectations, demonstrating the "next level" for the child, or using direct physical prompting. As the practitioner continues this shaping approach—an approach that the child soon learns will invariably include demands for successively higher levels of performance—he or she adjusts the reinforcement so that it is directly contingent on the child attaining this higher level (i.e., the practitioner withholds reinforcement previously offered for lower levels of performance the child already achieved.)

In addition to gradually modifying new behaviors, the practitioner and child can work as a team to have the behaviors generalize appropriately to similar activities, with variations in how the new, improved behaviors are used. After achieving a certain level of performance or after an extended session of shaping, the child often chooses to review and rehearse the behavior on his or her own. Thus, repetitive practice can follow formal shaping activities at intermittent periods throughout the day and over the course of the following days and weeks. While practice is occurring, some feedback to children is helpful, particularly to prevent loss of recently learned skills or to minimize developing idiosyncratic accommodations to complete a task (which later may take considerable effort to drop from the child's repertoire). Continuously building upon a child's recent achievements and eventually thinning or reducing the reinforcement schedule (particularly for older children who more readily recognize the inherent value and enjoyment related to new UE skills) become part of the cycle of this high-intensity therapy.

Although a written description of shaping may make it appear simple to enact, practitioners often need at least several weeks of intensive practice to become proficient in this technique. When a practitioner provides reinforcement that is time-delayed or generic and insufficiently specified and linked to actual moment-by-moment behavior, the shaping techniques are far less successful at producing the intended advances in a given skill or voluntary movement. Practitioners typically can benefit immensely from observing an expert P–CIMT therapist. In addition, they can refine their own competencies by receiving feedback on their administration of these techniques, either during in-person sessions or guided review of videotaped sessions.

An area of difficulty and controversy for some practitioners is that many children can and do creatively adapt to their physical and motoric impairments, commonly referred to as **compensatory movements**, which are those movements made to accomodate to an injury or disability that disrupt or prevent completing movements in the typical (i.e., nonimpaired) manner. The problem is that many of these adaptations limit the child's subsequent attainment of more complex or efficient levels of functional motor behavior. Moreover, these accommodations often add to the visible stigma of the child's disability. Whenever possible, practitioners should focus on shaping procedures that will allow a child to complete the UE "occupation" in as typical or normative a fashion as possible (taking the child's age into consideration). This encouragement and shaping of normal motor patterns also help facilitate subsequent bilateral or bimanual progress, in which the child will be able to use both UEs in a coordinated, supportive, or synergistic manner. However, practitioners also need to accept a child's atypical movements to some degree, so that the child experiences success. This acceptance is an important area for individualization; practitioners who received training that emphasized "normality" as the primary outcome goal often encounter less functional progress and experience difficulty in maintaining a child's level of enthusiasm, interest, and willingness to "try harder." Excellent sources for more details about the basic theory, principles, and practices used in applied

behavioral analysis (ABA) are the textbooks by Cooper (2007) and Alberto and Troutment (2012).

NATURAL ENVIRONMENTS

The fourth component of P–CIMT is learning functional skills in natural and diverse settings to promote their maintenance and generalization to other settings. The principle of learning in natural environments is not unique to P–CIMT, but almost all of the clinical trials and case histories emphasize that the treatment occurs in the child's home or a homelike setting, and often the therapy occurs while the child is playing, participating in daily activities, or engaging with peers, such as in a camp-like or school setting. In contrast, customary treatment often takes place in a clinic where the child has few opportunities to realize how the therapy sessions relate to the everyday rhythms and expectations that he or she experiences. Natural environments have long been shown to promote both generalization and maintenance of new behaviors, rather than learning and practice that occurs in unfamiliar or therapy-only settings (Cooper et al., 2007). Chapter 9, "Alternative Pediatric CIMT: Understanding the How and Why of Clinical Variations in Pediatric CIMT," discusses examples of clinic-based approaches that also engage children in home-based tasks to promote generalization of new behaviors.

TRANSITION PLANNING

The final component is formal transition planning for posttherapy activities that recognize the child's primary functional activities and the importance of continuing to gain both bilateral and unilateral competencies to support future development.

An interesting and somewhat distinctive feature of P–CIMT is that it almost always includes working closely with the child, the child's parents, and other adults (e.g., teachers, community therapists) to establish a way to promote continued use of the new UE skills. There are at least two compelling reasons for this transition planning:

1. Children primarily function using both of their arms and hands.
2. Many children have ambitious goals for improving their voluntary use of the impaired UE, so withdrawing high-intensity therapy can disappoint them.

With the impaired or less-functional UE being far more capable after intervention, there will be new opportunities to use this UE, along with the less- or unimpaired UE to achieve greater daily success. Sometimes P–CIMT includes a formal, multiday bilateral training period; other times, this phase occurs after the P–CIMT therapy ends as the child returns to his or her typical pattern of daily life. In the United States, almost all children with hemiparesis will continue to receive some form(s) of therapy and other assistance after receiving P–CIMT if they are participating in early intervention or special education programs (Batshaw, 2000). Having explicit plans and ideas for how to promote continued progress and prevent any regression toward non-use of the more-impaired UE is particularly important.

Many children who are verbal and engaged in educational and recreational activities have their own high goals for improving their voluntary use of the impaired UE. For these children, the withdrawal of the high-intensity therapy that produced rapid and observable improvement can sometimes be disappointing. Children thus often look forward to having a plan for how to "work hard" to continue to "get better." Many parents express high interest in learning to implement some of the shaping and reinforcement techniques as well as improving their ability to observe and encourage their child in effective use of the more-impaired UE. Practitioners can help parents and older children think about ways to reward their use of new skills in everyday activities. They often design plans to reinforce use of the more-impaired UE in everyday tasks by setting aside "special" activities that can be completed only with the weaker extremity. Even for adults recovering from a stroke, the feature of transition planning has been recognized as key to long-term improvements (e.g., Morris, Taub, & Mark, 2006).

SUPPLEMENTAL COMPONENTS OF P–CIMT

Table 7.1 on page 118 presents the five essential components of P–CIMT in terms that identify two acceptable variations that have been used in the reported scientific and clinical literature: (1) signature, or standard, P–CIMT and (2) modified P–CIMT. In addition, P–CIMT often includes several other treatment aspects that are likely to be valuable and often are used in many other forms of pediatric therapy, such as setting individual goals through collaborating with the child and parents; providing supportive instruction to parents to assist their child in using and refining new and more complex skills the child acquires; and identifying effective reinforcers, motivating activities, and appropriate rewards for the child (as well as learning about any other social, emotional, and health issues that should be considered over the course of P–CIMT).

Exhibit 7.1 lists many other components or features of P–CIMT therapy that are mentioned in published studies as being integrated with the other core elements. These features are not considered unique to P–CIMT and are unlikely to be sufficient by themselves to produce large and enduring functional improvements. Rather, they might be considered as child-friendly and promotive factors in almost any form of pediatric rehabilitation.

DEVELOPING A FIDELITY MEASURE OF P–CIMT

The science of pediatric rehabilitation is well supported by having systematic therapy protocols in the form of manualized treatment guidelines. This manualization of interventions promotes clarity in planning and implementing the therapy and facilitates establishing measures of adherence to the protocol. In other words, the manualization of P–CIMT interventions helps ensure that the delivery of the therapy remains true to the underlying philosophy, principles, and procedures for which there is evidence of efficacy with specific client populations. Although many practitioners once relied on their own clinical impressions and experiences as adequate to guide their work with clients, there is strong consensus that more rigorous evidence and documentation of the content of therapy, as well as dosage, are needed.

There is a high priority to develop valid and reliable measures for assessing the fidelity of implementation of P–CIMT that has produced measurable gains. Specifically, we propose that the five core elements (described earlier) form the centerpiece of a general fidelity measure, with additional and adjunctive components added as appropriate. These measures will also further a more rapid acceleration of clinical knowledge that can be shared, consistent with the idea of moving toward precision practice (see "Introduction" to this text) in a manner that incorporates advances from basic science, rigorous clinical trials, and ongoing clinical practice as new treatments move into large-scale implementation.

BECOMING QUALIFIED TO DELIVER EVIDENCE-BASED FORMS OF P–CIMT

In many fields of health care and rehabilitation, particular treatments require specialized training and sometimes certification. To date, no formal qualifications have been required for training and certification in the delivery of evidence-based P–CIMT. Some clinical groups, however, have developed training programs for both students (preservice training primarily in pediatric occupational therapy and pediatric physical therapy) and practitioners (often as part of continuing education available in professional workshops and training courses offered by experts in tested forms of P–CIMT).

The signature and modified forms of P–CIMT are distinctive as a multi-element treatment package; they extend beyond the rehabilitation techniques covered in the majority of pediatric occupational and physical therapy programs as well as the preparation of pediatric physiatrists, whether as doctors of medicine or doctors of osteopathic medicine.

Exhibit 7.1   Supplemental Components Often Included in P–CIMT Protocols

Common treatment features that accompany signature and modified P–CIMT include
- Setting treatment goals in a partnership that includes contributions from the child, the parents, and the practitioners
- Identifying rewards and motivators for the child that can be used in shaping and repetitive practice activities
- Setting times and places for the therapy that are "family friendly" and varied
- Including periods for free or unstructured play-based activities that readily permit practicing new and improved UE skills
- Having parents learn some of the techniques of P–CIMT and setting up activities for practice during nontherapy times
- Using technology in ways that facilitate treatment goals rather than distract from therapy goals
- Meeting with other professionals who provide clinical and other services to the child and family to help explain P–CIMT and to coordinate and share information.

Note: P–CIMT = pediatric constraint-induced movement therapy; UE = upper extremity.

Although not all of the essential treatment features are novel, their integration into a single program of treatment is novel. Perhaps the two most novel and demanding aspects of P–CIMT are its
1. High intensity, particularly when the sessions last 3 to 6 hours in duration and are provided 5 to 7 days per week for 2 to 6 weeks (and sometimes up to 10 weeks), and
2. Use of rigorous, skillful application of shaping (successive approximations to achieve a given neuromotor outcome) and repetitive practice techniques.

In addition, many different forms of constraint can be used for children, which require expertise in semirigid, flexible casting and splinting for children of different ages and with different clinical concerns.

Accordingly, many practitioners seeking to become qualified in P–CIMT can benefit from additional professional education and training opportunities, ranging from the study of written P–CIMT protocols or manuals to observational learning to formal course instruction. Ideally, for practitioners who have not been formally trained and supervised in P–CIMT as part of their preservice or in-service instruction (currently available at only a few institutions), receiving detailed feedback from more-experienced P–CIMT practitioners when they provide this therapy for the first several children would be extremely valuable.

For both signature and modified P–CIMT, the intervention has engaged practitioners who are trained and qualified in their locales. Practitioners usually are the direct providers of P–CIMT, although some studies have combined practitioner-delivered therapy with parent-delivered therapy, and some have relied extensively on parents delivering the therapy. (See Chapter 9, "Alternative Pediatric CIMT: Understanding the How and Why of Clinical Variations in Pediatric CIMT," and Chapter 10, "Group-Based Models of Pediatric CIMT: Special Camps, School-Based Treatment, and Home Environment Models," for more details about modified and alternative

forms of P–CIMT in which parents receive training and actively participate in the intervention.) Because P–CIMT has been applied and studied in many countries, differences exist in the preparation and designation of professionals who work in the field of pediatric rehabilitation. For example, in the United States, variations occur in each specialty area and most states in terms of standards for board certification and licensing, including how to administer and oversee the testing process and how to document continuing education credits and activities, usually following national guidelines (e.g., National Board for Certification in Occupational Therapy, Federation of State Boards of Physical Therapy). Similarly, degree-granting programs in rehabilitation receive accreditation appropriate for their discipline.

For rehabilitation professionals seeking specialized training in P–CIMT, the following strategies may be helpful:
- Study the written P–CIMT protocols and administration manuals that might be available in print (e.g., DeLuca, Echols, & Ramey, 2007), online through a clinic Web site (e.g., Cincinnati Children's Hospital Medical Center, Kennedy Kreiger Institute), or shared directly by scientists and practitioners who have evaluated a type of P–CIMT and produced evidence of its efficacy (through a well-controlled clinical trial) or effectiveness (through clinical reporting of progress monitoring of children receiving the therapy);
- Attend workshops and special courses about P–CIMT offered through major professional organizations at international, national, and regional meetings;
- Participate in formal, in-depth training that may be available, particularly training that affords opportunities to work directly with children and receive in-person feedback about application of techniques (e.g., the Pediatric Neuromotor Research Clinic in Birmingham, Alabama, offered a 40-hour course over 5 days in the implementation of ACQUIREc P–CIMT, a signature

form of P–CIMT, with feedback provided post training using a combination of videotaped therapy sessions and individualized consultation about therapy protocols); and

- Establish professional learning circles locally to exchange information and develop strategies for documenting the delivery of P–CIMT and measuring both its fidelity of implementation (i.e., adherence to the guidelines and parameters of the original protocol; see below) and its effects on children (e.g., measuring pre- and posttherapy competence of each child and including practitioner, parent, and child reports of changes and challenges).

FIDELITY OF TREATMENT: IMPORTANCE OF RECORDING P–CIMT AS DELIVERED TO INDIVIDUAL CHILDREN

Historically, most rehabilitation practitioners have documented the delivery of treatment in the terms required for reimbursement (particularly if a third-party or medical insurance payment is made) and in ways that provide useful clinical notations for the practitioner. No formal requirement or professional expectation exists to maintain **standardized treatment logs,** which are used to systematically document the times of therapy, therapy activities and their targeted goals, and observed progress. Similarly, clinical notes or logs have rarely been shared openly with parents or clients. A new frontier in personalized and participatory medicine, including rehabilitation, would include ways to share treatment progress notes and use them as a basis for ongoing adjustments to therapy and future planning for transition activities after P–CIMT ends.

The relatively new international journal *Implementation Science* (2013), launched in 2007, supports a growing concern that many research findings that could improve health and functional outcomes are not being implemented in a timely and effective manner to yield the intended benefits in routine health care clinical, organizational, and policy contexts. Thus, scientific methods are now being applied to study how to improve the "update" and "scale-up" from discoveries such as those represented in this book. (For two excellent resources about the field of implementation science, see Brownson, Colditz, & Proctor, 2012, and Kelly & Perkins, 2013.) The following quotation from *Implementation Science* (2013) underscores the urgent need in this field:

Biomedical, social science, organisational, and managerial research constantly produce new findings—but often these are not routinely translated into healthcare practice. Implementation research is the scientific study of methods to promote the systematic uptake of proven clinical treatments, practices, organisational, and management interventions into routine practice, and hence to improve health. In this context, it includes the study of influences on patient, healthcare professional, and organisational behavior in either healthcare or population settings.

The lack of routine uptake of research findings is strategically important for the development of healthcare because it clearly places an invisible ceiling on the potential for research to enhance health. Further, it is scientifically important because it identifies the behaviour of healthcare professionals and healthcare organisations as key sources of variance requiring improved empirical and theoretical understanding before effective uptake can be reliably achieved.

One key aspect of understanding how effectively new discoveries are translated into routine rehabilitation for large populations requires systematic documentation of how these discoveries are specifically used for individual clients. This documentation can be facilitated through the establishment of clinical research networks that involve partnerships among practitioners, clinics or organizations, and investigators. Even without a supportive infrastructure, individual practitioners and practices can develop their own methods for uniformly recording the ways in which they intend to implement (i.e., operationalize) each of the five essential components of P–CIMT and the extent to which the intended treatment plan is fulfilled, using a combination of daily therapy logs, photos or videotapes, and direct measures of treatment and treatment progress.

These documentation strategies benefit clients immensely when individual practitioners also record the challenges and obstacles encountered, and describe the ways they try to solve them. Frequently reviewing and sharing (usually in abstracted and condensed forms) these fidelity of implementation documents with others in a professional network increase the opportunities to accelerate learning about variations in effective implementation and may help prevent some of the difficulties anticipated or encountered. Table 7.2 provides key topics to cover when documenting P–CIMT treatment protocols and fidelity.

TENSION BETWEEN THE IDEAL AND PRACTICAL: STRATEGIES FOR PROVIDING SIGNATURE P–CIMT TO CHILDREN OF DIFFERENT AGES, TEMPERAMENTS, AND FUNCTIONAL LEVELS

The response from professionals to the early reports of case histories and the smaller scale randomized controlled

Table 7.2   KEY TOPICS TO COVER WHEN DOCUMENTING P–CIMT TREATMENT PROTOCOLS AND FIDELITY

P–CIMT ELEMENTS	KEY TOPICS DOCUMENTING THERAPY PROTOCOLS AND FIDELITY
1. Constraint of less-impaired UE	• Type of constraint • Duration of use • Schedule for removing and checking (only if full-time constraint is used)
2. High therapy dosage in concentrated period	• Duration of each therapy session • Total number of therapy sessions • Sessions per week and number of weeks (exact calendar schedule) • Summary • If any sessions were missed or shorter, were compensatory make-up sessions scheduled? If so, when did they occur?
3. Formal shaping and massed and varied repetitive task practice	• Therapy goals • Number and type of activities shaped • Types and schedules of reinforcement used • How often activities shaped • Number and types of activities practiced • How often activities practiced
4. Natural and diverse settings	• Settings in which treatment is provided
5. Transition and posttherapy planning	• Number of posttherapy unilateral activities identified to be completed with impaired UE • Number of posttherapy bilateral activities identified • Types of communication and future planning with parents and family • Types of communication, coordination, and future planning with other professionals treating the child

Note. P–CIMT = pediatric constraint-induced movement therapy; UE = upper extremity.

trials of signature P–CIMT was in many ways surprising. Rather than enthusiastically embracing the results, many practitioners responded with strong concerns and criticisms. Some comments included "This would be too demanding and stressful for both the children and the families," "The costs of this therapy would be excessive," and "We already have an inadequate workforce to serve young children with neuromotor disabilities, and this high-intensity treatment would mean that many children would not receive treatment at all."

These initial cautionary reactions represented an understandable tension for many dedicated practitioners who functioned within existing service delivery systems over which they had little control and that often were slow to change. In fact, the practical and logistical issues do not represent insurmountable challenges; similarly, the costs of high-intensity therapy that produces measurable improvement in outcomes can be well-justified on clinical and ethical grounds, whereas continuing the status quo of providing treatments of a type or dosage that does not produce comparable benefits is far more questionable.

As mentioned earlier in this chapter, providing high-intensity therapy of 3 hours or more per day for many days per week and multiple weeks is difficult, because the family and the child must find sufficient time to dedicate to this. Summers and school breaks often are excellent times for school-age children. However, even when children are attending a day program, practitioners and families often can find time sufficient for the therapy (such as from 3 p.m. to 6 or 8 p.m. on school days, or divided between an early morning session of 1 or 2 hours and then receiving the remaining therapy hours after school and during dinner and family evening times at home). Many families have succeeded in working closely with their child's school to have a 1-month break, obtaining school assignments in advance, some of which can be built into the P–CIMT therapy activities.

Practitioners have an undeniable need for maintaining high stamina, that is, the focused energy to remain engaged in providing therapy. They also must encourage the child's interest level and monitor for signs of fatigue or possible distress that would require shifting activities and communicate with the child's parents, who may be present for part or all of the lengthy therapy session. Stamina is needed to provide high-fidelity delivery of the signature form of P–CIMT. Clearly, the practitioner is required to be just as busy and engaged as the child is, sometimes for 6 hours a day or more. Therefore, the practitioner needs to be well rested, well prepared with ideas and supplies for the therapy activities, and well nourished (bringing food and beverages to the setting where the P–CIMT is given). Interruptions such as phone calls or e-mail exchanges are highly disruptive to therapy sessions, so the practitioner also needs to be sure communication with others is handled before or after therapy.

For one of the signature forms of P–CIMT, known as **ACQUIREc therapy** (DeLuca et al., 2007), practitioners often need to spend up to 8 hours in the child's home, because he or she needs to have breaks and child rest or nap times built into the full day. The ACQUIREc practitioner sometimes divides the 6 hours of therapy into 2 separate sessions, one provided in the morning and the other in the afternoon or early evening. For practitioners who have become accustomed to working in 1- or 2-hour sessions, with a break between sessions, providing high-intensity therapy is really a new endeavor. Fortunately, for many practitioners, after several months of this type of schedule, they report experiencing very high rewards through documenting the child's rapid progress, and find the schedule far easier. Not only can children become fatigued, bored, and frustrated, but also practitioners can if they are not well-prepared and mentored.

In addition to surmounting the stamina demands for individual practitioners, most clinics or organizations throughout the world have been designed to provide relatively brief (usually 1-hour) sessions to clients, which is the greatest barrier to widespread provision of high-intensity P–CIMT, thus making it administratively prohibitive to determine how a practitioner can be "reassigned" to work with only 1 or perhaps 2 children for many weeks, often all day. One solution is for P–CIMT practitioners can commit to certain time periods when they provide P–CIMT and in the other months, they can do follow-up or work with children who need relatively short-term therapy. Summer months are ideal for many school-based practitioners to offer P–CIMT to several children individually or to participate in local P–CIMT summer camps that last from 1 to 3 weeks in collaboration with other practitioners and supportive staff and volunteers.

Designating a specialty clinic within a larger pediatric rehabilitation clinic focused on serving children exclusively with forms of evidence-based P–CIMT (adhering to the five core components) has been ideal. Working business models are available, and practitioners can increasingly anticipate that insurance companies will reimburse fully for the forms of P–CIMT that conform to the tested protocols and for which the clinic collects evidence about effectiveness. Fortunately, the core component of delivering the therapy in natural environments means that practitioners do not need to occupy large amounts of space in formal clinics. Similarly, with the exception of the constraint supplies, many of the toys, games, and everyday activities for the long daily therapy sessions already exist in the child's home and in the community.

Becoming a P–CIMT specialist may be ideal for practitioners who prefer working only part-time—somewhere between 50% and 75% time—or for those who would like to have school vacations and summers off. They could schedule their work to accommodate their own personal or family calendars.

HOW TO KEEP A CHILD ENGAGED IN HIGH-INTENSITY THERAPY

For children who are naturally active, curious, and playful, the best form of P–CIMT feels a lot like their everyday lives. Of course, they are being asked to exert new effort and try new activities that are not easily achieved at first, but if an activity is truly interesting and fun, many children are naturally prepared to stick with it. No doubt, there are moments of frustration and a desire to take a rest. The practitioner's energy and good-natured encouragement contribute to a highly positive environment, for most of the time, for children.

Some children do better without their parents directly observing or participating, at least during the early phase of P–CIMT, although some do well with their parents. Parents often "sympathize" in ways that are emotionally challenging when they observe the practitioner engaged in what used to be called *forced use*. **Forced use** refers to the expectation that a child must use the more-impaired UE to complete a task, such as when a skilled practitioner repeatedly insists that the child continue to stay engaged with a task (e.g., "Keep reaching as far as you can, for just a few more times," "I know you are getting a little tired, but do you think you can try to do this again until you can pop 3 bubbles in a row? I will help you keep count," or "This is like getting ready for the Olympics. Let's see what happens if you do this again, just using your [right/left] hand to hit the drum"). Experienced P–CIMT practitioners share that this strong encouragement is very similar to what parents, teachers, and therapists encounter with children in almost all areas of life, when children themselves may show an ever-changing mix of eagerness to try some new and difficult tasks followed by wanting to go back to the old and easier way of doing things.

When practitioners plan for each day and week of therapy and also maintain logs of the activities they engage in and how they relate to the overall goals for a child, they become better prepared to introduce new and varied activities for both new learning and repetitive practice based on previous activities. Not surprisingly, even very young children can help shape the day and find new things to do that allow them to keep practicing without becoming overly fatigued or bored.

By building on the natural rhythms of the day and taking advantage of the season of the year, many forms of self-care and playful engagement can cause the day to fly by—especially when the practitioner has become highly familiar with how to apply the shaping techniques to almost any activity that occurs. Breaks are important, but they usually are not really breaks from therapy because they involve shifting activities, using different objects and reinforcers, moving to new places, and changing the tone—from more concentrated hard work to sometimes practice and review of something learned earlier or yesterday—or taking on one very difficult task before having a real rest period.

SUMMARY

P–CIMT appears to be a compelling approach to rehabilitation for children with hemiparesis; it often produces significant and clinically meaningful improvements in children's abilities to use their arm and hand in a relatively short time period. In addition, it has been demonstrated that P–CIMT can be implemented in a variety of community and clinical settings; however, there is an urgent need for P–CIMT as an entire treatment package of operationalized componential parts to be explicitly defined and systematically documented.

This chapter identified and operationalized the componential parts that, to date, are distinctive features of the P–CIMT package. The wide range of studies with varying levels of evidence are both the basis for and a demonstration of the need for these definitions. These contradictory yet complementary positions represent, for us, part of the overall scientific process in the development of P–CIMT. It is crucial that rehabilitation treatments follow a trajectory of scientific evidence as they are developed and tested in today's health care arena, which requires evidence-based practice with considerations for efficacy and timely implementation. We hope that this chapter provides guidance for defining the core components and underscores the importance of documentation of both the treatment planned and the treatment delivered.

REFERENCES

Alberto, P. A., & Troutman, A. C. (2012). *Applied behavior analysis of teachers* (9th ed.). Upper Saddle River, NJ: Pearson Education.

Barry, M. (2001). Evidence-based practice in pediatric physical therapy. *Physical Therapy, 9*(11), 39–51.

Batshaw, M. L. (Ed.). (2000). *When your child has a disability: The complete sourcebook of daily and medical care* (2nd ed.). Baltimore: Paul H. Brookes.

Blanton, S., Wilsey, H., & Wolf, S. L. (2008). Constraint-induced movement therapy in stroke rehabilitation: Perspectives on future clinical applications. *NeuroRehabilitation, 23,* 15–28.

Brady, K., & Garcia, T. (2009). Constraint-induced movement therapy (CIMT): Pediatric applications. *Developmental Disabilities Research Reviews, 15,* 102–111. http://dx.doi.org/10.1002/ddrr.59

Broman, S. H., & Michel, M. E. (Eds.). (1995). *Traumatic head injury in children.* Oxford, UK: Oxford Press.

Brownson, R. C., Colditz, G. A., & Proctor, E. K. (Eds.). (2012). *Dissemination and implementation research in health: Translating science to practice.* New York: Oxford University Press.

Butler, C., & Darrah, J. (2001). Effects of neurodevelopmental treatment (NDT) for cerebral palsy: An AACPDM evidence report. *Developmental Medicine and Child Neurology, 43,* 778–790.

Cooper, J. O. (2007). *Applied behavior analysis* (2nd ed.). Englewood Cliffs, NJ: Prentice Hall.

Cooper, J. O., Heron, T. E., & Heward, W. L. (2007). *Applied behavior analysis* (2nd ed.). Upper Saddle River, NJ: Pearson/Merrill-Hall.

DeLuca, S. C., Case-Smith, J., Stevenson, R., & Ramey, S. L. (2012). Constraint-induced movement therapy (CIMT) for young children with cerebral palsy: Effects of therapeutic dosage. *Journal of Pediatric Rehabilitation Medicine, 5,* 133–142. http://dx.doi.org/10.3233/PRM-2012-0206

DeLuca, S. C., Echols, K., Law, C. R., & Ramey, S. L. (2006). Intensive pediatric constraint-induced therapy for children with cerebral palsy: A randomized controlled crossover trial. *Journal of Child Neurology, 21,* 931–938. PMID: 17092457

DeLuca, S. C., Echols, K., & Ramey, S. L. (2007). *ACQUIREc therapy: A training manual for effective application of pediatric constraint-induced movement therapy.* Hillsborough, NC: Mindnurture.

Gillick, B. T., & Zirpel, L. (2012). Neuroplasticity: An appreciation from synapse to system. *Archives of Physical Medicine and Rehabilitation, 93,* 1846–1855.

Gordon, A. M., Charles, J., & Wolf, S. L. (2006). Efficacy of constraint-induced movement therapy on involved upper-extremity use in children with hemiplegic cerebral palsy is not age-dependent. *Pediatrics, 117,* e363–e373. http://dx.doi.org/10.1542/peds.2005-1009

Gordon, A. M., Hung, Y. C., Brandao, M., Ferre, C. L., Kuo, H-C., Friel, K., . . . Charles, J. R. (2011). Bimanual training and constraint-induced movement therapy in children with hemiplegic cerebral palsy: A randomized trial. *Neurorehabilitation and Neural Repair, 25,* 692–702.

Govaert, P., Ramenghi, L., Taal, R., De Vries, L., & deVeber, G. (2009). Diagnosis of perinatal stroke I: Definitions, differential diagnosis and registration. *Acta Paediatrica, 98,* 1556–1567. http://dx.doi.org/10.1111/j.1651-2227.2009.01461.x

Hoare, B. J., Imms, C., Carey, L., & Wasiak, J. (2007). Constraint-induced movement therapy in the treatment of the upper limb in children with hemiplegic cerebral palsy: A Cochrane systematic review. *Clinical Rehabilitation, 21,* 675–685.

Huang, H. H., Fetters, L., Hale, J., & McBride, A. (2009). Bound for success: A systematic review of constraint-induced movement therapy in children with cerebral palsy supports improved arm and hand use. *Physical Therapy, 89,* 1126–1141. http://dx.doi.org/0.2522/ptj.20080111

Kelly, B., & Perkins, D. F. (Eds.). (2012). *Handbook of implementation science for psychology in education.* Cambridge, UK: Cambridge University Press.

Implementation Science. (2013). *About* Implementation Science. Retrieved from http://www.implementation science.com/about

Michie, S., Fixsen, D., Grimshaw, J. M., & Eccles, M. P. (2009). Specifying and reporting complex behaviour change interventions: The need for a scientific method. *Implementation Science, 4,* 40. http://dx.doi.org/10.1186/1748-5908-4-40

Morris, D. M., Taub, E., & Mark, V. W. (2006). Constraint-induced movement therapy: Characterizing the intervention protocol. *European Journal of Physical and Rehabilitation Medicine, 42,* 257–268.

Özduman, K., Pober, B. R., Barnes, P., Copel, J. A., Ogle, E. A., Duncan, C. C., & Ment, L. R. (2004). Fetal stroke. *Pediatric Neurology, 30,* 151–162. http://dx.doi.org/10.1016/j.pediatrneurol.2003.08.004

Ramey, S. L., DeLuca, S. C., Case-Smith, J., & Stevenson, R. (2012). Caution is warranted in interpreting data from recent trial of modified constraint-induced therapy. *Developmental Medicine and Child Neurology, 54,* 477–479. http://dx.doi.org/10.111/j.1469-8749.2012.04240.x

Reiss, A. P., Wolf, S. L., Hammel, E. A., McLeod, E. L., & Williams, E. A. (2012). Constraint-induced movement therapy (CIMT): Current perspectives and future directions. *Stroke Research and Treatment, 2012,* 1–8. http://dx.doi.org/10.1155/2012/159391

Sakzewski, L., Ziviani, J., & Boyd, R. (2009). Systematic review and meta-analysis of therapeutic management of upper-limb dysfunction in children with congenital hemiplegia. *Pediatrics, 123,* e1111–e1122. 10.1542/peds.2008-3335.

Taub, E., Griffin, A., Nick, J., Gammons, K., Uswatte, G., & Law, C. R. (2007). Pediatric CI therapy for stroke-induced hemiparesis in young children. *Developmental Neurorehabilitation, 10,* 3–18.

STEPHANIE C. DeLUCA, PhD; SHARON LANDESMAN RAMEY, PhD; MARY REBEKAH TRUCKS, MS, OTR/L; REGGI LUTENBACHER, MS, OTR/L; and DORY AINSWORTH WALLACE, MS, OTR/L

8

The ACQUIREc Protocol: What We Have Learned From a Decade of Delivering a Signature Form of Pediatric CIMT

CHAPTER HIGHLIGHTS

- Component parts of the ACQUIREc therapy protocol
- ACQUIREc treatment goals
- Phase 1: Casting for ACQUIREc therapy
- Phase 2: ACQUIREc therapy in the child's natural environment
- Phase 3: ACQUIREc posttherapy transfer package
- Daily documentation of ACQUIREc
- Lessons learned from clinical experience implementing ACQUIREc therapy.

KEY TERMS

ACQUIREc
Asymmetrical weakness
Fading
Focused rigidity casting material
Hand-over-hand facilitation
Intangible reinforcement
Massed practice
Modeling
Movement
MR3 Cycle
Quadriplegia
Refinement
Reinforcement
Repetition
Shaping
Signature CIMT
Successive approximations
Tangible reinforcement
Transfer package

ACQUIREc is a form of pediatric constraint-induced movement therapy (P–CIMT) that has been rigorously tested in multiple randomized controlled trials (RCTs; see Case-Smith, DeLuca, Stevenson, & Ramey, 2012; DeLuca, Case-Smith, Stevenson, & Ramey, 2012; DeLuca, Echols, Law, & Ramey, 2006) and delivered to more than 400 children served by the former Pediatric Neuromotor Research Clinic at the University of Alabama at Birmingham (PNRC; DeLuca, Echols, & Ramey, 2007). The name *ACQUIREc therapy* (DeLuca et al., 2007) was created as a way to capture in one acronym the specific elements of the team's P–CIMT protocol, which contained several novel features. Today, this form of P–CIMT, first pilot tested in 1998 (see DeLuca, Echols, Ramey, & Taub, 2003; Echols, DeLuca, Ramey, & Taub, 2001; Echols, DeLuca, Taub, & Ramey, 2001), is referred to by others as "traditional" P–CIMT and conforms to the definition of a signature form of CIMT as proposed by Blanton,

Wilsey, and Wolf (2008). Specifically, **signature CIMT** involves constraint of the less-impaired upper extremity (UE) for at least 90% of waking hours, treatment for at least 2 consecutive weeks, intensive training for 3 or more hours per day 5 days per week, and a **transfer package**, or formal posttreatment plan, to increase the likelihood that the client will transfer gains made during treatment to use in everyday situations. To our knowledge, ACQUIREc therapy is the only tested and manualized P–CIMT protocol that conforms to this definition of signature CIMT.

The ACQUIREc acronym stands for the following key features:

- **A**cquisition of new motor and functional skills through
- **C**ontinuous practice and shaping to produce
- **Q**uality movement in the
- **U**pper extremity through
- **I**ntensive therapy that is
- **RE**inforced in the child's
- Everyday patterns and places.

The overall goal of ACQUIREc is to improve the functional competence of the weaker or impaired arm and hand in ways that support a child's everyday movement patterns and functional activities. The "c" at the end of ACQUIREc stands for constraint of the less-impaired or stronger arm and hand. This letter is lowercase to convey that although constraint of the stronger arm is an important portion of this treatment approach, it is part of a package of techniques that rely primarily on intensive therapy guided by specific behavioral and learning principles to stimulate, reinforce, encourage, and increase the child's functional use of the more impaired arm and hand in everyday tasks, patterns, and places. Each year, therapists help design T-shirts that remind them and others of what the acronym *ACQUIREc* stands for and wear the shirts while providing treatment.

The ACQUIREc form of P–CIMT was the first developed that explicitly sought to apply all of the principles used in the adult version of CIMT, using a structured or manualized protocol adapted specifically for very young children (starting in infancy) that could be replicated by others. The theoretical basis for these principles is the same as for the adult form of CIMT—namely, that

- Constraint of the unimpaired or less-impaired UE will facilitate the child's ability to concentrate on acquiring improved skills with the more-impaired UE
- Immediate and specific feedback (reinforcement) to the child about use of the more-impaired UE will reward successful behavior and rapidly help shape and refine movements and functional achievements
- Opportunity for **massed practice** (i.e., many repetitions in close temporal proximity) both during formal therapy sessions and throughout the day and night

outside of therapy (when the child is in natural settings and still wearing the constraint) will result in large and lasting improvements. (For additional background on general therapy principles closely related to P–CIMT, see Chapter 2, "Pediatric CIMT: History and Definition.")

The ACQUIREc protocol has been implemented since 1998 in a research clinic.[1] From the start, our clinical research team committed to providing evidence-based treatments that adhere to the same high standards for implementation as those in the closely monitored RCTs. All of the parents and children who were provided ACQUIREc treatment as voluntary, paying patients who sought this treatment were offered an opportunity to participate in the research assessment protocol before and after receiving ACQUIREc. (In the RCTs, however, all children received the therapy at no cost, and families were selected on the basis of prior clinical trial eligibility criteria rather than self-selected.) To date, 100% of the parents and children served clinically have provided written informed consent and assent (for minors old enough to understand the purpose of the research) to participate in the clinical research. Further, no one has ever withdrawn from research participation after providing initial consent.

This active research protocol helps the clinical team stay focused on maintaining all of the component parts of P–CIMT with systematic documentation about each child's daily treatment in terms of session duration, treatment activities, and progress and difficulties observed. In addition, all children receive a battery of standardized assessments before and after ACQUIREc therapy, and parents complete ratings of their children's use of the impaired UE. From its inception, the research clinic has had a publicly stated goal to contribute to the knowledge base about effective treatments and individual differences in response to the ACQUIREc therapy model. This goal is consistent with the need to build a larger clinical database to help inform the individualization of P–CIMT for children of different ages and with different clinical presenting characteristics.

DeLuca and colleagues (2007) wrote an administration manual for ACQUIREc treatment based on the findings from the first RCT and case histories (DeLuca et al., 2003; DeLuca

---

[1]Sharon Landesman Ramey was principal investigator for a grant that funded the opening of the Pediatric Neuromotor Research Clinic at the University of Alabama at Birmingham, which was founded in 1998. Following the clinic's inception, Stephanie DeLuca served as codirector and then director until the end of 2012, at which time the original research program ended. In 2013, DeLuca and Ramey opened a new research clinic in Roanoke as part of the Virginia Tech Carilion Research Institute. This clinic implements the same ACQUIREc therapy protocol and continues the collection of research data about children and families served. Two of the senior ACQUIREc therapists and coauthors of this chapter, Mary Rebekah Trucks and Dory Ainsworth Wallace, are part of the Roanoke clinic.

et al., 2006; Taub, Ramey, DeLuca, & Echols, 2004) so that full details of the treatment and its documentation could be made widely available. This write-up of the treatment protocol means that ACQUIREc can be replicated elsewhere. The administration manual has been used as the textbook for week-long training workshops provided to practitioners throughout the United States, supplemented by live demonstrations with children and hands-on practice by workshop participants. Subsequently, the ACQUIREc protocol was used in a three-site study that demonstrated that other sites (i.e., outside the site where ACQUIREc originated) could replicate the therapy with high fidelity and achieve comparable effect sizes (i.e., benefits; Case-Smith et al., 2012; DeLuca et al., 2012).

Finally, analysis of the PNRC clinical database (summarized in the "Lessons Learned" section at the end of this chapter) demonstrates that ACQUIREc therapy can be provided by licensed and certified master's- or doctoral-level pediatric occupational and physical therapists in a specialty clinic and can lead to the same types and magnitude of benefits as those reported from carefully controlled RCTs following the same therapy protocol. This chapter provides an abbreviated version of the administration manual, with updates based on clinical insights and new research and data analyses.

COMPONENT PARTS OF THE ACQUIREc THERAPY PROTOCOL

The formal components of ACQUIREc include full-arm, full-time constraint of the stronger arm and hand over 17 or 18 treatment days, with 6 hours of intensive therapy per day focused mostly on unilateral UE skills. This phase is followed by 3 treatment days with no constraint (i.e., cast removed) that involve a transfer skill component to integrate unilateral UE skills into a variety of bilateral or bimanual activities for use in everyday situations. All therapy takes place in natural settings, including the home or a homelike setting (e.g., a furnished home or apartment where the child and family live for 1 month) and a variety of community settings (e.g., early intervention program, school setting, park, store).

The ACQUIREc protocol is presented to families as consisting of three distinct phases:
1. Constraint of the child's stronger arm and hand through the creation of a long-arm cast that the child will wear continuously for about 3½ weeks,
2. Intensive therapy 6 hours daily for 5 consecutive weekdays over a 4-week period (total dosage = 120 hours), and
3. Joint development by the family (including the child) and the therapist of a transfer package to support maintenance and continued improvement of the child's UE functioning (both unilateral and bilateral).

Parents and clinicians new to the ACQUIREc therapy protocol are encouraged to think of these components as working synergistically and over time. Each child and family participates in a process that begins with reviewing the characteristics of the child, establishing initial treatment targets or goals, and committing to high levels of engagement by both the child and the parents in the therapy process.

INCLUSION AND EXCLUSION CRITERIA FOR ACQUIREc THERAPY

ACQUIREc therapy has been provided to many children and adolescents ranging in age from 12 months to 21 years. The main inclusion criterion for clinical treatment is **asymmetrical weakness** (i.e., *hemiparesis*, or weakness on one side of the body) with a pressing therapy goal to improve use of the arm and hand on the impaired (hemiparetic) side. In most cases, the children present with a physician's diagnosis of cerebral palsy, usually presumed to be the result of prenatal stroke or other prenatal or perinatal brain injury (see Chapter 4, "Motor Development and Physical Growth in Children With Cerebral Palsy," for more information about diagnostic classification).

Most diagnoses are considered hemiparetic or unilateral, although the ACQUIREc protocol has been used extensively with children whose primary diagnosis is **quadriplegia,** or severe involvement on both sides of the body. For most children with quadriplegia, one side of the body is somewhat more functional than the other, which guides the use of constraint and the focus of the first 18 days of intensive unilateral therapy. ACQUIREc therapy also has been implemented successfully with children who present with hemiparesis secondary to a later postnatal acquired or traumatic brain injury, hemispherectomy, arterial valve malformation, or brain injury secondary to surgeries such as tumor resection and heart surgery.

Approximately half of the children served over the past decade also have one or more comorbid diagnoses, including seizure disorder, cognitive delay, developmental delay, speech and language delay, autism, visual impairment, or severe behavior disorder. As a result, we now have an extensive database on children's participation levels and responses to ACQUIREc therapy, including more than 400 treatment epochs with pre- and posttreatment data gathered systematically on children and their families.

The following criteria necessitate exclusion of children from treatment:
- Age younger than 8 months; the protocol has not yet been adequately pilot tested with infants this young, and attention span and need for sleep are markedly different in early infancy compared with later infancy (Ramey & Ramey, 1999)

- Presence of an acute or chronic comorbid illness that could impair the child's ability to participate in the 6-hour daily therapy protocol
- Presence of severe cognitive and communicative impairments or cognitive level below that of a 6-month-old typically developing infant that prevent give-and-take interactions; these children usually also have comorbid health conditions that exclude their participation.

ACQUIREc therapy has been successfully implemented with children who have severe behavioral challenges, although these children require high levels of patience, innovation, and dedication from ACQUIREc therapists and commitment from the parents. The decision to implement a course of ACQUIREc therapy is made jointly, with input from one or more experienced pediatric therapists on the basis of prescreening information; from the parents and child, whenever the child can be included; and from the child's primary care physician or pediatric neurologist.

CLINIC ENROLLMENT MATERIALS FOR FAMILIES

To date, the PNRC has done little to recruit clients; parents usually contact the clinic by phone or e-mail or are referred by another health professional. The parents typically provide sufficient information to make the initial determination of their child's suitability for the ACQUIREc treatment program. If there is any question about a child's appropriateness for the therapy, the parents are asked to provide a video of their child for review. The ideal, however, is to conduct an in-person assessment for children whose families can travel to the clinic in advance.

In addition, parents complete and return an information packet before implementation of the ACQUIREc protocol to provide relevant information about the child and family. This packet contains demographic forms for the family to complete, a medical referral form to be completed by the child's primary care physician or pediatric neurologist, a request for copies of medical or therapy records that may be helpful in planning details of the ACQUIREc therapy, and information on housing in the clinic area if the family will need to relocate for the month of treatment.

In advance, the ACQUIREc therapist provides an in-depth explanation to parents, other caregivers, and children who are >5 years about the procedures that will occur throughout the treatment period. This explanation includes the treatment elements of ACQUIREc and the importance of individualizing the treatment goals and activities for each child and family. Parents are encouraged to contact other parents who have been through the ACQUIREc therapy process to hear about their experiences. Families and children are asked to come prepared to talk about their treatment goals.

In addition, alterations to the child's environment they think may be needed after treatment are completed so that the child will achieve maximum benefit.

ACQUIREc TREATMENT GOALS

ACQUIREc treatment goals are based on the age, developmental level, motor abilities, cognitive abilities, and motivation of the child. The goals are established in a collaborative process involving multiple people. Therapist goals are based largely on the child's abilities as observed during the pretesting session and refined over the first few days of therapy. Typically, the therapist identifies both component movement goals and everyday functional goals. Component goals are usually short-term goals centered on individual movements, and functional goals are typically longer-term goals that are often still achievable in the 4-week treatment program. The therapist plays an important role in goal setting because sometimes parents are not aware of how the child's use of the UE influences overall balance, posture, mobility, and coordination—that is, aspects of everyday movement that go beyond hand and finger skills.

Goals are also set by the child (if age appropriate) and parents. The child most often sets goals based on his or her areas of interest and activities he or she finds enjoyable and motivating. For instance, the therapist might ask the child both about activities that present difficulty as he or she completes schoolwork, gets dressed, or plays with family and friends and about favorite activities he or she would like to be able to do better. For many preschool and elementary school–age children, everyday self-help skills, such as dressing, bathing, and eating, may not be identified as therapy goals because the family has already developed compensatory techniques that work well, at least for this period in their lives. Also, some children understandably do not consider these activities to be fun, and they may not be motivated to engage in extended practice. Older children, however, may be more motivated to increase their independence and avoid embarrassment related to daily living skills.

Parent goals frequently focus on increasing the child's independence level in activities of daily living and having the child appear as "normal" as possible. Parents often insert new goals throughout the course of treatment as they notice their child making rapid improvements with the impaired arm and hand. Addition of goals is appropriate, and goal setting should be an ongoing process throughout ACQUIREc therapy. Finally, sometimes goals are nominated by other professionals (e.g., teachers, therapists, physicians) who know and work with the child on a regular basis. Table 8.1 lists examples of ACQUIREc goals for children of different ages.

Table 8.1   Age-Specific Examples of Goals for ACQUIREc Therapy

APPROXIMATE AGE RANGE	GOAL
18 months–3 years	• Increase active range of motion of weaker UE to functional limits. • Increase purposeful movement of the weaker UE with no verbal cues. • Increase recognition of the weaker arm and hand. • Increase gross grasp and use of weaker arm and hand with cause-and-effect toys. • Increase self-feeding to minimal assistance with finger foods and early utensil use. • Increase weight-bearing abilities, and crawl or use a walker with the weaker UE. • Use the more impaired UE to reach out to be picked up. • Increase spontaneity in using the more impaired UE.
3–5 years	• Perform a pincer grasp. • Increase fine motor skills for self-feeding. • Increase pointer isolation, such as for pushing buttons on toys. • Increase a consistent grasp for both unilateral and bilateral tasks (e.g., ability to carry a full cup across the room when setting the table for a meal). • Increase ability to carry items from place to place. • Increase dressing skills with both hands. • Increase involvement in hygiene activities (e.g., brushing teeth, washing hands or face, grooming hair).
6–8 years	• Cut with scissors or hold paper with the more-impaired UE. • Zip and unzip backpack using both UEs to increase independence and school readiness. • Hold down paper when writing or drawing with the more impaired UE to increase independence in writing and drawing activities. • Use hook-and-loop fastener to secure shoes (or, if achievable, tie shoelaces). • Increase independence with dressing (often including accessories, coats, hats, mittens). • Increase skills needed for participation in a sport or recreational activity (e.g., softball, swimming, martial arts, tennis).
10 years or older	• Increase all finger isolation and thumb mobility, especially to accomplish school-related tasks related to writing and reading. • Play video games or board games (approved by parents and therapist). • Increase functional independence in meal preparation and cleanup. • Increase skills within a car (e.g., turning on a radio, fastening a seat belt, adjusting windows, opening and closing doors). • Increase skills needed for participation in a sport or recreational activity (e.g., baseball, golf, pool, lacrosse, basketball, swimming, martial arts).

Note. UE = upper extremity.

ACQUIREc therapy, like all shaping procedures, succeeds only when the client has a high rate of positive experiences. Thus, setting appropriate goals is very important. ACQUIREc therapists can help children or parents think of goals in stages so that success throughout the process can be ensured. In the ACQUIREc therapy protocol, the therapist includes parent and child goals and does not discourage them as long as they involve age-appropriate, functional skills that are safe and appropriate for therapy. It is the therapist's job to help identify the key components of long-term therapy goals (e.g., playing baseball, dressing alone, packing and unpacking a schoolbag or backpack) that may not be fully attainable during the 4 weeks of treatment.

PHASE 1: CASTING FOR ACQUIREc THERAPY

Once the comprehensive assessment process is complete, the therapist applies the constraint on either the first day of treatment or the day before. The constraint is a cast fabricated in the clinic using **focused rigidity casting (FRC) material.** This lightweight material allows the rigidity of the constraint to be focused on the dorsal side of the arm to prevent movement of the elbow into extension and to maintain the hand and fingers in a neutral position (see Figure 8.1). The cast covers the entire arm from approximately 2 to 4 inches below the shoulder and underarm to slightly past the fingertips. It is important to cover the fingertips so the child does not use the fingertips to pick up objects. The elbow is placed in 90° of flexion, the wrist is neutral, and the hand is placed in a functional resting neutral position with the thumb facing up, as if the child were reaching to shake a person's hand. If the child is younger (with more fleshiness and less evident bony prominences), the therapist positions the elbow in a few more degrees of flexion to keep the cast from slipping off. The therapist might also slightly curl the fingers and thumb to keep the cast in place.

Figure 8.1   DIAGRAM AND PHOTO OF A LIGHTWEIGHT LONG-ARM CAST USED FULL-TIME IN ACQUIREc THERAPY.

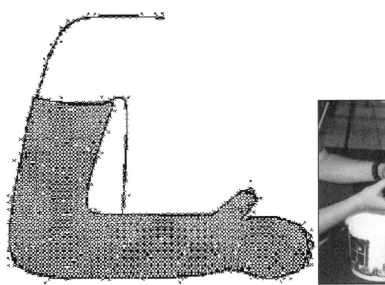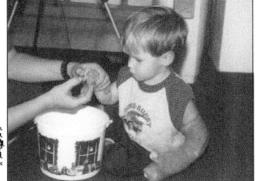

Source. S. DeLuca.

The cast is lined with a soft terry cloth–like stockinette followed by padding. Both stockinette and padding are applied before wrapping the casting tape to make the cast comfortable and decrease the possibility of skin breakdown. The following areas are specifically targeted with padding beyond the stockinette: thenar eminence (the muscle belly or ball of the thumb), palm of the hand, ulnar styloid (distal end of the forearm attached to the wrist), and the anterior and posterior portion of the elbow. The padding eliminates or limits pressure points that could cause skin breakdown. Additional padding is used depending on the needs of the child and the clinical judgment of the therapist.

The entire casting process takes approximately 30 to 45 minutes. During casting, some young children like to sit in a parent's lap, whereas older children may prefer sitting independently in a chair with a parent in the room. Children often enjoy either watching the casting process or choosing a movie to watch until the casting is completed. FRC material is easy to work with, even when a child is on a parent's lap. The casting process is done most efficiently by 2 therapists, one to assist in maintaining the correct position of the arm and hand during the casting process and the other to construct the cast itself. Once the casting tape is wrapped and set (FRC sets within minutes), it is univalved with scissors for easy removal during the weekly checkup periods. Additional padding and adhesive liner are placed on the edges of the cast after the therapist checks and trims the edges to prevent sharp points or ridges. If a spot is identified that is of concern, additional padding is applied.

The two therapists then replace the child's arm and hand in the cast. Often, one therapist holds the constructed cast open while the other therapist guides the child's fingers, thumb, and arm into the correct position. The cast is secured with casting tape, and self-adherent wrap (e.g., Coflex, Coban) is wrapped around the outside as the final layer to make the cast appear continuous and nonremovable. The use of a self-adherent wrap allows the child to choose a favorite color to cover the cast. Over time, as the self-adherent wrap covering the cast becomes dirty, the treating therapist can cut it off and apply a fresh color of the child's choice without having to remove the entire cast.

The cast remains on 24 hours a day to keep the child's focus on the impaired arm and hand (with presumed consistent input to the opposite side of the brain during this time). The cast being a constant also seems to encourage decreased input to the less involved (constrained) side and allows the child to settle more naturally into the treatment process focused on the daily use of the impaired arm and hand without questioning the removal and replacement of the cast for each therapy session.

Adjustment to having the cast on is different for every child but usually occurs within 24 to 48 hours. Parents are educated regarding cast removal in case of emergencies but are strongly encouraged to redirect the child when questions arise regarding removal of the cast. Young children are often told that the parent cannot remove the cast. If the cast gets wet or another problem with the cast arises, families are directed to call the treating therapist to discuss the situation.

The therapist then calls a supervising therapist who helps determine whether the cast needs to be removed. If the cast is removed, needed adjustments are made as quickly as possible to the cast (e.g., to avoid future occurrences of the irritation that led to the removal). If visible signs of irritation are present, appropriate treatment is applied immediately and, if necessary, a medical referral made. (A medical referral has been needed only once, for a small cut to the thumb that was easily treated; therapy continued on schedule.) In 400 treatment sessions at the PNRC clinic, only a handful of times has the cast needed to be removed and left off for more than a few hours to ensure that the irritation was reduced and healing progressing. When applied correctly and appropriately, a cast is a safe and effective tool, but the potential risks for harm we have noted make systematic monitoring vital. Any report of discomfort should be immediately addressed.

As a routine procedure, the ACQUIREc protocol calls for weekly removal of the cast, even when the child seems totally comfortable. During the cast removal process, it is advisable to have another therapist (i.e., not the child's primary treating therapist) remove the cast to check for skin integrity and to give the child a chance to bathe and dry the arm and practice bilateral activities for as long as 30 to 45 minutes. Then the univalved cast is reapplied. No lotion, powders, or ointments are applied during this time, because they could act as irritants once the cast is on (e.g., by caking or wadding up).

When the cast is permanently removed for the final 3 days of ACQUIREc therapy for work on bilateral activities, the child again has the arm and hand thoroughly bathed, and application of hypoallergenic lotion on the arm and hand is advised. Children with certain skin types experience peeling or flaking of the skin between the fingers, which is usually short lived and painless. Currently, we recommend that therapists document the casting process at the start with a photograph of the child's arm, the cast applied to the arm, and the cast alone. Weekly checks on the casted arm also can be documented with a photograph or short video. This documentation provides valuable supplementary evidence to the therapist's written notes.

PHASE 2: ACQUIREc THERAPY IN THE CHILD'S NATURAL ENVIRONMENT

SHAPING AS A STRUCTURED MEANS TO LEARNING

CIMT was derived in large part from ideas surrounding operant conditioning or training, as explained in other chapters, including the principles of shaping and successive approximations (e.g., Bijou & Baer, 1961; Skinner, 1953). **Shaping** refers to a well-documented technique that was scientifically studied as part of formal learning theory in the field of psychology, identifying the progressive acquisition of new behaviors through performance of successive acts that collectively represent the final target skill. The term *successive approximations* is used to capture the sequence of behaviors that come increasingly closer to the final targeted behavior or skill.

Key features of shaping through the procedures surrounding successive approximations are the division of the final target skill or behavior into incremental steps or parts (depending on the complexity of the behavior or skill) and the elicitation of the achievement of steps with immediate, direct, and definable rewards, starting with the basic or most primitive version of the behavior (or its component parts) and then increasing the expectations (criteria) for achievement to enable reinforcement across and within shaping sessions. In general, criteria for success (to receive the reward) are increased in very small ways at each level along the continuum of successive approximation. New criteria are developed only when the previous ones are being met, generally in about 70% to 80% of the repetitive attempts.

Shaping is focused on successful completion of discrete behavioral acts. Whereas learning naturally involves trial and error, shaping builds on the idea that the recognition of success creates an internal reinforcement for the participant in addition to the external reinforcers provided. In rehabilitation, this internal reinforcement is a highly effective motivator and is closely tied to the concepts undergirding motor learning theory (see Chapter 3, "Applying Occupation and Motor Learning Principles in Pediatric CIMT: Theoretical Foundations and Conceptual Framework"). Shaping is particularly well suited for behaviors that are multicomponent, complex, and developmental in nature. For example, a behavior such as reaching normally goes through many developmental stages in the first year of life (and beyond) as it becomes increasingly sophisticated and approximates its eventual mature adult form.

Many everyday examples of shaping can be found, even though they may not necessarily be labeled as a formal shaping process. For older children, for instance, learning a multifaceted and complex physical skill activity (e.g., ice skating, swimming, tennis, basketball, ballet dancing) or playing a musical instrument involves many sessions that use principles of shaping and successive approximation. (All of these skills have been included as therapy goals for children who have been treated with ACQUIREc therapy.) The child first learns a brand-new, often quite simple skill that gets practiced over and over, with monitoring and reinforcement from a coach, teacher, or parent, so it becomes more precise, stronger, faster, or more fluid and automatic. The child then extends the skill by a small step or adds a second component while continuing to practice and refine or integrate the first skill into a chain.

Children are encouraged to practice new skills very frequently, often with daily sessions, with lots of repetition. Over time, children become increasingly aware of the demands or standards for judging performance level and know that they will become more difficult to achieve. For children who train for the Olympics or for concert-level performance, it is not unusual to practice 4, 5, or 6 hours a day. These examples are not identical to the shaping that is used in ACQUIREc therapy, but they demonstrate that achieving high levels of performance for sensory–motor coordinated movement, even in children without neuromotor impairment, is likely to be easier using structured learning opportunities, training by an expert or mentor who can help a child realize increasingly higher levels of performance, and extensive shaping followed by massed practice until a behavior that initially was difficult to achieve becomes almost easy.

MASSED PRACTICE

Massed practice occurs after shaping and consists of many frequent, closely spaced *trials,* or enactments of the behavior, skill, or movement that is being learned. Extensive research documents the clear benefits of massed practice and shaping for many types of learning. Most theories suggest that the engagement of the central nervous system is quite different when the neural pathways related to the behavior are elicited frequently and in close temporal proximity; this process is discussed in other chapters. The ideas behind shaping and massed practice were specifically built into the ACQUIREc therapy protocol. In the training protocol for ACQUIREc therapists, the elements of shaping and massed practice are combined and labeled the *MR3 Cycle.*

ACQUIREc MR3 CYCLE

The **MR3 Cycle** (DeLuca et al., 2007) provides a framework that specifies the repeated steps used to induce the acquisition of new movement and functional ability with the weaker arm and hand. The acronym *MR3* stands for the sequence of **M**ovement, immediate and direct **R**einforcement, **R**epetition, and **R**efinement of the movement. The MR3 Cycle (Figure 8.2) is designed to support rapid and secure acquisition of a functional ability, task, or skill involving the weaker arm and hand, either alone or in combination with the other UE.

The **movement** portion of the cycle includes one or more movements that are voluntary and involuntary. The idea is to reinforce any and every type of movement that the child exhibits with the impaired UE that might be a beginning basis for the specific target behavior being shaped. At times in the initial segment of treatment, some children are completely unaware of their impaired UE and exhibit almost no volitional movement. For these children, any type of movement with the impaired UE is reinforced immediately by the treating therapist.

Reinforcement is a driving force that serves to motivate and improve learning and persistence in a task. Receiving immediate reinforcement for efforts made, big or small, increases the likelihood that a child will repeat the positive behavior or movement. Reinforcement for UE movements in the MR3 Cycle is prompt and comes in two different forms, tangible and intangible.

Tangible reinforcement for younger children is provided in the form of small rewards for hard work such as food snacks, colorful stickers, or little toys or objects. (Therapists always communicate in advance with parents about acceptable and healthy food rewards and always consider the safety of reward toys and snacks.) Over the course of a 6-hour therapy session, variety in types of rewards is valuable. Pushing a button on a toy and experiencing the reinforcement of seeing lights or hearing sounds is another effective reward that links UE behavior with immediate consequences.

Tangible rewards for older children can be staged by allowing them to earn points for small successes and accumulate enough points to earn a much larger tangible reward. Using a point or token system for children who can understand this concept can be a big motivator. These points can be visibly represented by small objects, such as poker chips, or by a tally written on a board. Parents often provide a larger reward (such as a special toy or game) that the child can receive when a certain number of points or tokens has been earned. For many children, turning in their earned points for the choice of a favorite activity later in the treatment day is as highly motivating as an immediate physical reward.

Intangible reinforcement is just as important and is used far more frequently in ACQUIREc therapy than tangible rewards. Verbal praise and positive facial expressions are the most frequently delivered forms of intangible reward and are used regularly throughout the day as the child exhibits desirable behavior. Examples of verbal praise include "Good job," "You did it," "Awesome!" and so on. The type and extent of verbal praise depend on the age and cognitive level of the child. For older children, the therapist might say "Good job," followed by a brief explanation of how the child completed the task at a better-than-before level. This feedback is something older children enjoy hearing, and it provides encouragement for further efforts. For young children, hand clapping, a hug, and a big smile are valued forms of reinforcement. Intangible rewards also can come in the form of singing a favorite song, getting to watch a favorite television show after therapy, receiving a hug from a sibling or caregiver, or getting a high five or thumbs-up from the therapist or a family member.

Regardless of the reward type, consistency must be used in its application for the child to fully benefit from the

Figure 8.2   ACQUIREc THERAPY MOVEMENT, REINFORCEMENT, REPETITION, AND REFINEMENT (MR3) CYCLE.

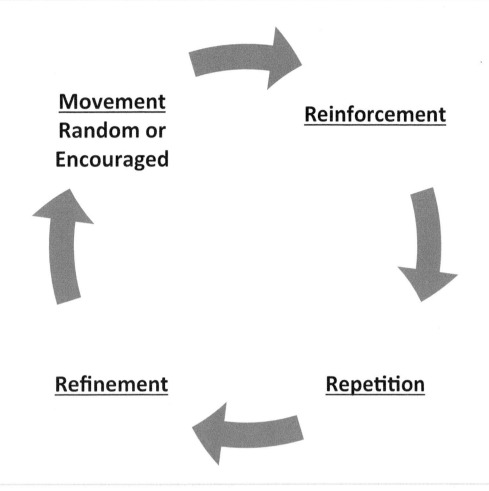

process. Part of building trust, and thus increasing the child's efforts in therapy, is to follow through with the rewards that are promised if the child consistently stays engaged and completes his or her portion of the work. It is important that reinforcement not be casual or given in a way that is not directly linked to behavior because it can confuse the child and usually is ineffective.

Repetition is a straightforward but powerful concept in the MR3 Cycle. The simple act of performing a movement or activity multiple times can lead to a great increase in a child's ability to perform a motor or functional skill or task. This concept applies to both very simple movements and very complex skills. Promoting the amount of repetition essential for progress requires creativity from the therapist because the attention of any child can change frequently throughout the day and throughout the activity. The therapist must be mindful of the child's level of attention and know when to end an activity or change it to maintain the child's attention and best efforts to achieve the maximum number of repetitions for the desired movement, skill, or task.

Each day, the therapist must choose certain movements or functional activities and determine different means of eliciting them in a manner that is fun, engaging, and challenging while remaining mindful of the importance of success for the child as the end result of any activity. Activities are chosen on the basis of the child's specific deficits, functional needs, and established therapeutic goals. A high rate of success is vital for a child, although moments of nonsuccess, frustration, or failed attempts are a natural part of the ACQUIREc therapy process. Encouragement to try again and demonstration, verbal guidance, and physical prompts to promote progress are companion behaviors that ACQUIREc therapists use with the MR3 Cycle. Maintaining the MR3 Cycle, which soon becomes familiar to the child over the 4 weeks of therapy, encourages the needed repetition and allows ample opportunities for the therapist and child to explore new and numerous movements en route to achieving success in functional UE activities. The goal is to reach the thresholds to construct a permanent movement and skill representation in the central nervous system.

Refinement, the third R in the MR3 Cycle, is implemented by the therapist throughout the ACQUIREc therapeutic process; it does not strictly follow repetition but rather typically occurs in the midst of repetition. An ACQUIREc therapist follows the general rule for shaping that once a child displays at least 75% to 80% proficiency, the challenge must be increased to continue to shape the child's emerging movements, behaviors, tasks, or skills. Because children are quick to adapt and often progress or develop at relatively fast rates, the therapist needs to be well prepared for the next levels for refinement for each therapy goal or type of functional activity. On occasion, the children surprise themselves and even the therapist by what they are able to do rapidly when given the opportunity, including the opportunity to problem solve and work through the learning process.

Although success is part of the end product, some struggle in the learning process is OK and sometimes necessary for the child to process what needs to be done. The final result still needs to be success, but if the child is determined to master a task, providing him or her the opportunity to do so in as independent a manner as possible is worthwhile. The internal sense of success is far greater for the child when the child can recognize variations and mistakes en route. Full implementation of the refinement portion of the MR3 Cycle requires the therapist to thoroughly understand the desired movement and functional activity so the child can be guided from one step to the next to increase his or her independence and success in the given movement or functional activity, often in very small and subtle ways.

Refinement should be implemented each day, but the amount of refinement on each particular day should be based on the ability and interest level of the child. It is important to share with parents that the child's ability may vary from one day to the next and that adapting activities to encourage success is very important. Newly emerging skills can fluctuate considerably, and the child may encounter small setbacks until he or she achieves much greater mastery and automaticity. (This is true for typically developing children as well as children with neuromotor impairments.) Shaping occurs not only within sessions for a particular child but also across days and multiple, interrelated tasks. When a therapist knows how tasks are similar and different in how they elicit particular movements, patterns of movements, skills, and behaviors, he or she is able to make modifications readily during the refinement phase.

Sample tasks are presented in Table 8.2, along with examples of how the MR3 Cycle is carried out within each movement, task, or skill. Each portion of the MR3 Cycle varies slightly depending on the child's age, developmental stage, level of ability, and motivating factors. In essence, almost the entire 6 hours of daily ACQUIREc therapy involve implementing the MR3 Cycle in bursts, with frequent shifts in what skills and activities are occurring.

Movements and Activities Used in ACQUIREc Therapy

Some common movements and patterns used to implement the MR3 Cycle on a clinical level are reaching, grasp–release of an object, and wrist extension. The targeted outcome of improving these movements through the MR3 Cycle is to increase the child's level of performance and self-initiation of voluntary UE behavior. Even though movement is a primary focus of the MR3 Cycle, functional activities are integral. For example, dressing is a primary functional skill almost all children practice during the MR3 Cycle. The movements involved in dressing are highly purposeful and must be appropriate for the child's current level.

Facilitation, Fading, and Modeling

The description of the MR3 Cycle and shaping may imply that progression in skills and tasks only occurs with independently initiated and volitional movements and skills accomplished by the child. However, therapists often use three well-known therapeutic techniques to assist in the shaping process:

1. **Hand-over-hand facilitation:** The therapist helps the child control the weaker UE by manually holding and manipulating the arm and hand to allow the child to accomplish the desired movement and function.
2. **Fading:** The therapist lessens the direct manual assistance he or she provides during a given task as the child demonstrates the ability to accomplish all or part of the task independently.
3. **Modeling:** The therapist shows exactly how he or she would like the child to accomplish the task. This demonstration is usually done side-by-side, with the same UE and orientation as the child, and is supported by clear verbal descriptions of what the therapist is doing.

Because ACQUIREc therapy was designed for implementation by licensed and highly experienced therapists, ACQUIREc therapists are able to readily and skillfully integrate these techniques with the MR3 Cycle. Throughout the cycle and during briefer play sessions, therapists also observe the child's UE task execution so that they can anticipate and minimize any compensatory movements that may cause later neuromotor or musculoskeletal problems secondary to these adaptations. Experience with parents who help extend the MR3 Cycles during nontherapy hours shows that they are unaware of many of the important and consequential aspects of body posture, alignment, and sequencing that ACQUIREc therapists routinely consider when they implement the therapy protocol with high fidelity. Case Examples 8.1 and 8.2 describe how these techniques are applied in ACQUIREc therapy.

Table 8.2 Examples of Applying the MR3 Cycle to Specific Therapy Goals

TARGET MOVEMENT	ACTIVITY TO CREATE REPETITION	REINFORCEMENT	WAYS TO REFINE MOVEMENT, SKILL, OR TASK
Reaching	Reach to be picked up Pop bubbles Turn light switch on and off Turn water on and off Activate toy Point to objects	Use verbal praise ("Good job!" "You did it!" "Yeah!") Activate a toy with lights or a song Provide a tangible reward (e.g., sticker)	Vary height for required reaching Vary location (e.g., below waist, across midline, shoulder height, above head) Vary assistance between verbal and physical cues Ask to reach without visual assistance (behind the head)
Grasp–release	Assemble large-knob puzzles Pick up and release animal figures, game pieces, or finger foods	Provide verbal praise Allow choice of object to grasp Save favorite toy or color for last grasp Play game after grasp of all pieces Provide favorite finger food to pick up	Vary size or weight of object Vary surface and height of grasp–release items Request use of various grasp types (tripod, pincer)
Wrist extension	Spread shaving cream on window or other vertical surface Close door, drawers, or cabinet with palmar surface of hand Scoop beans into container; vary angle of scoop to elicit extension Grasp–release magnets from a vertical magnetic surface Stabilize forearm and lift wrist as high as possible Go on a treasure hunt and bend over to grasp items	Allow choice of pictures or words to spell with shaving cream on window Hide favorite toy to find in drawer, then close to hide additional toys Hide motivating toys in beans to scoop; guess how many scoops to fill bucket or cover a favorite toy Play a spelling game or spell friends' names Use fun magnets Lift wrist up to touch favorite toy or favorite object Search motivating toys; let child take turn hiding toys	Vary verbal and physical cues Change angle of toy or working surface to require increased wrist extension Include grasp of smaller objects with combination of wrist extension

DEVELOPING A FULL-DAY INDIVIDUALIZED TREATMENT PROGRAM

When developing an individualized ACQUIREc therapy plan, the therapist considers the ability of the child at the beginning of the program and then blends in issues associated with the child's age and cognitive development, child and parent goals, and any unique considerations. With all children, the therapist uses the standard professional therapy techniques of shaping, facilitation, fading, massed practice, reinforcement, and cueing (verbal and tactile) throughout the day. General treatment activities for each day include stretching, sensory awareness, weight bearing, gross motor activities, fine motor activities, functional activities, and caregiver education (including a home program). During the 6-hour therapy sessions, the ACQUIREc therapist constantly adapts and changes to meet the needs and maintain the enthusiasm of the child, always seeking to find the just-right challenge. (See Chapter 7, "Operationalizing Pediatric CIMT: Guidelines for Transforming Basic Principles and Scientific Evidence Into Clinical Practice for Individual Children," for clinical suggestions about treatment and UE activities suitable for children of different ages; these apply to both the signature and modified forms of P–CIMT and are strongly endorsed in DeLuca and colleagues' [2007] ACQUIREc manual.)

Case Example

ACQUIREc THERAPY PROTOCOL SCENARIO: 1-YEAR-OLD CHILD WORKING ON TOY ACTIVATION

With a **1-year-old child,** the therapist holds up a fun musical toy and models the desired behavior by reaching and activating the toy in a way that is possible for the child to achieve. If the child does not readily imitate, the therapist offers verbal encouragement to try. If successive demonstrations and verbal prompts do not result in the child trying to activate the toy, then the therapist lifts the child's arm and uses the technique of hand-over-hand facilitation so the child can experience activating the toy. This facilitation is combined with a verbal cue such as "Arm up and hit it!" As soon as the facilitated effort results in any effort by the child—on his or her own—to activate the toy, the therapist reinforces the child with big smiles, clapping, and praise. The process is then repeated many times, with very brief rests between repetitions to allow the therapist to note if the child makes any self-initiated movement (no matter how small) toward the toy.

Note. UE = upper extremity.

Sometimes the therapist completes the child's partial efforts by activating the toy's sound so that the child clearly understands the cause-and-effect relationship. As the efforts progress, the therapist does not continue this completion on all trials but offers immediate reinforcement for all correct UE movements the child makes. Sometimes the therapist varies the activity, making it easier or more difficult (as part of successive approximations) to keep the child interested. Often, the therapist and child add their own sounds or variations in how the toy is used to build UE competence.

For very young children, activities that naturally provide immediate sensory consequences are highly successful and entertaining. Other examples include reaching out to pop soap bubbles, splashing during water play, and knocking over towers of blocks.

USING NATURAL ENVIRONMENTS

One of the most important reasons for success in implementing the high-intensity ACQUIREc protocol is that it is not conducted in a limited or artificial clinical setting. Therapists go to the child's everyday environments, including home, motel, or apartment; child care or child development center; grandparents' home; the playground; the zoo; a store; a restaurant; and the doctor's office. For some periods of the day, the therapist and child work alone quietly in a room, but just as often they are in busier places with other people and many distractions. This practice embeds the child's learning in the full range of places where he or she will be using the newly acquired skills after therapy ends.

Therapists and children adapt to therapy, and the MR3 Cycles unfold in a way that is not embarrassing to the children or intrusive to others. Many times, parents and other families join in, although not for the entire day. This emphasis on the child's natural environment brings a different feel to the therapy environment than that experienced in most clinical settings. For the child, therapy seems less invasive, as if another adult (a highly supportive and playful one!) has simply come into the child's life and is offering directions and new opportunities and experiences. Most children are accustomed

to adults directing them to some degree, especially when they are learning about new things. However, ACQUIREc therapy entails constant concentration on using the impaired arm and hand to improve function. The ACQUIREc 6-hour therapy protocol usually requires the therapist to be on the job for at least 7, and sometimes 8, hours for young children who have rest and nap times. In other words, the 6-hour dosage is for active therapy, not just being with the child. Any breaks or interruptions are not counted as part of the therapeutic dosage but qualify as needed professional time and clinical monitoring to deliver the full dosage.

PHASE 3: ACQUIREc POSTTHERAPY TRANSFER PACKAGE

In the first RCT of P–CIMT (Taub et al., 2004), the researchers did not systematically apply a bilateral transfer package for all children. In 2002, the PNRC added the bilateral phase as an integral, formal part of ACQUIREc therapy. This addition addressed the request of numerous parents for assistance in helping their children better integrate their newly acquired skills into daily life, which the therapists had already begun to

Case Example

ACQUIREc THERAPY PROTOCOL SCENARIO:
5-YEAR-OLD CHILD WORKING ON SELF-FEEDING WITH A UTENSIL

A **5-year-old girl** who can already feed herself with utensils is challenged by now eating using her hemiparetic arm and hand. Meals are incorporated into her ACQUIREc therapy each day. Casting has an immediate and strong effect on the child's ability to self-feed, so almost all children can benefit from snack and mealtime practice with their weaker UE. The therapist recognizes that the child is not likely to shift to the weaker UE as the primary arm and hand for eating after therapy ends, but this practice is a highly effective way to have the child learn and use a wide variety of refined arm, wrist, hand, and finger movements multiple times throughout the 4-week treatment period. Many meal-related behaviors have both UEs participating in different ways, and these behaviors can be practiced during the final 3 therapy sessions after the cast is removed. At first, children may show mild frustration related to eating and drinking, but they find this set of MR3 Cycles to be highly successful, fun, and varied.

The use of nonadapted (i.e., regular) spoons and forks is recommended whenever possible. At first, the therapist may use hand-over-hand facilitation to enable the child to initially grip the handle, raise the elbow, make scooping or stabbing motions, and bring the food to her mouth. The therapist explains verbally the movements

Note. UE = upper extremity.

that are needed to accomplish part of this multiphase task, for example, "Make sure you hold on tight with your grip," "Lift your elbow" (which helps many children succeed before they can later isolate just the wrist and hand motions used in eating), or "Turn your hand to scoop." The therapist also models using the utensil, but during actual feeding, the therapist tries to facilitate the child's ability to successfully eat and enjoy the food. As treatment progresses and the therapist notices skills developing in the child, he or she fades the assistance. Sometimes for children with very low ability to use a utensil at first, the meal can permit some finger feeding with utensils and still work to improve some general movements.

The therapist also uses observational skills and provides anticipatory guidance verbally, such as "Keep holding on tightly to your spoon," followed by "Great!" if the child does not loosen the grip or drop the spoon. Skilled pediatric therapists often use a variety of tactile cues in a timely way, such as gently tapping the child's elbow to help the child remember to lift while raising the spoonful of food to the mouth. Similarly, if the child gains the ability to scoop or stab with the utensil, the therapist fades assistance from direct facilitation with the hand to manipulation of the utensil only as an assist.

---

do in the last few days of the 20- or 21-day treatment protocol and in their posttreatment planning with families.

After children have acquired new and improved skills with their involved weaker UE, they can benefit from systematic shaping and practice to use these unilateral skills in their everyday execution of bilateral tasks. This phase is similar to the practice in piano lessons of first alternating between practice with the right and then the left hand, then combining the hands, and then returning to more advanced unimanual practice. Other repetitive task activities in which a similar process is used include playing tennis, basketball, and the drums, all of which have been used as ACQUIREc therapy activities. Children recognize that the same task is easier to perform with one hand than the other, thus they understand why they need to spend more time trying to improve their skill with the nondominant or more-impaired arm and hand. Further, many bilateral activities are included in the earlier phase of ACQUIREc therapy, even while the child is wearing the full-arm cast.

In the final 3 days of ACQUIREc, the therapist provides 18 hours of formal therapy with a central focus on using both arms and hands by continuing to demonstrate, shape, and practice while the child is engaged in bilateral tasks. This period is a natural time to remind the child of the progress he or she has made, perhaps by going back to an earlier activity the child worked on and showing how that skill has other uses. During this phase, the theme of ACQUIREc therapy—that the child is the active agent in (rather than the passive recipient of) therapy—surfaces very strongly. In addition, after 4 weeks, the therapist and child have formed a warm, reciprocal relationship that prepares the child for a positive transition to life without 6 hours of therapy and without spending almost every day with their own full-time therapist–playmate.

Home and school follow-up programs are very important in helping children maintain the benefits of ACQUIREc therapy. Many therapists were skeptical about how well children and families would follow a posttherapy plan. These plans have met with remarkable success with most, but not all, families, perhaps because of the high levels of investment the parents and children had already made and the tremendous progress they observed in a relatively short time. Thus, at the end of therapy, parents and children are highly motivated to think about how to maintain these gains and even improve on their progress.

The ACQUIREc posttherapy transfer package has two components: (1) a long list of specific tasks for parents and caregivers to continue working on after completing ACQUIREc and (2) written descriptions and demonstrations of the specific ways parents can help the child use his or her impaired arm and hand in everyday life. Therapists talk with the parents and, when appropriate, the children about everyday life. Families talk about current and future functional tasks appropriate for using the impaired arm and hand in a practice or strengthening mode.

For example, if a child's favorite dessert is frozen yogurt, the therapist might suggest that the parents require the child to use his or her weaker arm or hand when eating this treat. Another example is to require the child to open the drawer where his or her socks are kept using the impaired hand (sometimes using a visual reminder cue on the drawer). Therapists also ask parents to identify toys or computer games that are appropriate to designate for playing with the weaker arm and hand. These suggestions are provided in conjunction with behavioral guidelines to ensure that the rules surrounding use of the child's impaired arm and hand are nonnegotiable and consistently implemented (as in any positive behavioral program) and that the choices are realistic for the parent to implement on a daily basis, perhaps with help from other caregivers or family members.

Above all, the child is often the one who is most highly motivated to continue improving, which creates a strong beginning point for the posttherapy program. Parent rewards can, of course, be used, but these need to be selective and realistic. With the increasing availability of electronic devices, such as smart phones and tablets, that have videorecording capacity, parents and children can send evidence of progress to and seek feedback from ACQUIREc therapists, who can directly see the progress a child is making. Similarly, a therapist can send video examples to the family about new and more complex behaviors to focus on once the original transfer program is fulfilled.

DAILY DOCUMENTATION OF ACQUIREc

From the founding of the PNRC, the therapists made a commitment to high levels of documentation of ACQUIREc therapy for every child. In part, this effort supports the research mission of the clinic, but over the years, the therapists

have come to see that systematic and required documentation contributes the following benefits:

- Ability to supervise ACQUIREc therapists on the basis of detailed information about their behavior and their observations of each child
- Maintenance of high standards at the clinic because all therapists, and not just newly trained ones, know that documentation is part of their job description and that each treatment epoch will be carefully reviewed in real time (not just once every 6 or 12 months)
- Ability to provide evidence of their accrued knowledge that certain activities and approaches appear to work better with some children than with others, something that can happen only when consistent documentation is available on all children (as opposed to relying on clinical anecdotes and impressions alone).

Providing detailed documentation was not something that therapists initially embraced with enthusiasm. However, this requirement was made part of their 8-hour workday, with about 7 hours dedicated to being with the child and 30 to 45 minutes set aside for completing the daily log. Therapists thus feel compensated for this activity and understand how it helps fulfill the clinic's commitment that all children receive the high-quality, consistent form of ACQUIREc therapy for which families are paying. Another benefit is that the therapists themselves rely on these daily logs to be sure they are not overlooking any treatment components or goals they and the families have set. These logs facilitate the sharing of innovative ideas and problem solutions with other therapists and have prompted new research questions to be pursued in systematic study. Appendix 8.A, which is also on the flash drive included with this handbook, is the template for systematic documentation of ACQUIREc therapy and also is well suited for use with other forms of P–CIMT.

LESSONS LEARNED FROM CLINICAL EXPERIENCE IMPLEMENTING ACQUIREc THERAPY

The most important lesson from clinical experience at PNRC is that the signature form of P–CIMT can be effectively implemented in an ongoing, full-time clinical practice in a manner that produces similar types and magnitude of benefits for children and with a strong business model that can support its operations. Historically, clinical implementation of many efficacious intervention protocols has been highly variable, with many examples of failure to produce the high levels of benefits anticipated. This phenomenon is particularly true in areas such as preschool educational interventions and home-based visiting programs to improve parenting and child outcomes; RCTs have yielded great benefits, but community programs

Table 8.3 Comparison of Clinical Results With RCT Results

STUDY AND MEASURES	PRETREATMENT MEAN SCORE *(SD)*	POSTTREATMENT MEAN SCORE *(SD)*	CHANGE SCORE FROM PRE- TO POSTTREATMENT
RCT crossover study (DeLuca, Echols, Law, & Ramey, 2006)			
PMAL Quality of Use score	0.90 (0.62)	2.70 (0.97)	1.90
PMAL Frequency of Use score	0.80 (0.44)	2.80 (1.14)	2.00
EBS score	12.20 (5.64)	21.50 (4.45)	9.30
Clinic results			
PMAL Quality of Use score	0.99 (0.84)	2.89 (0.99)	1.90
PMAL Frequency of Use score	0.73 (0.52)	3.19 (1.16)	2.40
EBS score	9.98 (5.02)	20.91 (3.83)	10.93

Note. EBS = Emerging Behaviors Scale; PMAL = Pediatric Motor Activity Log; RCT = randomized controlled trial; SD = standard deviation.

have shown few or no detectable benefits (cf. Ramey, Sparling, & Ramey, 2012; Ramey & Ramey, 2007). Often, careful delivery of professional development or supplemental individualized training for professionals is needed to achieve high levels of fidelity in implementing programs in real-world settings (e.g., Ramey & Ramey, 2007).

Table 8.3 presents data from the first 3 years of clinical cases that enable comparison of the results with the first rigorous clinical trial sample using scores on the Emerging Behaviors Scale (EBS; DeLuca et al., 2007; Taub et al., 2004), which records the number of brand-new skills (from a list of 31) the child has displayed in two or more settings, and average parent ratings on the Pediatric Motor Activity Log, which asks how often and how well a child completes several age-appropriate tasks (Taub et al., 2004). The clinical sample included more children with a much wider age range than the original RCT of 2- to 6-year-olds and had some children with more severe and milder forms of initial UE impairment. Remarkably, the results are almost identical. (Neither the therapists nor the parents knew that these direct comparisons would be made.) For example, in the RCT, the children had a pretherapy mean of 12.2 of 31 skills on EBS, which increased to 21.5 skills post therapy. Children served by the clinic over the next decade had a pretherapy mean of 9.9 skills, which rose to 20.9 post therapy. Thus, the clinic sample displayed a greater magnitude of benefit than the sample of the originally published rigorous research trial.

Similarly, both the frequency of use and quality of movement of the UE, as rated by parents, showed large increases of almost identical magnitude for both the RCT study group and the clinical sample. On a scale of 0 to 4, parents in the research and clinic samples rated their children at 0.8 and 0.7, respectively, before therapy; at posttherapy, the corresponding ratings increased to 2.8 and 3.2. These results represent a

large effect size and meaningful everyday gains. Figure 8.3 displays the gain scores for the two groups on these measures. Researchers now routinely use many other assessments with the clinical sample, but some of the psychometrically robust tools, such as the Assisting Hand Assessment (Krumlinde-Sundholm, Holmefur, Kottorp, & Eliasson, 2007), were not yet available in 1999 when this research began.

In all of the research studies on ACQUIREc, the 6-month maintenance levels remained high; unfortunately, longer-term outcome data for the clinical population were not systematically obtained, primarily because most of the clinic children were from out of town (including foreign countries). Researchers have now had experience in providing repeated epochs of ACQUIREc (a topic discussed in general in Chapter 7, "Operationalizing Pediatric CIMT: Guidelines for Transforming Basic Principles and Scientific Evidence Into Clinical Practice for Individual Children"), and assessment data from a self-selected subgroup of returning children indicate that they have experienced relatively good levels of maintenance, although because they are older and thus acquiring new skills, making direct comparisons about maintenance can be challenging (see Chapter 16, "Research Priorities: Understanding and Transcending the Limits of Current Knowledge to Inform Best Practices in Pediatric CIMT," for a more detailed discussion of the need for future research related to assessment methods).

SUMMARY

One form of traditional or signature P–CIMT, ACQUIREc therapy, consists of high levels of constraint use throughout the day and night and 6 hours of daily therapy involving formal reinforcement and shaping procedures in natural

Figure 8.3 COMPARISON OF GAIN SCORES (POSTTHERAPY MINUS PRETHERAPY) FOR CLINICAL AND RESEARCH SAMPLES RECEIVING ACQUIREc TREATMENT.

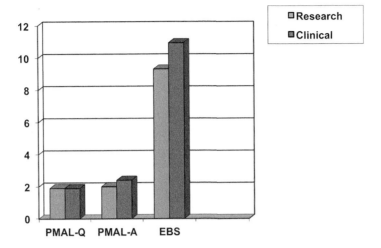

Note. EBS = Emerging Behaviors Scale; PMAL–A = Pediatric Motor Activity Log Amount of Use subscale; PMAL–Q = Pediatric Motor Activity Log Quality of Movement subscale.

environments, administered by licensed and highly qualified therapists trained to implement the criteria in the therapy protocol. Research has demonstrated that this therapy is feasible for use in clinical and community settings, that it can be replicated in other sites, and that it can produce remarkably equivalent types and amounts of benefits. Evidence obtained from detailed clinical therapy logs and pre- and posttherapy assessment data affirms that this form of pediatric rehabilitation has shown the following:

- High levels of acceptability by parents, children, and referring physicians and therapists
- Virtually no negative side effects or dropout because of the intensity of the 4-week treatment or the use of full-arm, full-time constraint for 18 consecutive days
- Significant and multiple benefits for a wide age and ability range of children, with very few children (several with many and severe comorbid conditions and one with severe dystonia) classified as low-level responders
- High levels of job satisfaction among ACQUIREc therapists despite very demanding work schedules (most ACQUIREc full-time therapists provide a 4-week therapy program to about 9 to 11 children per calendar year; the PNRC tries to stagger treatment sessions so that one therapist is available as a backup each week to help with any urgent conditions and with casting or assessment, if needed)
- Increasing success in receiving reimbursement from third-party payers for this high-intensity treatment on

the basis of scientific evidence the clinic and parents provide to insurance companies.

ACQUIREc is not the only form of P–CIMT treatment and may not be the best for all children. We look forward to an era when therapists will know more about how to combine traditional and modified forms of P–CIMT into a much larger plan to support a child's development from infancy to and through adulthood, taking advantage of other evidence-based medical and educational practices appropriate for many of the children diagnosed with hemiparesis. First and foremost, we see each child as a "total child," whose quality of life and positive engagement in the full range of functional occupations are the shared goals of parents, therapists, other clinicians, educators, and the child.

REFERENCES

Bijou, S. W., & Baer, D. M. (1961). *Child development I: A systematic and empirical theory.* New York: Appleton-Century-Crofts.

Blanton, S., Wilsey, H., & Wolf, S. L. (2008). Constraint-induced movement therapy in stroke rehabilitation: Perspectives on future clinical applications. *NeuroRehabilitation, 23,* 15–28.

Case-Smith, J., DeLuca, S. C., Stevenson, R., & Ramey, S. L. (2012). Multicenter randomized controlled trial of pediatric constraint-induced movement therapy: 6-month follow-up. *American Journal of Occupational Therapy, 66,* 15–23. http://dx.doi.org/10.5014/ajot.2012.002386

DeLuca, S. C., Case-Smith, J., Stevenson, R., & Ramey, S. L. (2012). Constraint-induced movement therapy (CIMT) for young children with cerebral palsy: Effects of therapeutic dosage. *Journal of Pediatric Rehabilitation Medicine, 5,* 133–142. http://dx.doi.org/10.3232/prm-2012-0206

DeLuca, S. C., Echols, K., Law, C. R., & Ramey, S. L. (2006). Intensive pediatric constraint-induced therapy for children with cerebral palsy: Randomized, controlled, crossover trial. *Journal of Child Neurology, 21,* 931–938. PMID: 17092457

DeLuca, S. C., Echols, K., & Ramey, S. L. (2007). *ACQUIREc therapy: A training manual for effective application of pediatric constraint-induced movement therapy.* Hillsborough, NC: MindNurture.

DeLuca, S., Echols, K., Ramey, S. L., & Taub, E. (2003). Pediatric constraint-induced movement therapy for a young child with cerebral palsy: Two episodes of care. *Physical Therapy, 83,* 1003–1013.

Echols, K., DeLuca, S., Ramey, S., & Taub, E. (2001). Constraint-induced movement therapy in the child with cerebral palsy. In Proceedings of the American Academy of Cerebral Palsy and Developmental Medicine. *Developmental Medicine and Child Neurology, 43*(Suppl.), 37.

Echols, K., DeLuca, S. C., Taub, E., & Ramey, S. (2001). Constraint-induced movement therapy in young children: A protocol and outcomes compared to traditional measures. *Pediatric Physical Therapy, 12,* 210.

Krumlinde-Sundholm, L., Holmefur, M., Kottorp, A., & Eliasson, A. C. (2007). The Assisting Hand Assessment: Current evidence of validity, reliability, and responsiveness to change. *Developmental Medicine and Child Neurology, 49*(4), 259–264.

Ramey, C. T., Sparling, J. J., & Ramey, S. L. (2012). *Abecedarian: The ideas, the approach, and the findings.* Los Altos, CA: Sociometrics Corporation.

Ramey, S. L., & Ramey, C. T. (1999). Early experience and early intervention for children "at risk" for developmental delay and mental retardation. *Mental Retardation and Developmental Disabilities Research Reviews, 5,* 1–10.

Ramey, S. L., & Ramey, C. T. (2007). Establishing a science of professional development for early education programs: The Knowledge Application Information Systems (KAIS) theory of professional development. In L. M. Justice & C. Vukelich (Eds.), *Achieving excellence in preschool language and literacy instruction* (pp. 41–63). New York: Guilford Press.

Skinner, B. F. (1953). *Science and human behavior.* New York: Free Press.

Taub, E., Ramey, S. L., DeLuca, S. C., & Echols, K. (2004). Efficacy of constraint-induced (CI) movement therapy for children with cerebral palsy. *Pediatrics, 113,* 305–312.

APPENDIX 8.A. DAILY THERAPY LOG FOR P–CIMT

Purpose: The P–CIMT daily therapy log serves as a guide for the therapist to document what occurred and to record observations about new emerging skills and progress the child makes, any difficulties or challenges that arise (that may require problem solving with the child, parents, or other professionals), and approximate time spent on shaping and repetitive practice. The first page is a summary of the session that the therapist completes soon after the P–CIMT session. The second page provides a standard format for documenting activities as they occur during the session. (*Note:* This form is well suited for use in an electronic format for a handheld or tablet device that can automatically record the time for starting and ending of discrete activities. Electronic devices can help provide useful supplemental material via photographs and brief videos that display progress the child demonstrates during the session.)

Child _____ Therapist _____

Start time _____ End time _____

Location(s) for therapy today _____

1. Overall rating of child engagement on a 4-point scale (1 = *very low,* 4 = *very high*) ___

2. Did any problems or challenges arise? If yes, describe these and how they were addressed. If follow-up is needed, indicate plans and assignment of responsibility.

_____
_____
_____

3. Was the parent or caregiver present during the treatment session? No___ Yes___ If yes, for how long? _____

4. Rate the level of parent or caregiver involvement (1 = *very low,* 4 = *very high*). Provide additional observations or ideas for follow-up with family, if appropriate.

_____

5. Were there any breaks or times when no therapy was provided? No ___Yes ___
If yes, describe what happened and approximate time when therapy was not provided. Indicate if the session was extended to compensate for any lost therapy time.

_____

6. Check which therapy goals were worked on today. (*Note:* For each child, a list of therapy goals is inserted here. When goals change, additions are noted and included here.)

Goal 1. _____

Goal 2. _____

Goal 3. _____

Goal 4. _____

Goal 5. _____

(Add other goals as necessary.) _____

7. Other comments or observations related to today's session _____

_____

(Continued)

Developed by Sharon L. Ramey, Mary Rebekah Trucks, Dory Ainsworth Wallace, and Stephanie DeLuca, Virginia Tech Carilion Research Institute Neuromotor Research Clinic. Used with permission.

DAILY ACTIVITY LOG

Instructions: For each session, complete this log to document activities in the order in which they occurred. Typically, the P–CIMT therapist takes a brief 1-min break to jot down notes and record times in the transition between activities.

Activity #__

Type of activity and location: _____
_____

Component movements or skills being worked on: _____
_____
_____

Observations about child progress, emerging skills, and any problems or difficulties encountered: _____
_____
_____

Approximate time spent on this activity: _____ min

Describe shaping details: _____
_____
_____
_____

Approximate proportion of session spent in shaping: _____min

Approximate time spent and/or number of repetitions completed: _____

Reinforcers used: _____
_____

Activity #__

Type of activity and location: _____
_____

Component movements or skills being worked on: _____
_____
_____

Observations about child progress, emerging skills, and any problems or difficulties encountered: _____
_____
_____

Approximate time spent on this activity: _____ min

Describe shaping details: _____
_____
_____
_____

Approximate proportion of session spent in shaping: _____min

Approximate time spent and/or number of repetitions completed: _____

Reinforcers used: _____
_____

(Note: Use duplicates of this page to document additional activities in this therapy session.)

PATTY COKER-BOLT, PhD, OTR/L; TERESSA GARCIA REIDY, MS, OTR/L; and ERIN NABER, PT, DPT

9

Alternative Pediatric CIMT: Understanding the How and Why of Clinical Variations in Pediatric CIMT

CHAPTER HIGHLIGHTS

- Background
- Modified treatment protocols
- Modification of the treatment environment.

This chapter discusses the differences between signature pediatric constraint-induced movement therapy (P–CIMT) and modified P–CIMT (mP–CIMT) and provides an overview of the evidence that supports the use of modified approaches for children with unilateral motor dysfunction. Subsequent chapters provide a deeper discussion of mP–CIMT approaches in the home, school, clinic, and camp-based environments.

BACKGROUND

Recent systematic reviews of P–CIMT help define the differences between signature forms of CIMT and modified approaches to this intensive therapy approach (Brady & Garcia, 2009; Hoare, Imms, Carey, & Wasiak, 2007; Huang, Fetters, Hale, & McBride, 2009). Constraint therapy provides several components that are packaged together to maximize rehabilitation efforts. The unique aspects of constraint therapy need to be considered, even in modified approaches. Modified CIMT approaches provide the essential elements of traditional CIMT, including restraint of the stronger unaffected upper extremity (UE); concentrated, massed practice of specific motor activities; and

KEY TERMS

Constraining glove
Continuous casting
Developmental disregard
Forced use
Intermittent constraint
Learned nonuse
Massed practice
Modified pediatric CIMT
Shaping
Signature, or traditional, pediatric CIMT

shaping of more-mature motor movement. The overall aim of both traditional P–CIMT and mP–CIMT is to reverse **developmental disregard** or **learned nonuse** of the affected extremity in children with unilateral motor weakness. *Developmental disregard* and *learned nonuse* refer to the process by which children with unilateral motor weakness learn to perform tasks primarily using their noninvolved or stronger arm while engaging in minimal to no use of the involved or weaker arm.

Systematic reviews of the published literature on CIMT highlight the similarities and differences between traditional and modified approaches. **Signature, or traditional, CIMT** has been defined as restraint of the unaffected upper limb combined with more than 3 hours of therapy per day (Brady & Garcia, 2009; Hoare et al., 2007; Huang et al., 2009). Massed practice and shaping of more-mature motor movement are provided for at least 2 consecutive weeks (14 to 21 days) by a professional with an understanding of rehabilitation techniques to improve motor function. In **massed practice,** the child performs many repetitions of the same or a highly similar behavior within a concentrated continuous time (i.e., high density of repetition with minimal rest intervals between repetitions). **Shaping** consists of a combination of strategies to prompt, reinforce, and continuously refine and improve behavior. Shaping for a given type of UE movement or skill begins with a functional behavioral assessment of both the task and the child's initial level of performance.

In contrast, **mP–CIMT** has been defined as restraint of the stronger unaffected upper limb combined with less than 3 hours per day of therapy involving specific motor task practice and shaping of the weaker affected UE by a professional with an understanding of rehabilitation techniques to improve motor function (Brady & Garcia, 2009; Hoare et al., 2007; Huang et al., 2009). Although the dosage of intensive task practice provided in an mP–CIMT program is probably the largest difference between it and signature P–CIMT, modified approaches also may differ in the type of restraint used, the environment in which the intervention is completed, or the person providing the motor skill practice. **Forced use** is defined as restraint of the stronger unaffected upper limb with no additional treatment of the affected upper limb, meaning that the cast itself is applied without regard to a plan for specific motor task practice or intensive therapy by a rehabilitation specialist.

mP–CIMTprograms provide the essential elements of the signature form of P–CIMT but may differ slightly in the provision of these components. The following sections provide a broad overview of the current research on mP–CIMT programs and highlight the variations in treatment protocols and therapeutic environments that have been studied.

MODIFIED TREATMENT PROTOCOLS

Current studies on mP–CIMT approaches highlight differences in treatment intervention protocols, which vary greatly, particularly in relation to the intensity of treatment and the duration of the program (i.e., *dosage*). The strongest support for the use of mP–CIMT approaches is provided by studies with randomized controlled trials (Aarts, Jongerius, Geerdink, van Limbeek, & Geurts, 2010; Boyd et al., 2010; Charles, Wolf, Schneider, & Gordon, 2006; de Brito Brandão, Mancini, Vaz, Pereira de Melo, & Fonseca, 2010; Eliasson, Krumlinde-Sundholm, Shaw, & Wang, 2005). These studies have explored the use of mP–CIMT approaches in children aged 2 to 16 years in a variety of treatment settings, including home, school, and camp programs. The type of restraint has included a cast, sling, or mitt.

In addition, the dosage of mP–CIMT has varied from several hours a day over several weeks to a few hours a day over several months. Many other published case studies and cohort trials on the use of mP–CIMT approaches have reported positive outcomes. However, limitations of several of these studies include small sample size or lack of randomization of participants to treatment or control groups. It is not clear what intensity of task practice and duration of mP–CIMT therapy are required to overcome learned nonuse.

Again, effective P–CIMT is a package of rehabilitation techniques that are used to maximize rehabilitation efforts. Before selecting an mP–CIMT treatment protocol, several factors should be considered, including dosage, type of constraint, age of the child, and treatment providers.

DOSAGE

Although the dosage, or intensity and duration, at which shaping and practice is provided to the child varies greatly in the literature, the essential component of concentrated practice in the weaker affected extremity is maintained. Signature P–CIMT involves approximately 6 hours of daily practice, 5 to 6 days per week, for 21 days (DeLuca, Echols, Law, & Ramey, 2006; Taub et al., 2007). Many times, mP–CIMT programs reduce the intensity of practice each day from 6 hours but may extend the program to more than 21 days. The intensity of shaping and practice in published mP–CIMT studies has varied widely in reported studies to meet the unique needs of the children enrolled in each mP–CIMT program (Huang et al., 2009). Authors of several published studies justified variations in duration of constraint and intensity of treatment as being necessary to create a "child-friendly" intervention, adjust to limitations in practitioner time, or fit the demands of the clinical treatment environment. The amount of time spent wearing a restraint on the stronger, nonaffected UE varied notably (e.g., 1 hour per day for 30 days, dosage = 30 hours; Coker, Lebkicher, Harris, & Snape, 2009) to 2 hours per day for 60 days (dosage = 60 hours; Eliasson et al., 2005; Eliasson, Shaw, Berg, & Krumlinde-Sundholm, 2011). The number of hours of formal repetitive task practice has ranged from 1 hour per day (Coker et al., 2009) to 3 hours per day (Charles & Gordon, 2005; Dickerson & Brown, 2007; Eliasson et al., 2005, 2011), depending on the age of the child and environment. The effective dosage provided in an mP–CIMT program that has been shown to change motor patterns has ranged from 30 hours to 124 hours.

Several reasons have been stated for why this level of intensity may not be ideal for all client populations, including age, cognitive ability, affected hand skills, educational needs, and family support (Brady & Garcia, 2009; Huang et al., 2009). The shortest reported mP–CIMT program lasted 5 consecutive days, during which children were engaged in task practice 6 hours each day (dosage = 30 hours; Coker, Karakostas, Dodds, & Hsiang, 2010), and the longest lasted 30 weeks (Miller & Hale, 2005). Others have reported a hybrid approach with partial CIMT and bimanual training (Aarts et al., 2010) or a gradual reduction in constraint-wearing schedule and treatment intensity in a multiphase model (Fergus et al., 2008).

One reason for modifying the duration of repetitive task practice is to accommodate the child's level of functioning. For example, to decrease frustration in a child with poor hand use, Eliasson and colleagues (2005) suggested reducing treatment time to 1 to 2 hours of daily practice. Because of structural and functional limitations, creating opportunities and presenting enticing activities for massed practice may be difficult for such children (Eliasson et al., 2005). In their study, Eliasson and colleagues reported that tailoring activities to suit each child's level of function while in turn considering his or her current functional abilities led to study participants reporting minimal frustration with the experience. Reduction in treatment hours also may limit fatigue for participants and, in turn, minimize their frustration (Assis, Massaro, Chamlian, Silva, & Ota, 2007; Gordon et al., 2007).

Modification of treatment duration could be beneficial for clients with impairments such as traumatic brain injury (Karman, Maryles, Baker, Simpser, & Berger-Gross, 2003; Miller & Hale, 2005) or hemispherectomy (de Bode, Fritz, Weir-Haynes, & Mathern, 2009) who may have cognitive limitations, increased fatigue, medication side effects, impaired emotional states, or behavioral concerns. de Bode and colleagues concluded that a 3-hour intervention model was optimal for clients with chronic UE dysfunction secondary to hemispherectomy. They suggested that reducing the duration of daily treatment mitigated boredom, fatigue, and frustration

secondary to diminished mental capacity and psychological disabilities.

Both mP–CIMT and traditional P–CIMT can require a large time commitment from families. Karman and colleagues (2003) noted,

> Young people present unique challenges to the goal of constant constraining and six hours per day of shaping activities. Children attend school, children should play and socialize, and younger children cannot be expected to perform tedious tasks for long periods. (p. 261)

To accommodate school-age children, some mP–CIMT protocols have been shortened to allow them to be carried out in the summer months, during school holidays, or after school (de Bode et al., 2009; Gordon et al., 2007; Martin, Burtner, Poole, & Phillips, 2008) to minimize disruption in the children's education. A shorter treatment duration may allow access to services for families traveling from rural areas; shorter durations of therapy can allow them to travel and stay for the intervention (Martin et al., 2008). Miller and Hale (2005) and Eliasson and colleagues (2011) described school-based models that modified the intensity of treatment to accommodate the school schedule.

For younger children who are not yet in school, a shorter, structured intervention and constraint time with prolonged duration of intervention may be beneficial and address their continued developmental changes in skill (Fergus et al., 2008). To accommodate their sleep–wake cycles, developmentally appropriate activity levels, and repertoire of play skills, the intensity of intervention constraint for young toddlers could be modified to 1 to 2 hours per day at home and in the clinic (Coker et al., 2009).

As children age, daily activities and play demands change. As growth occurs, motor skills and tone change. Different types of treatment throughout development could be considered and have shown to be beneficial (Charles & Gordon, 2007). A counterargument is that a minimal threshold of treatment intensity may exist. With a modified approach, the client does not receive as much training, which may not maximize client time, functional potential, or therapy visits. Further studies should examine a dosage–response threshold to determine the appropriate length of treatment (Case-Smith, DeLuca, Stevenson, & Ramey, 2012).

TYPE OF CONSTRAINT

Use of a restraint on the stronger, less-affected UE is an important component of implementing a constraint program. Several published mP–CIMT studies offer alternatives to using a cast as the restraint, with wide variation reported in selection of restraint type (Brady & Garcia, 2009; Huang et al., 2009). Many studies have selected the type of restraint on the basis of the child's age and temperament, treatment environment, and parental choice. The most common types of restraint are a full-arm cast, a cast that is bivalved and removed, a soft glove or mitt, a sling, or gentle physical restraint by the parent or practitioner.

A cast is commonly used to restrain the stronger, less-affected UE. First used in P–CIMT studies (DeLuca, Echols, Ramey, & Taub, 2003), the cast was a departure from the adult CIMT protocols, which used a soft glove mitt as the restraint. A cast applied at the start of an mP–CIMT program requires only one application, which eliminates the need for frequent removal and reapplication. Young children, such as toddlers and preschoolers, may respond best to a restraint that they cannot remove or slip off. In addition, each time a restraint is placed on a child may cause distress because the child is reminded of the overall (but temporary) loss of use of the stronger arm. A cast may be bivalved to allow for weekly removal to check for skin integrity (Taub, Ramey, DeLuca, & Echols, 2004). Casting of the less-involved and stronger extremity should be completed by someone specialized in correct placement of pediatric casts to reduce the likelihood of any potential harm to the child's arm and skin while the cast remains in place.

A soft mitt or glove, sling, or arm immobilizer splint (e.g., Pedi-Wrap) also can be used as a restraint during a mP–CIMT program. The goal of the restraint is to prevent automatic use of the stronger, less-affected UE while allowing a practitioner to shape movement patterns in the weaker, more-involved extremity. A soft mitt, sling, or wrap must eliminate the child's ability to flex the fingers and thumb (to prevent grasp) and reduce positive sensory feedback from spontaneous use of the stronger arm. The ability to use protective responses in the stronger arm remains intact, which may be very important for children with gait abnormalities. A **constraining glove** has been described in several mP–CIMT programs as a comfortable mitt or glove placed over a volar splint on the child's dominant hand, preventing finger and thumb movement (Coker et al., 2010; Eliasson et al., 2005, 2011). The hand can still be used for support and for protection during falls. A child-friendly approach for a mitt could be a puppet that fits over a volar-based splint (Coker et al., 2010; see Figures 9.1 and 9.2).

Children who are old enough to understand the use of the restraint may be more compliant with a soft mitt or sling restraint that is placed and removed each day at constraint therapy sessions. Fergus and colleagues (2008) noted that the use of a gentle restraint or glove may be preferable to a cast in the home setting for safety. Whereas a cast may limit children's protective responses, a mitten or glove can allow them to catch themselves if they fall. The use of a mitt or glove also may be preferable with small children because it allows for bilateral

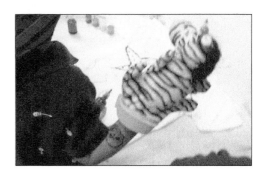

Figure 9.1 SOFT PUPPET RESTRAINT OVER A VOLAR-BASED HAND ORTHOTIC.

Source. P. Coker-Bolt.

weight bearing during transitional movements and crawling (Coker et al., 2009).

Some mP–CIMT studies have suggested that the restraint is not the most important feature of the intervention, although it is the most visible feature of CIMT approaches (Morris, Taub, & Mark, 2006; Naylor & Bower, 2005; Sterr & Freivogel, 2004). The literature on providing mP–CIMT without a restraint is limited, but one study attempted to provide intensive task practice and shaping of motor skills with minimal or no use of physical restraint. Naylor and Bower reported restraining the stronger, unaffected UE with gentle feedback and physical cues from an adult. Children were verbally encouraged to use their weaker hand in developmental play activities and were allowed to use both hands between activities. Unfortunately,

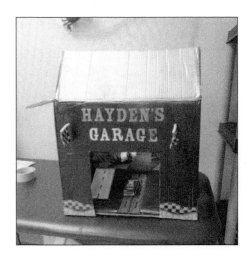

Figure 9.2 INCORPORATING A SOFT MITT PUPPET INTO AN mP–CIMT THEME HOUSE.

Source. P. Coker-Bolt.

this study provides only limited evidence to support an mP–CIMT program without use of a physical restraint. The pilot study data are from a cohort of 9 children aged 6 to 8 years. No control group was used, and no follow-up testing of participants was done to see whether gains made during the mP–CIMT program were maintained over time.

AGE OF CHILD

Adult CIMT protocols typically require participants to wear a soft mitt restraint for up to 90% of waking hours (Morris et al., 2006). During this time, intensive and specific motor skill practice is encouraged in the weaker, more affected UE. When applying principles of CIMT to a pediatric population, it is important to consider the age of the child, time spent awake, and attention level for participation in repetitive task practice. This section provides an overview of mP–CIMT for children aged younger than 1 year to adolescence and discusses implications for current practice.

An early study by Taub and colleagues (2004) included 18 children with hemiplegic cerebral palsy (CP) recruited and assigned randomly to receive either P–CIMT or conventional occupational and physical therapy. This study included 1 infant aged 7 months and 1 aged 10 months. The children participating in CIMT had the unimpaired limb casted with a lightweight fiberglass cast for 21 days. The study gave no specific information on how the infants under age 1 year tolerated intensive CIMT therapy or any specific descriptions of motor and functional gains seen in these infants following participation in the CIMT program.

Subsequent case studies have reported successful mP–CIMT approaches for infants under age 1 year (Bollea et al., 2007; Coker et al., 2009). The outcomes are encouraging and can help focus the direction of future studies on use of mP–CIMT with infants. Results should be viewed cautiously, however, and may not be generalizable to larger populations. Infants in these studies ranged from age 7 to 9 months, and mP–CIMT was implemented from 1 hour a day for 30 days to 4 hours a day for 2 months.

A possible explanation for the paucity of CIMT research with children less than age 1 year may be questions concerning the accuracy of the diagnosis of CP in children of that age. Diagnosis can be substantiated for a child under age 1 year by a medical history of prenatal stroke and marked clinical symptoms confirmed by magnetic resonance imaging.

Concern may exist that younger children cannot tolerate wearing the constraint and engaging in intensive task practice over several hours a day and that mP–CIMT will negatively affect the function of the unaffected arm, but these concerns have not been confirmed in the literature. Children less than age 1 year may actually demonstrate greater acceptance of the restraint and acquire new motor skills in the affected arm as part of the everyday, normal developmental process before learned nonuse occurs. Case Example 9.1 describes the use of mP–CIMT with a 9-month-old child.

CONTINUOUS VS. INTERMITTENT CONSTRAINT

Traditional P–CIMT protocols use a removable cast to constrain the unaffected UE. The child wears the cast 24 hours per day until the completion of the program. This type of constraint and wearing schedule are referred to as **continuous casting.** mP–CIMT programs often use **intermittent constraint,** which involves a less-intense wearing schedule and repeated removal of constraint.

When deciding on the use of continuous versus intermittent constraint, a practitioner should consider multiple factors. For infants or young toddlers who have limited waking hours, an intermittent constraint that accommodates nap schedules and can be worn for a reasonable number of waking hours (e.g., 1 or 2) may be preferable.

For older children who use their hands more actively during the day, continuous casting may afford greater opportunities to use their affected hand in daily activities and play. Case-Smith and colleagues (2012) stated,

> The theory guiding the use of continuous constraint is that young children are far more motivated to attempt to use their involved upper extremity when they cannot rely on their more functional (i.e., less involved or uninvolved extremity) to play, explore, or complete everyday tasks. (p. 20)

If a child is safe and caregivers minimize the frustration of using the restraint, continuous casting may be a good option.

Caregivers should be warned that a child who was independent before intervention may need additional assistance with activities of daily living (ADLs), such as toileting and self-feeding, during this intervention. For adolescents and teenagers, the ability to text or dial the phone in case of emergency may be limited if the fine motor coordination in their involved hand is compromised. In addition, a child using continuous constraint, especially one with diminished protective responses in his or her affected hand, may be at greater risk for sustaining injury in a fall (Glover, Mateer, Yoell, & Speed, 2002). It is the practitioner's job to evaluate the child to determine whether it is safe to use continuous casting and to take into account the child's frustration tolerance. With either method, activities should be modified to provide the just-right challenge to the affected UE when possible.

Although parents are often concerned whether a child will tolerate continuous constraint, in multiple studies, many children adapted well to the continuous constraint, did not

Case Example

mP–CIMT FOR AN INFANT

Johnny, age 6 months, was referred for occupational therapy and physical therapy because of weakness in his right arm and leg and delays in the attainment of developmental milestones. A diagnosis of hemiplegic CP was confirmed by a medical history of prenatal stroke revealed by marked clinical symptoms and confirmed by magnetic resonance imaging. The Peabody Developmental Motor Scale–2 (PDMS–2; Boulton et al., 1995) was administered at the initial occupational therapy evaluation and at follow-up. Johnny demonstrated fine motor skills for grasping, visual–motor skills in the 50th percentile, and an age equivalent of 5 months as measured by the PDMS–2. He was unable to use both hands for activities such as holding a bottle or toys or transferring objects from one hand to the other. He was able to sit with the support of a caregiver but was unable to roll, crawl, sit unsupported, stand using his hands as support, or use his affected right arm for protective responses.

Johnny received traditional therapy services of 1 hour of occupational therapy and 1 hour of physical therapy weekly for 3 months. On reevaluation, his scores on the PDMS–2 had declined, and he could complete only approximately 35% of motor tasks on the Gross Motor Function Measure–88 (GMFM–88; Russell, Rosenbaum, Avery, & Lane, 2002). At this time, Johnny's therapists decided to implement an mP–CIMT program and developed a specially designed protocol to meet the family's daily schedule. The protocol included daily constraint of the stronger hand with a resting hand splint and mitt and task practice and shaping of motor skills for 1 hour a day for 30 consecutive days, with therapists providing treatment in the clinic 4 days a week and family members providing treatment at home 3 days a week. Training for family members was provided before implementing the mP–CIMT program, and a manual was created to assist the family with the daily home-based constraint therapy sessions (Figure 9.3). Specific activities were developed for Johnny, including sensory play, repetitive reaching and batting of toys, grasp–release, and use of the affected extremity in weight bearing and protective positions.

Along with the PDMS–2 and GMFM–88 assessments, the therapist videotaped Johnny before implementing the constraint program, at the start of each week of the program, and at the end of the constraint program. The parents were asked to complete a daily log of constraint therapy sessions and to keep a list of

new motor skills observed when Johnny was not wearing the restraint (Appendix 9.A and on the flash drive). This log included a checklist of age-appropriate motor tasks that would occur around his developmental age.

After the end of the 30-day mP–CIMT program, Johnny demonstrated greater spontaneous use of his affected UE without needing physical cues from the therapist or parents and showed gains in both gross and fine motor skills. His scores on the PDMS–2 improved to within the average range, and scores on the GMFM–88 increased because he was able to complete approximately 56% of skills on this measure. Johnny demonstrated a functional grasp in the weaker hand and could bring his right hand to midline to transfer objects. He showed improved ability to bear weight with the arm, which increased his skills in crawling, pulling to stand, and cruising furniture with two hands.

Figure 9.3 EXAMPLE OF A TRAINING MANUAL FOR A FAMILY IMPLEMENTING AN mP–CIMT PROGRAM AT HOME.

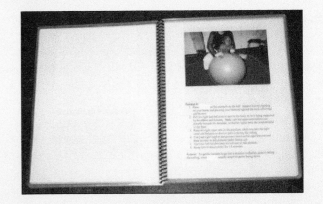

Source. P. Coker-Bolt.

Case Example

mP–CIMT FOR A TODDLER

Jane, an 18-month-old girl, was born at 26 weeks gestation. Her neonatal history was complicated by perinatal depression, severe hypotension, suspected sepsis, right intraparenchymal hemorrhage, left intraventricular hemorrhage, bilateral cerebellar hemorrhages, posthemorrhagic hydrocephalus, respiratory distress syndrome, chronic lung disease, and retinopathy (requiring laser surgery) of prematurity.

Functionally, Jane presented with left-sided hemiplegia. She sat unsupported with posterior pelvic tilt and postural asymmetries. She transitioned from sitting to prone. She did not pull to stand or maintain static standing balance with anterior support. She avoided weight-bearing positions through her left upper extremity (UE). She could visually track objects but did not dissociate her eye from head movements, and nystagmus was present. She babbled but did not say any clear words. She had limited active range of motion (AROM) at her shoulder and moved her

arm as a unit in shoulder abduction with the elbow flexed at 90°. She was at risk for contracture at her left elbow. She brought objects to her left hand to explore but did not have active grasp-release of items when placed in her hand. She tolerated AROM and stretching to her left UE.

Because of her limited mobility and cognitive level, slow growth and development, and decreased communication skills, Jane's therapist chose not to cast her or use a continuous constraint. Her therapist used an mP–CIMT approach for 30 days. Jane wore a stockinette on her right UE for 30 minutes daily during occupational therapy sessions and again at home for 30 minutes. Her caregivers reported back via a communication log. At the end of the mP–CIMT trial, Jane demonstrated increased active shoulder abduction, increased spontaneous use, and the ability to activate simple musical toys with her left UE. Therapy last 4 weeks.

---

resist its replacement after periodic skin checks, and found it not as frustrating as first anticipated (Case-Smith et al., 2012; Eliasson, Bonnier, & Krumlinde-Sundholm, 2003; Taub et al., 2007). For some children, the continuity of casting decreases attention to the dominant arm that might be associated with frequent removals and that might lead to behavioral outbursts, noncompliance, or both.

Intermittent constraint may, however, make treatment an option for clients who are typically not suited for P–CIMT with continuous casting. Clients with seizure disorders, behavior issues, skin issues, or orthopedic issues (e.g., arthritis, joint laxity) may not be able to tolerate continuous static positioning. Clients who are nonambulatory or have postural control issues may not be safe wearing a continuous constraint. For these clients, intermittent constraint provides an opportunity to participate in this intervention while minimizing risk. Case Example 9.2 describes the use of intermittent constraint with a toddler who has multiple areas of delay.

TREATMENT PROVIDERS

During traditional P–CIMT protocols, treatment is provided by trained therapists, but some mP–CIMT protocols are applied by nontherapists such as other trained professionals

(e.g., teachers, aides, nurses), students, or parents of the children participating in the CIMT program. Using these other caregivers may decrease the cost of the treatment and increase availability of the intervention for children who are uninsured or underinsured (Karman et al., 2003). It also increases the number of people who are available to apply the intervention, thus improving access to care in rural areas. Use of people who are already part of the child's natural environment, such as parents, day care providers, or teachers, may minimize disruption of the child's routine while completing the modified protocol. Fergus and colleagues (2008) reported that the involvement of caregivers in their mP–CIMT protocol contributed to the success of the intervention through improved motivation of the child.

Although using nontherapists can be advantageous, potential disadvantages to nontherapists guiding children through CIMT exist. One concern is that nontherapists may not have the knowledge required to provide appropriate shaping of new movements (Gordon et al., 2007; Karman et al., 2003). Although some studies have provided training to nontherapist providers, questions remain about fidelity of treatment (Case-Smith et al., 2012). Therapists also have access to modalities, such as electrical stimulation, that other caregivers would need special training to implement.

Another concern specific to parents as interventionists is the strain that this approach can place on the family. Glover and colleagues (2002) reported that the families were "at times exhausted" (p. 130) by the amount of attention and assistance their child required. They also noted that families had to change their usual routines and activities to accommodate the child's needs during the intervention. Because of this potential for stress and frustration, some studies have reported, parents showed decreased compliance with maintaining the restraint-wearing schedule and completing specific activities, which affected outcomes (Karman et al., 2003).

Several studies have proposed a hybrid model in which treatment is provided by a combination of therapists and other caregivers, with therapists providing ongoing training and support to caregivers throughout the protocol (Al-Oraibi & Eliasson, 2011; Coker et al., 2009; de Brito Brandão et al., 2010; Eliasson et al., 2005; Naylor & Bower 2005; Pierce, Daly, Gallagher, Gershkoff, & Schaumberg, 2002). Case Example 9.3 describes the use of a hybrid model for an older child doing a repeat mP–CIMT program. Hybrid models allow the benefits of the expertise of a therapist while maintaining the advantages of other caregivers providing some of the treatment; however, the optimal balance of therapist and caregiver has not been established. Further research is needed to compare the effects of type of interventionist on treatment outcomes.

Case Example

Case Example

9.3

REPEAT TRIAL OF mP–CIMT FOR AN OLDER CHILD

Seth, a 5-year-old boy, is participating in an mP–CIMT day program. Seth's birth at 36 weeks gestation was complicated by prenatal hydrocephalus seen on ultrasound; he was delivered by cesarean section. Neonatal computed tomography scan showed an intraventricular hemorrhage, and an intraventricular shunt was placed at age 2 weeks. He had motor impairment on the left side, including increased tone. He walked independently at about age 21 months. At age 4 years, he was diagnosed with a sensory processing disorder and pervasive development disorder. He had language delays and spoke in two- and three-word phrases. He had impairments in attention but was able attend to nonpreferred tasks for approximately 5 minutes at a time.

At age 5 years, he was referred to a clinic-based mP–CIMT day program. At that time, Seth was intermittently using his left UE as a gross assist. It was noted during his initial evaluation for the program that he had decreased efficiency opening his hand and during grasp–release. Seth was beginning to show interest in assisting with self-care tasks such as dressing but required total assistance at admission for most ADLs. He received 21 days of treatment (16 casted days and 5 bimanual days), including 3 hours of combined physical and occupational therapy services per day, 5 days a week. Seth's right UE was casted from axilla to fingertips in a univalved, waterproof cast. The cast was applied on Day 1 of the protocol and remained on until Day 16, at which time it was removed and bilateral tasks were addressed for the remaining treatment days. The

cast also was removed for 15 to 20 minutes each week to check his skin and allow the right UE time for AROM.

At reevaluation, Seth was initiating self-care tasks with greater frequency. He had improved grip strength and was carrying items in his left UE more often. His bilateral coordination improved as noted by his ability to open zipper-lock bags with greater efficiency and greater success cutting with scissors. He continued with occupational therapy services 3 to 4 times per month to address bilateral skills, sensory strategies, and self-care. Approximately 1 year after completing the day program, his mother asked if he would benefit from another admission to the constraint day program.

To help his response, his occupational therapist initiated a modified CIMT approach to brush up his skills. The therapist made a long arm cast for him to wear 1 hour per day at home and 1 hour per day during therapy. Seth's mother was provided a short checklist of activities and skills to work on each week with gradually increasing difficulty. She also encouraged him to use both arms during ADLs, play, and self-care when the cast was off by playing games that encouraged bimanual coordination and talking through dressing strategies with both hands. After 4 weeks, Seth's mother and teachers observed greater spontaneous use of his left UE. He built on the skills he had learned during his first CIMT admission. He had a functional pincer grasp and increased grip strength. He fastened zippers independently after setup and donned socks with both hands.

MODIFICATION OF THE TREATMENT ENVIRONMENT

Children attend signature P–CIMT programs in a home-based or simulated home-based environment. Home-based services afford the opportunity for practice in the child's natural environment, encouraging greater generalization of skills. In the home setting, the child's parents, siblings, and extended family have opportunities to be involved in treatment and therefore may carry over activities after formal therapy services end. Home-based services are not as disruptive to a child's routine, and the child may be more comfortable in familiar surroundings (Dickerson & Brown, 2007).

In contrast, children can participate in mP–CIMT programs in a variety of environments, including inpatient or other clinical settings, schools, day care centers, or other community centers. Treatment in a center-based setting has the advantages of centralizing therapy resources and allowing access to treatment by a larger number of participants. Such settings typically have greater availability of equipment that complements treatment, such as adaptive bikes, electrical stimulation, gaming systems, robotics, and virtual reality systems. Disadvantages of center-based services include transportation issues that may lead to missed visits and disruption of the school routine for older children and adolescents.

SUMMARY

mP–CIMT approaches provide the essential elements of signature CIMT, including restraint of the stronger, nonaffected UE; concentrated, massed practice of specific motor activities; and shaping of more-mature motor movement, which are packaged together to maximize rehabilitation efforts. In addition, the overall aim of both traditional P–CIMT and mP–CIMT is to reverse developmental disregard or learned nonuse of the affected extremity in children with unilateral motor weakness.

Practitioners considering an mP–CIMT approach should evaluate the current literature on modified approaches when determining the best approach for a specific client. They need to be particularly sensitive to maintaining the essential elements of P–CIMT, including intensity and task practice, which are prescribed over a shortened period of time compared with traditional pediatric rehabilitation. Future studies of mP–CIMT approaches should focus on the characteristics of the children (e.g., age, specific diagnoses) most likely to benefit from modified approaches. Also of interest is further examination of the type of training

required by parents and nontherapist professionals, who are increasingly being asked to contribute to mP–CIMT programs in home or school settings.

REFERENCES

Aarts, P. B., Jongerius, P. H., Geerdink, Y. A., van Limbeek, J., & Geurts, A. C. (2010). Effectiveness of modified constraint-induced movement therapy in children with unilateral spastic cerebral palsy: A randomized controlled trial. *Neurorehabilitation and Neural Repair, 24,* 509–518.

Al-Oraibi, S., & Eliasson, A. C. (2011). Implementation of constraint-induced movement therapy for young children with unilateral cerebral palsy in Jordan: A home-based model. *Disability and Rehabilitation, 33,* 2006–2012.

Assis, R. D., Massaro, A. R., Chamlian, T. R., Silva, M. F., & Ota, S. M. (2007). Constraint-induced movement therapy for a child with hemiplegic cerebral palsy: Case report. *Acta Fisiatrica, 14,* 62–65.

Bollea, L., Rosa, G. D., Gisondi, A., Guidi, P., Petrarca, M., Giannarelli, P., & Castelli, E. (2007). Recovery from hemiparesis and unilateral spatial neglect after neonatal stroke: Case report and rehabilitation of an infant. *Brain Injury, 1,* 81–91.

Boulton, J. E., Kirsch, S. E., Chipman, M., Etele, E., White, A. M., & Pape, K. E. (1995). Reliability of the Peabody Developmental Gross Motor Scale in children with cerebral palsy. *Physical and Occupational Therapy in Pediatrics, 15,* 37–52.

Boyd, R., Sakzewski, L., Ziviani, J., Abbott, D. F., Badawy, R., Gilmore, R., . . . Jackson, G. D. (2010). INCITE: A randomised trial comparing constraint induced movement therapy and bimanual training in children with congenital hemiplegia. *BMC Neurology, 10,* 4.

Brady, K., & Garcia, T. (2009). Constraint-induced movement therapy (CIMT): Pediatric applications. *Developmental Disabilities Research Reviews, 15,* 102–111.

Case-Smith, J., DeLuca, S. C., Stevenson, R., & Ramey, S. L. (2012). Multicenter randomized controlled trial of pediatric constraint-induced movement therapy: 6-month follow-up. *American Journal of Occupational Therapy, 66,* 15–23. http://dx.doi.org/10.5014/ajot.2012.002386

Charles, J., & Gordon, A. M. (2005). A critical review of constraint-induced movement therapy and forced use in children with hemiplegia. *Neural Plasticity, 12,* 245–261; discussion 263–272.

Charles, J. R., & Gordon, A. M. (2007). A repeated course of constraint-induced movement therapy results in further improvement. *Developmental Medicine and Child Neurology, 49,* 770–773.

Charles, J. R., Wolf, S. L., Schneider, J. A., & Gordon, A. M. (2006). Efficacy of a child-friendly form of constraint-induced movement therapy in hemiplegic cerebral palsy: A randomized control trial. *Developmental Medicine and Child Neurology, 48,* 635–642.

Coker, P., Karakostas, T., Dodds, C., & Hsiang, S. (2010). Gait characteristics of children with hemiplegic cerebral palsy before and after modified constraint-induced movement therapy. *Disability and Rehabilitation, 32,* 402–408. http://dx.doi.org/10.3109/09638280903171592

Coker, P., Lebkicher, C., Harris, L., & Snape, J. (2009). The effects of constraint-induced movement therapy for a child less than one year of age. *NeuroRehabilitation, 24,* 199–208. http://dx.doi.org/10.3233/NRE-2009-0469

de Bode, S., Fritz, S. L., Weir-Haynes, K., & Mathern, G. W. (2009). Constraint-induced movement therapy for individuals after cerebral hemispherectomy: A case series. *Physical Therapy, 89,* 361–369.

de Brito Brandão, M., Mancini, M. C., Vaz, D. V., Pereira de Melo, A. P., & Fonseca, S. T. (2010). Adapted version of constraint-induced movement therapy promotes functioning in children with cerebral palsy: A randomized controlled trial. *Clinical Rehabilitation, 24,* 639–647.

DeLuca, S. C., Echols, K., Law, C. R., & Ramey, S. L. (2006). Intensive pediatric constraint-induced therapy for children with cerebral palsy: Randomized, controlled, crossover trial. *Journal of Child Neurology, 21,* 931–938. PMID: 17092457

DeLuca, S. C., Echols, K., Ramey, S. L., & Taub, E. (2003). Pediatric constraint-induced movement therapy for a young child with cerebral palsy: Two episodes of care. *Physical Therapy, 83,* 1003–1013. PMID: 14577827

Dickerson, A. E., & Brown, L. E. (2007). Pediatric constraint-induced movement therapy in a young child with minimal active arm movement. *American Journal of Occupational Therapy, 61,* 563–573. http://dx.doi.org/10.5014/ajot.61.5.563

Eliasson, A. C., Bonnier, B., & Krumlinde-Sundholm, L. (2003). Clinical experience of constraint induced movement therapy in adolescents with hemiplegic cerebral palsy: A day camp model. *Developmental Medicine and Child Neurology, 45,* 357–359.

Eliasson, A. C., Krumlinde-Sundholm, L., Shaw, K., & Wang, C. (2005). Effects of constraint-induced movement therapy in young children with hemiplegic cerebral palsy: An adapted model. *Developmental Medicine and Child Neurology, 47,* 266–275.

Eliasson, A. C., Shaw, K., Berg, E., & Krumlinde-Sundholm, L. (2011). An ecological approach of constraint induced movement therapy for 2–3-year-old children: A randomized control trial. *Research in Developmental Disabilities, 32,* 2820–2828.

Fergus, A., Buckler, J., Farrell, J., Isley, M., McFarland, M., & Riley, B. (2008). Constraint-induced movement therapy for a child with hemiparesis: A case report. *Pediatric Physical Therapy, 20,* 271–283.

Glover, J. E., Mateer, C. A., Yoell, C., & Speed, S. (2002). The effectiveness of constraint induced movement therapy in two young children with hemiplegia. *Pediatric Rehabilitation, 5,* 125–131.

Gordon, A., Connelly, A., Neville, B., Vargha-Khadem, F., Jessop, N., Murphy, T., & Ganesan, V. (2007). Modified constraint-induced movement therapy after childhood stroke. *Developmental Medicine and Child Neurology, 49,* 23–27.

Hoare, B., Imms, C., Carey, L., & Wasiak, J. (2007). Constraint-induced movement therapy in the treatment of the upper limb in children with hemiplegic cerebral palsy: A Cochrane systematic review. *Clinical Rehabilitation, 21,* 675–685.

Huang, H. H., Fetters, L., Hale, J., & McBride, A. (2009). Bound for success: A systematic review of constraint-induced movement therapy in children with cerebral palsy supports improved arm and hand use. *Physical Therapy, 89,* 1126–1141.

Karman, N., Maryles, J., Baker, R. W., Simpser, E., & Berger-Gross, P. (2003). Constraint-induced movement therapy for hemiplegic children with acquired brain injuries. *Journal of Head Trauma Rehabilitation, 18,* 259–267.

Martin, A., Burtner, P. A., Poole, J., & Phillips, J. (2008). Case Report—ICF-level changes in a preschooler after constraint-induced movement therapy. *American Journal of Occupational Therapy, 62,* 282–288. http://dx.doi.org/10.5014/ajot.62.3.282

Miller, R., & Hale, L. (2005). Constraint-induced movement therapy for a youth with a chronic traumatic brain injury. *New Zealand Journal of Physiotherapy, 33,* 85–90.

Morris, D. M., Taub, E., & Mark, V. W. (2006). Constraint-induced movement therapy: Characterizing the intervention protocol. *Europa Medicophysica, 42,* 257–268.

Naylor, C. E., & Bower, E. (2005). Modified constraint-induced movement therapy for young children with hemiplegic cerebral palsy: A pilot study. *Developmental Medicine and Child Neurology, 47,* 365–369.

Sterr, A., & Freivogel, S. (2004). Intensive training in chronic upper limb hemiparesis does not increase spasticity or synergies. *Neurology, 63,* 842–844.

Pierce, S. R., Daly, K., Gallagher, K. G., Gershkoff, A. M., & Schaumburg, S. W. (2002). Constraint-induced therapy for a child with hemiplegic cerebral palsy: A case report. *Archives of Physical Medicine and Rehabilitation, 83,* 1462–1463.

Russell, D., Rosenbaum, P., Avery, L., & Lane, M. (2002). *Gross Motor Function Measure (GMFM–66 and GMFM–88) user's manual.* London: Mac Keith Press.

Taub, E., Griffin, A., Nick, J., Gammons, K., Uswatte, G., & Law, C. R. (2007). Pediatric CI therapy for stroke-induced hemiparesis in young children. *Developmental Neurorehabilitation, 10,* 3–18.

Taub, E., Ramey, S. L., DeLuca, S., & Echols, K. (2004). Efficacy of constraint-induced movement therapy for children with cerebral palsy with asymmetric motor impairment. *Pediatrics, 113,* 305–312.

APPENDIX 9.A. PARENT REPORT LOG USED DURING AN mP–CIMT PROGRAM FOR AN INFANT

Date _____

Amount of time spent in splint _____

What was the child doing while wearing the splint (e.g., playing with toys, feeding)?

_____

Activity	Check for Yes
Supported self while sitting with right hand (fingers open with hand on floor)	
Supported self while on stomach up on elbows	
Supported self on all fours	
Passed a toy from right hand to left hand	
Clapped	
Brought hands together	
Held bottle with both hands	
Picked up a toy with right hand	
Batted at a toy with right hand	
Fully straightened right arm when reaching out for a toy while sitting	
Fully straightened right arm when reaching for a toy while lying on back	
Released a toy from right hand	
Banged a toy with right hand (e.g., keys of a toy piano, drum)	
Grasped and shook a toy (e.g., beads) with right hand	
Reached for an object (e.g., cell phone) with right hand while lying on stomach	
Rolled from back to stomach toward right side	
Rolled from stomach to back toward right side	
Rolled from back to stomach toward left side	
Rolled from stomach to back toward left side	
Held a rattle with right hand and shook it	
Moved toward left side on hands, on belly (pivot-on-prone)	
Moved toward right side on hands, on belly (pivot-on-prone)	

Comments:

_____

_____

_____

New motions or actions with the right hand:

_____

_____

_____

_____

_____

Note. Courtesy of P. Coker-Bolt. Used with permission.

ANN-CHRISTIN ELIASSON, PhD, and
PATTY COKER-BOLT, PhD, OTRL

10

Group-Based Models of Pediatric CIMT: Special Camps, School-Based Treatment, and Home Environment Models

CHAPTER HIGHLIGHTS

- Using constraint-induced movement therapy (CIMT) in children's daily environment: ECO–CIMT model
- Agenda for using ECO–CIMT in the daily environment: The 10-step model
- Application of ECO–CIMT: Case example
- Group- and camp-based models
- Groups, camps, and observational learning
- Research on group- and camp-based P–CIMT models
- Delivery of group- or camp-based P–CIMT models
- Example of a P–CIMT camp model: Camp Hand 2 Hands.

KEY TERMS

Assisting Hand Assessment
Child centered
Dynamic Systems Theory
ECO–CIMT
Ecological Systems Theory
Motor learning
Social group approach
Task-specific training

Two programs that use modified or alternative pediatric constraint-induced movement therapy (P–CIMT) approaches have treated children successfully over the past decade: (1) a home-based model from Sweden and (2) a group-based camp program in South Carolina. This chapter provides information supporting the benefits of these modified P–CIMT approaches and describes how these programs vary from signature P–CIMT (see Chapter 8, "ACQUIREc Protocol: What We Have Learned From a Decade of Delivering a Signature Form of Pediatric CIMT," this volume) yet maintain the essential elements of intensive dosage of treatment, repetitive task practice, and shaping techniques.

Ecological P–CIMT, known as *ECO–CIMT,* is a treatment model that takes place in the daily environments of children with cerebral palsy (CP)—that is, in the home and preschool environments. It is especially useful for younger children beginning at age 18 months. The primary practitioner trains and provides supervision to the parents and preschool teacher before the treatment starts, commonly during one evening session. This training ensures that the parents and teacher understand what they should be doing and the background that guides the treatment model. Parents and preschool teachers are responsible for providing the training on a daily basis. The child's primary therapist meets weekly with the child and is responsible for treatment planning, continually adjusting the plan according to the child's interests and abilities throughout the training period.

During ECO–CIMT, children wear a comfortable fabric glove with a built-in volar splint made from stiff plastic on the dominant hand. The glove prevents them from flexing their fingers and thumb, prohibiting the ability to grasp. They can, however, use the dominant hand for support.

The ECO–CIMT model is consistent with Bronfenbrenner and Morris's (1998) Ecological Systems Theory of child development, Dynamic Systems Theory as discussed by Thelen and Smith (1996), and the principles of motor learning (Smith & Wrisberg, 2001). **Ecological Systems Theory** looks at a child's development within the context of the environment, which comprises various systems, including interactions in personal relationships. **Dynamic Systems Theory** is an approach to the study of development that looks at the interaction of multiple body systems over time.

EVIDENCE BASE FOR THE ECO–CIMT MODEL

ECO–CIMT has been demonstrated to be effective starting with children as young as age 18 months. The model, described by Eliasson, Krumlinde-Sundholm, Shaw, and Wang (2005), was tested in a controlled clinical trial and then replicated in a randomized controlled trial (Eliasson, Shaw, Berg, & Krumlinde-Sundholm, 2011). The control groups in both trials received ordinary treatment. The effect size was high and similar between studies (1.16 and 1.26, respectively).

The same protocol was used in somewhat older children in a study from Jordan, in which a positive effect was found when ECO–CIMT was compared with intensified neurodevelopmental training (Al Oraibi & Eliasson, 2011). This study also demonstrated that a 2-day workshop was enough for practitioners who had never heard of CIMT; that is,

they were able to provide training that produced comparable benefits (i.e., was similarly effective) to those described in earlier studies.

Other studies have evaluated the implementation of P–CIMT in daily environments. In some studies, daily treatment was provided at a lower intensity but over a longer time period (Lin et al., 2011; Rostami & Malamiri, 2012; Wallen et al., 2011), whereas in others, children received up to 6 hours per day for at least 3 weeks (Case-Smith, DeLuca, Stevenson, & Ramey, 2012; DeLuca, Echols, Law, & Ramey, 2006). All of these treatment approaches were grounded in the understanding that what children learn in their natural environments has the potential to be maintained readily because the initial learning and practice are embedded in daily activities with a variety of physical and social supports for this new learning. Only one study directly compared the effects of therapy delivered in the child's natural environment (home) versus another environment (clinic; Rostami & Malamiri, 2012). Although all participants showed significant improvements in posttest measures, the children in the home-based therapy continued to show significant changes at follow-up testing, but the children treated in the clinic environment did not.

ADAPTATION OF CIMT TO THE DAILY ENVIRONMENT

As emphasized in Section I of this book, which provides a history of both CIMT for adult stroke patients and P–CIMT, practitioners must think about which elements of CIMT would be the most appropriate and influential to include in an adapted form provided in a group context. In Sweden, a team of researchers first adapted the reported forms of CIMT, observed the effects, and continued to make modifications based on observations.

The team reasoned that 6 hours of daily training might be difficult for very young children, who have relatively shorter attention spans and spend more time in activities such as eating and sleeping than do older children. Most importantly, many parents and preschool teachers might find it difficult to provide a 6-hour therapy program each day, given their many other responsibilities. Therefore, the team began providing the ECO–CIMT model for 2 hours per day, usually divided into two sessions. This reduced intensity worked well in both the home and school environments, and compliance with this model was high. The overall period for the treatment was extended from 2 or 3 weeks to 8 weeks, which provided additional time for training and supervision of the teachers and parents.

The second modification concerned the constraint used for the dominant hand. One of the key components of signature CIMT is to facilitate the use of the nondominant, or hemiplegic, hand by using a constraint for the nonhemiplegic hand. The research evidence to date is not adequate to support the use of any particular type of constraint or duration of use. Thus, the team chose a simple glove that somewhat prevented the children from grasping and was fairly comfortable. This constraint was used only during the training periods. The aim was to enable the hemiplegic hand to become far more capable by requiring the child to depend on that side while the dominant side was temporarily limited by the constraint glove.

The team members assumed that the glove would encourage the children to use the hemiplegic hand, which in turn would become more capable. The children could use the gloved hand when needed to lift and carry big and heavy objects, to engage in activities requiring two hands, or to keep their balance, but they could not use it for grasping objects. Allowing children wearing the constraint glove to use their dominant hand as a shovel or support made it easier to engage them in fun and meaningful activities. In addition, by respecting the children's reaction to the constraint and giving explanations in response, practitioners promoted their compliance with wearing the glove, even in very young children.

The third modification concerned the practices and theories for training. Repetition and shaping are key elements in signature CIMT. Younger children find repetition to be a common and fun aspect of play. If tasks are of interest, young children do not mind repeating a game over and over, especially if they feel they are getting better. Shaping requires vigorous adult engagement in the form of providing children with immediate information and feedback so they can be more successful in enacting a task or an activity.

The theories used to guide the ECO–CIMT therapy model all highlight the importance of the complex interactions among the active child and persons, objects, and symbols in their immediate environment. The model is **child centered** in that children do interesting things with people who care about them. Bronfenbrenner and Morris's (1998) observation that unconditional love and time spent with a child are the two most important agents giving energy for development was an important guideline in the design of ECO–CIMT. From this perspective, parents and preschool teachers are very important contributors to the success of the program.

The Dynamic Systems Theory is an ecological model postulating that motor development hinges on children's ability to construct a solution to a motor problem (Thelen & Smith, 1996). This theory highlights the importance of children's self-initiated activity, which has always been a key element of ECO–CIMT. From the Dynamic Systems Theory perspective, development is driven by children's unique characteristics and capacity to explore a situation, through which they discover new and more adaptive forms; thus, children do not use "right" or "wrong" movements when performing the selected activities. Dynamic Systems Theory emphasizes the importance of a rich natural environment in which a wide variety of situations are encountered that facilitate the learning process.

Finally, **motor learning** principles focus on the understanding of how people learn and perform skilled motor activities through a series of steps. The child's natural caregivers organize level-appropriate tasks and provide feedback. Another key element is that children should engage in meaningful activities at "just the right level"; this principle forms the basis for planning and performing treatment in ECO–CIMT. Through motor learning, the child is capable of achieving skilled behavior, and through repetitive training, a degree of automation can be expected. These assumptions are the basis of the expectation that ECO–CIMT will help prevent developmental disregard and improve hand function in children with unilateral CP.

The theories included in ECO–CIMT are well known and are used, with slight variations, in other pediatric training programs, including functional training and goal-directed training, as well as in family-centered services (King, Teplicky, King, & Rosenbaum, 2004; Löwing, Bexelius, & Carlberg, 2010; Mastos, Miller, Eliasson, & Imms, 2007). Furthermore, preschool teachers are usually well educated in theories of child development, although practitioners need to specify how these theories are applied to the one-handed training required for P–CIMT.

The team made an additional adaptation to Swedish children, society, and health care in terms of who should do the training and where it should take place. The original adult CIMT models were based on having a specialist deliver the therapy, often in a hospital or rehabilitation setting; signature P–CIMT was provided in the child's home. The adapted model for Sweden is based on the fact that almost all young children are in full-time child care while parents work, so having teachers deliver training makes sense. Parents' time at home with the child is limited, making two 1-hour sessions at home both feasible and economical. The possible disadvantage is that teachers and parents may be less skilled than trained practitioners in helping a child with hemiparesis learn new motor skills and functional activities and in minimizing interfering or compensatory movements the child has already adopted. Parents and preschool teachers are given a diary to record training hours and add comments, which the practitioner reviews and incorporates in the weekly supervision sessions. The quality of the training depends very much on effective supervision, education, trust, and communication.

AGENDA FOR USING ECO–CIMT IN THE DAILY ENVIRONMENT: THE 10-STEP MODEL

It is important to systematically approach the ECO–CIMT model step by step. Experience shows that careful preparation before training begins is vital for success. This section describes each step, grouped into three phases: (1) preparation, (2) execution, and (3) conclusion.

PREPARATION PHASE

1. *Discuss with the family factors involved in a decision on training sessions.* Make sure the parents are informed about the principles of, and commitment required for, this intensive training method. A mature and carefully considered decision is the basis for successful results. Explain why you think CIMT may benefit the child and how he or she may be able to improve through the training program. Discuss the family's expectations of the program. Explain what is required from parents and others, such as preschool teachers. Clarify the importance of the preschool's involvement, if applicable, and ensure that appropriate and responsible personnel are available.

2. *Decide to use CIMT.* All parties should understand the decision to start the ECO–CIMT program and their roles in implementing the treatment plan. If the child is old enough and able to understand, involve him or her in the process.

3. *Consider the practitioner's schedule.* An ECO–CIMT program requires careful scheduling for the process to run smoothly. It is recommended that two practitioners are involved to allow for creative discussion and backup for the weekly supervision. Preparation time is needed to provide information to parents and staff and to make the glove, as well as for assessment and treatment planning.

4. *Provide information to the parents and preschool.* It is beneficial to hold an information meeting for families and staff to present broader information about the training and diagnosis and about children with unilateral CP. This information also can be provided on an individual basis if necessary. Information is needed to create the right expectations. Be very practical during the meeting, addressing questions such as what to do, how to play with the child, and what will happen during therapy. To increase motivation, use video recordings and pictures as examples of what other children have achieved with CIMT. Present ideas based on the assumption that activities at "just the right level" are important to motivate a lot of repetition.

5. *Meet with the child for the initial assessment.* The initial assessment meeting is the child's starting point for ECO–CIMT and might include, for example, the Assisting Hand Assessment (AHA; Krumlinde-Sundholm, Holmefur, Kottorp, & Eliasson, 2007) or a video recording of the child performing several activities requiring bimanual or unimanual involvement. (Be sure to use the same toys in the before-treatment and after-treatment videos.) To make a glove, trace the noninvolved hand. Talk to the child in an age-appropriate way about what is going to happen the next time you meet. Decide on the exact date to start the training program.

6. *Prepare for the first training session.* Treatment planning is preferably based on analysis of the assessment video recording. Choose three or four aspects of hand function in which you believe the child could improve. Think about activities that are possible to use for training in the child's environment and about what you know about the child's interests. Discuss how to grade activities to make games easier or more complex and to adjust the level of challenge. Already having several ideas in mind makes it easier to make appropriate suggestions to families and school.

EXECUTION PHASE

7. *Start training.* The primary practitioner should be present at the first training session. The starting day is important. Choose activities that you know the child can do with the hemiplegic hand and that he or she likes to do; the session has to be fun. Make sure that the glove fulfills its purpose—namely, to prevent grasping—but otherwise is fairly comfortable. Introduce a diary in which parents and staff are to record the actual time of each training session and key therapy activities. The diary should be used for the weekly supervision meetings to discuss the latest developments and occurrences and also for setting goals for the forthcoming week. If training with the glove on does not seem to be going well, it may be necessary to discontinue the program. Try it for a week, but stop after that if the child does not accept the glove. A common problem is that children are given activities that are too difficult to result in success. Likewise, some children are extremely reluctant or skeptical at first, but it usually does not last for long. Take the glove off while the child feels positively toward it.

8. *Execute CIMT, and supervise once per week.* Meet with the child, parents, and staff in the child's environment. Review the previous week, using the diary; discuss what went well and what did not. Attend the training session that the parent or teacher provides that day, participate in the activities, and contribute new ideas. Allocate time at the end of the session to plan activities for the following week. Give a pep talk. Be positive, encouraging, and understanding, and help the parents or staff be creative.

CONCLUSION PHASE

9. *Conduct a follow-up assessment after the training sessions conclude.* Carry out the same assessment as before the training. Analyze the results using the video, the AHA, and any other tests. Write up a report for the child's record.

10. *Provide results and feedback to the family and preschool.* It is important to have a closing meeting with the family and preschool to allow everyone an opportunity to discuss what went well and what did not. It is crucial to communicate the results thoroughly because everyone involved made a large effort.

APPLICATION OF ECO–CIMT: CASE EXAMPLE OF VIKTOR

TREATMENT PLANNING

Treatment planning should be based on the practitioner's analysis of the child's behavior and reports from the parents and teachers. The **Assisting Hand Assessment,** an observation-based test designed for children with congenital unilateral disability in the arm and hand, measures how effectively they use their affected hand in bimanual activities and is very useful in treatment planning. The AHA has been found to produce valid measures for children aged 18 months to 12 years and has excellent inter- and intrarater reliability (Holmefur, Aarts, Hoare, & Krumlinde-Sundholm, 2009; Krumlinde-Sundholm et al., 2007). For the child, the test involves an approximately 15-minute, semistructured videorecorded play session with toys requiring bimanual use. The AHA is scored on 22 items with a 4-point rating scale, resulting in a raw score of 22 to 88 points.

For **Viktor, a 2-year-old boy who almost never used one hand,** the results of the AHA before treatment showed 6% assisting hand function (26 points), meaning that Viktor did not try to grasp objects, not even those that were easy to grasp. He could, however, hold a toy in his hand if someone else placed it there. He also could independently place objects in his hemiplegic hand but did so only a few times during the assessment. Viktor typically chose not to use the hemiplegic hand and rarely initiated any movements. Usually his arm lay still on the table. He had limited spontaneous range of motion (ROM) and often asked an adult for help with a task. Viktor is used in this example because he had a severe problem, and when a child has severely decreased hand function, it is important to select easy activities. Often when activities are too difficult, the child does not like to participate.

IMPORTANT ASPECTS OF HAND FUNCTION TO BE TRAINED

On the basis of the AHA results and what the practitioner knew about Viktor, the following actions were identified as important:

- Reaching for objects (e.g., moving his arm and touching the objects, banging and flinging objects)
- Holding something in his hand (e.g., actively and steadily holding an object)
- Holding an object against something
- Problem solving during play (e.g., learning various strategies to solve a task, finding out that the same task can be done in several ways)
- Grasping simple objects, if possible (e.g., discovering how his hand works).

IMPORTANT CONSIDERATIONS WHEN SELECTING GAMES

When planning Viktor's training, it was important to

- Choose games that Viktor enjoyed and that attracted him.
- Choose games that included the aspects of hand function in the preceding list.
- Choose games that could be carried out with one hand and that were appropriate to Viktor's everyday environment.
- Avoid games that were too difficult. It was important for Viktor to be able to succeed at the tasks set; otherwise he would tire, and it would be difficult to continue the training program.

The following are examples of some games that Viktor enjoyed and that stimulated him to use his hand and arm in various ways:

- *Water play.* Water play can be varied and includes turning the faucet on and off, running the arm through the water stream, filling the sink with water, pouring and stirring water, and using soap to wash and rinse the hand. Training involved Viktor choosing to use his hand, initiating movement and discovering the position of his hand and arm in relation to his body, discovering that he was able to do things with his hand, and engaging in goal-oriented reaching in different directions.
- *Finger painting.* First, the practitioner encouraged Viktor to get paint by taking his hand and placing it in a jar; then the practitioner held the jar so he could put his hand in himself. Training involved Viktor using his hand and arm, reaching, orienting, and controlling his hand and arm in goal-directed actions.
- *Decorating a frame.* A ready-made cardboard frame can be used for this activity. The glue can be scraped out of the container with a craft stick, but fingers also can be

used. The practitioner placed previously cut out pieces of tissue paper in the frame. Viktor was told to grasp the pieces of paper from the practitioner's hand, which is much easier than from the table. Training involved Viktor learning how to open his hand and how to pick up pieces of paper and crunch them up to make them easy to grasp.

The following are examples of other games mainly intended to increase the movement repertoire of the arm:

- *Knocking over blocks.* An adult builds a tower on the child's weak side so that the child naturally uses the hemiplegic hand. Training involves initiating movements and goal-directed reaching.

- *Driving cars down a slide.* An adult places the cars on the track; the child gets to push them down. Training involves initiating movements and goal-directed reaching and pushing away.

- *Finger play and action songs.* An adult sings a song and does the corresponding hand movements for such songs as "Itsy Bitsy Spider," "Where Is Thumbkin?" or "Twinkle Twinkle Little Star." The adult helps the child adapt movements to what is possible for him or her to manage independently. Training involves varying arm and finger movements.

- *Paging through a book with cardboard pages.* An adult helps the child turn the pages by lifting a little at one edge and letting the child do the rest. The adult lets the child point with one finger or the whole hand and tell about the pictures. Training involves doing simple grasping and accurate pointing.

- *Throwing a ball.* Large balls are good for this activity because the child must use both hands without grasping. To avoid having the child kick the ball, the task can be to throw the ball at a specific place. Training involves timing goal-directed arm movements and coordinating hands.

- *Finding hidden objects.* An adult places objects under a towel or small blanket that is easy to grasp. The adult helps the child take the towel in his or her hand and lets him or her independently pull it away to reveal the hidden object. Objects can also be hidden behind cushions that can be pushed away with an arm or under upside-down containers that the child can knock over with his or her hand. If simple grasping is possible, the adult can hide an object that is easy to grip (e.g., wire ball, key ring with many objects on it). Training involves doing simple grasping and controlling arm movements.

- *Pressing buttons on toys.* An adult shows the child an electronic toy with keys or buttons and gets the child to press the different buttons to play a melody or start an action. Training involves initiating movements, pressing, building strength, and orienting hand movements.

RESULTS

Viktor improved to 18% assisting hand function (from 26 to 34 points raw score). This improvement is considerable and is well above the smallest detectable difference for the AHA, which is 4 points raw score. After the training, he started to use his hand more often, and he initiated use of the hand, albeit with a delay. He almost always approached an object with the hemiplegic hand. He still did not grasp objects, but he could stabilize them. Even if this action was somewhat ineffective, it was enough to allow him to manipulate the objects with the other hand, raising his score for coordination. By the end of the training, he also had started to problem solve and sometimes changed strategies to be more successful.

GROUP- AND CAMP-BASED MODELS

Group-based models of P–CIMT have been explored in several research studies. In signature P–CIMT programs, children participate in individual therapy, but in some modified P–CIMT programs, children participate in group therapy sessions with similar-age peers. These modified programs may use a combination of individual and group therapy sessions (Aarts et al., 2012; Juenger et al., 2007; Kuhnke et al., 2008; Walther et al., 2009), or the children may exclusively participate in group sessions throughout the protocol (Boyd et al., 2010; Charles & Gordon, 2007; Gordon, Charles, & Wolf, 2006).

No studies published to date compare outcomes of group-based versus individual intervention in P–CIMT; however, group therapy has a number of proposed benefits for the children participating in these programs. The group environment may be more natural for older children who attend school, and peers can provide each other with support and motivation. Eliasson, Bonnier, and Krumlinde-Sundholm (2003) noted that the group allowed children to "support and collaborate with each other when they encountered difficulties" (p. 358).

Group therapy may provide a motivating environment and is typically less expensive than individual therapy, decreasing program costs and allowing more children to be treated at the same time, thus improving access to P–CIMT in clinics that have waiting lists for this intervention. Individual P–CIMT places greater demands on therapy personnel, clinic space, and pediatric equipment than group-based models, which may mitigate these demands and reduce organizational barriers to providing P–CIMT in busy pediatric clinics. Although several studies have been published on group-based models of P–CIMT, limited evidence is available to aid in determining the optimal intensity or duration for group protocols or the elements in the therapy environment that can maximize a child's response to group-based treatment.

Although using a group-based P–CIMT approach has several advantages, potential disadvantages exist. In group environments, the practitioner's attention is divided among the children in the group, and specific feedback and shaping may not be provided in the same way as in individual approaches. This divided focus may lead to the children in group treatment completing tasks with increased compensatory movements and less precise shaping of motor skills. It has been suggested that children should be grouped by age, motor skill ability, and cognitive level (Bonnier, Eliasson, & Krumlinde-Sundholm, 2006; Boyd et al., 2010; Coker, Karakostas, Dodds, & Hsiang, 2010; Eliasson et al., 2003). Gordon, Charles, and Wolf (2005) reported that a 2:1 child-to-practitioner ratio was ideal to maximize the advantages of a group-based P–CIMT approach while allowing close monitoring of the children as they completed activities.

GROUPS, CAMPS, AND OBSERVATIONAL LEARNING

Several studies of group-based models have explored the outcomes of implementing P–CIMT in a camp setting. Camps specially designed to meet the physical and emotional needs of children on the basis of their medical diagnosis have been found to have therapeutic effects for children with neuromuscular conditions and chronic illnesses (Epstein, Stinson, & Stevens, 2005; Gaskell, 2007; Moons et al., 2006). These quantitative and qualitative studies have found that children who participated in therapeutic camps increased their motor skill abilities for overall coordination, hand strength, and dexterity (Bonnier et al., 2006; Eliasson et al., 2003).

Camp-based programs are a natural fit for the summertime, when most children have a break from daily school routines and families are looking for fun, socially engaging enrichment programs. Camps can help children with disabilities become more confident in their motor abilities, improve coping skills, develop better social interactions, and improve emotional responses to injury and illness (Epstein et al., 2005; Gaskell, 2007; Moons et al., 2006). Additional effectiveness research on camp programs is needed that uses comparison group designs and appropriate sample sizes to allow for more rigorous statistical analysis.

Studies have reported motor-learning benefits from group therapy with peers; children benefit from observation of and interaction with peers, and observational learning can be an effective means to teach many types of motor skills (Crompton et al., 2007; Lepage et al., 2012; McNevin, Wulf, & Carlson, 2000). A peer model does not have to be an expert performer, and the observation of a variety of peer performers potentially has a beneficial effect on learning (Lee & White,

1990; Lepage et al., 2012; McCullagh, Weiss, & Ross, 1989; McNevin et al., 2000).

Several behavioral studies have shown that motor performance can be influenced positively by concomitant observation of simple movement (Avenanti, Bolognini, Maravita, & Aglioti, 2007; Brass, Bekkering & Prinz, 2001; Brass, Bekkering, Wohlschläger, & Prinz, 2000; Crompton et al., 2007; Mattar & Gribble, 2005; Press, Cook, Blakemore, & Kilner, 2011). Observations of a peer's actions can support the formation of motor memory and influence subsequent motor performance. For example, Mattar and Gribble (2005) showed that participants observing a video depicting another person learning a motor task performed better than participants who were asked to perform similar movements (motor practice) without observing the video.

Positive consequences for motor performance also were seen by combining action observation and motor practice, the combined effects of which were stronger than action observation alone (Stefan et al., 2005). Taken together, available studies show that observation of others' actions can facilitate motor learning and produce changes that resemble those elicited by actual practice of a repeated movement (Mattar & Gribble, 2005; Press et al., 2011; Stefan et al., 2005).

RESEARCH ON GROUP- AND CAMP-BASED P–CIMT MODELS

Several studies of camp-based P–CIMT programs have outlined essential elements of using a **social group approach,** which entails the development of skills specifically related to interaction with peers in a social setting (Aarts et al., 2012; Bonnier et al., 2006; Boyd et al., 2010; Coker et al., 2010; Eliasson et al., 2003; Sakzewski et al., 2011). These camp-based models have been used to provide P–CIMT to preshool-age children as young as 3 years and to adolescents aged 13 to 18 years.

One of the first published camp-based P–CIMT models, by Bonnier and colleagues (2006), was implemented with 9 adolescents described as having mild-to-moderate hemiplegic CP. A splint that fixed the thumb against the index finger prevented finger and wrist movement. The modified P–CIMT program included 7 hours of daily camp activities offered 5 days per week for 2 weeks (dosage = 70 hours). The daily camp program included recreational activities that the participants completed while wearing the constraint splint. The activities varied each camp day and consisted of age-appropriate games such as disc, golf, mountain climbing, basketball, boules (lawn bowling), baseball, volleyball, canoeing, and water games, as well as various fine motor board, dice, and card games.

All activities were completed in a group, which Bonnier and colleagues (2006) believed was important for motivation and support during failures and challenging tasks. The adolescents also participated in daily tasks such as meal preparation and cleanup and performed hand manipulation activities each morning. Hand manipulation activities were selected to allow participants to practice general aspects of hand function, allowing specific task training and practice of skills that the adolescents might not normally have tried with the affected extremity.

Several assessments, including subtests of the Bruininks–Oseretsky Test of Motor Proficiency (BOTOP; Bruininks, 1978), the Jebsen–Taylor Hand Function Test (JTHFT; Taylor, Sand, & Jebsen, 1973), and the Assessment of Motor and Process Skills (AMPS; Kirkley & Fisher, 1999), and measures of strength and in-hand dexterity were completed before and after camp and at a 5-month follow-up. Results of posttreatment assessment showed significantly improved hand function for dexterity, coordination, precision, and manipulative abilities but not for grip strength. Statistically significant changes were seen in scores on the BOTOP, JTHFT, and in-hand manipulation skills, which continued to be at the same level or above pretest values at the 5-month follow-up but not on the AMPS or grip strength. Bonnier et al. (2006) believed that the adolescents greatly benefited from training together in a group of similar-age peers who had approximately the same functional limitations. The participants appeared to be less frustrated when failing at a task and wanted to make additional efforts when working with others in the group.

A pirate-themed camp model studied by Aarts and colleagues (2010, 2012) combined a modified P–CIMT approach with **task-specific training**—that is, training related to a specific activity and upper-extremity (UE) movement—provided over an 8-week period. The P–CIMT portion was provided in the first 6 weeks with groups of 6 children participating in activities 3 hours per day, 3 days per week (dosage = 54 hours). The last 2 weeks focused on bimanual training integrating new skills into daily life activities. The modified P–CIMT program used a sling for constraint of the stronger extremity, included repetitive task practice and shaping of movements in the affected arm and hand, and applied behavioral procedures in the home environment to encourage the habit of using the weaker extremity in daily activities.

The first phase with the group format was an important part of implementation of this program and provided healthy competition between peers and modeling of movement activities. Aarts et al. (2010, 2012) described the group format as positive for the children's motivation to participate in activities, promote attention to pirate-themed games, and maintain appropriate temperament during times of frustration. They noted positive emotional expressions when the children engaged in play tasks with same-age peers and hypothesized that the group environment may enhance the

likelihood that children will repeat activities while absorbed in group play.

The physical environment was arranged and decorated to reflect the pirate theme. Children were told to pretend that their nonaffected arm was injured during a play pirate activity and that a sling had to be worn to rest the arm. Children had to learn how to use the weaker but "uninjured" arm to complete pirate tasks. Practitioners provided feedback and instructions about the children's performance to enhance the quality of movement, and home activities were provided to help parents transfer new skills into daily tasks. The Canadian Occupational Performance Measure (Cusick, Lannin, & Lowe, 2007; Law et al., 2005), Goal Attainment Scaling (GAS; Kiresuk, Smith, & Cardillo, 1994), ROM, the AHA (Krumlinde-Sundholm et al., 2007), the ABILHAND–Kids (Arnould, Penta, Renders, & Thonnard, 2004), the Melbourne Assessment2 of Unilateral Upper Limb Function (Randall, Johnson, & Reddihough, 2010), and the Video Observations Aarts and Aarts to Determine Developmental Disregard (Houwink, Geerdink, Steenbergen, Geurts, & Aarts, 2013) were used to assess changes in performance after participation in the camp.

Children in the camp program met most goals outlined in the GAS, and improvements were noted on most motor skill tests following completion of the pirate camp program, except for the Melbourne Assessment and ROM measures (Aarts et al., 2010, 2012). For tasks that did not require use of the affected hand (i.e., that could be completed with one hand only), children continued to use the nonaffected hand, demonstrating continued signs of developmental disregard. At the end of the camp experience, children performed their new "pirate skills" for parents and were presented with a certificate of achievement. A video of each child's performance and overall motor gains was provided to families to promote maintenance of skills after the program ended.

Delivering P–CIMT during a camp-based program has many benefits, most of which were highlighted in these published studies. Children are motivated by peers who challenge their motor skills and support them when difficulties arise using the weaker UE in life tasks. Camps provide a sense of belonging, cohesiveness, and camaraderie, allowing children to endure frustrating activities. Camps offer a place where play and friendship become principal in the delivery of therapy, reinforcement, and positive feedback on performance.

DELIVERY OF GROUP- OR CAMP-BASED P–CIMT MODELS

To optimize children's engagement in group P–CIMT interventions, day camps can be held in community facilities, schools, or outpatient rehabilitation centers. Camps are ideal for summertime programming and may allow busy clinics to provide a modified P–CIMT program for a wide age range of children while maximizing clinician time and therapy space.

Several key factors must be considered when deciding to implement a group- or camp-based P–CIMT program:

- Occupational and physical therapy practitioners trained in the principles of P–CIMT should be responsible for evaluating clients and planning and organizing daily treatment activities.
- Pre- and postintervention evaluation of each child should be completed by the lead occupational or physical therapy practitioner before and after the camp program.
- Staff members and others who are not formally trained practitioners can assist with the delivery of activities to provide an appropriate staff-to-child ratio. The studies reviewed in the preceding section reported successful use of therapy student volunteers, parents, and sports recreation staff to help ensure a ratio of 2 to 3 students per staff member.
- All staff should be trained in the theory supporting P–CIMT and the importance of the essential therapy elements, including repetitive task practice, shaping of more mature motor skills, and scaffolding to optimize success during tasks.
- A specific daily camp schedule should be developed that emphasizes age-appropriate play activities and themes. Play and planned group activities can be used as the medium for providing specific task practice that brings forth emotional responses and taps into the children's inner drive to participate and succeed.
- Documentation procedures should be developed to allow staff to summarize motor changes seen in children after each day of participation in camp. Procedures should include filling out task-specific record sheets that include type of task, number of repetitions, and how well the child performed each task.
- A program of activities to be used at home and school should be developed to help children transfer new skills into everyday activities. This program should be developed in collaboration with family members and caregivers. Home and school programs should focus on continued practice of new skills learned at camp, including ways to incorporate new skills into bimanual activities that occur naturally during daily tasks.

EXAMPLE OF A P–CIMT CAMP MODEL: CAMP HAND 2 HANDS

Faculty members in the Occupational Therapy Department at the Medical University of South Carolina developed

Figure 10.1   HOUSES USED FOR STORAGE OF CONSTRAINT MITTS.

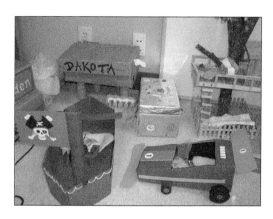

Source. A. Eliasson and P. Coker-Bolt.

and first implemented a camp-based P–CIMT program in 2001 and since then have provided this modified group program to more than 100 preschool-age children (aged 3 to 6 years; Coker et al., 2010). The camp P–CIMT program is embedded in an elective course for graduate students enrolled in occupational and physical therapy programs and provides children with 6 hours of specific task training over 5 consecutive camp days (dosage = 30 hours). The constraint is a resting hand splint covered with a puppet mitt. The constraint and puppet are consistent with the camp theme, and children wake the puppet up at the start of each camp day (and don the restraint) and put the puppet to bed at the end of each camp day (Figure 10.1 shows theme-based houses where puppets "sleep").

Therapy students spend 9 weeks planning theme-based camp activities, reviewing the research evidence about P–CIMT, learning principles of constraint therapy, and practicing a variety of hands-on and other treatment techniques for children with unilateral motor weakness. Table 10.1 describes the training provided to students before they participate in Camp Hand 2 Hands. A team of 1 occupational therapy and 1 physical therapy student works with each child who attends Camp Hand 2 Hands, a ratio of 2 students to 1 child.

A specific Camp Hand 2 Hands daily schedule has been developed based on a typical preschool day that allows both individual and group activities and breaks for a snack and meals (Table 10.2). The camp environment is changed somewhat each day to highlight the age-appropriate and child-friendly camp themes; theme-based days that have been popular with preschool-age children include Holiday Day, Disney Day, Zoo or Safari Day, Western Day, All Around Town Day, Rock Star Day, International or Around the World Day, Olympics Day, Field Day, Pirate Day, Cartoon Day, When I Grow Up Day, and Carnival Day. Pictures of theme-based activities appear

Table 10.1　STUDENT AND STAFF TRAINING SESSIONS BEFORE CAMP HAND 2 HANDS

SESSION	DISCUSSION TOPIC	ACTIVITY
1 and 2	Overview of CIMT and P–CIMT and essential elements (i.e., repetitive task practice and shaping)	Students review the research on P–CIMT and discuss levels of evidence and the outcomes of the most current studies.
3 and 4	Group- and theme-based treatment approaches for children	Students work in teams to develop daily themes for the camp and create a list of needed camp supplies.
5	Assessment and goal setting	Students review preschool-age developmental tasks and discuss functional goals and measurement tools used for children with unilateral motor weakness.
6	Social play and behavior management strategies for children	Students work through case scenarios of behavioral challenges that may be encountered during therapy and camp sessions and discuss possible ways to encourage and motivate participation in tasks.
7	Documentation and discharge planning	Students review examples of camp documentation and discharge and home activities from prior camp years.
8	Case presentation and review of preliminary information on children attending camp	Students work through video case scenarios from previous camps and review enrollment information and parent goals for children attending the current camp.

Note. CIMT = constraint-induced movement therapy; P–CIMT = pediatric constraint-induced movement therapy.

Table 10.2　SAMPLE SCHEDULE FOR A 6-HOUR P–CIMT CAMP FOR PRESCHOOL-AGE CHILDREN

TIME	ACTIVITY	TIME	ACTIVITY
9:00–9:10	Greet campers as they arrive, talk to parents, and prepare for the day	12:00–12:30	Lunch (campers bring their own)
9:10–9:30	Group time: music, story, movement activity to introduce daily camp theme	12:30–1:00	Story time and bathroom
9:30–10:30	Theme-based centers and individual and small-group activities	1:00–2:15	Theme-based centers and individual and small-group activities
10:30–10:50	Snack time and bathroom	2:15–2:45	Snack time and bathroom
10:50–11:15	Theme-based large-group activity	2:45–3:00	Group time, music, and daily wrap-up (parents begin arriving)
11:15–12:00	Theme-based centers and individual and small-group activities		

Note. P–CIMT = pediatric constraint-induced movement therapy.

Figure 10.2   EXAMPLES OF CAMP ENVIRONMENTS THAT INCORPORATE THEME DAYS: (a) OUTER SPACE DAY AND (b) AROUND THE WORLD DAY.

(a)

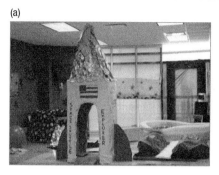

(b)

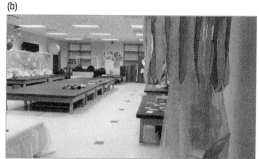

Source. A. Eliasson and P. Coker-Bolt.

in Figures 10.2 and 10.3. A detailed schedule of activities for Beach Day is provided in Appendix 10.A.

A 1-year study was conducted to evaluate the outcomes of participation in the Camp Hand 2 Hands programs. The outcome measures included the Pediatric Motor Activity Log (Taub, Ramey, DeLuca, & Echols, 2004), the Child Arm Use Test (Taub et al., 2004), the Pediatric Evaluation of Disability Inventory (PEDI; Haley, Coster, Ludlow, Haltiwanger, & Andrellos, 1992), and the GAITRite Walkway (CIR Systems, Clifton, NJ). Children were tested 1 week before camp, 1 week

Figure 10.3   EXAMPLES OF THEME-BASED ACTIVITIES: (a) ACTIVITY FOR CARNIVAL DAY, (b) OBSTACLE COURSE FROM CAMPING DAY, (c) POPCORN SNACK FROM CIRCUS DAY, AND (d) BUILD-YOUR-OWN CASTLE FROM FAIRY TALE DAY.

a
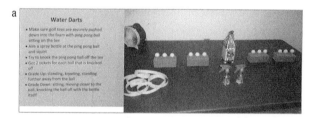

b
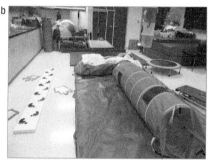

c
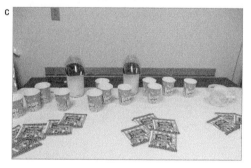

d
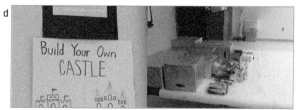

Source. A. Eliasson and P. Coker-Bolt.

Figure 10.4 CHANGES IN SCORES ON THE HOW OFTEN AND HOW WELL SUBSCALES OF THE PEDIATRIC MOTOR ACTIVITY LOG (PMAL) AT PRETEST (1 WEEK BEFORE CAMP), POSTTEST (1 WEEK AFTER CAMP), AND 6-MONTH FOLLOW-UP.

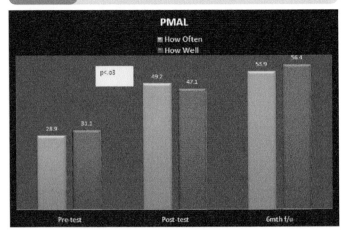

Source. A. Eliasson and P. Coker-Bolt.

Figure 10.6 CHANGES IN SCORES ON THE PEDIATRIC EVALUATION OF DISABILITY INVENTORY (PEDI) AT PRETEST (1 WEEK BEFORE CAMP), POSTTEST (1 WEEK AFTER CAMP), AND 6-MONTH FOLLOW-UP.

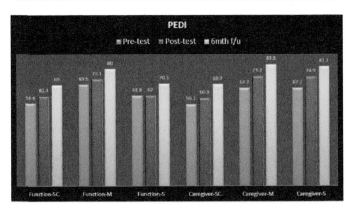

Source. A. Eliasson and P. Coker-Bolt.

after camp, and 6 months following the completion of camp. Statistically significant changes were seen in all measures, and gains were maintained at the 6-month follow-up (Figures 10.4, 10.5, and 10.6). Changes in the temporal and spatial aspects of gait are discussed in more detail in Chapter 16, "Research Priorities: Understanding and Transcending the Limits of Current Knowledge to Inform Best Practices" (see also Coker et al., 2010).

SUMMARY

This chapter has provided examples of widely used modified or alternative P–CIMT approaches that maintain the five core features of signature P–CIMT but modify the type of constraint or treatment setting while maintaining a high dosage of concentrated therapy using systematic shaping and repetitive practice to refine motor skills. It is important to continue to study the long-lasting effects of these modified and alternative approaches for children with unilateral motor weakness of different ages and varying medical diagnoses.

Figure 10.5 CHANGES IN SCORES ON THE HOW OFTEN AND HOW WELL SUBSCALES OF THE CHILD ARM USE TEST (CAUT) AT PRETEST (1 WEEK BEFORE CAMP), POSTTEST (1 WEEK AFTER CAMP), AND 6-MONTH FOLLOW-UP.

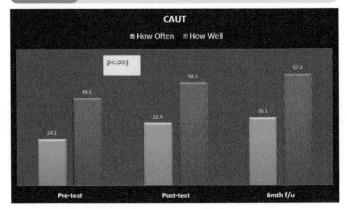

Source. A. Eliasson and P. Coker-Bolt.

REFERENCES

Aarts, P. B., Jongerius, P. H., Geerdink, Y. A., van Limbeek, J., & Geurts, A. C. (2010). Effectiveness of modified constraint-induced movement therapy in children with unilateral spastic cerebral palsy: A randomized controlled trial. *Neurorehabilitation and Neural Repair, 24,* 509–518.

Aarts, P. B., van Hartingsveldt, M., Anderson, P. G., van den Tillaar, I., van der Burg, J., & Geurts, A. C. (2012). The pirate group intervention protocol: Description and a case report of a modified constraint-induced movement therapy combined with bimanual training for young children with unilateral spastic cerebral palsy. *Occupational Therapy International, 19,* 76–87.

Al Oraibi, S., & Eliasson, A. C. (2011). Implementation of constraint-induced movement therapy for young children with unilateral cerebral palsy in Jordan: A home-based model. *Disability and Rehabilitation, 33*, 2006–2012.

Arnould, C., Penta, M., Renders, A., & Thonnard, J. L. (2004). ABILHAND–Kids: A measure of manual ability in children with cerebral palsy. *Neurology, 63*, 1045–1052.

Avenanti, A., Bolognini, N., Maravita, A., & Aglioti, S. M. (2007). Somatic and motor components of action simulation. *Current Biology, 17*, 2129–2135.

Bonnier, B., Eliasson, A. C., & Krumlinde-Sundholm, L. (2006). Effects of constraint-induced movement therapy in adolescents with hemiplegic cerebral palsy: A day camp model. *Scandinavian Journal of Occupational Therapy, 13*, 13–22.

Boyd, R., Sakzewski, L., Ziviani, J., Abbott, D. F., Badawy, R., Gilmore, R., . . . Jackson, G. D. (2010). INCITE: A randomised trial comparing constraint induced movement therapy and bimanual training in children with congenital hemiplegia. *BMC Neurology, 10*, 4.

Brass, M., Bekkering, H., & Prinz, W. (2001). Movement observation affects movement execution in a simple response task. *Acta Psychologica, 106*, 3–22.

Brass, M., Bekkering, H., Wohlschläger, A., & Prinz, W. (2000). Compatibility between observed and executed finger movements: Comparing symbolic, spatial, and imitative cues. *Brain and Cognition, 44*, 124–143.

Bronfenbrenner, U., & Morris, P. A. (1998). The ecology of developmental processes. In W. Daman & R. M. Lerner (Eds.), *Handbook of child psychology: Vol. 1: Theoretical models of human development* (pp. 993–1028). New York: Wiley.

Bruininks, R. H. (1978). *Bruininks–Oseretsky Test of Motor Proficiency: Examiner's manual.* Circle Pines, MN: American Guidance Service.

Case-Smith, J., DeLuca, S. C., Stevenson, R., & Ramey, S. L. (2012). Multicenter randomized controlled trial of pediatric constraint-induced movement therapy: 6-month follow-up. *American Journal of Occupational Therapy, 66*, 15–23. http://dx.doi.org/10.5014/ajot.2012.002386

Charles, J. R., & Gordon, A. M. (2007). A repeated course of constraint-induced movement therapy results in further improvement. *Developmental Medicine and Child Neurology, 49*, 770–773.

Coker, P., Karakostas, T., Dodds, C., & Hsiang, S. (2010). Gait characteristics of children with hemiplegic cerebral palsy before and after modified constraint-induced movement therapy. *Disability and Rehabilitation, 32*, 402–408. http://dx.doi.org/10.3109/09638280903171592

Crompton, J., Imms, C., McCoy, A. T., Randall, M., Eldridge, B., Scoullar, B., & Galea, M. P. (2007). Group-based task-related training for children with cerebral palsy: A pilot study. *Physical and Occupational Therapy in Pediatrics, 27*, 43–65.

Cusick, A., Lannin, N. A., & Lowe, K. (2007). Adapting the Canadian Occupational Performance Measure for use in a paediatric clinical trial. *Disability Rehabilitation, 29*, 761–766.

DeLuca, S. C., Echols, K., Law, C. R., & Ramey, S. L. (2006). Intensive pediatric constraint-induced movement therapy for children with cerebral palsy: Randomized, controlled, crossover trial. *Journal of Child Neurology, 11*, 931–938. PMID: 17092457

Eliasson, A. C., Bonnier, B., & Krumlinde-Sundholm, L. (2003). Clinical experience of constraint induced movement therapy in adolescents with hemiplegic cerebral palsy: A day camp model. *Developmental Medicine and Child Neurology, 45*, 357–359. PMID: 12729152

Eliasson, A. C., Krumlinde-Sundholm, L., Shaw, K., & Wang, C. (2005). Effects of constraint-induced movement therapy in young children with hemiplegic cerebral palsy: An adapted model. *Developmental Medicine and Child Neurology, 47*, 266–275. PMID: 15832550

Eliasson, A. C., Shaw, K., Berg, E., & Krumlinde-Sundholm, L. (2011). An ecological approach of constraint induced movement therapy for 2–3-year-old children: A randomized control trial. *Research in Developmental Disabilities, 32*, 2820–2828. http://dx.doi.org/10.1016/j.ridd.2011.05.024

Epstein, I., Stinson, J., & Stevens, B. (2005). The effects of camp on health-related quality of life in children with chronic illnesses: A review of the literature. *Journal of Pediatric Oncology Nursing, 22*, 89–103.

Gaskell, S. (2007). The challenge of evaluating rehabilitative activity holidays for burn-injured children: Qualitative and quantitative outcome data from a Burns Camp over a five-year period. *Developmental Neurorehabilitation, 10*, 149–160.

Gordon, J., Charles, J., & Wolf, S. L. (2005). Methods of constraint-induced movement therapy for children with hemiplegic cerebral palsy: Development of a child-friendly intervention for improving upper-extremity function. *Archives of Physical Medicine and Rehabilitation, 86*, 837–844.

Gordon, A. M., Charles, J., & Wolf, S. L. (2006). Efficacy of constraint-induced movement therapy on involved upper-extremity use in children with hemiplegic cerebral palsy is not age-dependent. *Pediatrics, 117*, e363–e373.

Haley, S. M., Coster, W. J., Ludlow, L. H., Haltiwanger, J. T., & Andrellos, P. J. (1992). *Pediatric Evaluation of Disability Inventory (PEDI): Development, standardization and administration manual.* Boston: New England Medical Center Hospitals, and PEDI Research Group.

Holmefur, M., Aarts, P., Hoare, B., & Krumlinde-Sundholm, L. (2009). Test–retest and alternate forms reliability of the Assisting Hand Assessment. *Journal of Rehabilitation Medicine, 41,* 886–891.

Houwink, A., Geerdink, Y. A., Steenbergen, B., Geurts, A. C., & Aarts, P. B. (2013). Assessment of upper-limb capacity, performance, and developmental disregard in children with cerebral palsy: Validity and reliability of the revised Video-Observation Aarts and Aarts module: Determine Developmental Disregard (VOAA–DDD–R). *Developmental Medicine and Child Neurology, 55,* 76–82.

Juenger, H., Linder-Lucht, M., Walther, M., Berweck, S., Mall, V., & Staudt, M. (2007). Cortical neuromodulation by constraint-induced movement therapy in congenital hemiparesis: An fMRI study. *Neuropediatrics, 38,* 130–136.

King, S., Teplicky, R., King, G., & Rosenbaum, P. (2004). Family-centered service for children with cerebral palsy and their families: A review of the literature. *Seminars in Pediatric Neurology, 11,* 78–86.

Kiresuk, T., Smith, A., & Cardillo, J. (1994). *Goal Attainment Scaling: Applications, theory, and measurement.* Hillsdale, NJ: Lawrence Erlbaum.

Kirkley, K. N., & Fisher, A. G. (1999). Alternate forms reliability of the Assessment of Motor and Process Skills. *Journal of Outcome Measures, 3*(10), 53–70.

Krumlinde-Sundholm, L., Holmefur, M., Kottorp, A., & Eliasson, A. C. (2007). The Assisting Hand Assessment: Current evidence of validity, reliability, and responsiveness to change. *Developmental Medicine and Child Neurology, 49,* 259–264.

Kuhnke, N., Juenger, H., Walther, M., Berweck, S., Mall, V., & Staudt, M. (2008). Do patients with congenital hemiparesis and ipsilateral corticospinal projections respond differently to constraint-induced movement therapy? *Developmental Medicine and Child Neurology, 12,* 898–903.

Law, M., Baptiste, S., Carswell, A., McColl, M., Polatajko, H., & Pollock, N. (2005). *Canadian Occupational Performance Measure* (3rd ed.). Ottawa: CAOT Publications ACE.

Lee, T. D., & White, M. A. (1990). Influence of an unskilled model's practice schedule on observational motor learning. *Human Movement Science, 9,* 349–367.

Lepage, J. F., Morin-Moncet, O., Beaulé, V., de Beaumont, L., Champoux, F., & Théoret, H. (2012). Occlusion of LTP-like plasticity in human primary motor cortex by action observation. *PLoS ONE, 7,* e38754.

Lin, K. C., Wang, T. N., Wu, C. Y., Chen, C. L., Chang, K. C., Lin, Y. C., & Chen, Y. J. (2011). Effects of home-based constraint-induced therapy versus dose-matched control intervention on functional outcomes and caregiver

well-being in children with cerebral palsy. *Research in Developmental Disabilities, 32,* 1483–1491.

Löwing, K., Bexelius, A., & Carlberg, E. B. (2010). Goal-directed functional therapy: A longitudinal study on gross motor function in children with cerebral palsy. *Disability and Rehabilitation, 32,* 908–916.

Mastos, M., Miller, K., Eliasson, A. C., & Imms, C. (2007). Goal-directed training: Linking theories of treatment to clinical practice for improved functional activities in daily life [Case reports]. *Clinical Rehabilitation, 21,* 47–55.

Mattar, A. A., & Gribble, P. L. (2005). Motor learning by observing. *Neuron, 46,* 153–160.

McCullagh, P., Weiss, M. R., & Ross, D. (1989). Modeling considerations in motor skill acquisition and performance: An integrated approach. In K. Pandolf (Ed.), *Exercise and sport science reviews* (pp. 475–513). Baltimore: Williams & Wilkins.

McNevin, N., Wulf, G., & Carlson, C. (2000). Rehabilitation training on motor learning: Implications for physical effects on attentional focus, self-control, and dyads. *Physical Therapy, 80,* 373–385.

Moons, P., Barrea, C., Suys, B., Ovaert, C., Boshoff, D., Eyskens, B., . . . Sluysmans, T. (2006). Improved perceived health status persists three months after a special sports camp for children with congenital heart disease. *European Journal of Pediatrics, 165,* 767–772.

Press, C., Cook, J., Blakemore, S. J., & Kilner, J. (2011). Dynamic modulation of human motor activity when observing actions. *Journal of Neuroscience, 31,* 2792–2800.

Randall, M. J., Johnson, L. M., & Reddihough, D. S. (2010). *The Melbourne Assessment 2 of Unilateral Upper Limb Function: Test administration manual.* Melbourne, Australia: Royal Children's Hospital.

Rostami, H. R., & Malamiri, R. A. (2012). Effect of treatment environment on modified constraint-induced movement therapy results in children with spastic hemiplegic cerebral palsy: A randomized controlled trial. *Disability and Rehabilitation, 34,* 40–44.

Sakzewski, L., Ziviani, J., Abbott, D. F., Macdonell, R. A., Jackson, G. D., & Boyd, R. N. (2011). Participation outcomes in a randomized trial of 2 models of upper-limb rehabilitation for children with congenital hemiplegia. *Archives of Physical Medicine and Rehabilitation, 92,* 531–539.

Smith, R. A., & Wrisberg, C. A. (2001). *Motor learning and performance: A problem-based learning approach* (Vol. 2). Baltimore: Human Kinetics Publisher.

Stefan, K., Cohen, L. G., Duque, J., Mazzocchio, R., Celnik, P., Sawaki, L., . . . Classen, J. (2005). Formation of a motor memory by action observation. *Journal of Neuroscience, 25,* 9339–9346.

Taub, E., Ramey, S. L., DeLuca, S., & Echols, K. (2004). Efficacy of constraint-induced movement therapy for children with cerebral palsy with asymmetric motor impairment. *Pediatrics, 113,* 305–312. PMID: 14754942

Taylor, N., Sand, P. L., & Jebsen, R. H. (1973). Evaluation of hand function in children. *Archives of Physical Medicine and Rehabilitation, 54,* 129–135.

Thelen, E., & Smith, L. B. (1996). *A dynamic systems approach to development of cognition and action.* Cambridge, MA: MIT Press.

Wallen, M., Ziviani, J., Naylor, O., Evans, R., Novak, I., & Herbert, R. D. (2011). Modified constraint-induced therapy for children with hemiplegic cerebral palsy: A randomized trial. *Developmental Medicine and Child Neurology, 53,* 1091–1099.

Walther, M., Juenger, H., Kuhneke, N., Wilke, M., Brobeck, V., Berweck, S., . . . Mall, V. (2009). Motor cortex plasticity in ischemic perinatal stroke: Transcranial magnetic stimulation and functional MRI study. *Pediatric Neurology, 3,* 171–178.

APPENDIX 10.A. SCHEDULE FOR BEACH DAY

TIME	ACTIVITIES	SUPPLIES NEEDED	INSTRUCTIONS
		Morning	
9:10–9:30	Circle time (group): Minnow, Minnow, Shark	None	Have all the children sit in a circle. One child is the shark, and the others are the minnows. Play this game like Duck, Duck, Goose.
9:30–10:30	Centers and activities		
	Feed the dolphins	8 buckets Beanbags Tricycles	Before the game begins, scatter 8 buckets (these are the dolphins) around the hallway. Make sure the buckets are at least 4 feet apart and not in a straight line. Tell the children they are in charge of feeding the dolphins. They need to get on their "jet skis" (tricycles) and ride into the "ocean" (hallway). The children ride the tricycles down the hallway, placing a "fish" (bean bag) into each dolphin's mouth. *Grade down:* • Push the tricycle for the child so he or she can focus on throwing the fish into the dolphin's mouth. • If the child cannot ride the tricycle, have him or her "swim" (walk) through and place the fish in the dolphin's mouth. *Grade up:* • Tell the children they cannot get close to the dolphin or they will get bitten, and make the children throw the fish into the bucket from 2 feet away.
	Soccer	Soccer ball or kickball Pool Soccer goal	Have the children stand in the pool. Tell the children to try and kick the ball to the other side of the pool as quickly as possible. (You can tell them to kick as quickly as possible so they don't get bitten by a shark!) You also can stand at the other end of the pool and have the children kick the ball to you. *Grade down:* • Give the child a larger ball to kick, or stand closer to the child in the pool so he or she doesn't have to kick the ball as far. • If the water makes it too difficult, play soccer outside of the pool, and have the child try and kick the ball to you. *Grade up:* • Give the child a smaller ball to kick, or have the child kick to one side and then the other.

(Continued)

APPENDIX 10.A. SCHEDULE FOR BEACH DAY *(Cont.)*

TIME	ACTIVITIES	SUPPLIES NEEDED	INSTRUCTIONS
	Fishing	Blue sheet with paper fish taped to it Dowels with string and clothespin attached	Children stand 1–2 feet away from the "fishing hole" (blue sheet with fish). They use their affected extremity to cast the "fishing pole" (dowel with string and clothespin) over the hole. The children wait for a tug on the rod indicating that they have caught a fish and then use the affected arm to pull in the pole with the fish. Each child does this activity 5 times in a row. After getting the fish, the child opens the clothespin with affected hand and puts the fish in the fish bucket. *Grade down:* • Use a large chip clip if the child is having problems releasing the fish from the clothespin. • Use a larger fish on the chip clip. • Use a paperclip with a large fish so the child can slide the fish out of the pole without having to pinch down. • Use a shorter pole if the child is having difficulty getting the pole over the hole. *Grade up:* • Attach a smaller fish to the clothespin for the child. • Use a smaller clothespin with a larger fish. • Use a smaller clothespin with a smaller fish.
	Decorating visors	Visors Puff paint, squeeze paint, stencils, glitter paint Stick-on eyes, pipe cleaners, stickers, sponges, flowers, fuzzy balls—things to glue on with glue gun	Have children decorate their visor as they wish. *Grade down:* • Have the child paint the visor with a sponge or fingers. *Grade up:* • Have the child put stickers on the visor.
	Sorting goldfish	Colored paper goldfish Cups	Children sort the different colors of goldfish into individual cups with their affected hand. *Grade down:* • Have the child pick up any 10 goldfish and place them in the cup. *Grade up:* • Have the child use tweezers or tongs to pick up goldfish or place the goldfish in a smaller cup.
	Modified cornhole— fish feeding	Board with 4 different-sized holes, each with a fish painted beside it Beanbags	Children stand 3 feet away from board and "feed the fish" by tossing a beanbag into each of the 4 holes. Each child gets 5 attempts to feed the fish, then switches with another camper or student practitioner to have a turn, then tries again. *Grade down:* • Decrease the distance the child stands from the board. • Have the child sit on a bench or stool while throwing the beanbags. • Encourage the child to feed only the fish that is next to the largest opening in the board. *Grade up:* • Increase the distance the child stands from the board. • Change the child's base of support to stand with feet together or stand on one leg. • Balance on a Swiss ball or T-seat while throwing the beanbags. • Encourage the child to feed only the fish that is next to the smallest opening in the board.

(Continued)

APPENDIX 10.A. SCHEDULE FOR BEACH DAY *(Cont.)*

TIME	ACTIVITIES	SUPPLIES NEEDED	INSTRUCTIONS
10:30–10:50	Snack time	Multicolored goldfish crackers (i.e., edible snack)	Have children separate a cup of goldfish by colors before eating.
10:50–11:15	Circle time (group): Dressing relay	Hats Sunglasses Flipflops T-shirts Flower leis	Have children run to where the clothing is, put it on, and go back to tag the next person in their group. This continues until a group finishes first.
11:15–12:00	Centers and activities		
	Decorate fish	Paper or cardboard fish Art supplies (e.g., paint, markers)	Have children decorate their fish as they wish. *Grade down:* • Gradually decrease the incline on which the child decorates the fish. • Use thicker markers, paint brushes, and larger items to decorate the fish. • Allow the child to sit on a stable surface to decrease the amount of trunk control required. *Grade up:* • Have the child decorate the fish on a vertical surface. • Have the child use skinny markers, thin paintbrushes, or smaller items to decorate the fish. • Require the child to sit on a bolster or stand to increase the amount of trunk control required.
	Treasure hunt	Trunk full of sand with prizes buried inside	Children search for buried treasure in a trunk full of sand. *Grade down:* • Have larger objects hidden in the sand right below the surface. • Allow the child to use the hand to dig. *Grade up:* • Have smaller objects hidden deeper in the sand. • Require the child to use a shovel or rake instead of the hand.
	Nemo obstacle course	Paper or cardboard rocks and jellyfish on floor Decorations representing a sunken ship, shark, and Nemo Beanbags Bolster swing Tape for finish line	Children pretend they are Marlin looking for his son Nemo. They get through the swarm of jellyfish by hopping from rock to rock over the jellyfish using alternating feet. They "swim" to the sunken ship on the scooter board. They feed the shark by standing behind a taped line and using their involved extremity to toss 2 fish into the shark's mouth. They get past the shark by holding on to a bolster swing for 30 seconds. They finish by running to the finish line and find Nemo at the end of the course. *Grade down:* • Decrease distance between rocks for shorter hops. • Decrease distance from the taped line to the shark's mouth. *Grade up:* • Increase distance between rocks for longer hops. • Increase distance from the taped line to the shark's mouth.

(Continued)

APPENDIX 10.A. SCHEDULE FOR BEACH DAY *(Cont.)*

TIME	ACTIVITIES	SUPPLIES NEEDED	INSTRUCTIONS
	Squirt bottle beach ball game	Pool partially filled with water Water squirt toy Beach balls	Children use a water gun in their involved extremity to push the ball from one side of the pool to the other. The goal is to get the beach ball across the pool 5 times within the allotted time. *Grade down:* • Have the child use his or her hand to push the ball across pool against the resistance of the water. *Grade up:* • Use smaller balls as targets. • Have the child try to get the ball across the pool 10 times within the allotted time.
12:00–12:30	Lunch		
Afternoon			
12:30–1:00	Storytime and bathroom	Fish and beach books	Read books as children listen.
1:00–2:00	Centers and activities		
	Miniature golf	Minigolf course Minigolf clubs	Children do one-handed putting with the puppet hand stabilizing the club. They start 5 feet from the hole and putt the ball toward the hole. Children should stand perpendicular to the hole to encourage trunk rotation during putting and should use the base of support that is comfortable for them. Practitioners watch for even weight bearing between the feet and a proper hold on the golf club to encourage supination and wrist extension. *Grade down:* • Have the child move close to hole. • Help the child hold on to the club. *Grade up:* • Have the child move further from hole. • Have the child decrease the base of support if the chosen one is wider than normal.
	Picture frames	Frames Art supplies	Children decorate frames with provided supplies. Objects are situated around the table to encourage reaching. This activity can be modified depending on the needs of each child so that reach is done with proper biomechanics. *Grade down:* • Have the child use big objects for decorating. • Have the frame flat on the table. • Have the child use a stable, supportive chair while decorating. *Grade up:* • Have the child decorate on a more vertical surface (i.e., prop up the frame). • Have the child use smaller decorations. • Ask the child to use specific colors or objects. • Have the child decorate while standing or while sitting on a ball.

(Continued)

APPENDIX 10.A. SCHEDULE FOR BEACH DAY *(Cont.)*

TIME	ACTIVITIES	SUPPLIES NEEDED	INSTRUCTIONS
	Badminton	Badminton net, rackets, and birdies	A child is on one side of the net, and a practitioner is on the other. The practitioner tosses the child a birdie, and the child aims to hit it back over the net using the badminton racket at least 10 times successfully. *Grade down:* <ul><li>Throw a ball instead of a birdie over the net.</li><li>Decrease distance between the child and the net.</li></ul> *Grade up:* <ul><li>Hit the birdie back and forth 15–20 times.</li><li>See if the child can keep the birdie going back and forth.</li><li>Increase distance between the child and the net.</li></ul>
2:00–2:15	Circle time (group): Limbo	Limbo bar Music	Have the children line up and go under the limbo bar one at time, lowering it each time.
2:15–2:45	Sand cup for snack	Clear plastic cups Vanilla pudding Vanilla sandwich cookies Nemo gummy snacks Blue food coloring Spoons	Children put the pudding into the cup, squeeze 3 drops of food coloring into the pudding, and stir with a spoon. Then they crush the vanilla sandwich cookies to be the sand and add it to the cup. Finally, they put Nemo gummies into the cup.
2:45–3:00	Group time, music, daily wrap-up		

Source. A. Eliasson and P. Coker-Bolt. Used with permission.

TERESSA GARCIA REIDY, MS, OTR/L; PATTY COKER-BOLT, PhD, OTR/L; and DORY AINSWORTH WALLACE, MS, OTR/L

11

Adapting Pediatric CIMT for Children With Brachial Plexus Injuries, Traumatic Brain Injury, and Hemispherectomy and Other Surgical Interventions

CHAPTER HIGHLIGHTS

- Brachial plexus injuries
- Traumatic brain injury
- Hemispherectomy and other surgical interventions.

The mechanisms of motor and cognitive control and the neural adaptations that accompany motor skill training are not dependent on a disease or disorder, but they rely on rehabilitation approaches that enable better reaching, grasping, and upper-body movement. The sensorimotor networks engaged in improving motor performance and used during pediatric constraint-induced movement therapy (P–CIMT) are highly integrated with other systems that represent aspects of cognition, working memory, error detection and correction, reward and motivation, and responsiveness to verbal and physical cues.

The essential components of P–CIMT, including intensive task-oriented training and shaping, can be used with populations of patients who have unilateral motor weakness other than children with cerebral palsy (CP). Recent studies have investigated the use of P–CIMT with diverse populations, including children recovering from brachial plexus injury, traumatic brain injury, and hemispherectomy. This chapter explores the literature on the use of P–CIMT with diverse populations and provides case examples to highlight how constraint therapy has improved the overall function of children with unilateral motor disabilities.

KEY TERMS

Anatomical hemispherectomy
Arterial venous malformations
Axonmetesis
Brachial plexus palsy
Contusion
Diffuse injury
Diffuse axonal injury
Erb–Duchenne palsy
Erb–Klumpke palsy
Erb's palsy
Focal injury
Frontal lobes
Functional hemispherectomy
Hemispherectomy
Intractable epilepsy
Intractable epileptiform abnormalities
Klumpke's palsy
Neurological recovery
Neuroma
Neuropraxia
Neurotmesis
Postganglionic injury
Preganglionic injury
Shoulder dystocia
Traumatic brain injury
Tumor resection

BRACHIAL PLEXUS INJURIES

BACKGROUND AND MECHANISM OF INJURY

Brachial plexus palsy is weakness related to insult or injury to nerves in the brachial plexus; the incidence is reported to be 0.4 to 4.0 per 1,000 births (Pham, Kratz, Jelin, & Gelfand, 2011). It is most commonly associated with **shoulder dystocia,** which occurs when the infant's anterior shoulder becomes trapped behind the mother's symphysis pubis during delivery. During delivery, a corrective maneuver to provide lateral traction of the head and facilitate movement of the infant through the birth canal can stretch the brachial plexus, leading to injury in 4% to 40% of cases (Doumouchtsis & Arulkumaran, 2009). This forcible separation of the head and neck from the shoulder may create long-term clinical issues and a spectrum of possible injuries to the plexus.

Brachial plexus palsies are classified in two ways: (1) by anatomical location and (2) by degree of nerve injury and neuropathic injury (Benjamin, 2005; Kwazneski, Iyer, Panthaki, & Armstrong, 2009; McGillicuddy, 2011; Pham et al., 2011). Upper root injury, or **Erb–Duchenne palsy,**

involves damage to spinal nerves C5 and C6. This type of brachial plexus injury, also referred to as **Erb's palsy,** results in paralysis of the shoulder muscles, the elbow flexors, and the forearm supinators. If the C7 nerve is involved, the wrist and finger extensors also are paralyzed.

Injury to lower spinal roots, commonly C8 to T1, is referred to as **Klumpke's palsy.** This type of palsy is characterized by weakness of the triceps, forearm pronators, and wrist flexors, with the classic physical presentation of a paralyzed hand with no individual digit or thumb movement. These pure lower-root injuries with isolated distal hand weakness are rare.

The third type of palsy based on anatomical location is **Erb–Klumpke palsy.** This type of brachial plexus injury involves injury to the complete plexus from C5 to T1, with total sensory and motor deficits of the entire upper extremity (UE). The child presents with a flaccid UE with little to no active movement in the shoulder, elbow, forearm, wrist, fingers, and thumb. Horner's syndrome also may be present (Benjamin, 2005; Kattan & Borschel, 2011; Pham et al., 2011; Piatt, 2005; Table 11.1).

Brachial plexus palsies also can be classified by neuropathic injury (Piatt, 2005). **Preganglionic injury** is a proximal lesion of the spinal roots, also known as *root avulsion*. This is the

Table 11.1   Types of Brachial Plexus Palsy: Sensory Deficits and Clinical Presentation

TYPE	NERVE ROOTS	AFFECTED NERVES	SENSORY DEFICITS	CLINICAL PRESENTATION	ASSOCIATED PROBLEMS
Upper: Erb–Duchenne	C5, C6, possibly C7	Shoulder • Dorsal scapular • Suprascapular • Lateral pectoral • Long thoracic Upper arm • Musculocutaneous Forearm • Radial and median Wrist or fingers • Median Diaphragm • Phrenic	Radial side of deltoid, forearm, and hand; medial side of hand unaffected	Shoulder adducted and internally rotated, arm adducted Elbow extended Forearm pronated Wrist and fingers flexed—"waiter's tip" Possible diaphragm paralysis	Shoulder dislocation and "winged scapula" Osseous deformity Limb-length disparity Forearm deformity
Lower: Klumpke's	C8 to T1, possibly C7	Forearm • Radial • Ulnar • Thoracodorsal Hand and wrist • Median and radial Medial pectoral	Ulnar side of forearm and hand	Forearm Wrist and fingers Miosis and ptosis	Limb-length disparity Horner's syndrome
Complete: Erb–Klumpke	C5 to T1 (full plexus)	Complete plexus (all nerves)	Entire arm	Flaccid paralysis of arm Miosis and ptosis	Limb-length disparity Possible Horner's syndrome

most severe type of injury and usually occurs at the nerve rootlet near the spinal cord. These lesions occur proximal to the dorsal root ganglia. **Postganglionic injury** is a more distal spinal lesion and may be complete axonmetesis, neurotmesis, neuroma, neuropraxia, or a combination of Erb's palsy, Klumpke's palsy, and Erb–Klumpke palsy (Kwazneski et al., 2009; Pham et al., 2011). The least severe injury is a **neuropraxia,** or stretch injury. This type of conduction block may resolve spontaneously over a few hours or weeks with no permanent structural damage to the nerve. An **axonmetesis** is an injury to the axons as well as connective tissues. If only the axons are disrupted, they may regrow with full recovery. A **neurotmesis** is a complete nerve rupture. Scar tissues may form between the proximal and distal nerve ends and become a **neuroma**. It is difficult to achieve full recovery with this type of injury without surgical intervention to excise the neuroma and construct a patch graph to reconnect the proximal and distal nerve ends (Benjamin, 2005; Kattan & Borschel, 2011; Pham et al., 2011; Piatt, 2005).

TREATMENT CONSIDERATIONS FOR BRACHIAL PLEXUS INJURIES

Surgical intervention remains an area of current research interest. Some physicians advise surgical intervention by age 3–6 months if antigravity biceps function is absent, whereas other physicians prefer to wait for possible spontaneous recovery of movement until age 9–10 months (Benjamin, 2005; Kozin, 2011; Pham et al., 2011). Approximately 10% of infants born with brachial plexus palsies require some type of surgical intervention, including nerve grafting and transfer or secondary reconstruction of the shoulder, forearm, wrist, or hand (Benjamin, 2005; Bisinella & Birch, 2003; Kozin, 2011). At this time, no randomized controlled trials have been conducted of conservative versus surgical treatment for severe cases of brachial plexus palsy. Current studies are considering the optimal surgical treatment approach to use for different types of brachial plexus injuries and critical time periods for considering this type of medical intervention.

Therapy services for an infant with birth-related brachial plexus palsy typically are initiated before the infant is discharged from the hospital. Early therapy referrals are to prevent or reduce the possibility of joint contractures in the shoulder, elbow, forearm, and wrist; to maintain range of motion (ROM) in UE joints; and to instruct caregivers on proper positioning and exercises for the affected arm (see Case Example 11.1).

Passive ROM typically is initiated within the first week after birth and no later than age 3 weeks. Sometimes a wrist orthotic is indicated to maintain the wrist in extension if the infant presents with Erb's palsy (Benjamin, 2005; Kwazneski et al., 2009; Piatt, 2005). Caregivers often are provided exercises

and developmental positions for play that can be incorporated into treatment sessions and home activities. Early exercise programs remain an essential component of a rehabilitation approach for children with brachial plexus palsy to maintain joint ROM, improve muscle strength, and prevent possible future contractures and joint deformities (Murphy et al., 2012; Ramos & Zell, 2000; Shenaq, Bullocks, Dhillon, Lee, & Laurent, 2005).

The phase of **neurological recovery** is the time it takes for the initial neurological injury or the reconstructed plexus to recover or plateau in recovery (Murphy et al., 2012; Price, Tidwell, & Grossman, 2000; Shenaq et al., 2005). This phase usually lasts at least 5 to 6 years. During this time, the overall goal of therapy is to maintain full passive ROM of all joints, primarily through an ongoing and consistent rehabilitation program. Timing of treatment is important. Because most children realize neurological recovery over a number of years, the delay in normal muscle function and the presence of muscle imbalance across any UE joint can have a profound impact on the growing skeleton and overall function. Thus, if the injury is ignored, the child may be left with permanent musculoskeletal abnormalities that may require surgical intervention later in life (Kozin, 2011; Kwazneski et al., 2009; Price et al., 2000; Sheffler, Lattanza, Hagar, Bagley, & James, 2012).

Weakness and disuse of the affected UE are common consequences of birth-related brachial plexus injury. Children recovering from brachial plexus palsy find it difficult to move the affected arm against gravity and demonstrate the same issues with developmental learned nonuse noted in children with hemiplegic CP (Brady & Garcia, 2009; Murphy et al., 2012; Taub, Ramey, DeLuca, & Echols, 2004).

Recent neuroimaging studies using functional magnetic resonance imaging have shown that patients with unilateral motor weakness such as brachial plexus injury, upper-limb amputation, and spinal cord injury showed no brain activation in attempts to complete motor tasks with the weaker affected extremity (Malessy, Bakker, Dekker, Van Duk, & Thomeer, 2003; Yoshikawa, Hayashi, Tajiri, Satake, & Ohtomo, 2012). Restriction and recovery of neural input–output activity occur over several months in children with brachial plexus palsy, suggesting a multistage brain reorganization process that may coincide with recovery of arm function.

Recent pilot studies on the recovery of arm function in adults and children with brachial plexus palsy suggested that improved motor function in a patient's affected limb could be related to the degree of peripheral plasticity and neural activation in the brain (Santamato, Panza, Ranieri, & Fiore, 2011; Yoshikawa et al., 2012). Intensive rehabilitation programs could not only enhance the recovery of functional movement in the affected limb but also could lead to long-lasting cortical reorganization.

Case Example

P–CIMT FOR A CHILD WITH ERB–KLUMPKE PALSY

Jenny was born at full term by standard vaginal delivery and weighed just over 9 pounds at birth. Shortly after delivery, it was noted that Jenny had a completely flaccid left arm with no shoulder, elbow, forearm, wrist, or digit movement. The neurologist diagnosed her with left-sided Erb–Klumpke brachial plexus palsy.

Jenny was referred to occupational therapy services at age 2 months, and customary therapy services were initiated twice a week to provide passive ROM exercises and educate the family on home programs and positions for play. At age 6 months, Jenny underwent electromyography (EMG), which revealed abnormal signaling in the left arm with mild reinnervation of the upper trunk (C5 and C6) and complete denervation of the distal trunk (C8 to T1). The findings indicated likely superimposed evulsion of the lower cervical and upper thoracic roots, and Jenny underwent a lengthy neurosurgery at age 7 months to repair the evulsion. This surgery included dissection of a large neuroma involving the upper and middle trunk and three patch graphs from C7 to C8 roots. Occupational therapy began again shortly after surgery.

Eight months after the surgery, a repeat EMG revealed that the left medial and ulnar nerve sensory studies were normal, yet persistent proximal muscle weakness was present with reduced signal activation. Distally, there was now a weak signal in the first dorsal interosseous activating the abductor pollicis brevis. The occupational therapy practitioner noted significant clinical improvement in Jenny's shoulder and elbow movement and emerging wrist and finger flexion. Jenny could abduct the shoulder to 90° and could almost bring her left hand to her mouth. Although she was able to flex her wrist and fingers, she was unable to hold and sustain a grasp on toys or objects.

An mP–CIMT program was implemented 10 months after Jenny's neurosurgery, when the occupational therapy practitioner determined that clinical changes in motor activation and strength were significant enough to allow participation in task-oriented practice. The modified program was implemented 1 hour per day for 30 consecutive days (dosage = 30 hours), and a specially

designed protocol was developed to meet the infant's and family's daily schedule (Coker, Lebkicker, Harris, & Snape, 2009). The protocol included daily constraint of the stronger hand with a resting hand splint and puppet mitt, practitioners provided task practice and shaping of motor skills in the clinic 4 days a week, and family members provided therapy at home 3 days a week. Family members were trained before implementing the modified program, and a specific plan was created to assist the family with the home-based constraint therapy sessions. Special activities were developed for the child, including sensory play, repetitive reaching and batting of toys, grasping and releasing, and use of the affected extremity in weight-bearing and protective positions.

Goals for the program included increasing isolated shoulder flexion, external rotation, elbow flexion, and left-hand grasp strength to allow Jenny to better use both hands during play and self-care tasks. For shoulder movement, the goal was to increase active range and improve proximal strength in the scapula while reducing compensatory trunk movement. The practitioner complemented the mP–CIMT program with kinesiotaping for the scapula, shoulder, and wrist. The kinesiotaping was applied during a weekly session with the primary therapist.

After the 30-day program, Jenny demonstrated increased spontaneous use of her left arm in daily tasks and play. She started using both hands to remove her shirt, shoes, and socks and was able to hold a plate with her left hand while spoon-feeding with the right hand. Jenny also was able to use both hands to carry large toys and to steer a toddler tricycle around corners. When Jenny turned age 4 years, she participated in a modified camp-based P–CIMT program that provided 30 hours of P–CIMT over 1 week. After this additional trial, Jenny was able to hold paper to cut with scissors and was beginning to use both hands to fasten large buttons and manage zippers. At age 5 years, Jenny did not require any additional orthopedic surgeries for the shoulder and was completing preschool-age tasks at the same level as her peers.

Three pilot case studies provided emerging evidence on the use of modified P–CIMT with children recovering from brachial plexus palsy (Buesch et al., 2009; Santamato et al., 2011; Vaz et al., 2010). A single-case study by Buesch and colleagues (2009) investigated the use of a modified P–CIMT program for two children ages 10 and 12 years. The 10-year-old child presented with muscular atrophy in the shoulder girdle, upper arm, and forearm with reduced strength. No surgical intervention was discussed for this child. The 12-year-old child had undergone a tendon transfer at age 10 years and presented with muscle weakness in the shoulder, forearm, and hypothenar eminence. Both children appeared to have adequate finger function and grip strength.

A modified P–CIMT program was provided 6 hours per day for 3 weeks for the 10-year-old patient and 4 hours per day for 4.5 weeks for the 12-year-old patient (dosage = 126 hours for each case). The constraint was a forearm splint worn on the affected hand, and the intervention was completed in a community setting by the patients' parents, who were provided a checklist of one-handed activities. The parent diaries for the intervention period revealed that both children had shorter periods of modified P–CIMT than was suggested by the study protocol, although the study report did not provide the exact amount of constraint therapy intervention. The Melbourne Assessment of Unilateral Upper Limb Function (Melbourne Assessment; Johnson et al., 1994; Randall, Carlin, Chondros, & Reddihough, 2001; Randall, Johnson, & Reddihough, 1999), the Assisting Hand Assessment (AHA; Krumlinde-Sundholm, Holmefur, & Eliasson, 2007), and the Nine-Hole Peg Test (NHPT; Smith, Hong, & Presson, 2000) were used as outcome measures. The children demonstrated improvements on both the Melbourne Assessment and the AHA.

The authors reported difficulty with compliance in wearing the restraint and with adherence to the study protocol. They offered no information on the type of training provided to the families or whether consistent and subsequent follow-up sessions were provided to support the families in implementing the one-handed practice sessions during the P–CIMT program. This study highlights important considerations for providing either a signature or modified P–CIMT program. How is training provided to a nontherapist who is asked to conduct intensive task practice? How is compliance monitored to ensure that essential elements of a P–CIMT program are being provided (e.g., intensive task practice, shaping)? Answers to both of these questions could provide insight into why the children and families had issues with compliance with the prescribed constraint therapy protocol.

In 2010, Vaz and colleagues reported the results of a single-case study of a child with Erb–Duchenne palsy. The child was able to reach and hold objects with her weaker UE, but the parents reported that she demonstrated limited spontaneous use of her arm during everyday tasks. The child had movement of her shoulder but used several trunk compensations during reach tasks and did not have active elbow movement. Although the child had active grasp, she would drop objects because of hand weakness.

A modified P–CIMT program of 30-minute training sessions daily for 14 weeks (dosage = 49 hours) was initiated. The constraint was described as "restriction . . . attained by dressing the child with a jumper, closing the opening of the left sleeve and tying it on the child's back with and elastic band" (Vaz et al., 2010, p. 161). The only assessment used was the Todder Arm Use Test (TAUT; Taub et al., 2004). At the end of the intervention, the child demonstrated improvements in willingness to use the affected arm and ability to complete most tasks on the TAUT.

Santamato and colleagues (2011) described a case series with two girls with Erb–Duchenne palsy ages 6 and 7 years using the modified protocol described by Vaz and colleagues (2010). Both children were described as having the ability to move the shoulder and elbow but not with complete ROM. The children had marked biceps hypertrophy and were unable to fully extend the elbow. Each child was treated with intramuscular botulinum toxin injections in the involved UE, specifically in two sites in the biceps and two sites in the pectoralis muscle. Following injections, the involved UE was provided passive ROM, and the elbow was casted for 10 days to increase elbow extension. After treatment of the affected arm, a modified P–CIMT program was implemented.

The mP–CIMT program included daily training sessions of 30 minutes each day for a period of 2 months (dosage = 30 hours). The constraint was a jumpsuit with a hook-and-loop closure, with the nonaffected arm placed under the jumpsuit parallel to the chest. The assessment measures included three measures commonly used for children with brachial plexus injuries—the Gilbert–Raimondi score for elbow function, the Raimondi hand score, and the Mallet Scale (Reading, Laor, Salisbury, Lippert, & Cornwall, 2012)—as well as the NHPT. At the end of the mP–CIMT program, the children demonstrated improvements in all three brachial plexus measures and the NHPT.

SUMMARY AND NEXT DIRECTIONS

Children with brachial plexus palsy may benefit from an intensive therapy approach such as P–CIMT, which could be a promising intervention to help strengthen muscles in the affected UE and improve spontaneous use of the weaker arm in everyday tasks. Although case reports have provided preliminary evidence, questions remain regarding several key issues, including

- Age at which to implement P–CIMT,
- Minimum amount of movement required in the child's affected UE,
- Intensity and dosage required for long-lasting functional change,
- Best assessments for measuring structural and functional changes, and
- Use of complementary therapies before, during, or after P–CIMT (e.g., botulinum toxin therapy).

The case presentations used various modified P–CIMT approaches with children who had different patterns of UE weakness and functional ability. From these case reports, it is difficult to determine which type of brachial plexus palsy and amount of functional movement are necessary to benefit from P–CIMT. In addition, the total dosage of the modified approaches ranged from 30 to 126 hours, and limited follow-up information was provided to indicate whether changes seen after P–CIMT were long-lasting.

The time to initiate P–CIMT and age of child are critical issues in birth-related brachial plexus injuries. Most longitudinal studies of children born with brachial plexus injuries have determined that the delay in normal muscle function and muscular imbalance across shoulder, elbow, and wrist joints affect skeletal and muscle growth and overall function in daily tasks (Kozin, 2011; Kwazneski et al., 2009; Price et al., 2000; Sheffler et al., 2012). Could a P–CIMT program implemented early in life prevent or change the trajectory of musculoskeletal abnormalities that may require surgical intervention later in a child's life? Current studies do not answer this question or the question of whether complementary therapies, such as intramuscular botulinum toxin therapy or casting, should be implemented before constraint programs are started. Further investigations are needed to determine reproducibility of the case reports in larger case series or randomized controlled trials.

TRAUMATIC BRAIN INJURY

BACKGROUND AND MECHANISM OF INJURY

According to the Centers for Disease Control and Prevention (2010), 35,136 children between ages 0 and 14 years were hospitalized for a brain injury from 2002 to 2006. With timely medical treatment, survival rates have greatly improved, but residual mental, cognitive, emotional, and physical deficits may persist, depending on the severity of injury (Anderson, Godfrey, Rosenfeld, & Catroppa, 2011).

Traumatic brain injury (TBI) is an injury to the head that results in a change in consciousness or specific neurological signs (Christensen, 1996). TBI is also referred to as acquired brain injury; both are broad terms that describe a vast array of injuries that occur to the developing brain after birth. Children with TBI present with a specific set of traits that are unique to this type of injury and that differentiate TBI from congenital disorders of hemiplegia. These characteristics are determined by the child's developmental level at time of insult, type of injury, and distribution of injury (Christensen, 1996).

TBI can be described as mild, moderate, or severe. The level of injury is defined by the severity and duration of acute initial loss of consciousness, usually measured by the Glasgow Coma Scale, and the duration of coma and posttraumatic amnesia (Christensen, 1996). Anderson and colleagues (2011) confirmed previous reports that a direct correlation exists between severity of injury and adaptive behavior: Children with more severe injuries have greater functional deficits. In addition, TBI can be described as either a **focal injury,** with damage to a specific region or structure of the brain, or a **diffuse injury,** with damage affecting many areas.

Two major types of injury to the brain are (1) contusion and (2) diffuse axonal injury (Christensen, 1996). **Contusion** is bruising to brain tissue that occurs when force is applied to the skull, usually from an object moving at low velocity for a short duration. Damage occurs not only at the location where the head was struck but also 180° opposite the location, where the brain makes contact with the opposite side of the skull. When a high-velocity, long-duration force makes contact with the skull, contusion occurs because the brain decelerates on the bony prominences at the base of the skull (Christensen, 1996). **Diffuse axonal injury** is usually the result of relatively long-duration trauma that involves rotational forces, such as a severe car accident. Mechanical forces on the axons disrupt the transmission of signals throughout the brain. Additional injury to the brain can occur from hemorrhaging or swelling during and after these types of injuries. TBI can further be complicated by concurrent injuries, such as cardiac arrest or hypoxia resulting from shock at the time of injury.

TBI affects many areas of the brain, especially the **frontal lobes,** or the area of the brain located at the front of each cerebral hemisphere that is the center of executive functioning. Therefore, patients with TBI often have impairments in areas of cognition, including attention, processing, problem solving, perception, and reasoning. Memory impairments are among the most common impairments after TBI (Gerrard-Morris et al., 2010). A study by Anderson and colleagues (2011) of participants 10 years after a severe childhood TBI found that slow processing speed was most detrimental to day-to-day functioning. Impairments in this area interrupt a child's ability to follow directions, can affect test taking and academic work, and impair vocational abilities.

Difficulty in understanding written and oral language, reading comprehension, aphasia, and apraxia are common in TBI (Slomine & Locascio, 2009). Oral–motor deficits that result from TBI include dysarthria (Guo & Togher, 2008) and impaired breath control that affects the length of utterances during speech. Feeding and nutrition issues may arise because of oral–motor paralysis and dysphagia, and patients may require altered food consistencies to help them safely swallow (Morgan, Ward, & Murdoch, 2004).

Psychiatric disorders are common after severe TBI and may be characterized by one or more of the following symptoms: impulsivity, perseveration, aggression, depression, and altered inhibition (Anderson et al., 2011). Sensory processing also may be affected. Head injury can result in full or partial hearing loss, impaired tactile discrimination of the impaired or both UEs, and visual impairments. Visual impairments common in this population include convergence or divergence insufficiency, cranial nerve involvement, optic atrophy, and visual field cuts (Christensen, 1996).

Motor impairments in children with mild TBI may resolve almost completely within 3 years post injury (Jaffe, Polissar, Fay, & Liao, 1995). Subtle differences in speed and dexterity may persist in the chronic stages (Chaplin, Deitz, & Jaffe, 1993). Children with moderate to severe TBI typically have more long-lasting motor deficits that may include ROM limitations, decreased strength, ataxia, spasticity and tonal changes, and abnormal sensation. Long-term motor deficits may lead to irreversible muscle shortening and contractures. Other common orthopedic issues include subluxations, growth disturbances, scoliosis, and limb-length discrepancies (Christensen, 1996).

TREATMENT CONSIDERATIONS FOR TBI

Brain injuries limit neuroplasticity and new learning because of many factors that occur at the time of injury, including diffuse axonal injury, swelling, hemorrhaging, and the excitatory neurotoxic cascade (i.e., alterations in the normal activity of the nervous system that may cause damage to nervous system tissue in the brain). With this damage, fewer intact areas are available for recruitment, leading to greater disconnection between areas of the brain and cognitive impairment (Brady & Garcia, 2009).

Following a TBI, the child typically receives acute occupational therapy services in an intensive inpatient rehabilitation program, where the focus is on cognitive and motor rehabilitation embedded in functional tasks. The child may learn adaptive strategies to successfully perform activities of daily living (ADLs) and instrumental activities of daily living. Depending on the rate of recovery and level of cognitive ability postinjury, CIMT may be used in the intensive inpatient rehabilitation setting.

Research on the use of CIMT in the acute phase is extremely limited. One study in rats found that restraint of the limb ipsilateral to the cortical impairment immediately after injury caused hypothermia, which in turn caused greater cortical damage (DeBow, McKenna, Kolb, & Colbourne, 2004). The researchers hypothesized that if the rats were using their impaired limb to assist with mobility in the acute phase, they were activating an area of the brain that required a period of rest to restore function, thereby causing greater damage to the brain.

Another study examined the effect of CIMT on patients with stroke in the subacute phase of recovery (Treger, Aidinof, Lehrer, & Kalichman, 2012). They reported increased blood flow to the damaged hemisphere in participants who used their affected hand to perform eating and grasping tasks. The participants who used their affected hand while their dominant hand was restricted had a significant increase in blood flow. No change was reported in healthy controls.

Studies examining the effect of CIMT on adults with TBI are limited to date. Most studies on the adult population have used a modified CIMT (mCIMT) approach, and no studies have looked at the outcomes of CIMT offered during the acute or immediate recovery phase of injury. Page and Levine (2003) used an mCIMT protocol with 3 adults 5 hours per day, 3 times per week, for 10 weeks and found improvements more than 1 year after TBI.

Shaw and colleagues (2005) conducted a larger study with 22 adult participants an average of 9 years post injury who had average scores on memory and verbal comprehension testing. Their CIMT intervention lasted for 2 weeks, 6 hours per day, and used a mitt as a constraint. They found significant improvements on all measures (Motor Activity Log [Taub et al., 1993], the Wolf Motor Function Test [Wolf et al., 2001], Fugl-Meyer Motor Performance Assessment [Fugl-Meyer, Jääskö, Leyman, Olsson, & Steglind, 1975]) at 1 month and at 2 years post treatment. Performance had declined at 2 years, but scores were noted to be above pretreatment levels. Additionally, the authors observed that patients with TBI had a lower rate of adherence to restraint and that rate of adherence correlated with improvement.

One study examined the duration of restraint needed to improve fine motor coordination in 9 adult participants with acquired brain injury (6 stroke, 3 TBI; Cho et al., 2005). All participants were compliant with the restraint-wearing schedule. The authors identified 2 to 5 weeks of restraint as ideal for the participants and recommended regular intervals of assessment to monitor progress and need for the restraining device. The authors also recommended discontinuing use of the restraint when fine motor progress plateaus.

Four studies have examined CIMT in the pediatric population with TBI (Table 11.2). The first, by Karman, Maryles, Baker, Simpser, and Berger-Gross (2003), included

7 patients ages 7 to 17 years with acquired brain injuries resulting in hemiparesis (3 TBI, 4 stroke). Patients were 4 weeks to 2 years post injury. The constraining device used was a mitt, and intervention lasted 6 hours per day for 2 weeks. Five participants showed improvement on outcome measures after CIMT (including the Actual Amount of Use Test—Amount of Use and Quality of Use; Chen, Wolf, Zhang, Thompson, & Winstein, 2012), whereas 2 did not. The authors noted that parent compliance with the home program was lacking for 2 patients. These parents did not support their child's practice with the paretic hand, and the children were often observed not using their mitts. One of the parents actively interfered with therapy, often taking the mitt off in an attempt to shield the patient from difficult work. This study illustrates the importance of parental involvement in CIMT.

Second, Cimolin and colleagues (2012) examined the efficacy of CIMT intervention for 10 weeks in which the unaffected arm was restrained during therapy 3 hours a day, 7 days per week, using a fabric glove with built-in splint. Participants were 10 children ages 8 to 12 years with hemiplegia secondary to TBI. No child had lesions in the cerebellum, basal ganglia, or brainstem.

The outcomes of intervention included improvements on the Gross Motor Function Measure (Brunton & Bartlett, 2011), the Quality of Upper Extremity Skills Test (DeMatteo et al., 1992), and the Besta scales (Fedrizzi, Oleari, Inverno, Dal Brun, & Bono, 1994). Kinematic improvements included reaching, hand-to-mouth movement, smoothness, and precision of movements. Limitations of the study include the small number of participants and lack of a control group of matched children with hemiplegia who did not receive CIMT.

Third, Gordon and colleagues (2007) used a resting hand splint worn for 2 hours daily during therapy sessions for 4 weeks with 6 children ages 6 to 15 years with hemiparesis resulting from ischemic stroke. Participants had lesions in the cerebral cortex, basal ganglia, and internal capsule. They noted that the majority of participants had no significant improvement on the battery of sensory–motor function assessments or quality of movements. Improvement was reported on specific functional goals quantified using Goal Attainment Scaling (Krasny-Pacini, Hiebel, Pauly, Godon, & Chevignard, 2013). One participant made significant gains on the Melbourne Assessment.

Table 11.2 STUDIES OF CIMT FOR CHILDREN WITH TBI

STUDY	PARTICIPANTS	DOSAGE AND SETTING	RESTRAINT	ASSESSMENTS	OUTCOMES
Cimolin et al. (2012)	N = 10 8–12 years	3 hours/day, 7 days/week, 10 weeks Restraint of unaffected arm during therapy	Fabric glove with built-in splint	GMFM, QUEST, Besta scales, kinematic measures of reaching, hand-to-mouth movement	Improvements on all measures
Gordon et al. (2007)	N = 6 with childhood stroke 6–15 years	2 hours/day, 4 weeks	Resting hand splint	MAUUL, GAS	No change on battery of sensory–motor function assessments No change on quality of movements Increased functional goals quantified using GAS
Karman, Maryles, Baker, Simpser, & Berger-Gross (2003)	N = 7 7–17 years	6 hours/day, 2 days/week Inpatient setting	Mitt	AAUT	5 participants had significant changes, 2 did not
Reidy et al. (2012)	N = 29 1.6–19.1 years	3–6 hours/day, 21 days Outpatient clinic	Continuous cast	QUEST, MAUUL, AHA, COPM	Statistically significant changes on all measures

Note. AAUT = Actual Amount of Use Test; AHA = Assisting Hand Assessment; CIMT = constraint-induced movement therapy; COPM = Canadian Occupational Performance Measure; GAS = Goal Attainment Scaling; GMFM = Gross Motor Function Measure; MAUUL = Melbourne Assessment of Unilateral Upper Limb Function; QUEST = Quality of Upper Extremity Skills Test.

Fourth, Reidy and colleagues (2012) used clinic-based CIMT for patients with congenital ($n = 21$) and acquired hemiparesis ($n = 8$) from TBI, tumor resection, and hemispherectomy. Intervention was 3 to 6 hours of therapy daily for 21 days using a long-arm continuous cast, 24 hours a day. Statistically significant gains were made on the Melbourne Assessment, Quality of Upper Extremity Skills Test (except the Protective Extension subtest), the AHA, and the Canadian Occupational Performance Measure (COPM; Law et al., 2005; Verkerk, Wolf, Louwers, Meester-Delver, & Nollet, 2006). The effect sizes varied from .46 to .70, indicating a moderate effect.

Occupational therapy practitioners must keep in mind several considerations when implementing CIMT with children recovering from a head injury, including attention to task, visual deficits, motor planning impairments, and impulsivity and safety issues. Because TBI is acquired, this patient population is slightly older on average than patients with congenital hemiparesis and may need to balance educational needs with intensive therapy needs. Patients who were developing typically before the injury may have a level of familiarity with ADL completion and with using their affected UE in bimanual tasks.

Type of injury, level of cognitive damage, and stage of recovery and rehabilitation inform the method of instruction. Shaping activities may need to be done in small doses or on a rotating basis to maintain the patient's attention if it has been affected by the injury. For children with a short attention span or impulsivity, a routine of activities or a picture schedule may be a helpful behavior management technique to promote practice of a component skill at a high level of repetition. Setting up the environment to limit distractors also may be helpful.

Diffuse axonal injury impairs the speed of processing directions and feedback. Practitioners should factor the patient's receptive communication skills into the way they phrase or deliver directions. Practitioners should be mindful of the number of steps a patient can easily follow before giving directions and during cueing. Children with moderate to severe TBI may prefer simple, one-step directions. Multimodal delivery of instruction may help the child understand directions and execute tasks more easily and fully. Visual impairments or field cuts also affect the choice of materials to present. Practitioners should pay attention to the background of objects or placement within an available visual field when setting up the treatment environment and presenting tasks during intervention.

During motor activities, more acute patients may have developed fewer compensatory movement patterns and may have fewer contractures compared with more chronic patients who may have well-established compensatory patterns and resulting overuse injuries. Monitoring for subluxations or orthopedic deformities in the affected UE and trunk is advised. When setting up the treatment environment, practitioners should take into account a patient's level of impulsivity and safety awareness. Memory deficits may require a high level of repetition before a skill or concept is solidified, retained, or generalized.

Executive functioning skills may be greatly affected in children with frontal lobe damage. Before selecting a task, practitioners should be aware of the problem-solving, sequencing, and organizational requirements. Practitioners may need to carefully grade tasks to limit frustration with activities. If the patient has decreased inhibition or social awareness, he or she may have a low threshold for frustration tolerance. Fine motor intervention is also a great opportunity to incorporate problem-solving strategies or motor planning. For example, while building a block tower, the patient can be directed to copy a sequence of colors.

Because inhibition and psychosocial impairments are common in children with TBI, it may be beneficial to implement a behavior management plan early in treatment. Strategies include, but are not limited to, use of positive reinforcement (e.g., prize box, stickers) for task completion, a timer, a visual schedule, choice in therapeutic activities, and clear visual and verbal cues of expectations and rules (see Case Example 11.2).

SUMMARY AND NEXT DIRECTIONS

Occupational therapy practitioners must consider how the long-term deficits related to moderate to severe TBI affect a child's participation in daily activities, social interactions, and engagement in therapy sessions. TBI may lead to slower processing speeds, and central nervous system (CNS) deficits may influence the manner in which treatment is delivered. Goals in outpatient programs address specific areas of concern such as improving tone, ROM, and coordination. CIMT may be used in this setting to combat chronic disuse of the UE or limitations in ROM and strength. Further studies are needed to examine the physiological effects of CIMT, especially in children, and to determine whether CIMT can be started safely in the acute phase of recovery.

HEMISPHERECTOMY AND OTHER SURGICAL INTERVENTIONS

BACKGROUND AND MECHANISM OF INJURY

Surgical interventions that affect the CNS include

- Correction for **arterial venous malformations**—surgery to correct an abnormal connection between arteries and veins that bypasses the capillary system, most common in the CNS

Case Example

P–CIMT FOR A CHILD WITH TBI

Mark was a 7-year-old child with a TBI from a motor vehicle accident 3 years previously. Mark sustained a right parietal fracture with intraparenchymal hemorrhage and right tibial and right fibular fractures. He had resultant neurological deficits, including left hemiparesis, swallow dysfunction, and dysarthria. He had diffuse axonal injury and therefore slow processing. His receptive language was impaired, and he benefited from clear, concise directions. His parents reported that he learned best through demonstration and that he had difficulty organizing his materials for school and recalling his homework assignments. During his initial evaluation for the CIMT program, he had difficulty sustaining and focusing his attention for more than 8 or 9 minutes. He was easily distracted by external stimuli, including other people and objects of preference (Table 11.3).

Mark had difficulty sequencing dressing tasks; for example, he put his shoe on before his sock and donned his shirt backward. During fine motor testing, Mark had difficulty changing strategies when he was unable to complete a task. He required assistance to open containers during lunch and required assistance with all fasteners. When he tried to open his lunch box zipper with his right UE, it often slipped.

Mark had significant flexor tone throughout his left UE and decreased active ROM and left UE strength. He had full passive ROM and could use gross grasping patterns to pick up objects from a tabletop. At admission, Mark's Manual Ability Classification System level was 3 (Eliasson et al., 2006).

Mark required minimal verbal cues or physical prompts to initiate use of his left hand during functional bimanual tasks such

Table 11.3   MARK'S DEFICITS SECONDARY TO TBI

IMPAIRMENT	TYPE	COMPENSATORY STRATEGIES AND INTERVENTIONS
Left hemiparesis	Motor	Reduced task demands, compensatory dressing techniques, adaptive equipment
High flexor tone in left upper extremity	Motor	Bracing, taping, stretching, electrical stimulation
Decreased fine motor control	Motor	Reduced task demands, built-up handles
Gait abnormalities	Motor	Supervision during mobility and dynamic standing balance, lower-extremity brace
Slow processing speed	Cognitive	Increased time to complete activities, simple directions
Difficulty with problem solving	Cognitive	Reduced task demands, assistance with parts of task, talking through of steps, indirect or direct verbal cues
Perseveration	Cognitive	Redirection, schedule sheet, provision of choices for appropriate topics
Decreased attention	Cognitive	Schedule, timer, reduced task demands, reduced distractions in the environment, alternation between gross and fine motor tasks
Difficulty with multistep directions	Cognitive, language	Verbal cues, reduced task demands, picture directions for tasks, checklists, simple directions
Language comprehension difficulties	Cognitive, language	Picture directions, reduced task demands, simple one-step directions
Dysarthria	Oral–motor	Increased time for response or repeated responses
Decreased short-term and long-term memory	Cognitive	Presentation of one direction at a time, strategies to compensate for lack of working memory such as checklists and reminders using electronic devices

(Continued)

Case Example 11.2 P–CIMT FOR A CHILD WITH TBI *(Cont.)*

as holding a cup during a pouring task or supporting a piece of paper during a writing or scissoring task. He had difficulty catching and throwing balls of various sizes in his left hand during sports activities. He also occasionally lost his balance during dynamic activities requiring maximal excursion out of midline. Mark required verbal cues to stay on task during functional activities secondary to decreased attention and impulsiveness.

Mark required one-on-one attention from the practitioner because of his distractibility. His treatment team decided that individual therapy would be more beneficial than group-based intervention. Mark's family was very supportive and willing to give him the extra help he would need at home while wearing a long-arm cast continuously. His mother also agreed with the practitioner that because of Mark's learning difficulties, he would need high repetition of practice and opportunities to generalize the skills learned in the clinic, which would be provided by wearing the cast at home each day after the program. After considering all these factors, the team and parents decided that Mark would participate in 3 hours of daily on-site P–CIMT intervention in an outpatient clinic.

To aid his success, Mark's practitioner provided him with daily visual schedules of session activities. Mark chose from a variety of therapeutic options and put them in the order he preferred. Mark also benefited from a timer to show him how much time was left until the next activity. Frequent simple reminders to stay on task were helpful when Mark began to get distracted or perseverated on an inappropriate topic.

One of Mark's preferred activities was building with Lego© blocks. The practitioner modified this activity on the basis of Mark's strengths and impairments in the following ways:

- *Organizing, sequencing, and planning*
  - Mark sorted pieces by shape and color into containers while grasping them from various surfaces (e.g., table, practitioner's fingertips or palm). He then released them into labeled containers at various heights.
  - Mark had difficulty reading the directions for the Lego kit. The practitioner presented one picture at a time and covered up nonpertinent sections of the project so he could focus on the salient information. When he had difficulty, the practitioner first demonstrated what needed to be done and then had Mark imitate the actions.
  - After completing the directions with the kit, the practitioner had Mark design his own Lego project. He typed out the directions, working on isolated finger movements or pointing and clicking with an adaptive mouse.
- *Memory*
  - Before taking a break from the Lego project, the practitioner asked Mark to recall the steps he had already completed.

- While Mark was building, the practitioner used simple phrases to elicit greater ROM when reaching and fewer compensations. Instead of giving him lots of detailed feedback, the practitioner repeatedly stated, "Move your arm, not your body" when he reached.
- *Attention*
  - It was hard for Mark to concentrate, especially when the directions were complicated. When needed, the practitioner had him work in a quiet environment with his back to the other children in the therapy gym.
  - After a few steps, Mark had difficulty attending. The practitioner alternated activities. Mark sorted Legos, cleaned up extra pieces, and went on a Lego scavenger hunt throughout the room.
- *Motor planning*
  - Mark sometimes had difficulty coordinating his body for reaching and grasping tasks. Some strategies the practitioner tried were talking through the plan of action in simple phrases, having Mark practice component movements, and facilitating visualization of tasks.

Before starting therapy and immediately after, Mark's practitioner administered standardized testing—specifically, the Melbourne Assessment and the AHA—to measure his progress with UE skills. The Melbourne Assessment is a standardized measure that assesses ROM, fluidity of movement, accuracy, and object manipulation through a series of unilateral activities. It is designed for children with neurological impairment ages 5 to 15 years. All sessions are videotaped for scoring by a trained occupational or physical therapist. Mark's score on the Melbourne Assessment was 35 at admission and 38 at discharge.

The AHA is a criterion-referenced tool developed specifically for children with hemiplegia ages 18 months to 12 years. The AHA assesses bimanual function in the context of natural play with age-appropriate toys. Some of the components of bimanual function assessed include initiation of use of the affected hand, reaching, manipulation, flow of bimanual performance, grasp patterns, stabilization of objects with the affected hand, and calibration when manipulating objects with the affected hand. The videotaped structured observation is administered and scored by a certified rater. A change of 4 points or more on retesting indicates a significant change. Mark's score on the AHA was 31 at admission and 37 at discharge.

Mark's practitioner also found it important to identify goals that Mark and his family had during treatment and to find a way to measure them. The practitioner decided to use the COPM, which is a semistructured interview completed by parents or caregivers that is used to identify their priorities for the child's participation in the areas of self-care, productivity, and leisure. The parent identifies problem areas and assigns a numerical value to current performance and satisfaction with that perfor-

(Continued)

Case Example 11.2 P–CIMT FOR A CHILD WITH TBI *(Cont.)*

mance. Current performance is rated on a scale of 1 to 10, with 1 = *not able to do it* and 10 = *able to do it extremely well.* Satisfaction also is rated on a scale of 1 to 10, with 1 = *not satisfied at all* and 10 = *extremely satisfied.* A change of 2 points is considered clinically significant (Law et al., 2005).

Table 11.4 presents the most important problems identified by Mark's family and his COPM scores at admission and discharge. Mark's performance with complicated fine motor tasks such as fasteners did not show much improvement, but his ability to open containers did. His mother's satisfaction with his ability to hold objects during ADLs improved slightly. Gross UE skills such as ball-handling skills and swimming showed larger improvements.

Mark also had some success in achieving goals set by his practitioner. Goals that Mark achieved during the program included the following:

- Mark will initiate stabilizing and holding paper on a flat surface using his left hand during scissoring and coloring 75% of the time during craft activities.
- Mark will grasp and carry a lightweight bucket approximately 25 feet in 3 of 5 trials.
- Mark will pick up a medium lightweight ball using his bilateral UEs from the floor and place it in a net at 90° of shoulder flexion.

- Mark will point to a preferred object in a book by initiating second digit finger extension on the left hand in 3 of 5 trials.
- Mark will maintain a grasp on a parachute with his bilateral UEs while shaking it with team members for 60 seconds in 2 of 3 trials.
- Mark will throw a medium lightweight ball overhand using bilateral UEs in 4 of 5 trials.
- Mark will ride an adapted tricycle 100 feet around 6 cones while steering the bike with both hands.

Mark made progress toward the following goals but was unable to achieve them while he was in the program:

- Mark will actively weight bear through his left UE without collapsing at the shoulder in prone for 5 minutes in 3 of 5 trials. Status: Ongoing, achieved for ~3 minutes once.
- Mark will release 8 of 10 1-inch blocks into a large container, demonstrating improved finger extension. Status: Ongoing, achieved 5 of 10 times with increased time and compensatory strategy of shaking hand to release object in 50% of trials.

Table 11.4 Mark's Goals Identified Using the Canadian Occupational Performance Measure

OCCUPATIONAL PERFORMANCE PROBLEM	INITIAL PERFORMANCE SCORE	INITIAL SATISFACTION SCORE	DISCHARGE PERFORMANCE SCORE	DISCHARGE SATISFACTION SCORE
Fastening and unfastening buttons	1	1	1	1
Opening containers	3	1	6	5
Holding activity of daily living objects in left hand to assist with activity	4	3	4	4
Completing scissoring task with bilateral hands	2	1	2	1
Ball handling during sports activities	3	3	7	6
Swimming (dog paddling)	2	1	7	7
Total of above scores	15	10	27	24
Score (total ÷ number of problems)	2.5	1.6	4.5	4.0
Change	—	—	+2.0	+2.4

Note. — = not applicable.

- **Tumor resection**—surgical removal of a tumor
- **Hemispherectomy**—removal of all or part of one cerebral hemisphere, most commonly done to treat a seizure disorder.

This section focuses on hemispherectomy, but many treatment issues are also relevant to any surgical process resulting in hemiparesis or asymmetrical motor impairment.

Of children diagnosed with epilepsy, an estimated 10% to 25% have **intractable epilepsy,** or recurrent uncontrolled seizure activity that is resistant to drug therapy (Hindi-Ling et al., 2011; Kim et al., 2008; Mathern, 2010). Hemispheric surgery techniques are used both for patients with intractable epilepsy and for those with **intractable epileptiform abnormalities,** or uncontrolled seizure activity secondary to another CNS diagnosis or lesion.

Surgical intervention for intractable seizure activity is almost always reserved for patients who present with unilateral hemispheric seizure activity, but some hemispherectomies are now performed palliatively for children and adults who have bilateral seizure activity (Ciliberto et al., 2012). Numerous surgical procedures are used, but globally, hemispherectomies can be classified as either anatomical or functional and as partial or complete (Hindi-Ling et al., 2011; Kim et al., 2008; Spencer & Huh, 2008). An **anatomical hemispherectomy** involves resection of the lobes where the seizure activity is believed to originate, and in **functional hemispherectomy,** the lobe or hemisphere with the identified seizure activity is disconnected from other CNS areas but the tissue remains in place (Dijkerman, Vargha-Khadem, Polkey, & Weiskrantz, 2008; Kim, Osburn, & Cohen-Gadol, 2009). Complete hemispherectomy is removal of the entire hemisphere, and partial hemispherectomy is removal of only part of the hemisphere.

The goal of hemispherectomy is to eliminate or drastically reduce seizure activity, and numerous studies have documented the success of these procedures (e.g., Limbrick et al., 2009; Mathern, 2010). Improvements in surgical techniques have resulted in reduced complications (Flack, Ojemann, & Haberkern, 2008). Often these surgeries result in other benefits for patients, including increased cognitive and overall motor performance (Flack et al., 2008; Limbrick et al., 2009; Mathern, 2010; Samargia & Kimberley, 2009).

Although in some respects, this overall increased motor performance seems counterintuitive, it is believed to occur because the absence of seizure activity allows the nonseizing areas of the brain to function in a more typical manner (Flack et al., 2008; Holt & Mikati, 2011). In addition, almost all motor actions, even those originating in the contralateral hemisphere, have ipsilateral pathways (Dijkerman et al., 2008). Similarly, motor impairments secondary to hemispherectomy are rarely limited to contralateral functions but almost always involve ipsilateral manifestations (Dijkerman et al., 2008). Also note that motor functions are often kept on the contralateral side (Dijkerman et al., 2008; Govindan, Chugani, Luat, & Sood, 2010), indicating that the patients may already have been using ipsilateral portions of the CNS to produce these motor functions.

TREATMENT CONSIDERATIONS FOR HEMISPHERECTOMY AND OTHER SURGICAL INTERVENTIONS

Several clinical demonstrations indicate that children undergoing hemispherectomy and other surgical procedures can benefit from P–CIMT when the resulting motor impairment secondary to the procedure involves asymmetrical impairment involving the UEs. Practitioners must recognize, however, that the motor dysfunction and impairment secondary to these surgical procedures, which often appear similar to those in children with hemiparetic CP, present a very different clinical case, and practitioners must consider alterations in treatment given the different etiology.

Motor outcomes secondary to hemispherectomy are varied and multifactorial and are dependent on factors such as primary and secondary etiology, age at time of surgery, type of surgical procedure, surgical complications, and presurgical level of functioning. Understanding of the postsurgical treatment needs of children who undergo hemispherectomy, however, is limited (Fritz et al., 2011). Hemispherectomies often are believed to have better developmental outcomes when performed in younger children because of the availability of neural plastic mechanisms (Flack et al., 2008; Samargia & Kimberley, 2009), but research is needed that addresses how motor outcomes might be altered by behavioral treatment techniques such as physical and occupational therapy. Various amounts of hemiplegia are expected, and the general approach often is to anticipate and plan for whatever hemiplegia manifests by teaching unilateral functional skills. These treatments often are prescribed, but little evidence is available about their efficacy in improving motor outcomes.

P–CIMT treatment activities must be tailored to match these children's developmental level at the start of therapy, and practitioners often must consider aspects of motor and developmental control that are not addressed in more routine cases of hemiparesis secondary to CP. For example, hand and arm function in children who have undergone hemispherectomy must be developed concordantly with other skills to enable them to control the core postural muscles in the trunk and maximize their functional possibilities. In addition to postural control, therapy should focus on sensory processing, because both are critical foundations for most movement abilities (see Case Example 11.3).

Case Example

P–CIMT FOR A CHILD RECOVERING FROM HEMISPHERECTOMY

Kelly, age 3½ years, had spastic CP secondary to in-utero stroke. She had had severe brain swelling at birth and multiple delivery complications. Later, Kelly was diagnosed with infantile spasms and right-side hemiparesis. The continued occurrence of severe seizure activity eventually led to a left hemispherectomy and placement of a ventriculoperitoneal shunt. Surgery resulted in 25% visual loss and decreased verbal skills. The surgery greatly reduced but did not eliminate seizure activity. After surgery, Kelly demonstrated severe impairments in multiple developmental domains and continued severe right-side hemiplegia.

Kelly began P–CIMT 2 years after the hemispherectomy. Although Kelly had made numerous functional gains throughout the postsurgical period, she presented at the start of P–CIMT with significant motor, cognitive, and functional limitations. Kelly's gross motor impairments included decreased head and neck control and decreased trunk control, and she was non–weight bearing through the right UE. She demonstrated no established means of mobility by crawling or walking, no ability to push to sit from the right side, and no right-side reflexive or protective activity involving the arm and hand. In general, she displayed a lack of awareness of her right UE regarding all sensory input and had significant language and cognitive delays.

Kelly's visual impairment compromised her ability to track and focus on toys within her environment. She had mild-to-moderate tone throughout her right side. Her right arm rested in extension and moved actively less than half the active ROM in all shoulder movements. She was unable to demonstrate movement of the forearm toward supination or active finger movement, and her wrist was flexed. Overall, her interaction with the environment, including family members, was minimal. Kelly expressed excitement and happiness only through smiling and screaming. She did not communicate through speaking or signing and had delayed cognitive processing skills.

Kelly's P–CIMT treatment followed the ACQUIREc therapy protocol (see Chapter 8, "ACQUIREc Protocol: What We Have Learned From a Decade of Delivering a Signature Form of Pediatric CIMT"). Treatment was conducted for 21 days, 6 hours each day, in a home setting (the family rented an apartment near the treatment center). Kelly wore a long arm cast as a constraint 24 hours a day, 7 days a week, for the first 18 days. The ACQUIREc treatment process for Kelly after the hemispherectomy was similar to that used with any child with hemiparesis, but her impairment was significantly greater than that of most children with right-sided hemiparesis secondary to CP with more global involvement. In fact, Kelly had global developmental delays across all major areas of development.

All P–CIMT treatments are individualized to match the child's starting developmental level. For Kelly, treatment began with activities to help her develop global awareness, core (trunk) motor abilities, and basic skills with the right UE; learn sensory information; and develop perceptual skills. For most children, including those with more typical hemiparesis, these types of activity are focused on in infancy and the early toddler months. P–CIMT for more traditional diagnoses often is used with more developmentally advanced children and focuses primarily on UE motor skills, with other developmental areas or core motor abilities being of only ancillary concern. Kelly's case demonstrates how P–CIMT can be modified to meet the developmental needs and individual abilities of children who have had a surgical procedure such as hemispherectomy.

Treatment for Kelly's gross motor skills started with a focus on the development of head and neck control using activities such as moving motivating toys (e.g., that produce light or sound) in various planes in her proximal visual field, providing verbal and tactile cues to maintain an upright head position during play, and varying trunk support through use and removal of adaptive seating. Trunk control and strengthening were addressed during static weight bearing through quadruped positioning, with the head in a neutral position and with Kelly using her right arm for support. These activities also assisted and encouraged head control, neck stability, and strengthening and awareness of the right arm and hand. At the beginning of treatment, these activities involved full assistance and facilitation, and weight-bearing positioning was later combined with practice in transitioning skills by pushing to sit from quadruped and eventually to crawling from one toy to another with transitional body placement between toys.

During play, Kelly often was positioned on elevated surfaces such as a bench or stepstool to encourage increased trunk activation. Trunk rotation was encouraged by elevating the toys or moving them around the environment. The practitioner manipu-

(Continued)

Case Example 11.3 P–CIMT FOR A CHILD RECOVERING FROM HEMISPHERECTOMY *(Cont.)*

lated the placement of toys in proximal positions at the beginning of treatment, often with full trunk support, and in more distal positions as treatment progressed to behaviorally shape Kelly's skills within and across days. This progression focused on and forced dynamic sitting balance, encouraged greater proficiency in reaching with the right UE, and required greater trunk stability and control.

Sensory activities were crucial to increase Kelly's awareness of her right side and encourage motor abilities in the right arm and hand. Sensory techniques used during treatment included play in beans, water, and shaving cream and constant tactile cueing with immediate reinforcement of appropriate sensory responses; sensory awareness was required during all activities. Visual cues and scanning and tracking tasks involved moving objects throughout Kelly's visual field and were combined with auditory reinforcement through verbal praise and music.

The right UE was most directly targeted in the area of reaching. The practitioner initially encouraged reaching using sensory (visual and tactile) input applied to the right arm and hand to increase Kelly's awareness and understanding both of their existence and of her own ability to directly manipulate them. This encouragement is often crucial for children whose CNS lesions are so large or global that the children fail to understand that they can actively manipulate their involved extremity, often termed *developmental disregard.* Kelly's lack of awareness of her own ability to effect the action of an extremity was an extreme case of developmental disregard.

To develop Kelly's awareness of her right UE, the practitioner placed toys proximally in the space on the right side of her body. At the start of treatment, the practitioner facilitated successful attempts to enable Kelly to make direct contact with the toy; facilitation was faded and the need for verbal and tactile cues

decreased in subsequent days as Kelly's skills in reaching developed. For example, once Kelly reached for toys in a direct proximal position on the right side with 75% consistency, the practitioner began to move toys into different planes, requiring Kelly to develop other skills involved in reaching, including perceptual realization of the new placement of the toy, with the goal of increasing Kelly's motor-planning abilities. Through this process, Kelly also developed the ability to follow multiple steps during activities to receive the rewards associated with the activity.

Kelly's progress with gross motor abilities was displayed in increased head control; increased core strength for sitting balance; increased weight bearing and tolerance through the right side; and increased ability to push to sit from and sit up straight on an elevated surface, which allowed her to begin to explore her environment more independently. She also developed the ability to independently reach to activate cause-and-effect toys, to be picked up by caregivers, and to give high fives at midline with emerging reaching across midline. She also developed some combined reaching, cognitive, and perceptual–motor planning as demonstrated by her ability to reach into and out of large containers with her right UE.

Overall, Kelly had increased spontaneous use and awareness of her right UE (with decreased cueing required) and demonstrated better awareness and control of her core trunk abilities, indicating a better awareness of that entire side of her body. P–CIMT also helped Kelly develop her visual tracking of objects during play and emerging communication skills through the signs for "more" and "all done." Although neither communication nor visual abilities are the targets of P–CIMT, they are indirectly worked on during the therapeutic process. P–CIMT activities have strong motor components but have additional advantages in many developmental domains.

SUMMARY AND NEXT DIRECTIONS

Hemispherectomy is a radical surgical procedure undertaken because of severe intractable seizure activity, and children often experience severe impairments after surgery. Case studies reported in the literature (e.g., de Bode, Fritz, Weir-Haynes, & Mathern, 2009) suggest that P–CIMT can be an effective treatment for children after hemispherectomy. The advent of new neuroimaging techniques, increased understanding of neural plasticity (Flack et al., 2008; Samargia & Kimberley, 2009), and new therapies such as P–CIMT (de Bode et al., 2009) and other intensive approaches (Fritz et al., 2011) has raised new questions about how therapeutic efforts might interact to produce better motor outcomes.

REFERENCES

Anderson, V., Godfrey, C., Rosenfeld, J., & Catroppa, C. (2011). 10 years outcome from childhood brain injury. *International Journal of Developmental Neuroscience, 9,* 1–8.

Benjamin, K. (2005). Injuries to the brachial plexus: Mechanisms of injury and identification of risk factors (Part 1). *Advances in Neonatal Care, 5*(4), 181–189.

Bisinella, G. L., & Birch, R. (2003). Obstetric brachial plexus lesions: A study of 74 children registered with the British Paediatric Surveillance Unit (March 1998–March 1999). *Journal of Hand Surgery, 28,* 40–45.

Brady, K., & Garcia, T. (2009). Constraint-induced movement therapy (CIMT): Pediatric applications. *Developmental Disabilities Research Review, 15,* 102–111.

Brunton, L. K., & Bartlett, D. J. (2011). Validity and reliability of two abbreviated versions of the Gross Motor Function Measure. *Physical Therapy, 91,* 577–588.

Buesch, F. E., Schlaepfer, B., de Bruin, E. D., Wohlrab, G., Ammann-Reiffer, C., & Meyer-Heim, A. (2009). Constraint-induced movement therapy for children with obstetric brachial plexus palsy: Two single-case series. *International Journal of Rehabilitation Research, 33,* 187–192.

Centers for Disease Control and Prevention. (2010). *Traumatic brain injury in the United States: Emergency department visits, hospitalizations and deaths 2002–2006.* Retrieved from http://www.cdc.gov/traumaticbraininjury/pdf/blue_book.pdf

Chaplin, D., Deitz, J., & Jaffe, K. M. (1993). Motor performance in children after traumatic brain injury. *Archives of Physical Medicine and Rehabilitation, 74,* 161–164.

Chen, S., Wolf, S. L., Zhang, Q., Thompson, P. A., & Winstein, C. J. (2012). Minimal detectable change of the Actual Amount of Use Test and the Motor Activity Log: The EXCITE Trial. *Neurorehabilitation and Neural Repair, 26,* 507–514.

Cho, Y. W., Jang, S. H., Lee, Z. I., Song, J. C., Lee, H. K., & Lee, H. Y. (2005). Effect and appropriate restriction period of constraint-induced movement therapy in hemiparetic patients with brain injury: A brief report. *NeuroRehabilitation, 20,* 71–74.

Christensen, J. R. (1996). Pediatric traumatic brain injury. In A. J. Capute & P. J. Accardo (Eds.), *Developmental disabilities in infancy and childhood: Vol. 1. Neurodevelopmental diagnosis and treatment* (2nd ed., pp. 189–198). Baltimore: Paul H. Brookes.

Ciliberto, M. A., Limbrick, D., Powers, A., Titus, J. B., Munro, R., & Smyth, M. D. (2012). Palliative hemispherectomy in children with bilateral seizure onset. *Journal of Neurosurgery in Pediatrics, 9,* 381–388.

Cimolin, V., Beretta, E., Piccinini, L., Turconi, A. C., Locatelli, F., Galli, M., & Strazzer, S. (2012). Constraint-induced movement therapy for children with hemiplegia after traumatic brain injury: A quantitative study. *Journal of Head Trauma Rehabilitation, 27,* 177–187.

Coker, P., Lebkicker, C., Harris, L., & Snape, J. (2009). The effects of constraint induced movement therapy for a child less than one year of age. *NeuroRehabilitation, 24,* 199–208. http://dx.doi.org/10.3233/NRE-2009-0469

de Bode, S., Fritz, S. L., Weir-Haynes, K., & Mathern, G. W. (2009). Constraint-induced movement therapy for individuals after cerebral hemispherectomy: A case series. *Physical Therapy, 89,* 361–369.

DeBow, S. B., McKenna, J. E., Kolb, B., & Colbourne, F. (2004). Immediate constraint-induced movement therapy causes local hyperthermia that exacerbates cerebral cortical injury in rats. *Canadian Journal of Physiology and Pharmacology, 82,* 231–237.

DeMatteo, C., Law, M., Russell, D., Pollock, N., Rosenbaum, P., & Walter, S. (1992). *QUEST: Quality of Upper Extremity Skills Test manual.* Hamilton, Ontario: Neurodevelopmental Research Unit, Chedoke Campus, Chedoke–McMasters Hospital.

Dijkerman, H. C., Vargha-Khadem, F., Polkey, C. E., & Weiskrantz, L. (2008). Ipsilesional and contralesional sensorimotor function after hemispherectomy: Differences between distal and proximal function. *Neuropsychologia, 46,* 886–901.

Doumouchtsis, S. K., & Arulkumaran, S. (2009). Are all brachial plexus injuries caused by shoulder dystocia? *Obstetric and Gynecological Survey, 64,* 615–623.

Eliasson, A. C., Krumlinde-Sundholm, L., Rösblad, B., Beckung, E., Arner, M., Ohrvall, A. M., & Rosenbaum, P. (2006). The Manual Ability Classification System (MACS) for children with cerebral palsy: Scale development and evidence of validity and reliability. *Developmental Medicine and Child Neurology, 48,* 549–554.

Fedrizzi, E., Oleari, G., Inverno, M., Dal Brun, A., & Bono, R. (1994). Motor performance assessment in children with cerebral palsy. In E. Fedrizzi, G. Avanzini, & P. Crenna (Eds.), *Motor development in childhood* (pp. 51–58). London: John Libbey.

Flack, S., Ojemann, J., & Haberkern, C. (2008). Cerebral hemispherectomy in infants and young children. *Paediatric Anaesthesia, 18,* 967–973.

Fritz, S. L., Rivers, E. D., Merlo, A. M., Reed, A. D., Mathern, G. D., & De Bode, S. (2011). Intensive mobility training postcerebral hemispherectomy: Early surgery shows best functional improvements. *European Journal of Physical and Rehabilitation Medicine, 47,* 569–577.

Fugl-Meyer, A. R., Jääskö, L., Leyman, I., Olsson, S., & Steglind, S. (1975). The post-stroke hemiplegic patient: I. A method for evaluation of physical performance. *Scandinavian Journal of Rehabilitative Medicine, 7,* 13–31.

Gerrard-Morris, A., Taylor, H. G., Yeates, K. O., Walz, N. C., Stancin, T., Minich, N., & Wade, S. L. (2010). Cognitive development after traumatic brain injury in young children. *Journal of the International Neuropsychological Society, 16,* 157–168.

Gordon, A., Connelly, A., Neville, B., Vargha-Khadem, F., Jessop, N., Murphy, T., & Ganesan, V. (2007). Modified constraint-induced movement therapy after childhood stroke. *Developmental Medicine and Child Neurology, 49,* 23–27.

Govindan, R. M., Chugani, H. T., Luat, A. F., & Sood, S. (2010). Presurgical prediction of motor functional loss using tractography. *Pediatric Neurology, 43,* 70–72.

Guo, Y. E., & Togher, L. (2008). The impact of dysarthria on everyday communication after traumatic brain injury: A pilot study. *Brain Injury, 22,* 83–98.

Hindi-Ling, H., Kipervasser, S., Neufeld, M. Y., Andelman, F., Nagar, S., Chistik, V., . . . Kramer, U. (2011). Epilepsy surgery in children compared to adults. *Pediatric Neurosurgery, 47,* 180–185.

Holt, R. L., & Mikati, M. A. (2011). Care for child development: Basic science rationale and effects of interventions. *Pediatric Neurology, 44,* 239–253.

Jaffe, K. M., Polissar, L., Fay, G. C., & Liao, S. (1995). Recovery trends over three years following pediatric traumatic brain injury. *Archives of Physical Medicine and Rehabilitation, 76,* 17–26.

Johnson, L. M., Randall, M. J., Reddihough, D. S., Oke, L. E., Bryt, T. A., & Bach, T. M. (1994). Development of a clinical assessment of quality of movement for unilateral upper-limb function. *Developmental Medicine and Child Neurology, 36,* 965–973.

Karman, N., Maryles, J., Baker, R. W., Simpser, E., & Berger-Gross, P. (2003). Constraint-induced movement therapy for hemiplegic children with acquired brain injuries. *Journal of Head Trauma Rehabilitation, 18,* 259–267.

Kattan, A. E., & Borschel, G. H. (2011). Anatomy of the brachial plexus. *Journal of Pediatric Rehabilitation Medicine, 4,* 107–111.

Kim, D. L., Osburn, L. L., & Cohen-Gadol, A. A. (2009). A novel method for confirmation of hemispherectomy disconnection during hemispherectomy surgery. *Pediatric Neurosurgery, 46,* 71–75.

Kim, S. K., Wang, K. C., Hwang, Y. S., Kim, K. J., Chae, J. H., Kim, I. O., & Cho, B. K. (2008). Epilepsy surgery in children: Outcomes and complications. *Journal of Neurosurgery Pediatrics, 1,* 277–283.

Kozin, S. H. (2011). The evaluation and treatment of children with brachial plexus birth palsy. *Journal of Hand Surgery, 36,* 1360–1369.

Krasny-Pacini, A., Hiebel, J., Pauly, F., Godon, S., & Chevignard, M. (2013). Goal Attainment Scaling in rehabilitation: A literature-based update. *Annals of Physical Rehabilitation and Medicine, 56,* 212–230.

Krumlinde-Sundholm, L., Holmefur, M., & Eliasson, A. C. (2007). *Assisting Hand Assessment manual, research version 4.4.* Stockholm: Karolinska Institute, Neuropediatric Research Unit, Astrid Lindgren Children's Hospital.

Kwazneski, D. R., Iyer, R. C., Panthaki, Z., & Armstrong, M. B. (2009). Controversies in the diagnosis and treatment of pediatric brachial plexus injuries. *Journal of Craniofacial Surgery, 20,* 1036–1038.

Law, M., Baptiste, S., Carswell, A., McColl, M., Polatajko, H., & Pollock, N. (2005). *Canadian Occupational Performance Measure* (4th ed.). Ottawa, Ontario: CAOT Publications ACE.

Limbrick, D. D., Narayan, P., Powers, A. K., Ojemann, J. G., Park, T. S., Bertrand, M., & Smyth, M. D. (2009). Hemispherectomy: Efficacy and analysis of seizure recurrence. *Journal of Neurosurgery Pediatrics, 4,* 323–332.

Malessy, M. J., Bakker, D., Dekker, A. J., Van Duk, J. G., & Thomeer, R. T. (2003). Functional magnetic resonance imaging and control over the biceps muscle after intercostal–musculocutaneous nerve transfer. *Journal of Neurosurgery, 98,* 261–268.

Mathern, G. W. (2010). Cerebral hemispherectomy: When half a brain is good enough. *Neurology, 75,* 1578–1580.

McGillicuddy, J. E. (2011). Neonatal brachial plexus palsy: Historical perspective. *Journal of Pediatric Rehabilitation Medicine, 4,* 99–101.

Morgan, A., Ward, E., & Murdoch, B. (2004). Clinical progression and outcome of dysphagia following paediatric traumatic brain injury: A prospective study. *Journal of Head Trauma Rehabilitation, 18,* 359–376.

Murphy, K. M., Rasmussen, L., Hervey-Jumper, S. L., Justice, D., Nelson, V. S., & Yang, L. J. (2012). An assessment of the compliance and utility of a home exercise DVD for caregivers of children and adolescents with brachial plexus palsy: A pilot study. *Physical Medicine and Rehabilitation, 4,* 190–197.

Page, S., & Levine, P. (2003). Forced use after TBI: Promoting plasticity and function through practice. *Brain Injury, 17,* 675–684.

Pham, C. B., Kratz, J. R., Jelin, A. C., & Gelfand, A. A. (2011). Child neurology: Brachial plexus birth injury: What every neurologist needs to know. *Neurology, 77,* 695–697.

Piatt, J. H., Jr. (2005). Birth injuries of the brachial plexus. *Clinics in Perinatology, 32,* 39–59, v–vi.

Price, A., Tidwell, M., & Grossman, J. A. (2000). Improving shoulder and elbow function in children with Erb's palsy. *Seminars in Pediatric Neurology, 7,* 44–51.

Ramos, L. E., & Zell, J. P. (2000). Rehabilitation program for children with brachial plexus and peripheral nerve injury. *Seminars in Pediatric Neurology, 7,* 52–57.

Randall, M., Carlin, J. B., Chondros, P., & Reddihough, D. (2001). Reliability of the Melbourne Assessment of Unilateral Upper Limb Function. *Developmental Medicine and Child Neurology, 43,* 761–767.

Randall, M., Johnson, I., & Reddihough, D. (1999). *The Melbourne Assessment of Unilateral Upper Limb Function: Test administration manual.* Melbourne, Australia: Royal Children's Hospital.

Reading, B. D., Laor, T., Salisbury, S. R., Lippert, W. C., & Cornwall, R. (2012). Quantification of humeral head deformity following neonatal brachial plexus palsy.

Journal of Bone and Joint Surgery (American), 94(18), e136(1–8).

Reidy, T. G., Naber, E., Viguers, E., Allison, K., Brady, K., Carney, J., . . . Pidcock, F. (2012). Outcomes of a clinic-based pediatric constraint-induced movement therapy program. *Physical and Occupational Therapy in Pediatrics, 32,* 355–367. http:/dx.doi.org/10.3109/01942638.2012.694991

Samargia, S. A., & Kimberley, T. J. (2009). Motor and cognitive outcomes in children after functional hemispherectomy. *Pediatric Physical Therapy, 21,* 356–361.

Santamato, A., Panza, F., Ranieri, M., & Fiore, P. (2011). Effect of botulinum toxin type A and modified constraint-induced movement therapy on motor function of upper limb in children with obstetrical brachial plexus palsy. *Children's Nervous System, 27,* 2187–2192.

Shaw, S. E., Morris, D. M., Uswatte, G., McKay, S., Meythaler, J. M., & Taub, E. J. (2005). Constraint-induced movement therapy for recovery of upper-limb function following traumatic brain injury. *Journal of Rehabilitation Research and Development, 42,* 769–778.

Sheffler, L. C., Lattanza, L., Hagar, Y., Bagley, A., & James, M. A. (2012). The prevalence, rate of progression, and treatment of elbow flexion contracture in children with brachial plexus birth palsy. *Journal of Bone and Joint Surgery, 94,* 403–409.

Shenaq, S. M., Bullocks, J. M., Dhillon, G., Lee, R. T., & Laurent, J. P. (2005). Management of infant brachial plexus injuries. *Clinics in Plastic Surgery, 32,* 79–98, ix.

Slomine, B., & Locascio, G. (2009). Cognitive rehabilitation for children with acquired brain injury. *Developmental Disabilities Research Reviews, 15,* 133–143.

Smith, Y. A., Hong, E., & Presson, C. (2000). Normative and validation studies of the Nine-Hole Peg Test with children. *Perceptual Motor Skills, 90,* 823–843.

Spencer, S., & Huh, L. (2008). Outcomes of epilepsy surgery in adults and children. *Lancet Neurology, 7,* 525–537.

Taub, E., Miller, N. E., Novack, T. A., Cook, E. W., 3rd, Fleming, W. C., Nepomuceno, C. S., . . . Crago, J. E. (1993). Technique to improve chronic motor deficit after stroke. *Archives of Physical Medicine and Rehabilitation, 74,* 347–354.

Taub, E., Ramey, S. L., DeLuca, S., & Echols, K. (2004). Efficacy of constraint-induced movement therapy for children with cerebral palsy with asymmetric motor impairment. *Pediatrics, 113,* 305–312. PMID: 14754942

Treger, I., Aidinof, L., Lehrer, H., & Kalichman, L. (2012). Modified constraint-induced movement therapy improved upper limb function in subacute poststroke patients: A small-scale clinical trial. *Topics in Stroke Rehabilitation, 19,* 287–293.

Vaz, D. V., Mancini, M. C., do Amaral, M. F., de Brito Brandão, M., de França Drummond, A., & da Fonseca, S. T. (2010). Clinical changes during an intervention based on constraint-induced movement therapy principles on use of the affected arm of a child with obstetric brachial plexus injury: A case report. *Occupational Therapy International, 17,* 159–167.

Verkerk, G. J., Wolf, M. J., Louwers, A. M., Meester-Delver, A., & Nollet, F. (2006). The reproducibility and validity of the Canadian Occupational Performance Measure in parents of children with disabilities. *Clinical Rehabilitation, 20,* 980–988.

Wolf, S. L., Catlin, P. A., Ellis, M., Archer, A. L., Morgan, B., & Piacentino, A. (2001). Assessing Wolf Motor Function Test as outcome measure for research in patients after stroke. *Stroke, 32,* 1635–1639.

Yoshikawa, T., Hayashi, N., Tajiri, Y., Satake, Y., & Ohtomo, K. (2012). Brain reorganization in patients with brachial plexus injury: A longitudinal functional MRI study. *Scientific World Journal, 2012,* 501751.

TERESSA GARCIA REIDY, MS, OTR/L; ERIN NABER, PT, DPT; and PATTY COKER-BOLT, PhD, OTR/L

12

Novel and Complementary Therapy Strategies: Critical Issues and Opportunities for Combining With Pediatric CIMT

CHAPTER HIGHLIGHTS

- Electrical stimulation
- Therapeutic taping
- Yoga-based therapy
- Aquatic therapy
- Therapeutic use of rehabilitation robotics, virtual reality, and gaming systems
- Botulinum toxin therapy.

KEY TERMS

Aquatic therapy

Botulinum toxin therapy

Complementary and alternative medicine

Functional electrical stimulation

Gaming technology

Kinesiology taping

Neuromuscular electrical stimulation

Physical agent modality

Rehabilitation robotics

Rigid taping

Therapeutic electrical stimulation

Virtual reality

Yoga

Yoga therapy

Rehabilitation planning for a client often spans infancy through adulthood. The overall goal of therapy intervention is to reduce functional limitations and facilitate optimal performance in daily life activities. Therapy strategies are selected to produce meaningful, optimal change in a child's motor skills that will enhance the child's future success in life experiences. Therapy should be goal directed and should engage a child in age-appropriate, meaningful activities that allow for adaptation and change in motor repertoires.

As appropriate, multiple treatment modalities should be considered part of the therapy tool chest to improve motor skills, enhance movement patterns, and increase overall skill and function. The selection of treatment modalities typically is based on a practitioner's advanced training or clinical experience; many times, selection of a modality does not rely on strong scientific evidence to support its use. A recent survey of occupational and physical therapy practitioners revealed that most used special treatment modalities on the basis of whether they had received special training or had the necessary time to implement the modality in a clinical setting (Saleh et al., 2008).

Few randomized controlled trials are available to support the use of the modalities mentioned in this chapter, and most evidence reported here is based on case study reports or noncontrolled pre- and postintervention studies. A recent review of physical therapy techniques targeting lower limb function in children with cerebral palsy (CP) noted that therapy interventions targeting problems at the body function and structure level generally influenced the level of impairment without greatly affecting the child's activity or overall participation (Franki et al., 2012).

This chapter discusses novel and complementary intervention strategies used by occupational and physical therapy practitioners to treat children with neuromotor disorders and addresses the compatibility of these strategies with pediatric constraint-induced movement therapy (P–CIMT). The chapter provides a broad overview of current treatment modalities that clinicians use to improve selective control of muscles, promote anticipatory upper- and lower-extremity movements, and force output that could lead to improved function in everyday life, especially if paired with P–CIMT. Readers should consider the information in this chapter in terms of how these therapeutic modalities affect the overall rehabilitation plan for a child and his or her family.

Rigorously designed studies of the effects of these treatment modalities and their long-term outcomes for multisystem impairments and overall function in children with neuromotor disorders are lacking to date. More in-depth examination is needed of how the treatment modalities are currently being applied and measured and of what effects are seen on long-term abilities.

ELECTRICAL STIMULATION

The therapeutic use of a peripherally applied electrical stimulus to depolarize nerve axons is a physical agent modality (PAM) recognized by the American Occupational Therapy Association (AOTA):

> The American Occupational Therapy Association . . . asserts that physical agent modalities . . . may be used by occupational therapists and occupational therapy assistants in preparation for or concurrently with purposeful and occupation-based activities or interventions that ultimately enhance engagement in occupation. AOTA further stipulates that PAMs may be applied only by occupational therapists and occupational therapy assistants who have documented evidence of possessing the theoretical background and technical skills for safe and competent integration of the modality into an occupational therapy intervention plan. (AOTA, 2012, p. S78)

A **physical agent modality** is an intervention that produces a response in soft tissue through the use of light, water, temperature, sound, or electricity. Practitioners using PAMs should be fully educated and trained in their indicated use and contraindications. They also should contact their state licensing or regulatory boards to obtain information about state guidelines for use of PAMs.

With PAMs involving electricity, a stimulus can be delivered in a variety of ways. Threshold electrical stimulation, sometimes called **therapeutic electrical stimulation,** refers to the application of an electrical stimulus below the threshold necessary to elicit muscular contraction. **Neuromuscular electrical stimulation** is application of a stimulus sufficient to elicit a muscular contraction. **Functional electrical stimulation** is coordinated application of a stimulus to elicit a muscle contraction during a functional task. A photo of a client undergoing neuromuscular electrical stimulation is presented in Figure 12.1. Although a few studies (e.g., Kerr, McDowell, & McDonough, 2004) have investigated the use of electrical stimulation in hemiplegia, its use as an adjunct to CIMT has not been reported in the literature.

Initial reports of the combination of CIMT with electrical stimulation were case studies of adults with hemiplegia. In 2005, Fritz, Chiu, Malcolm, Patterson, and Light published a case report of a 72-year-old man who, 10 years earlier, had

Figure 12.1 NEUROMUSCULAR ELECTRICAL STIMULATION APPLIED TO WRIST EXTENSORS WITH SPLINTING TO BLOCK HYPEREXTENSION AT THE METACARPOPHALANGEAL JOINTS.

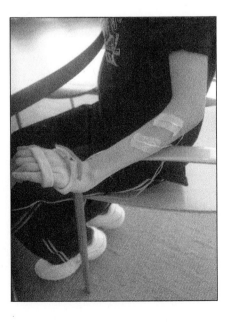

Source. Kennedy Kreiger Institute, Baltimore.

experienced a left-brain ischemic stroke resulting in right hemiparesis. He had impaired wrist and finger extension and did not meet minimum motor criteria for CIMT. Subsequently, he began a program of functional electrical stimulation to augment wrist extension. The functional electrical stimulation was paired with CIMT for 3 hours of a 6-hour daily CIMT session for 10 days. Two days after completing CIMT, he showed improvement in overall scores for the Fugl-Meyer Assessment of Sensorimotor Recovery After Stroke (Fugl-Meyer, Jääskö, Leyman, Olsson, & Steglind, 1975), Wolf Motor Function Test (Wolf et al., 2001), the Actual Amount of Use Test (Taub et al., 1993), and the Box and Block Test (Mathiowetz, Volland, Kashman, & Weber, 1985), as well as improvements in the Motor Activity Log score (van der Lee, Beckerman, Knol, de Vet, & Bouter, 2004) and Stroke Impact Scale score (Duncan, Bode, Min Lai, & Perera, 2003).

In a study reporting on functional electrical stimulation combined with CIMT, Page and Levine (2006) described a case series of 6 adults with stroke who did not meet minimum motor criteria for CIMT. The participants were a subset of participants already enrolled in a trial of electromyographically monitored stimulation who showed significant improvement after the stimulation. The participants used a NeuroMove NM900 electromyographically monitored stimulation device (Zynex NeuroDiagnostics, Lone Tree, CO) for 35 minutes twice daily on weekdays for 8 weeks. Electrodes were placed on wrist extensors and the activity of these muscles monitored. Stimulation was delivered only once a threshold was achieved. The authors reported that adherence to the protocol was high, and at the end of the intervention, participants had a mean change of 0.3 on the Action Research Arm Test (ARAT; Lyle, 1981), which the investigators characterized as a nominal change. Although the authors noted that the participants showed no functional changes, they found that participants did show an improved ability to initiate wrist extension, reflected in a 4.1-point increase in the mean Fugl-Meyer Assessment score. This improvement was sufficient to qualify them for a modified CIMT (mCIMT) protocol.

The mCIMT component was a 10-week intervention that included 30 minutes of structured therapy in an outpatient setting 3 days per week with a focus on shaping and functional task use, as well as an additional 5 hours of daily restraint with a sling and mitt on weekdays at home. After the mCIMT intervention, participants showed a mean increase of 14.5 points in the Fugl-Meyer Assessment score and a mean increase of 11.4 points in the ARAT score. Improvement also was reflected in the participants' self-reports, which revealed an increased ability to complete functional tasks, such as writing (Page & Levine, 2006).

Only one study has investigated the combination of electrical stimulation with a P–CIMT program. In 2012, Xu, Wang, Mai, and He published the results of a randomized controlled trial in which 68 children with hemiplegia aged 2 to 14 years received 2 weeks of modified P–CIMT (mP–CIMT), modified P–CIMT plus electrical stimulation, or occupational therapy without use of electrical stimulation or constraint. Electrical stimulation to the wrist and finger extensors was delivered by a MyoTrac Infiniti (Thought Technology, Montreal, Quebec) dual-channel neuromuscular electrical stimulation unit for 20 minutes, 5 times per week. Unlike the two studies mentioned previously, Xu and colleagues' protocol incorporated electrical stimulation but not functional electrical stimulation because the children were not engaged in a functional task while they completed the electrical stimulation program.

Xu et al.'s (2012) mP–CIMT intervention consisted of the use of a constraint splint for 3 hours per day, 5 days per week, during occupational therapy sessions at a children's hospital for the 2-week intervention period. Therapy sessions consisted of structured play and functional activities, with practitioners shaping new motor patterns and providing reinforcement for gains in targeted skills. The group of children receiving occupational therapy without electrical stimulation or constraint also attended occupational therapy sessions for 3 hours per day, 5 days per week, for the same intervention period. These sessions were based on principles of neurodevelopmental treatment and motor learning and used strengthening, stretching, and coordination training. Participants in each group were assessed at 2 weeks, 3 months, and 6 months after treatment. At the 6-month follow-up assessment, the group receiving constraint therapy plus electrical stimulation had a significantly ($p < .05$) greater improvement in Upper Extremity Functional Test (Carroll, 1965) scores than the other two groups, as well as significant increases in the visual–motor integration section of the Peabody Developmental Motor Scales (Folio & Fewell, 2000).

These promising findings in adult populations and the preliminary work in the pediatric population suggest that further research is needed to determine the optimal application of functional electrical stimulation before, during, and after a P–CIMT program and to examine the possible long-term functional outcomes of these combined interventions. Table 12.1 summarizes the considerations in using electrical stimulation as an adjunct to P–CIMT, and Case Example 12.1 describes the use of therapeutic electrical stimulation with P–CIMT for an 11-year-old boy.

THERAPEUTIC TAPING

Two types of therapeutic taping are used in rehabilitation: (1) rigid taping and (2) kinesiology taping. Practitioners use **rigid taping** to limit movement around a joint or to protect a joint during functional movement, whereas they use flexible, elastic

Table 12.1   PROS, CONS, AND APPLICATION TO P–CIMT PROGRAMS OF SELECTED COMPLEMENTARY THERAPY INTERVENTIONS

INTERVENTION	PROS	CONS AND CAUTIONS	APPLICATION TO P–CIMT
Electrical stimulation	Promotes strengthening Facilitates motor learning May ultimately make constraint programs accessible to clients who initially do not meet minimum motor criteria	May be difficult for some children to tolerate Is supported by few well-controlled trials in children Requires monitoring of skin, especially for children with sensory impairment Requires careful assessment of appropriateness, especially for children with impaired cognition or communication	Can be part of a home program to promote strength and encourage use in the affected hand Can be applied during massed practice and shaping to enhance performance of motor movements
Rehabilitation robotics, virtual reality, and gaming technology	Promotes repetitive task practice Could be used to target specific motor movements (e.g., shoulder flexion, supination) May have a high level of sensitivity, depending on the device, enabling activation even by children with limited AROM, which in turn can lead to increased self-efficacy Enables age-appropriate activity that can be done with peers or as a home exercise program Can simulate real-world activities Provides possible secondary benefits in visual–perceptual and visual–motor skills	May exclude participation by clients with AROM limitations (controller-based or glove-based games) Is not supported by adequate research (game systems) Requires monitoring for compensatory movements May require adaptation of controllers Requires seizure and shunt precautions Requires monitoring to prevent repetitive motion disorders	Allows greater opportunities for massed practice May be a possible home program activity for carryover of skills acquired during P–CIMT
Botulinum toxin therapy	Can reduce spasticity in combination with other therapies Is less invasive than surgical intervention	Produces a temporary effect May inadvertently spread to muscles near the injected muscle Requires monitoring of skin if used in combination with casting	May be tested with serial casting to gain range before P–CIMT

Note. AROM = active range of motion; P–CIMT = pediatric constraint-induced movement therapy.

Case Example

Case Example 12.1

USE OF THERAPEUTIC ELECTRICAL STIMULATION AS AN ADJUNCT TO P–CIMT

Luke was an 11-year-old boy with a history of hemiplegia following a traumatic brain injury at age 3 years. He presented with greatly decreased wrist and finger extension strength, limiting his ability to grasp with his affected upper extremity (UE). He was referred by his physiatrist to receive P–CIMT.

Before applying the constraint, Luke's outpatient practitioner elected to use electrical stimulation to strengthen his involved UE. Using a portable electrical stimulation device, the practitioner triggered the functional electrical stimulation to Luke's wrist and finger extensors to assist with opening

his hand to grasp small objects on a tabletop during therapy sessions.

Given Luke's response to this treatment modality, the practitioner ordered him a device for home use and trained him and his parents to use the device for 30 minutes per day at home. After 6 weeks of daily functional electrical stimulation, Luke's AROM improved, allowing him to actively open his hand to grasp small objects without the assistance of the stimulation. Luke then started a P–CIMT protocol, and his practitioner continued to include electrical stimulation in his home program and his therapy program.

kinesiology taping to facilitate improved movement patterns (Yasukawa, Patel, & Sisung, 2006). Kinesiology taping allows free range of movement of a joint, and rigid taping restricts movement of a joint (Kase, 2000).

Therapeutic taping was first used by athletes and then transferred for use in rehabilitation clinics with clients across the lifespan. Kase (2000) defined four major functions of kinesiology taping: (1) to support a weakened muscle, (2) to improve circulation, (3) to reduce pain, and (4) to improve joint alignment.

When applying kinesiology tape, the amount of stretch can be important for specific muscle tapings (Kase, 2000). For clients with chronic muscle weakness, such as those enrolled in a CIMT program, kinesiology tape should be applied with light tension from origin to insertion to enhance muscle contraction (Kase, Martin, & Yasukawa, 2006). Overstretching the tape can reduce the positive effects (Kase et al., 2006). Advanced training in kinesiology taping and rigid taping is available through continuing education courses (see Appendix 12.A for resources).

Taping techniques may be used alone or in conjunction with CIMT programs. Flexible kinesiology taping can help facilitate improved muscle activation during repetitive task practice. In conjunction with P–CIMT programs, kinesiology taping may improve a child's ability to initiate a movement and assist in aligning an upper-body joint, improving the quality and smoothness of movement. Being able to move the affected limb with greater ease may increase a child's willingness to engage in repetitive task practice and shaping activities (Figure 12.2). Rigid and flexible taping techniques can protect joints or reduce compensatory movements.

Rigid taping techniques should be used with caution because they restrict movement. In addition, both flexible and rigid taping may form a barrier impeding appropriate tactile sensory feedback, especially if the taping is across the child's palm.

Evidence to support the use of therapeutic taping is limited and includes a few case reports or small cohort studies without control groups. In a pediatric acute inpatient setting, Yasukawa and colleagues (2006) reported statistically significant gains on the Melbourne Assessment of Unilateral Upper Limb Function (Randall, Johnson, & Reddihough, 2010) after a 3-day taping intervention. Participants had a variety of acquired diagnoses, including traumatic brain injury, spinal cord injury, encephalitis, cardiovascular accident, and brain tumor.

In a case study with a 2-year-old client recovering from brachial plexus palsy, Walsh (2010) reported the use of kinesiology taping to target affected shoulder subluxation. After the taping intervention, improved alignment and function were reported. In fact, a planned reconstructive surgery on the child was cancelled because of the positive effects of taping; however, not all studies of therapeutic taping have noted this success. A study of 18 children with quadriplegic CP found no improvements on standardized measures after therapeutic rigid taping for postural control (Footer, 2006).

A study investigating the bioelectrical activity of the vastus medialis muscle in healthy adults found an increase in muscle recruitment 24 hours after kinesiology tape placement and continued effects for an additional 48 hours after application (Słupik, Dwornik, Białoszewski, & Zych, 2007). To date, no studies have specifically investigated the effect of combining therapeutic taping with P–CIMT protocols. Case Example 12.2 describes one possible use of kinesiology taping as an adjunct to P–CIMT.

Figure 12.2   USE OF KINESIOLOGY TAPING TO IMPROVE THUMB ABDUCTION NEEDED FOR GRASP–RELEASE.

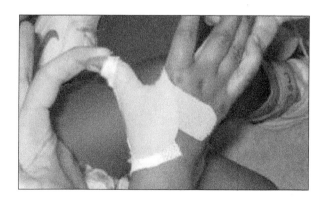
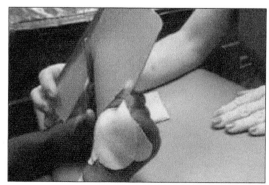

Source. P. Coker-Bolt.

Case Example

USE OF KINESIOLOGY TAPING AS AN ADJUNCT TO P–CIMT

Nina was a 5-year-old girl with right hemiplegia attending a 3-hour per day, clinic-based P–CIMT program. Every time Nina reached to point, she maintained her wrist in a flexed position, and she often kept her thumb adducted and in her fist. She had tightness and spasticity in her wrist flexors.

Nina's practitioner implemented the use of waterproof kinesiology tape to her thumb web space to increase thumb abduction. The practitioner also applied tape to her wrist extensors to improve wrist alignment. The tape stayed on for 2 to 3 days and was reapplied 4 times during Nina's course of P–CIMT. Between reapplications of the kinesiology tape, the skin surface was not taped to allow any skin irritation to resolve.

Although Nina did not achieve full active wrist extension, her wrist approximated neutral more often when engaging in P–CIMT repetitive task practice and shaping requiring forward reach and grasp. The thumb web space taping also improved her ability to easily grasp a cracker when eating her snack.

YOGA-BASED THERAPY

Yoga is an ancient Indian practice designed to unite the mind, body, and spirit. These three areas are addressed through a combination of movement, body positions (asanas), mindfulness, breathing, and meditation. **Yoga therapy,** as defined by the International Association of Yoga Therapists, is "the process of empowering individuals to progress toward improved health and well-being through the application of the philosophy and practice of yoga" (Taylor, 2007, p. 3).

Over the past several years, the use of complementary and alternative medicine (CAM) approaches, including yoga, has become more popular. The National Center for Complementary and Alternative Medicine (2008) defined **CAM** as "a group of diverse medical and health care systems, practices, and products that are not generally considered part of conventional medicine." The 2007 National Health Interview Survey of 9,000 children and teens found that 12% of respondents had used some form of CAM in the past 12 months (Barnes, Bloom, & Nahin, 2008); 2% of respondents had participated in some form of yoga practice in the past 12 months, and 4% of respondents had used CAM to address musculoskeletal issues.

The evidence to support the use of yoga by people with hemiplegia is limited and requires further evaluation (Galantino, Galbavy, & Quinn, 2008). Many published studies on the outcomes of yoga therapy report results from both adults and children, and most lack an adequate control group and follow-up outcome data. The yoga therapy interventions in these studies are often poorly defined and use different dosages.

Despite these limitations, emerging evidence indicates that yoga may be a promising intervention to address musculoskeletal and neuromuscular impairments in children with hemiplegia. Table 12.2 lists possible uses for yoga as an adjunct to P–CIMT, and Case Example 12.3 describes its use with a 6-year-old boy.

Several studies have reported an increase in grip strength following participation in a yoga program (Dash & Telles, 2001; Mandanmohan, Jatiya, Udupa, & Bhavanani, 2003; Raghuraj, Nagarathna, Nagendra, & Telles, 1997; Telles, Dash, & Naveen, 2009). Changes in UE coordination also have been reported. Telles, Hanumanthaiah, Nagarathna, and Nagendra (1993, 1994) found that following a 10-day daily yoga program, adult and child participants demonstrated fewer errors on a steadiness test consisting of inserting a stylus into various sized holes compared with control participants who did not participate in yoga practice. In addition, two studies reported finger-tapping speed improvements in adults and children following participation in a yoga program (Dash & Telles, 1999; Telles et al., 2009).

Further studies have evaluated fine motor skills following a yoga program. Subramanya and Telles (2009) noted improvements in men completing psychomotor tasks, including letter copying and circle dotting, following meditation, which was not seen with control sessions in which the same participants did not participate in meditation before completing the task. Lynton, Kligler, and Shiflett (2007) reported improvements on the O'Connor Tweezer Dexterity Test (Lafayette Instrument Company, Lafayette, IN) for three adults diagnosed with stroke who participated in 1.5 hours of yoga 2 times per week for 12 weeks. Another study (Bastille & Gill-Body, 2004)

Table 12.2 Addressing P–CIMT Goals During Yoga Therapy

EXAMPLE THERAPEUTIC GOAL	WAYS TO ADDRESS THROUGH YOGA THERAPY	EXAMPLE POSES OR ACTIVITY
Improved weight bearing of involved UE during floor transfers	• Yoga asanas in quadruped and prone prop • Transitions between floor and standing poses	• Cat, cow • Cobra (upward-facing dog) • Downward-facing dog
Improved shoulder elevation and AROM to reach into kitchen cupboard with involved UE	• Yoga asanas with shoulders flexed or abducted	• Warrior 1 and 2 • Sun salutation • Prone trunk extension with shoulder flexion
Improved grip strength to maintain grasp on lunch tray with bilateral UEs	• Yoga mudras (hand positions) with hands to midline in wrist extension • Weight bearing in wrist extension	• *Anjali* mudra (prayer position at midline)
Improved body awareness to maintain involved UE on tabletop during activities	• Copying of body positions • Activities for relaxation	• Progressive muscle relaxation • Deep breathing
Decreased tone in involved UE to tolerate resting hand splint overnight	• Activities for relaxation	• Deep breathing • Progressive muscle relaxation

Note. AROM = active range of motion; P–CIMT = pediatric constraint-induced movement therapy; UE = upper extremity.

Case Example

Case Example 12.3

USE OF YOGA AS AN ADJUNCT TO P–CIMT

Grayson was a 6-year-old boy with right hemiplegia secondary to a neonatal stroke. His mother reported that he had difficulty picking up toys with his right UE and had trouble stabilizing his paper on a tabletop. He also was unable to get up off the floor if he was holding something in his left hand.

Grayson was enrolled in a 23-day P–CIMT camp with 3 other children. On initial evaluation, the practitioner found that he had decreased ability to bear weight through his involved UE; weakness in his wrist, finger, and elbow extensors; and increased tone in his involved UE flexors.

During the P–CIMT camp, Grayson and the other campers completed 30 minutes per day of yoga therapy. Yoga sessions started with asanas with a focus on body awareness, UE weight bearing, and strengthening. During the yoga sessions, campers played games such as pretending to walk like different animals, moving fast and slow through asanas, and copying

positions done by their peers. Initially, the campers needed verbal and visual cues to complete the activities without bumping into each other, but with time the practitioner was able to fade these cues. At the end of each session, the practitioner cued campers to complete breathing exercises, and then the children lay in supine position for guided muscle relaxation. At first it was difficult for the campers to lie still without talking, so the practitioner used props such as eye bags and quiet music to help the campers learn to keep their bodies still during the relaxation phase.

Following the P–CIMT camp with daily yoga therapy, Grayson demonstrated improvements in all of his goals. His mother also noted that he was having an easier time getting to sleep at night and was able to pay attention to tasks for longer periods. He continued to participate in a yoga program at home with a DVD.

Table 12.3 THERAPEUTIC PROPERTIES OF WATER

PROPERTY	THERAPEUTIC BENEFIT
Buoyancy	Water assists in supporting the client's weight.
Viscosity	Water can be used to provide resistance to movement because water has more viscosity than air.
Hydrostatic pressure	Pressure of the water on the body at rest when submerged can improve sensory awareness and joint position sense.
Water temperature	Warm water can assist in decreasing muscle tone.

found that some adults with hemiparesis demonstrated improvements in performance on the Berg Balance Scale (Berg, Wood-Dauphinee, & Williams, 1995; Berg, Wood-Dauphinee, Williams, & Maki, 1992), Timed Movement Battery (Creel, Light, & Thigpen, 2001), and Stroke Impact Scale (Duncan et al., 2003) after completion of an 8-week yoga program, but these results were not observed with all participants. Although these studies provide early indications that yoga may be beneficial for children with hemiplegia, more rigorously designed studies with randomized controlled trials are needed to better understand the outcomes of yoga intervention.

AQUATIC THERAPY

Aquatic therapy is the scientific practice of physical or occupational therapy in an aquatic environment by trained practitioners. This therapy addresses treatment, rehabilitation, prevention, health, wellness, and fitness in an aquatic environment. The unique properties of the aquatic environment (Table 12.3) enhance treatments for clients across the age span with musculoskeletal, neuromuscular, cardiovascular or pulmonary, and integumentary diseases, disorders, or conditions (Aquatic Physical Therapy Section, n.d.). The specific properties of water provide an environment that may be helpful in addressing the strength and mobility limitations associated with hemiplegic CP (Ondrack & Thorpe, 2007).

Although water may be an ideal environment for therapy for children with CP, limited research supports the benefit of this intervention. In a review of available evidence on the use of aquatic therapy for children with CP, Kelly and Darrah (2005) concluded that further evidence was needed to determine its effectiveness for these children. In 2011, Gorter and Currie reviewed the evidence since the 2005 review and concluded that it remained limited. Studies included in both reviews had methodological flaws, including lack of control groups and randomization of participants. No studies have evaluated the effects of aquatic therapy specifically for children with hemiplegia, although these children were included in the intervention groups of some of the studies.

Despite the limited evidence for the effectiveness of aquatic therapy for children with hemiplegia, practitioners can use water as a tool to address the goals of these children. For some children, the aquatic environment may be more motivating or interesting than land for participating in therapy. Suggested ways to use the pool to address the goals of children in P–CIMT programs are summarized in Table 12.4, and Case Example 12.4 describes the use of aquatic therapy for a girl with hemiplegia.

Table 12.4 ADDRESSING P–CIMT GOALS DURING AQUATIC THERAPY

EXAMPLE THERAPEUTIC GOAL	WAYS TO ADDRESS THROUGH AQUATIC THERAPY	EXAMPLE ACTIVITY
Improved ability to reach across midline to doff sock on unaffected side	• Use buoyancy of water to support affected UE while reaching	• Use affected UE to reach across water surface for floating toys
Improved shoulder extension strength to pull to stand at a surface	• Use water to resist shoulder extension • Use water buoyancy to support movement of sit to stand	• Push beach ball underwater • Sit to stand with UE support on side of pool
Improved body awareness to maintain involved UE on tabletop during activities	• Use hydrostatic pressure of water on submerged UE to improve joint position sense	• Reach toward submerged toys • Move UE through water at variable speeds
Decrease involved UE tone to tolerate PROM	• Use warmth of water to relax muscle tone	• Submerge involved UE for swim strokes before stretching

Note. P–CIMT = pediatric constraint-induced movement therapy; PROM = passive range of motion; UE = upper extremity.

Case Example

USE OF AQUATIC THERAPY AS AN ADJUNCT TO P–CIMT

Gemma was an 8-year-old girl with right hemiplegic CP secondary to interventricular hemorrhage. Her parents reported that she had more tone and tightness in her involved arm than she used to, and she was having trouble using both hands to carry her lunch tray at school. Gemma loved to play in her family's backyard pool in the summer, but she tended to keep her involved arm out of the water and walked around the pool instead of swimming.

Gemma was enrolled in a modified P–CIMT protocol in which her involved UE was casted for 3 1-hour sessions per week for 8 weeks. In addition, her practitioner decided to complete 1 session per week in the pool. A removable waterproof cast was fabricated for Gemma to use for aquatic therapy sessions.

Gemma practiced carrying toys across the pool on a floating kickboard and reaching for toys floating on the water surface. She also worked on swimming with a float supporting her trunk. As she got stronger, her practitioner removed the support of the float and encouraged her to swim on her own for longer and longer distances.

Gemma's parents noted that her involved UE was more relaxed after her pool sessions, and she was starting to swim more often than she walked in the pool. At her discharge evaluation, she showed improved ability to carry her lunch tray without spilling. Her practitioner suggested pool activities in Gemma's home exercise program so that her parents could continue to use their home pool to strengthen their daughter's arm in a fun and motivating way.

THERAPEUTIC USE OF REHABILITATION ROBOTICS, VIRTUAL REALITY, AND GAMING SYSTEMS

Mainstream technology is advancing at a rapid pace. As a result, technological applications are increasingly being used in clinical settings to enhance rehabilitation outcomes. Current technologies can be broadly categorized into three types: (1) rehabilitation robotics, (2) virtual reality, and (3) gaming technology (see Table 12.1).

Rehabilitation robotics is the use of robotic devices to restore or improve function in a person with a disability. Robotics can be used as part of a prosthetic, an assistive device for some functional task, or a therapeutic tool. Therapeutic robotics may help promote massed practice during a CIMT program. Because most devices allow progressively more challenging settings or game play, under a practitioner's supervision they can provide a level of challenge appropriately tailored to the child.

Virtual reality is the use of a simulated environment experienced through the senses of sight and sound that is controlled by a person's movement. **Gaming technology** includes commercially available videogame systems that can

be used in the clinical environment in ways that are integrated with a planned therapy.

REHABILITATION ROBOTICS

Robotic devices come in all shapes and sizes, ranging from large stationary devices with both gross and fine motor components to glove-based systems with small wireless sensors. Robotic therapy provides a means for repetitive practice of target movements, such as reaching in space (Fasoli et al., 2008) or grasp–release (Carmeli, Peleg, Bartur, Elbo, & Vatine, 2010). These devices typically use robotic arms, joysticks, or other controllers to measure the client's performance of the targeted movement (Figures 12.3, 12.4, and 12.5). Most robotic devices are connected to a computer so clients can receive feedback from the game graphics on a screen or monitor (Figure 12.6).

Early studies demonstrated that clients using robotic devices in therapy sessions are motivated by and make positive gains after intervention with both stationary (Fasoli et al., 2008; Frascarelli et al., 2009) and glove-based devices (Carmeli et al., 2010). Fasoli and colleagues (2008) reported on use of the InMotion 2 robot (Interactive Motion Technologies, Watertown, MA) with 12 children with hemiplegia resulting from CP or acquired brain injury aged 4 to 12 years. Intervention

(A) ARMEO® POWER ROBOTIC ARM EXOSKELETON. (B) ARMEO® SPRING EXOSKELETON WITH INTEGRATED SPRING MECHANISM. (C) ARMEO® BOOM.

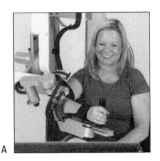 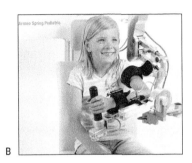 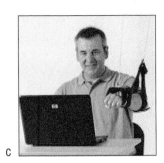

Source. Hocoma Ag, Volketswil, Switzerland.

consisted of 2 1-hour sessions per week for 8 consecutive weeks. During each session, the child completed 640 repetitive, goal-directed reaching movements in a planar field with his or her affected UE. Participants continued to receive established therapies in the community. The Fugl-Meyer Assessment (Fugl-Meyer et al., 1975) upper-limb subtest; the Quality of Upper Extremity Skills Test (QUEST; DeMatteo et al., 1992), an isometric elbow strength test; and the Modified Ashworth Scale (MAS; Bohannon & Smith, 1987) were administered during two baseline evaluations, after 4 weeks of intervention, after 8 weeks of intervention (at discharge from the robotic training), and at 1 month posttreatment.

Statistically significant improvements and moderate to large effect sizes were reported on the QUEST and the Fugl-Meyer Assessment. The MAS and isometric elbow strength testing had statistically significant improvements but small to moderate effect sizes. The authors reported that robotic training had a positive effect on ROM and coordination of the upper limb and a slight effect on strength and spasticity. On questionnaires, parents reported that the quantity and

quality of spontaneous use of the participants' affected arm increased during the study and, although lower at 1 month follow-up, were still greater than pretreatment levels (Fasoli et al., 2008).

Frascarelli and colleagues (2009) conducted further research with the InMotion 2 robot with a shorter duration, higher weekly intervention dosage of 1 hour, 3 times per week for 6 weeks, with 12 children with hemiplegia aged 5 to 16 years. In addition to the Fugl-Meyer Assessment, the Melbourne Assessment of Unilateral Upper Limb Function (Randall et al., 1999), and the MAS, the authors reported use of robot-based assessments to track trajectories and target accuracy and fluidity of movement. This study also reported statistically significant changes and moderate-to-large effect sizes on standardized measures. Parent questionnaires also reported improved UE movement patterns and performance of activities of daily living. Statistically significant changes on the robot-based assessments for close and far reaching were reported, as well as improvements in the trajectory, speed, and level of jerk and coordination of movements from

HANDTUTOR™ BY MEDITOUCH.

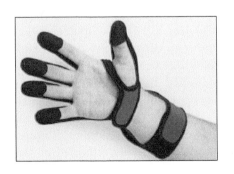 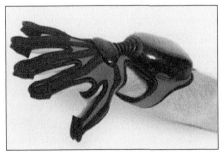 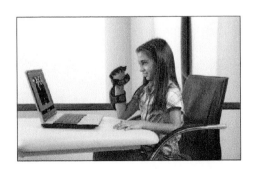

Source. Meditouch, Netanya, Israel.

Figure 12.5 3D TUTOR™ BY MEDITOUCH.

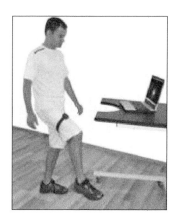
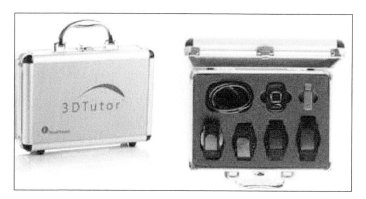

Source. Meditouch, Netanya, Israel.

the first to the last day of intervention. The authors reported secondary gains in postural and head control.

Further studies are needed on the long-term effects of robotics with children with CP. Studies with adults with chronic stroke using the InMotion 2 have reported sustained gains at testing 3 years after robotic training (Volpe et al., 1999).

Distal-based systems that promote repetitive practice of fine movements also are showing promising results. A recent parallel-group randomized controlled trial by Hwang, Seong, and Son (2012) with 17 adults at least 3 months post stroke reported positive effects using the Amadeo System (Tyromotion, Graz, Austria). During intervention, participants' individual fingers were connected to the device via a magnetic disc secured to each finger with tape. Movements at the elbow and shoulder were restricted with strapping to ensure that the device captured distal

movement only. The movement of the fingers was projected on a screen. The device was calibrated for each participant and helped them achieve their full PROM after they attempted movement.

Participants were randomized into full intervention, consisting of 20 sessions of robot-assisted movement over 4 weeks, or half-intervention, which consisted of 10 sessions over 2 weeks of passive therapy followed by 10 sessions over the next 2 weeks of active, robot-assisted intervention. A battery of assessments was performed at baseline and at 2-week intervals after training was initiated (Weeks 2, 4, and 8). The battery included the wrist and hand portion of the Fugl-Meyer Assessment, the Jebsen–Taylor Hand Function Test (Taylor, Sand, & Jebsen, 1973), the Nine-Hole Peg Test (Mathiowetz, Weber, Kashman, & Volland, 1985), a hand motor subscale of the Stroke Impact Scale, grip and pinch testing, and ROM of the metacarpophalangeal joints. Statistically

Figure 12.6 SCREEN SHOTS OF A HANDTUTOR™ GAME. (A) REHABILITATION EXERCISE INVOLVING TRACKING A TARGET AND (B) EVALUATION SOFTWARE SETTINGS AND FEEDBACK.

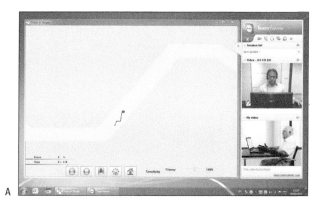
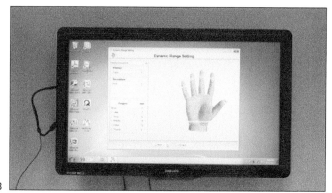

A   B

Source. Meditouch, Netanya, Israel, and Kennedy Krieger Institute, Baltimore.

significant improvements were noted for both groups on all the fine motor tests, the Fugl-Meyer Assessment, and the Jebsen–Taylor test, with the full-intervention group demonstrating a greater level of improvement than the half-intervention group. Results on the Stroke Impact Scale were not reported. The researchers concluded that "four-week rehabilitation using a novel robot that provides individual finger synchronization resulted in a dose-dependent improvement in hand function in subacute to chronic stroke patients" (Hwang et al., 2012, p. 700).

To our knowledge, no reports have been published of studies combining robotics with P–CIMT, although one can imagine a variety of interesting ways to combine these approaches. Robotics also could be used to achieve some of the intensity that otherwise may seem impossible or not reimbursable for the signature forms of P–CIMT by using robotics when active therapy (shaping and massed practice) from a clinician is not provided.

VIRTUAL REALITY

In a therapeutic environment, use of virtual reality could be combined with robotics. A few single-case studies have reported promising results from use of virtual reality to target reaching and gross motor skills in children with CP.

A few smaller studies have discussed rehabilitation using virtual environments for children with CP. Three studies used three-dimensional video-capture systems to address gross motor and reaching movements in children with CP (Chen et al., 2007; Reid, 2002; You et al., 2005). All studies indicated that participants demonstrated carryover of skills to real-world use, and one study reported significant changes in cortical activation via functional magnetic resonance imaging (You et al., 2005).

A study by Fluet and colleagues (2010) reported use of virtual reality combined with a robotic device in a pediatric setting with training 1 hour a day, 3 days a week for 3 weeks. Three intervention groups were compared, including one group using device training without postural restraint, a second group using device training while secured with a chest strap to a specialized chair, and a third group using device training without chest strapping with an additional 5 hours of CIMT and intensive bimanual training. Participants in the CIMT group wore a lightweight cast on their unaffected extremity daily for 6 hours except during the 30- or 60-minute virtual reality sessions. Although all three groups showed significant changes, the CIMT group made the largest gains in pinch and grip strength, most likely because of the fine motor training provided during CIMT.

A study by Brien and Sveistrup (2011) assessed mobility and balance of 4 adolescent boys before and after participating in a virtual reality–based intervention. The participants had diplegic CP or choreoathetosis. The study was a single-subject, multiple-baseline design using the following outcomes: Community Balance and Mobility Scale (Howe, Inness, Venturini, Williams, & Verrier, 2006), the 6-Minute Walk Test (Butland, Pang, Gross, Woodcock, & Geddes, 1982), the Timed Up and Down Stairs (Zaino, Marchese, & Westcott, 2004), and the Gross Motor Function Measure Dimension E (Russell et al., 1989). Intervention consisted of 5 consecutive days of 90-minute virtual reality sessions. The authors reported statistically significant improvements in all adolescents' performance on the Community Balance and Mobility Scale and the 6-Minute Walk Test.

GAMING TECHNOLOGY

In recent years, gaming devices that require gross motor activity to successfully operate have become commercially available and are quickly being incorporated into clinical rehabilitation programs. Research on the use of these devices in rehabilitation is limited to small case reports. Deutsch, Borbely, Filler, Huhn, and Guarrera-Bowlby (2008) reported positive changes in mobility, postural control, and visual perception in an adolescent with spastic diplegia after using the Nintendo Wii™ for 11 sessions. Figure 12.7 shows how the Wii remote can be adapted for use in rehabilitation.

A study with 8 adults with bilateral spastic CP at Gross Motor Functional Classification Scale Level I or II (Palisano et al., 1997) reported that playing Wii Sports provided moderate-

Figure 12.7 ADAPTIVE CUFF AND GRIP ADAPTATION USING SELF-ADHERENT WRAP ON THE NINTENDO WII™ REMOTE.

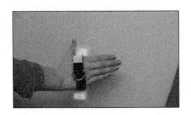 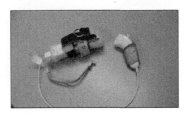 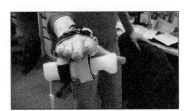

Source. Kennedy Krieger Institute, Baltimore.

intensity exercise (Hurkmans, van den Berg-Emons, & Stam, 2010). Intervention consisted of 2 15-minute sessions of either Wii tennis or Wii boxing played while standing. The participants chose the order of play and were allowed a 10-minute rest break between games to return their heart rate to baseline. Gas exchange before and after intervention was measured to calculate oxygen uptake and energy expenditure expressed in metabolic equivalent of task (MET). During game play, the participants achieved MET levels ranging from 3 METs (moderate intensity activity) to 6 METs (vigorous intensity activity).

Another study examined use of the EyeToy, a digital camera for the PlayStation 2 (Sony, New York), with children with CP and reported up to a 13% increase in UE function on standardized measures in the intervention group compared with a 1% to 2% increase in the control group (Jannink et al., 2008). The control group maintained their regular physical therapy program, whereas the intervention group used an EyeToy game as part of their physical therapy. Each group had the same duration and intensity of intervention—30 minutes, 2 times per week for 6 weeks. A study by Sandlund, Waterworth, and Häger (2011) using the EyeToy reported success on standardized measures and physical activity monitors using a home-based intervention of 4 weeks. The authors also reported a high level of motivation by participants to complete the intervention. This study reported qualitatively that children felt motivated and satisfied during intervention sessions.

Wade and Porter (2012) reported similar positive feedback from family members in their study of 13 pediatric participants who used a pressure detection pad to control games with postural movements. One participant reported that the device allowed him more opportunities to play with his father, and others reported improved ability to participate in classroom activities with peers.

Use of gaming devices should be viewed with caution. Supervision by a practitioner trained in the principles of P–CIMT is necessary to carefully monitor for compensatory movement patterns and adapt the task to best fit the client's needs. A study with typically developing boys measured energy expenditure while playing active video games and found that game play should not replace traditional fitness routines and recommendations (White, Schofield, & Kilding, 2011). Although energy expenditure rates may not be the same for clients with CP (Hurkmans et al., 2010), further studies with new game systems and persons with hemiplegia are needed to understand the potential value added by gaming technology.

When choosing a device or gaming system to use with a child, a practitioner should consider multiple factors. The age and cognitive ability of the child determine his or her capacity to follow directions and play the games associated with the device. The size of the child's arm and hand may prohibit use of a robotic device that was created for adult use. Baseline level of motor function should determine the level of additional support or adaptations a device may require for the participant to hold the device. Visual–perceptual capacities may pose a challenge or add additional frustration to game play. Games with high contrast or solid backgrounds may be easier for the child at first. During intervention, practitioners should monitor for compensatory movements that could cause repetitive use injuries, and rest should be provided at intervals. Monitoring muscle fatigue and providing the appropriate challenge based on the child's occupational performance are the responsibility of the practitioner.

AREAS FOR FUTURE RESEARCH

Robotics, virtual reality, and commercially available gaming systems may be effective complements to P–CIMT because they can provide motivation and additional opportunities for massed practice. Future research should examine the use of these technologies in conjunction with P–CIMT programs, including an appraisal of which systems best complement a P–CIMT program and what candidates are best suited for this combination of therapy approaches. One of the greatest challenges in using commercially available gaming systems such as the Wii in P–CIMT programs is the complexity of the children's games. Children using their weaker, affected UE may demonstrate slow response or frequent inaccuracy in movement patterns, leading to errors and failure that may increase frustration and lead to refusal to participate in massed practice. Clients who have active seizures or shunts may be contraindicated for some gaming and virtual reality systems, and use of gaming systems should be discussed with the child's physician.

BOTULINUM TOXIN THERAPY

Botulinum toxin therapy involves the intramuscular injection of botulinum toxin, a naturally occurring neurotoxin produced by *Clostridium botulinum* bacteria, to achieve localized reduction of spasticity. Table 12.1 summarizes the considerations in using botulinum toxin therapy as an adjunct to P–CIMT.

As noted in a review by Barnes (2003), several serotypes are known that target various components of the SNARE protein complex, which plays an important role in the nerve–muscle signaling that occurs at the neuromuscular junction. Vesicles within a nerve terminal filled with acetylcholine, a neurotransmitter, must fuse with the cell wall to release their contents into the synaptic cleft before binding to a receptor site on muscle to enable muscle contraction. Because the SNARE protein complex is needed for vesicular fusion, disruption of this complex by botulinum toxin ultimately inhibits muscle contraction and weakens the muscle.

In the 1980s, a purified form of botulinum toxin type A, now known as *onabotulinumtoxinA*, was approved by the U.S. Food and Drug Administration (FDA) for the treatment of blepharospasm and strabismus. Subsequently, it was approved for the treatment of cervical dystonia and, in 2010, for the treatment of spasticity in the flexor muscles of the elbow, wrist, and fingers in adults. Other formulations of botulinum toxin type A have been approved by the FDA, including abobotulinumtoxinA for the treatment of cervical dystonia and incobotulinumtoxinA for the treatment of blepharospasm and cervical dystonia. Risks are associated with administration of botulinum toxin, and since 2009, the FDA has required a boxed warning on all botulinum toxin products sold in the United States "to highlight that botulinum toxin may spread from the area of injection to produce symptoms consistent with botulism" (FDA, 2009).

This therapy has been shown to reduce spasticity, but the direct effects of the toxin are no longer seen after 2 to 4 months. Repeat doses of botulinum toxin typically are given no more frequently than every 3 months. Antibody formation could limit the effectiveness of future botulinum toxin injections if given to the same person more frequently than this recommended time frame.

Although no formulation of a purified botulinum toxin has been approved by the FDA for the treatment of spasticity in children or for the treatment of lower extremity spasticity, botulinum toxin injections have been used off-label for this purpose. In 2010, the Quality Standards Subcommittee of the American Academy of Neurology and the Practice Committee of the Child Neurology Society (Delgado et al., 2010) published a practice parameter on the pharmacological treatment of spasticity in children and adolescents with CP that assessed 148 studies, 20 of which were randomized controlled trials. Many of the studies assessed only the lower extremity. Specific adverse events, all transient and not requiring hospitalization, were reported in 17 studies. A decision to use botulinum toxin injections in children should be made after careful consideration by the client's physician; the authors cautioned that "severe generalized weakness may occur" but concluded that "for localized/segmental spasticity that warrants treatment, botulinum toxin type A should be offered as an effective and generally safe treatment" (Delgado et al., 2010, p. 338). Case Example 12.5 describes the use of botulinum toxin therapy in a 10-year-old boy with right hemiplegia that enabled the therapeutic use of a gaming system.

A few studies have investigated the use of botulinum toxin injection as an adjunct to CIMT. As was the case with the early CIMT literature, the earliest studies mentioning use of the two treatments together involved adults with stroke. In 2003, Page, Elovic, Levine, and Sisto reported the case of a 44-year-old man who had sustained a stroke and who undertook an mCIMT consisting of "half hour, structured activity sessions three times a week for 10 [weeks] with restraint of the affected hand and arm 5 days [per week] during 5 [hour] periods" (p. 78). They found positive changes in the Fugl-Meyer Assessment score and the ARAT (Lyle, 1981) score (statistical measures for significance were not reported) after the constraint program. OnabotulinumtoxinA was administered to the flexor digitorum superficialis, flexor pollicis longus, and pronator teres 2 weeks after termination of constraint, and the client's finger extension and grasp improved, resulting in further increases in his Fugl-Meyer and ARAT scores 4 weeks after botulinum toxin injection. His spasticity returned to baseline after 4 months, but "he subsequently had repeat injections with similar results" (Page et al., 2003, p. 79).

Sun and colleagues (2006) reported the case of a 52-year-old man who was recovering from a stroke and who did not initially meet inclusion criteria for a CIMT program because "he had only approximately 8 degrees of active wrist extension and minimal finger extension of less than 10 degrees" (p. 1389). He subsequently underwent injection of abobotulinumtoxinA to the biceps, flexor digitorum superficialis, flexor digitorum profundus, flexor carpi radialis, and flexor carpi ulnaris. He then "received a 4-week mCIMT program consisting of 2 hours of training each day 3 times weekly" (Sun et al., 2006, p. 1391). Comparing baseline with posttreatment testing, he showed gains in scores on the Motor Activity Log, Wolf Motor Function Test, ARAT, and Fugl-Meyer Assessment. At a follow-up evaluation 3 months later, he showed a decline in Motor Activity Log and Fugl-Meyer scores, but at 6 months, he again showed gains in scores for all assessments when compared with baseline. Statistical measures for significance were not reported, but the authors noted that the patient "reported making much progress in the functional use of the involved upper extremity" (Sun et al., 2006, p. 1393).

Levy and colleagues (2007) investigated whether the use of botulinum toxin type A combined with exercise therapy would allow people who had experienced a stroke but who did not meet the minimum motor criteria of 10° of volitional wrist extension, digit extension, and thumb abduction to attain these criteria and participate in a CIMT program consisting of constraint therapy 6 hours a day, 5 days per week for 2 weeks. Four of 12 participants were able to achieve the criteria, a finding that was statistically significant. In addition, the ability to extend three digits against gravity before botulinum toxin injection was found to be predictive of the ability to meet the minimal motor criteria. The participants who were able to meet the criteria and participate in CIMT initially showed modest improvement in scores on the Wolf Motor Function Test, Motor Activity Log, and Box and Blocks Test, but these gains regressed to near baseline values by 24 weeks after injection.

In 2010, Sun and colleagues conducted a randomized controlled trial comparing abobotulinumtoxinA injection

Case Example

USE OF BOTULINUM TOXIN THERAPY AND A GAMING SYSTEM AS ADJUNCTS TO P–CIMT

Mitchell was a 10-year-old boy with right hemiplegia as a result of an acquired brain injury during infancy. He had considerably increased tone in his right bicep. At rest, he maintained his right arm in approximately 60° of flexion, wrist in slight flexion, and hand fisted. His outpatient occupational therapy practitioner had applied splinting, heat, myofascial release, and passive stretching to his right bicep with little success. His mother was concerned about skin irritation and breakdown in his antecubital region.

Mitchell tolerated a neoprene resting hand splint at night and a wrist cock-up splint during the day. He could actively move into 100° of elbow extension, and with effort he could be passively ranged to 175°. He was at high risk for developing a contracture at his elbow. He used the tone in his hand functionally to maintain grasp on containers while opening them with his left hand.

The occupational therapy practitioner consulted with Mitchell's physiatrist and discussed administering therapeutic botulinum toxin injections to his bicep paired with serial casting to gain range before starting an mCIMT program. The physiatrist and occupational therapy practitioner agreed that at this time, therapeutic botulinum toxin injections should not be done to any of his hand muscles because they might limit his functional abilities.

After botulinum toxin injections to his biceps and 3 rounds of serial casts, Mitchell was able to extend his arm actively to 100° and passively could be ranged to 175° with minimal effort.

A 4-week CIMT program with 3 hours of daily therapy was trialed over the summer. His occupational therapy practitioner focused on use of robotic devices that required him to reach toward a target when activating games on a laptop. Other activities included playing games on a touch-screen tablet. The games were motivating to Mitchell because, despite his fisted hand, he could still activate the games easily. The practitioner modified the task to increase the challenge by positioning devices farther away and in various planes to encourage greater AROM of his right arm.

Using a universal cuff on the Wii remote, Mitchell played games that required him to shake the remote, thus flexing and extending his elbow at a high rate of repetition. He also enjoyed playing Xbox Kinect games that required him to reach to targets to pop bubbles and collect coins. He played a driving simulation game that required him to reach toward the TV with sustained shoulder flexion. He liked the reward of earning points and winning games. Because he and his brother had an Xbox at home, Mitchell also got in some extra practice after therapy sessions and on the weekends. He enjoyed being able do something fun with his older brother, and Mitchell's mother was happy to see him engaged in age-appropriate peer play when his friends came over.

At the conclusion of the CIMT program, Mitchell gained an additional 60° of AROM in his right elbow. He continued to use the Xbox Kinect as a home exercise program.

plus a CIMT program to abobotulinumtoxinA injection plus a conventional therapy program for adults. The CIMT program consisted of 2 hours of training a day for 3 days a week and restraint of the unaffected UE for at least 5 hours a day for 3 months. The conventional therapy program consisted of 1 hour of physical therapy and 1 hour of occupational therapy (using a neurodevelopmental approach) 3 times a week for 3 months. Twenty-nine participants who met minimum motor criteria at baseline completed the study, and outcome scores for the Modified Ashworth Scale, the Motor Activity Log, and the ARAT were compared. All participants showed improved (decreased) spasticity, and participants in the group receiving the CIMT showed significantly more improvement in Motor Activity Log and ARAT scores at 3 months and 6 months post injection.

Literature addressing the use of therapeutic botulinum toxin in conjunction with P–CIMT is sparse. Park, Rha, Lee, Yoo, and Chang (2009) prospectively studied children with spastic hemiplegic CP who received either onabotulinumtoxinA plus traditional therapy provided in an inpatient hospital setting or onabotulinumtoxinA plus a mCIMT regimen. The mCIMT regimen consisted of immobilization of the unaffected limb with an orthosis during waking hours for 3 weeks, with 1 day off per week, and physical and occupational therapy consisting of play-based activities based on motor learning principles for 1 hour a day during their 3-week hospital stay. Further information regarding the amount of time the constraint was applied was not provided. The groups were compared on the Modified Ashworth Scale score, Tardieu Scale score (Numanoğlu & Günel, 2012), Upper Limb Physician's Rating Scale (ULPRS) score (Park, Sim, & Rha, 2011), and Pediatric Motor Activity Log score (revised as described by Wallen, Bundy, Pont, & Ziviani, 2009). Both groups showed improvement in Modified Ashworth Scale, Tardieu, and ULPRS scores 3 weeks after the intervention, but no significant differences were found between the groups on these measures. The group receiving the onabotulinumtoxinA plus the mCIMT regimen, however, showed statistically significant improvement on the How Often and How Well scales of the Pediatric Motor Activity Log, whereas the group receiving onabotulinumtoxinA plus traditional therapy did not.

Eliasson, Shaw, Pontén, Boyd, and Krumlinde-Sundholm (2009) prospectively studied children with spastic hemiplegic CP who participated in an mCIMT program provided in a day camp setting. Constraint therapy was provided for 7 hours a day over a 9-day period. Five of the 16 children who participated received onabotulinumtoxinA before starting the camp. Because of the small sample size, parametric statistical tests between the two groups were impossible, but individual results were reported. Measures included the Melbourne Assessment of Unilateral Upper Limb Function (which assesses changes in the quality of movement); the Jebsen–Taylor Hand Function Test; the Assisting Hand Assessment (Krumlinde-Sundholm, Holmefur, Kottorp, & Eliasson, 2007); grip strength; two-point discrimination; and several trained tasks, including block stacking, disc golf score, and a pen shift task. The authors noted that "the only measure in which a trend was seen that could be related to effects from [botulinum toxin type A] was the Melbourne Assessment" (Eliasson et al., 2009, p. 329)—all 5 children who had received the onabotulinumtoxinA plus the mCIMT regimen showed an initial improvement on this measure, whereas children who received only the mCIMT regimen without onabotulinumtoxinA did not. However, this improvement did not persist at the follow-up assessment 6 months later. The authors acknowledged that not every child will show improvement in hand function after a constraint program but noted that the day camp model "may provide social and personal benefits for participants such as meeting new friends and learning a lot about themselves and their disability" (Eliasson et al., 2009, p. 323).

Research into the use of therapeutic botulinum toxin injections as an adjunct to mCIMT in the pediatric population is ongoing. Hoare and colleagues (2010) described methods for a randomized controlled trial of children with spastic hemiplegic CP. The trial aimed to compare a group receiving onabotulinumtoxinA followed by a mCIMT regimen with a group receiving onabotulinumtoxinA followed by a bimanual occupational therapy program. The mCIMT regimen consisted of wearing a neoprene glove on the nonaffected hand for 3 hours per day, 7 days a week. The primary outcome measure chosen was the Assisting Hand Assessment; other

outcome measures included the Modified Ashworth Scale, modified Tardieu Scale, QUEST Movement and Grasps subscales, the Canadian Occupational Performance Measure (Law et al., 2005), Goal Attainment Scaling (Kiresuk, Smith, & Cardillo, 1994), Pediatric Evaluation of Disability Inventory (Haley et al., 1992), and Pediatric Motor Activity Log. At the time of this writing, results had not yet been published.

Limitations to current studies combining use of onabotulinumtoxinA with P–CIMT include variability in the amount or dosage of onabotulinumtoxinA used based on the experience of the physician providing the intervention and on the presentation of the affected extremity. It has not been determined which upper-body muscle group (i.e., elbow flexor, wrist flexor, thumb adductor) may demonstrate the best functional outcomes after onabotulinumtoxinA injection. Future studies should define inclusion criteria to help determine which children would most benefit from onabotulinumtoxinA before participation in a P–CIMT program.

SUMMARY

This chapter provides a partial list of promising therapies and techniques that could be combined with P–CIMT for some children to increase initial performance levels, promote engagement in P–CIMT during treatment, or expand P–CIMT goals into other times and places, including the post-P–CIMT phase, during which maintenance and extension of benefits are important. The adjunctive therapies and approaches identified range from those that exert a direct effect on neuromuscular activity to those that could be considered motivating, engaging, and expanding.

When practitioners implement combined therapies, they should collect data from baseline and posttreatment assessments and on the child's and family's responses to these combinations to help advance the knowledge base. Because children with unilateral CP often are engaged in continuous efforts to increase their skills and functional levels of engagement, a more systematic knowledge base about sequential treatments and combined and coordinated therapies could be highly valuable.

REFERENCES

American Occupational Therapy Association. (2012). Physical agent modalities. *American Journal of Occupational Therapy, 66*(6 Suppl.), S78–S80. http://dx.doi.org/10.5014/ajot.2012.66S78

Aquatic Physical Therapy Section. (n.d.). *About aquatic physical therapy.* Retrieved from http://www.aquaticpt.org/about-aquatic-physical-therapy.cfm

Barnes, M. (2003, May). Botulinum toxin—Mechanisms of action and clinical use in spasticity. *Journal of Rehabilitation Medicine,* pp. 56–59.

Barnes, P. M., Bloom, B., & Nahin, R. L. (2008). Complementary and alternative medicine use among adults and children: United States, 2007. *National Health Statistics Reports, 10*(12), 1–23.

Bastille, J. V., & Gill-Body, K. M. (2004). A yoga-based exercise program for people with chronic poststroke hemiparesis. *Physical Therapy, 84,* 33–48.

Berg, K., Wood-Dauphinee, S., & Williams, J. I. (1995). The Balance Scale: Reliability assessment with elderly residents and patients with an acute stroke. *Scandinavian Journal of Rehabilitation Medicine, 27,* 27–36.

Berg, K. O., Wood-Dauphinee, S. L., Williams, J. I., & Maki, B. (1992). Measuring balance in the elderly: Validation of an instrument. *Canadian Journal of Public Health, 83*(Suppl. 2), S7–S11.

Bohannon, R. W., & Smith, M. B. (1987). Inter-rater reliability of a Modified Ashworth Scale of muscle spasticity. *Physical Therapy, 2,* 206–208.

Brien, M., & Sveistrup, H. (2011). An intensive virtual reality program improves functional balance and mobility of adolescents with cerebral palsy. *Pediatric Physical Therapy, 23,* 258–266.

Butland, R. J., Pang, J., Gross, E. R., Woodcock, A. A., & Geddes, D. M. (1982). Two-, six-, and 12-minute walking tests in respiratory disease. *British Medical Journal (Clinical Research Edition), 284,* 1607–1608.

Carmeli, E., Peleg, S., Bartur, G., Elbo, E., & Vatine, J.-J. (2010). HandTutor™ enhanced hand rehabilitation after stroke: A pilot study. *Physiotherapy Research International, 16,* 191–200.

Carroll, D. (1965). A quantitative test of upper extremity function. *Journal of Chronic Diseases, 18,* 479–491.

Chen, Y. P., Kang, L. J., Chuang, T. Y., Doong, J. L., Lee, S. J., Tsai, M. W., . . . Sung, W. H. (2007). Use of virtual reality to improve upper-extremity control in children with cerebral palsy: A single-subject design. *Physical Therapy, 87,* 1441–1457.

Creel, G. L., Light, K. E., & Thigpen, M. T. (2001). Concurrent and construct validity of scores on the Timed Movement Battery. *Physical Therapy, 81,* 789–798.

Dash, M., & Telles, S. (1999). Yoga training and motor speed based on a finger tapping task. *Indian Journal of Physiology and Pharmacology, 43,* 458–462.

Dash, M., & Telles, S. (2001). Improvement in hand grip strength in normal volunteers and rheumatoid arthritis patients following yoga training. *Indian Journal of Physiology and Pharmacology, 45,* 355–360.

Delgado, M. R., Hirtz, D., Aisen, M., Ashwal, S., Fehlings, D. L., McLaughlin, J., . . . Vargus-Adams, J.; Quality Standards Subcommittee of the American Academy of Neurology and the Practice Committee of the Child Neurology Society. (2010). Practice parameter: Pharmacologic treatment of spasticity in children and adolescents with cerebral palsy (an evidence-based review): Report of the Quality Standards Subcommittee of the American Academy of Neurology and the Practice Committee of the Child Neurology Society. *Neurology, 74,* 336–343.

DeMatteo, C., Law, M., Russell, D., Pollock, N., Rosenbaum, P., & Walter, S. (1992). *QUEST: Quality of Upper Extremity Skills Test manual.* Hamilton, Ontario: Neurodevelopmental Research Unit, Chedoke Campus, Chedoke-McMasters Hospital.

Deutsch, J. E., Borbely, M., Filler, J., Huhn, K., & Guarrera-Bowlby, P. (2008). Use of a low-cost, commercially available gaming console (Wii) for rehabilitation of an adolescent with cerebral palsy. *Physical Therapy, 88,* 1196–1207.

Duncan, P. W., Bode, R. K., Min Lai, S., Perera, S., & Glycine Antagonist in Neuroprotection Americas Investigators. (2003). Rasch analysis of a new stroke-specific outcome scale: The Stroke Impact Scale. *Archives of Physical Medicine and Rehabilitation, 84,* 950–963.

Eliasson, A. C., Shaw, K., Pontén, E., Boyd, R., & Krumlinde-Sundholm, L. (2009). Feasibility of a day-camp model of modified constraint-induced movement therapy with and without botulinum toxin A injection for children with hemiplegia. *Physical and Occupational Therapy in Pediatrics, 29,* 311–333.

Fasoli, S. E., Fragala-Pinkham, M., Hughes, R., Hogan, N., Krebs, H. I., & Stein, J. (2008). Upper limb robotic therapy for children with hemiplegia. *American Journal of Physical Medicine and Rehabilitation, 87,* 929–936.

Fluet, G., Qiu, Q., Kelly, D., Parikh, H., Ramirez, D., Saleh, S., & Adamovich, S. V. (2010). Interfacing a haptic robotic system with complex virtual environments to treat impaired upper extremity motor function in children with cerebral palsy. *Developmental Neurorehabilitation, 13,* 335–345.

Folio, M. R., & Fewell, R. R. (2000). *Peabody Developmental Motor Scales* (2nd ed.). Austin, TX: Pro-Ed.

Footer, C. (2006). The effects of therapeutic taping on gross motor function in children with cerebral palsy. *Pediatric Physical Therapy, 18,* 245–252.

Franki, I., Desloovere, K., De Cat, J., Feys, H., Molenaers, G., Calders, P., . . . Van Broeck, C. (2012). The evidence-base for conceptual approaches and additional therapies targeting lower limb function in children with cerebral palsy: A systematic review using the *ICF* as a framework. *Journal of Rehabilitation Medicine, 44,* 396–405.

Frascarelli, F., Masia, L., DiRosa, G., Cappa, P., Petrarca, M., Castelli, E., & Krebs, H. I. (2009). The impact of robotic rehabilitation in children with acquired or congenital movement disorders. *European Journal of Physical and Rehabilitation Medicine, 45,* 135–141.

Fritz, S. L., Chiu, Y. P., Malcolm, M. P., Patterson, T. S., & Light, K. E. (2005). Feasibility of electromyography-triggered neuromuscular stimulation as an adjunct to constraint-induced movement therapy. *Physical Therapy, 85,* 428–442.

Fugl-Meyer, A. R., Jääskö, L., Leyman, I., Olsson, S., & Steglind, S. (1975). The post-stroke hemiplegic patient: I. A method for evaluation of physical performance. *Scandinavian Journal of Rehabilitation Medicine, 7,* 13–31.

Galantino, M. L., Galbavy, R., & Quinn, L. (2008). Therapeutic effects of yoga for children: A systematic review of the literature. *Pediatric Physical Therapy, 20,* 66–80.

Gorter, J. W., & Currie, S. J. (2011). Aquatic exercise programs for children and adolescents with cerebral palsy: What do we know and where do we go? *International Journal of Pediatrics, 2011.* http://dx.doi.org/10.1155/2011/712165.

Haley, S. M., Coster, W. J., Ludlow, L. H., Haltiwanger, J. T., & Andrellos, P. J. (1992). *Pediatric Evaluation of Disability Inventory (PEDI): Development, standardization and administration manual.* Boston: New England Medical Center Hospitals, Inc., and PEDI Research Group.

Hoare, B. J., Wallen, M. A., Imms, C., Villanueva, E., Rawicki, H. B., & Carey, L. (2010). Botulinum toxin A as an adjunct to treatment in the management of the upper limb in children with spastic cerebral palsy (update). *Cochrane Database Systematic Review,* CD003469.

Howe, J. A., Inness, E. L., Venturini, A., Williams, J. I., & Verrier, M. C. (2006). The Community Balance and Mobility Scale—A balance measure for individuals with traumatic brain injury. *Clinical Rehabilitation, 20,* 885–895.

Hurkmans, H. L., van den Berg-Emons, R. J., & Stam, H. J. (2010). Energy expenditure with cerebral palsy playing Wii sports. *Archives of Physical Medicine and Rehabilitation, 91,* 1577–1581.

Hwang, C. H., Seong, J. W., & Son, D. S. (2012). Individual finger synchronized robot-assisted hand rehabilitation in subacute to chronic stroke: A prospective randomized clinical trial of efficacy. *Clinical Rehabilitation, 26,* 696–704.

Jannink, M. J., van der Wilden, G. J., Navis, D. W., Visser, G., Gussinklo, J., & Ijzerman, M. (2008). A low-cost video game applied for training of upper extremity function in children with cerebral palsy: A pilot study. *Cyberpsychology and Behavior, 11,* 27–32.

Kase, K. (2000). *Illustrated kinesio-taping* (3rd ed.). Albuquerque, NM: Ken'i Kai Information.

Kase, K., Martin, P., & Yasukawa, A. (2006). *Kinesio Taping® in pediatrics: Fundamentals and whole body taping.* Albuquerque, NM: Kinesio Taping Association.

Kelly, M., & Darrah, J. (2005). Aquatic exercise for children with cerebral palsy. *Developmental Medicine and Child Neurology, 47,* 838–842.

Kerr, C., McDowell, B., & McDonough, S. (2004). Electrical stimulation in cerebral palsy: A review of effects on strength and motor function. *Developmental Medicine and Child Neurology, 46,* 205–213.

Kiresuk, T., Smith, A., & Cardillo, J. (1994). *Goal Attainment Scaling: Applications, theory, and measurement.* Hillsdale, NJ: Erlbaum.

Krumlinde-Sundholm, L., Holmefur, M., Kottorp, A., & Eliasson, A. C. (2007). The Assisting Hand Assessment: Current evidence of validity, reliability, and responsiveness to change. *Developmental Medicine and Child Neurology, 49,* 259–264.

Law, M., Baptiste, S., Carswell, A., McColl, M., Polatajko, H., & Pollock, N. (2005). *Canadian Occupational Performance Measure* (3rd ed.). Ottawa: CAOT Publications ACE.

Levy, C. E., Giuffrida, C., Richards, L., Wu, S., Davis, S., & Nadeau, S. E. (2007). Botulinum toxin A, evidence-based exercise therapy, and constraint-induced movement therapy for upper-limb hemiparesis attributable to stroke: A preliminary study. *American Journal of Physical Medicine and Rehabilitation, 86,* 696–706.

Lyle, R. C. (1981). A performance test for assessment of upper limb function in physical rehabilitation treatment and research. *International Journal of Rehabilitation Research, 4,* 483–492.

Lynton, H., Kligler, B., & Shiflett, S. (2007). Yoga in stroke rehabilitation: A systematic review and results of a pilot study. *Topics in Stroke Rehabilitation, 14,* 1–8.

Mandanmohan, J., Jatiya, L., Udupa, K., & Bhavanani, A. B. (2003). Effect of yoga training on handgrip, respiratory pressures and pulmonary function. *Indian Journal of Physiology and Pharmacology, 47,* 387–392.

Mathiowetz, V., Volland, G., Kashman, N., & Weber, K. (1985). Adult norms for the Box and Block Test of manual dexterity. *American Journal of Occupational Therapy, 39,* 386–391. http://dx.doi.org/10.5014/ajot.39.6.386

Mathiowetz, V., Weber, K., Kashman, N., & Volland, G. (1985). Adult norms for the Nine Hole Peg Test of finger dexterity. *Occupational Therapy Journal of Research, 5,* 24–33.

National Center for Complementary and Alternative Medicine. (2008). *What is complementary and alternative medicine?* Retrieved July 31, 2012, from http://nccam.nih.gov/health/whatiscam

Numanoğlu, A., & Günel, M. K. (2012). Intraoberver reliability of Modified Ashworth Scale and modified Tardieu Scale in the assessment of spasticity in children with cerebral palsy. *Acta Orthopaedica et Traumatologica Turcica, 46,* 196–200.

Ondrak, K. S., & Thorpe, D. E. (2007). Physiologic responses of adolescents with CP when walking on land and in water: A case series. *Journal of Aquatic Physical Therapy, 15*, 10–15.

Page, S. J., Elovic, E., Levine, P., & Sisto, S. A. (2003). Modified constraint-induced therapy and botulinum toxin A: A promising combination. *American Journal of Physical Medicine and Rehabilitation, 82*, 76–80.

Page, S. J., & Levine, P. (2006). Back from the brink: Electromyography-triggered stimulation combined with modified constraint-induced movement therapy in chronic stroke. *Archives of Physical Medicine and Rehabilitation, 87*, 27–31.

Palisano, R., Rosenbaum, P., Walter, S., Russell, D., Wood, E., & Galuppi, B. (1997). Gross Motor Classification System for cerebral palsy. *Developmental Medicine and Child Neurology, 39*, 214–223.

Park, E. S., Rha, D. W., Lee, J. D., Yoo, J. K., & Chang, W. H. (2009). The short-term effects of combined modified constraint-induced movement therapy and botulinum toxin injection for children with spastic hemiplegic cerebral palsy. *Neuropediatrics, 40*, 269–274.

Park, E., Sim, E. G., & Rha, D. W. (2011). Effect of upper limb deformities on gross motor and upper limb functions in children with spastic cerebral palsy. *Research in Developmental Disabilities, 32*, 2389–2397.

Raghuraj, P., Nagarathna, R., Nagendra, H. R., & Telles, S. (1997). Pranayama increases grip strength without lateralized effects. *Indian Journal of Physiology and Pharmacology, 41*, 129–133.

Randall, M. J., Johnson, L. M., & Reddihough, D. S. (2010). *The Melbourne Assessment 2 of Unilateral Upper Limb Function: Test administration manual.* Melbourne, Australia: Royal Children's Hospital.

Reid, D. T. (2002). Benefits of a virtual play rehabilitation environment for children with cerebral palsy on perceptions of self-efficacy: A pilot study. *Pediatric Rehabilitation, 5*, 141–148.

Russell, D. J., Rosenbaum, P. L., Cadman, D. T., Gowland, C., Hardy, S., & Jarvis, S. (1989). The Gross Motor Function Measure: A means to evaluate the effects of physical therapy. *Developmental Medicine and Child Neurology, 31*, 341–352.

Saleh, S. A., El-Kemery, T. A., Farrag, K. A., Badawy, M. R., Sarkis, N. N., Sliman, F. S., & Mangoud, H. J. (2008). Actual vs. best practices for young children with cerebral palsy: A survey of paediatric occupational and physical therapists in Quebec, Canada. *Developmental Rehabilitation, 11*, 60–80.

Sandlund, M., Waterworth, E. L., & Häger, C. (2011). Using motion interactive games to promote physical activity and enhance motor performance in children with cerebral palsy. *Developmental Neurorehabilitation, 14*, 15–21.

Słupik, A., Dwornik, M., Białoszewski, D., & Zych, E. (2007). Effect of Kinesio Taping on bioelectrical activity of vastus medialis muscle: Preliminary report. *Ortopedia, Traumatologia, Rehabilitacja, 9*, 644–651.

Subramanya, P., & Telles, S. (2009). Performance on psychomotor tasks following two yoga-based relaxation techniques. *Perceptual and Motor Skills, 109*, 563–576.

Sun, S. F., Hsu, C. W., Hwang, C. W., Hsu, P. T., Wang, J. L., & Yang, C. L. (2006). Application of combined botulinum toxin type A and modified constraint-induced movement therapy for an individual with chronic upper-extremity spasticity after stroke. *Physical Therapy, 86*, 1387–1397.

Sun, S. F., Hsu, C. W., Sun, H. P., Hwang, C. W., Yang, C. L., & Wang, J. L. (2010). Combined botulinum toxin type A with modified constraint-induced movement therapy for chronic stroke patients with upper extremity spasticity: A randomized controlled study. *Neurorehabilitation and Neural Repair, 24*, 34–41.

Taub, E., Miller, N. E., Novack, T. A., Cook, E. W., Fleming, W. C., Nepomuceno, C. S., . . . Crago, J. E. (1993). Technique to improve chronic motor deficit after stroke. *Archives of Physical Medicine and Rehabilitation, 74*, 347–354.

Taylor, M. J. (2007, December). What is yoga therapy? An IAYT definition. *Yoga Therapy in Practice*, p. 3.

Taylor, N., Sand, P. L., & Jebsen, R. H. (1973). Evaluation of hand function in children. *Archives of Physical Medicine and Rehabilitation, 54*, 129–135.

Telles, S., Dash, M., & Naveen, K. V. (2009). Effect of yoga on musculoskeletal discomfort and motor functions in professional computer users. *Work, 33*, 297–306.

Telles, S., Hanumanthaiah, B., Nagarathna, R., & Nagendra, H. R. (1993). Improvement in static motor performance following yogic training of school children. *Perceptual and Motor Skills, 76*, 1264–1266.

Telles, S., Hanumanthaiah, B. H., Nagarathna, R., & Nagendra, H. R. (1994). Plasticity of motor control systems demonstrated by yoga training. *Indian Journal of Physiology and Pharmacology, 38*, 143–144.

U.S. Food and Drug Administration. (2009). *Information for healthcare professionals: OnabotulinumtoxinA marketed as Botox/Botox Cosmetic), AbobotulinumtoxinA (marketed as Dysport) and RimabotulinumtoxinB (marketed as Myobloc).* Retrieved from http://www.fda.gov/Drugs/DrugSafety/PostmarketDrugSafetyInformationforPatientsandProviders/DrugSafetyInformationforHealthcareProfessionals/ucm174949.htm

van der Lee, J. H., Beckerman, H., Knol, D. L., de Vet, H. C., & Bouter, L. M. (2004). Clinimetric properties of the Motor Activity Log for the assessment of arm use in hemiparetic patients. *Stroke, 35*, 1410–1414.

Volpe, B. T., Krebs, H. I., Hogan, N., Edelsteinn, L., Diels, C. M., & Aisen, M. L. (1999). Robot training enhanced motor outcome in patients with stroke maintained over 3 years. *Neurology, 53,* 1874–1876.

Wade, W., & Porter, D. (2012). Sitting playfully: Does the use of a centre of gravity computer game controller influence the sitting ability of young people with cerebral palsy? *Disability and Rehabilitation: Assistive Technology, 7,* 122–129.

Wallen, M., Bundy, A., Pont, K., & Ziviani, J. (2009). Psychometric properties of the Pediatric Motor Activity Log used for children with cerebral palsy. *Developmental Medicine and Child Neurology, 51,* 200–208.

Walsh, S. F. (2010). Treatment of a brachial plexus injury using kinesiotape and exercise. *Physiotherapy Theory and Practice, 26,* 490–496.

White, K., Schofield, G., & Kilding, A. E. (2011). Energy expended by boys playing active video games. *Journal of Science and Medicine in Sport, 14,* 130–134.

Wolf, S. L., Catlin, P. A., Ellis, M., Archer, A. L., Morgan, B., & Piacentino A. (2001). Assessing Wolf Motor Function Test as outcome measure for research in patients after stroke. *Stroke, 32,* 1635–1639.

Xu, K., Wang, L., Mai, J., & He, L. (2012). Efficacy of constraint-induced movement therapy and electrical stimulation on hand function of children with hemiplegic cerebral palsy: A controlled clinical trial. *Disability and Rehabilitation, 34,* 337–346.

Yasukawa, A., Patel, P., & Sisung, C. (2006). Pilot study: Investigating the effects of Kinesio Taping in an acute pediatric rehabilitation setting. *American Journal of Occupational Therapy, 60,* 104–110. http://dx.doi.org/10.5014/ajot.60.1.104

You, S. H., Jang, S. H., Kim, Y. H., Kwon, Y. H., Barrow, I., & Hallett, M. (2005). Cortical reorganization induced by virtual reality therapy in a child with hemiparetic cerebral palsy. *Developmental Medicine and Child Neurology, 47,* 628–635.

Zaino, C. A., Marchese, V. G., & Westcott, S. L. (2004). Timed Up and Down Stairs Test: Preliminary reliability and validity of a new measure of functional mobility. *Pediatric Physical Therapy, 16,* 90–98.

APPENDIX 12.A. TRAINING AND OTHER RESOURCES FOR ADJUNCTIVE TREATMENT MODALITIES

Electrical Stimulation

- **Physical Agent Modality Credentialing for the Occupational Therapy Practitioner:** http://www.pampca.org/

Therapeutic Taping

- **Kinesio Taping®:** http://www.kinesiotaping.com/

Yoga-Based Therapy

- **YogaKids:** http://yogakids.com/
- **Yoga for the Special Child:** http://www.specialyoga.com/
- **Integrated Movement Therapy:** http://samaryacenter.org/
- **International Association of Yoga Therapists:** http://www.iayt.org/
- *The Kids' Yoga Deck: 50 Poses and Games,* by Annie Buckley (San Francisco: Chronicle Books)
- *Samarya Yoga Deck,* by M. L. Kenny (Seattle, WA: Samarya Center; http://www.samaryacenter.org/)

- **YogaKids DVDs, books, and games** (New Buffalo, MI: YogaKids; http://yogakids.com/)
- **Yoga Pretzels yoga cards,** by T. Guber, L. Kalish, S. Fatus (Cambridge, MA: Barefoot Books)

Aquatic Therapy

- **Aquatic Therapy and Rehabilitation Institute Certification:** http://www.atri.org/ATRICertification.htm
- **Aquatics Section of the American Physical Therapy Association:** http://www.aquaticpt.org/

Therapeutic Use of Rehabilitation Robotics, Virtual Reality, and Gaming Systems

The best source of research on this emerging area of rehabilitation is presentations at conferences of the following professional organizations:

- **American Academy of Cerebral Palsy and Developmental Medicine:** www.aacpdm.org
- **American Academy of Physical Medicine and Rehabilitation:** http://www.aapmr.org
- **American Occupational Therapy Association:** www.aota.org
- **American Physical Therapy Association:** www.apta.org

ANDREW M. GORDON, PhD

13

Intensive Bimanual Training Approaches to Upper-Extremity Rehabilitation in Children With Cerebral Palsy

KEY TERMS

Asymmetrical bimanual movements
Bimanual coordination
Cerebral palsy
Corticospinal projections
Corticospinal terminations
Corticospinal tract
Developmental disuse
Functional training
Hand–arm bimanual intensive therapy
Learned nonuse
Motor cortex
Neuroplasticity
Part-task practice
Pruning
Reorganization
Self-determination theory
Spastic hemiplegia
Spatial–temporal coordination
Symmetrical bimanual movements
Traditional constraint-induced movement therapy without transfer
Transcranial magnetic stimulation
Unilateral damage
Verbal prompting
Whole-task practice

Cerebral palsy (CP) is the most common cause of severe physical disability during development (see Chapter 4, "Motor Development and Physical Growth in Children With Cerebral Palsy"). **Spastic hemiplegia,** with motor impairments mainly affecting just one side of the body, is among the most common forms of CP. The resulting impaired hand function is one of the most disabling symptoms of hemiplegia, affecting daily function.

As highlighted throughout this book, constraint-induced movement therapy (CIMT) and its modifications have completely changed the outlook for upper-extremity (UE) training in children with hemiplegia. Before its application to this population, treatment focused largely on the negative symptoms of CP (e.g., spasticity, contractures), and little evidence was available for any effective functional treatment approaches. It is now known that hand function in children with CP does improve as they become older (Eliasson, Forssberg, Hung, & Gordon, 2006; Eliasson, Krumlinde-Sundholm, et al., 2006; Fedrizzi, Pagliano, Andreucci, & Oleari, 2003; Hanna et al., 2003; Holmfur, Krumlinde-Sundholm, Bergstrom, & Eliasson, 2010) and that they can learn new and increasingly complex motor skills (Duff & Gordon, 2003; Gordon & Duff, 1999; Krebs et al., 2012; Shumway-Cook, Hutchinson, Kartin, Price, & Woollacott, 2003; Valvano & Newell, 1998; see Kantak, Sullivan, & Burtner, 2008, for a review).

An important recognition was that learning occurred only after considerable practice (Duff & Gordon, 2003; Gordon & Duff, 1999). For example, typically developing children learn to scale their fingertip forces during grasping after lifting a given object just 1 or 2 times (Forssberg et al., 1992). In contrast, children with unilateral CP fail to do so initially (Eliasson, Gordon, & Forssberg, 1992), but they can do so after 20 to 25 lifts of the object (Gordon & Duff, 1999). These findings about the benefits of high levels of practice led my colleagues and me to seek an intensive intervention to provide the necessary practice, and CIMT as done with adults with hemiplegia secondary to stroke was a logical choice and had supporting evidence. Charles, Lavinder, and Gordon (2001) conducted the first case studies of modified CIMT provided to children with CP in the late 1990s.

In this chapter, I identify what could be potential limitations of certain forms of CIMT, particularly what might be thought of as **traditional CIMT without transfer**—that is, replicating what is done with adult patients with chronic stroke, focusing solely on unilateral practice. Central to the development of bimanual training approaches is the recognition that bimanual impairments underlie most of the major functional limitations children (and adults) experience. After outlining the rationale for intensive bimanual training, I describe one form of intensive bimanual training that my colleagues and I developed to address these limitations—**hand–arm bimanual intensive therapy (HABIT)**—and present data on its efficacy. Finally, I discuss theme-based approaches to intensive UE training in general, describe the neural basis for bimanual training, and provide some guidance on selecting a unimanual versus a bimanual approach.

RATIONALE FOR INTENSIVE BIMANUAL TRAINING

Since the turn of the current century, more evidence for the efficacy of pediatric CIMT (P–CIMT) has accumulated than for any other UE treatment approach. It is safe to say that P–CIMT has the potential to benefit many children with hemiplegia. The intensity of training is likely a primary factor producing improvement, thus my colleagues and I began to consider alternative high-intensity treatment approaches that could produce equal or perhaps even greater benefits than some of the traditional forms of CIMT.

First, in contrast to adults with hemiplegia, among whom CIMT was developed to overcome **learned nonuse** (i.e., failure to use the affected UE because of the greater ease in using the stronger UE) secondary to stroke-induced impairment, children with hemiplegia must overcome **developmental disuse,** or failure to use their involved UE because they never learned how to use it for many tasks and may need to learn how to use it for the first time. Thus, my colleagues and I focused our treatment on motor learning and developmental issues.

Second, my colleagues and I wanted to include a wide array of activity and practice opportunities, regardless of a child's initial starting skills. We also wanted to ensure high levels of success during therapy sessions and avoid frustration resulting from inability to successfully use the affected UE unimanually.

Third, in humans, development of the **corticospinal projections** (i.e., axons that conduct signals from the brain to the spinal cord) that control unimanual UE abilities is incomplete at birth, with connectivity continuing to increase during the first year of life and perhaps well beyond (see Eyre, Taylor, Villagra, Smith, & Miller, 2001). Studies of corticospinal development in the kitten, for example, have indicated that refinement and maintenance of the final **corticospinal terminations** (i.e., completed connections with the spinal cord) are activity dependent (i.e., movement is required; Martin, Choy, Pullman, & Meng, 2004). Whether brief periods of constraint can cause problems in very early human development similar to those observed in animals is unknown, but the conservative approach my colleagues and I took was to avoid the possible risk associated with constraining (i.e., preventing movement of) the noninvolved UE for long periods with very young infants (e.g., during the 1st year of life). This approach creates opportunities to consider modified constraint approaches as well as use of nonconstraint treatments that could produce notable developmental benefits.

Finally, children with hemiplegia have impairments in **spatial–temporal coordination,** or sequencing and use of the two hands within space and time (e.g., Hung, Charles, & Gordon, 2004, 2010; Islam, Gordon, Forssberg, Sköld, & Eliasson, 2011; Steenbergen, Hulstijn, de Vries, & Berger, 1996; see also Gordon & Steenbergen, 2008; Utley & Steenbergen, 2006), as well as global impairments in motor planning (Steenbergen, Verrel, & Gordon, 2007). Problems with bimanual tasks can be among the most frustrating (Sköld, Josephsson, & Eliasson, 2004). Adult CIMT in its traditional form focuses solely on improving unimanual dexterity; for children, P–CIMT approaches sometimes include transfer packages to bridge the child's unimanual skills to become part of bimanual performance (Aarts, Jongerius, Geerdink, van Limbeek, & Geurts, 2010; Case-Smith, DeLuca, Stevenson, & Ramey, 2012; Taub et al., 2007).

My colleagues' and my philosophy has been that the goal of UE rehabilitation should be to increase functional independence by improving use of both hands in cooperation (Sköld et al., 2004). A type of therapy referred to as ***functional training,*** or therapy with an emphasis on practicing motor skills, has been shown to improve functional skills (e.g., Ahl, Johansson, Granat, & Carlberg, 2005; Gorter, Holty, Rameckers, Elvers, & Oostendorp, 2009; Ketelaar, Vermeer, Hart, van Petegem-van Beek, & Helders, 2001; Verschuren, Ketelaar, Gorter, Helders, & Takken, 2009). For example, Ketelaar et al. compared a group receiving physical therapy with an emphasis on functional training relevant to caregiver goals with a reference group receiving physical therapy that had an emphasis on normalization of movements in 55 children (aged 2 to 7 years) with CP over 18 months. The functional training group had greater improvements in the self-care and mobility domains of the Pediatric Evaluation of Disability Inventory (PEDI; Haley, Coster, Ludlow, Haltiwanger, & Andrellos, 1992) than did the physical therapy group, supporting the principle of specificity of practice (Thorndike, 1914; see Gordon & Magill, 2012). Along these lines, such principles of motor learning would imply that the best way to achieve improved bimanual skills would be to practice them directly. This rationale led my colleagues and me to develop a formalized approach to bimanual training that maintains the part-task practice (i.e., shaping), skill progression, and intensity of CIMT but does so without restraint of the less-affected UE.

HAND–ARM BIMANUAL INTENSIVE THERAPY

To motivate children, participation in therapy must be fun, which is consistent with the recent emphasis on functional training and practice of predefined goals in therapeutic environments (Ahl et al., 2005; Bower, Michell, Burnett, Campbell, & McLellan, 2001; Ketelaar et al., 2001; Law et al., 1998; Øien, Fallang, & Østensjø, 2010). HABIT aims to improve the amount and quality of involved hand use during bimanual activities (see Charles & Gordon, 2006). My colleagues and I based HABIT on

- Basic science work delineating the mechanisms of hand impairments in CP,
- Our intuition that the key ingredient in the effectiveness of CIMT is intensity of practice, and
- Specificity of training consistent with defined learning principles.

Thus, HABIT retains the intensive structured practice of P–CIMT but engages the child in improving bimanual activities. Typically, HABIT is provided 6 hours per day for 10 to 15 days (60–90 hours). Activities that necessitate coordination of both UEs are used.

Bimanual training is one of many strategies frequently used by occupational therapy practitioners and physical therapists (see Eliasson, 2007; Hoare, Imms, Rawicki, & Carey,

2010) and is sometimes used after removal of a constraint (e.g., Aarts et al., 2010; Case-Smith et al., 2012; Cohen-Holzer, Katz-Leurer, Reinstein, Rotem, & Meyer, 2011). HABIT differs from conventional physical and occupational therapy approaches in key ways, however. The intensity of HABIT is much higher than that of conventional therapies, providing ample practice using principles of motor learning and principles of **neuroplasticity,** whereby neuroplastic changes are theoretically induced by progressing task complexity and reward (e.g., Kleim et al., 2002; Nudo, 2003). HABIT is also far more structured than conventional therapy, combining ingredients gleamed from CIMT (e.g., shaping) and clear rules about activity selection and skill progression. The focus is on how the UE performs at the endpoint of the movement.

HABIT includes specific bimanual activities involving performance of play or functional activities (Charles & Gordon, 2006). The choice of activities is not as important as the movements they elicit. Movement impairments of the involved UE and bimanual coordination impairments are determined before and early during the intervention. Bimanual activities are then chosen that target these deficits and engage the child in activities with increasingly complex bimanual behaviors. Task demands are graded to ensure success, and the task is made more difficult once the child achieves successful performance on 70% of the trials. Examples of these activities and how they can be used to work on specific targeted movements and graded to change their difficulty are provided in Table 13.1.

Before the start of each task, the practitioner provides directions to the child specifying how the child will use each hand during the activity (often providing a choice) to prevent the child from using compensatory strategies (e.g., performing the task unimanually with the less-affected UE). Despite its structure, HABIT is also conducive to active problem solving, given the increased degree of freedom associated with the use of two hands. Positive reinforcement and knowledge of results are used to motivate the child's engagement and performance (often with tangible rewards as well as praise) and to reinforce target movements. Rather than the practitioner offering repeated **verbal prompting,** or cueing of the child to use the affected UE or not to use the stronger UE (to which children usually attenuate, as experienced by their parents), he or she halts the activity if the child does not adhere to the directions; the practitioner then playfully asks the child something such as "Which hand is used for that activity?" This approach actively involves the child in performing the movement as required.

HABIT is conducted in groups of children to provide social interaction, modeling, and encouragement. This day camp model is fun and makes it easy to motivate children. A 1:1 interventionist–child ratio is maintained in the day camp model to carefully structure the environment and ensure that

Table 13.1   Hand–Arm Bimanual Intensive Therapy Activities

ACTIVITY CATEGORY	TYPE OF INVOLVED HAND USE	GRADED CONSTRAINTS
Manipulative games and activities	Stabilizer, manipulator, active–passive assist, symmetrical and asymmetrical movements	Changing spatial–temporal constraints of the task; for symmetrical tasks, increasing the frequency with which the task is completed within a fixed time period
Card games	Stabilizer, manipulator, active–passive assist, symmetrical and asymmetrical movements	Changing spatial–temporal constraints of the task; for symmetrical tasks, increasing the frequency with which the task is completed within a fixed time period
Video games	Manipulator, active assist, symmetrical movements	Changing temporal constraints of the task, sitting on a fitness ball, taping the grip
Functional tasks	Stabilizer, manipulator, active–passive assist, asymmetrical movements	Progressing among stabilizer, manipulator, active–passive assist, or symmetrical and asymmetrical movements
Whole upper extremity	Stabilizer, manipulator, active–passive assist, symmetrical and asymmetrical movements	Progressing among stabilizer, manipulator, active–passive assist, or symmetrical and asymmetrical movements; sitting on a fitness ball
Arts and crafts	Stabilizer, manipulator, active–passive assist, symmetrical and asymmetrical movements	Progressing among stabilizer, manipulator, active–passive assist, symmetrical and asymmetrical movements; placing items on Dycem nonslip material (Dycem Limited; Warwick, RI); building up objects with tape

the child uses both hands at all times. Two types of practice are used in HABIT. First, during performance of **whole-task practice,** activities are continuously performed for a minimum of 15 to 20 minutes in the context of playing a game or performing a functional activity. Targeted movements and spatial–temporal coordination are practiced within the context of completing the activity. Second, **part-task practice** (often referred to as *shaping* in the psychology literature) involves practicing a targeted movement repeatedly in isolation.

Both **symmetrical bimanual movements,** such as putting game pieces away with both hands simultaneously, and **asymmetrical bimanual movements,** such as transferring items between the hands, are practiced. Although a strong theoretical basis built on neurophysiological principles exists for providing symmetrical practice (Cauraugh & Summers, 2005; Stinear & Byblow, 2004), children's interest and motivation (unlike those of adults) can seldom be sustained with only one type of movement.

Functionally, the hands also need to be used in a variety of ways during everyday life, including asymmetrical (e.g., opening a bottle) or sequential (e.g., shoe tying) movements. Task difficulty is altered by increasing speed or accuracy requirements or by using tasks that require more skilled use of the involved UE (e.g., moving from activities in which the involved UE is used as a passive stabilizer to those in which it is used as an active assist, and then to those in which it is used as an active manipulator; see Krumlinde-Sundholm & Eliasson, 2003; Krumlinde-Sundholme, Holmefur, Kottorp, & Eliasson, 2007).

The first published study of such a bimanual training approach was a small randomized clinical trial of HABIT (Gordon, Schneider, Chinnan, & Charles, 2007) with 20 children with hemiplegic CP between the ages of 3.5 and 14.0 years. In this study, 10 children who received 60 hours of HABIT were compared with a delayed-treatment control group who continued their usual and customary care over the study period. The Assisting Hand Assessment (AHA; Holmefur et al., 2010; Krumlinde-Sundholm & Eliasson, 2003; Krumlinde-Sundholme et al., 2007) was the primary outcome measure. The AHA measures and quantifies the effectiveness with which a child with unilateral disability uses the affected (assisting) hand during bimanual activities. Gordon et al. (2007) also placed accelerometers, which quantify the time spent moving, on the children's wrists during administration of the AHA to measure precisely the frequency of use of each UE (see Uswatte et al., 2006).

The changes in the AHA scores from before and immediately after treatment were compared for the two groups. The AHA scores showed significant increases for the children in the bimanual HABIT group but not for those in the control

Figure 13.1 (A) MEAN AHA UNIT SCORES. (B) ACCELEROMETRY DATA INDICATING PERCENTAGE OF TIME THE MORE-AFFECTED HAND MOVED DURING THE AHA TEST BEFORE AND AFTER CIMT AND HABIT.

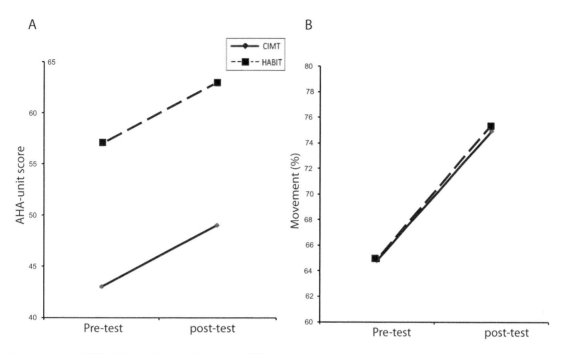

Note. Data adapted from Gordon et al. (2007). AHA = Assisting Hand Assessment; CIMT = constraint-induced movement therapy; HABIT = Hand–Arm Bimanual Intensive Training.

group. However, scores for the treatment group decreased by 1 month posttest, although they remained significantly higher than at pretest (Gordon et al., 2007). Data from accelerometers children wore yielded a percentage of total task time the involved UE was used during performance of the AHA. Use of the involved UE increased (with the increase sustained at the follow-up) for children who received HABIT but not for the control group. Interestingly, the change in the amount of use of the involved UE did not correlate with the change in AHA scores, emphasizing that quality and quantity of movement may change (and be maintained) independently.

It is important to note that the control group in the Gordon et al. (2007) study, as well as in most studies of P–CIMT, received treatment at a markedly different intensity (usual and customary care schedules). Furthermore, the study did not allow examination of treatment specificity (i.e., the exact therapy activities and goals). Using a small quasi-randomized study design, however, Gordon et al. (2008), in their first attempt to examine specificity of training, compared another group of 10 children who received 60 hours of HABIT with a group that received an equivalent dose of P–CIMT using only a cotton sling to constrain the less-affected UE during treatment sessions (see Charles, Wolf, Schneider, & Gordon,

2006; Gordon, Charles, & Wolf, 2005). Overall, Gordon et al. (2008) found similar positive changes in manual dexterity on the Jebsen–Taylor Test of Hand Function (JTTHF; Jebsen, Taylor, Trieschmann, Trotter, & Howard, 1969), quality of bimanual hand use on the AHA, and amount of movement as measured by accelerometers. These results indicate that treatment intensity likely contributes to P–CIMT benefits, because an equal amount of HABIT produced similar outcomes (Figure 13.1).

In a larger randomized trial of HABIT and P–CIMT, Gordon et al. (2011) randomly assigned 42 children (ages 3.5–10.0 years) to receive 90 hours of either HABIT or P–CIMT with a sling worn during therapy sessions. The primary outcomes were unimanual dexterity (JTTHF) and quality of bimanual hand use (AHA). Secondary outcome measures included accelerometry and UE impairment (Grasp and Dissociated Movements subtests of the Quality of Upper Extremity Skills Test [QUEST]; DeMatteo et al., 1992). Gordon et al. also used Goal Attainment Scaling (Kiresuk, Smith, & Cardillo, 1994) to quantify progress on one functional and one play goal defined by caregivers, children, or both before group assignment. Goals were assessed for appropriateness on the basis of age and current abilities and scaled by a physical

Figure 13.2 (A) MEAN ± SEM TIME TO COMPLETE THE 6 TIMED ITEMS (WRITING EXCLUDED) OF THE JTTHF BEFORE AND AFTER CIMT AND HABIT. FASTER TIMES CORRESPOND TO BETTER PERFORMANCE. (B) MEAN ± SEM AHA UNIT SCORES; HIGHER SCORES REPRESENT BETTER PERFORMANCE.

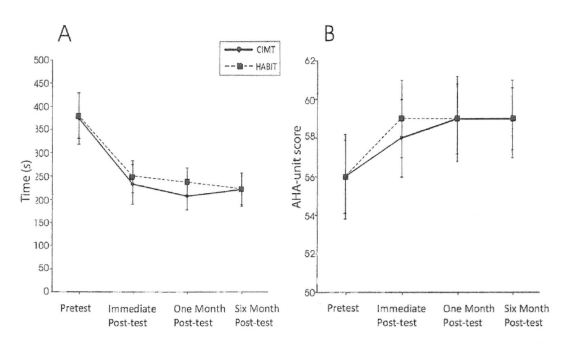

Source. From "Bimanual Training and Constraint-Induced Movement Therapy in Children With Hemiplegic Cerebral Palsy: A Randomized Trial," by A. M. Gordon, Y. C. Hung, M. Brandao, C. L. Ferre, H.-C. Kuo, K. Friel, . . . J. R. Charles, 2011, *Neurorehabilitation and Neural Repair, 25,* p. 698. Copyright © 2011 by SAGE. Adapted with permission.

Note. AHA = Assisting Hand Assessment; CIMT = constraint-induced movement therapy; HABIT = Hand-Arm Bimanual Intensive Training; JTTHF = Jebson–Taylor Test of Hand Function; SEM = standard error of the mean.

therapist. The goals were practiced as much as 30 minutes per day. Gordon et al. embedded practiced movements into fun activities, providing interventionists with considerable latitude as to how much training (if at all) to conduct within the 30-minute limit on the basis of the child's interest. The P–CIMT group did not practice bimanual goals; instead, they practiced unimanual movement components making up the unilateral goals. Goal attainment was rated by the caregiver and verified by a physical therapist.

Figure 13.2 shows that both groups had similar and significant changes on the JTTHF and AHA. Similar findings were seen for the accelerometry and the QUEST (not shown). Thus, these findings are consistent with the conclusion that intensity rather than therapeutic focus or ingredients (unimanual vs. bimanual) is the important factor in producing these outcomes. More important, unlike the Gordon et al. (2008) study involving 60 hours of bimanual training, the end-of-treatment improvements after an increase to a therapy dose of 90 hours (Gordon et al., 2011) were maintained 6 months later. Similar findings showing benefits

from high-intensity therapy, P–CIMT, or bimanual training were reported by Sakzewski and colleagues (Sakzewski, 2012; Sakzewski, Ziviani, Abbott, et al., 2011a, 2011b; Sakzewski, Ziviani, & Boyd, 2011) and by Facchin et al. (2011), with the latter study being a multisite trial.

Treatment specificity effects did appear for the goal attainment outcomes (Gordon et al., 2011). The majority of goals were bimanual (the remaining goals were unimanual with the paretic hand). Both groups achieved or exceeded their expected level of goal performance; however, the HABIT group made greater progress than the CIMT group. Approximately 20% of the identified goals were not practiced in either group during the interventions or at home because of changes in the children's interests. Interestingly, these unpracticed goals also improved more for the HABIT participants. Thus, the skills these children acquired during HABIT may have allowed faster learning by means of transfer of bimanual activities.

In a separate study of goal achievement using the Canadian Occupational Performance Measure (COPM; Carswell et al., 2004; Law et al., 1990) and self-care performance using the PEDI,

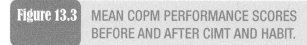

Figure 13.3 MEAN COPM PERFORMANCE SCORES BEFORE AND AFTER CIMT AND HABIT.

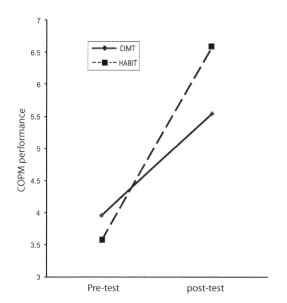

Note. Data plotted from de Brito Brandão, Gordon, and Mancini (2012). CIMT = constraint-induced movement therapy; COPM = Canadian Occupational Performance Measure; HABIT = Hand-Arm Bimanual Intensive Training.

16 children with CP received 90 hours of HABIT or P–CIMT (de Brito Brandão, Gordon, & Mancini, 2012). Both groups showed significant improvements in self-care performance (PEDI functional skills and independence) and progress on goals (COPM satisfaction and performance). However, caregivers of children who received HABIT perceived greater improvements on goal performance (Figure 13.3), again suggesting specificity of training for performance of specific goals established by parents. One study (Sakzewski, 2012) suggested improvements in child social well-being after receiving CIMT as reported by parents; the nuances of parents' perceptions of their child's well-being and function need further study.

These studies (de Brito Brandão et al., 2012; Sakzewski, 2012) focused on changes in clinical performance and caregiver perception of goal achievement. Whether CIMT or bimanual training affects the spatial–temporal coordination of the two hands is not known. Hung, Casertano, Hillman, and Gordon (2011) therefore examined the kinematics of a bimanual task with 20 children with hemiplegia who received 90 hours of either HABIT or CIMT. **Bimanual coordination,** or ability to coordinate use of both UE, was assessed by having participants open a drawer with one hand and manipulate its contents with the other hand while three-dimensional movement kinematics were recorded (see Wiesendanger & Serrien, 2004). After treatment, the HABIT group showed greater improvements in bimanual coordination as indicated

by greater movement overlap (percentage of time with both hands engaged in the task) and better goal synchronization (reduced time differences between the two hands completing the task goals). Both groups had greater movement overlap time of the two hands and shorter duration of goal synchronization after treatment, but the children in the HABIT group exhibited greater improvement. These results suggest that bimanual training improves the spatial–temporal control of the two hands and are also in agreement with the principles of practice specificity and high intensity.

THEME-BASED UPPER-EXTREMITY TRAINING APPROACHES

Several P–CIMT and bimanual training approaches have used a theme to increase children's engagement in the intervention, consistent with **self-determination theory,** which posits that "consideration of innate psychological needs for competence, autonomy, and relatedness" is required to maximize motiva-tion (Deci & Ryan, 2000, p. 227). For example, Boyd et al. (2010) compared P–CIMT with bimanual training in the context of day camps, conducted at a community sporting facility, with a novel circus theme. The day camp used circus activities provided by professional trainers in 2-hour workshops and included a low ropes course. Improvements were seen for both groups in bimanual performance, unimanual capacity, and participation and goal performance (Sakzewski, Ziviani, Abbott, et al., 2011a, 2011b; Sakzewski, Ziviani, & Boyd, 2011). Similarly, Aarts and colleagues (2010; Aarts, Jongerius, Geerdink, & Geurts, 2011; Crajé, Aarts, Nijhuis-van der Sanden, & Steenbergen, 2010) used a combined CIMT–bimanual training approach with a pirate theme and also found significant changes on the AHA and ABILHAND–Kids (Arnould, Penta, Renders, & Thonnard, 2004) and in goal attainment.

Green and colleagues (2013) used a magic theme–based variation of HABIT to investigate the effects across cultures (Israel and England) and among participants with more severe hand impairments (Manual Ability Classification System [MACS] Level III; Eliasson, Krumlinde-Sundholm, et al., 2006). Twenty-three children with hemiplegia (aged 7 to 15 years) participated in one of three 2-week camps. Both sites used the same repertoire of magic tricks, introduced at similar stages. The camps included individualized support for learning and practice of magic tricks; fine and gross bimanual motor play; and theatrical studies, which included fabrication of items such as costumes and props for the magic show (using both hands). Significant improvements were seen on the AHA and the Children's Hand-Use Experience Questionnaire (Sköld,

Hermansson, Kumlinde-Sundholm, & Eliasson, 2011). Severity of impairment and country did not influence the findings.

Theme-based approaches have the potential to motivate and maintain participants' interest, assuming they are drawn to the theme. Presumably, these approaches are also attractive to caregivers, likely aiding in study recruitment. Some of our projects have varied themes each day (Gordon et al., 2007, 2008, 2011). No direct comparisons of theme-based and non-theme-based interventions have been made, but across studies, the theme-based studies appear to have improvements similar to those of others studies. In my view, the attractiveness of the activities and the skill of the interventionists in motivating and shaping children's UE functions are likely the most important factors for success.

NEURAL BASIS OF BIMANUAL TRAINING

Unilateral damage to motor areas results in a failure of the affected **corticospinal tract (CST),** which consists of bundles of nerve cells that carry motor commands from the brain to the spinal cord, to establish and maintain normal terminations (i.e., connections) in the spinal cord (Eyre et al., 2007; see Martin, Chakrabarty, & Friel, 2011, for reviews). Normal termination is presumed to require activity-dependent competition between the two hemispheres of the developing motor system. In typical development, the CST bilaterally projects from each **motor cortex** (i.e., the part of the brain that generates nerve impulses that control the voluntary muscles) at birth and undergoes **pruning,** or selective reduction in terms of neural connections, into a more mature contralateral projection pattern during the first few years of life (Eyre et al., 2001).

Unilateral damage to the motor cortex, as often occurs with hemiplegic CP (particularly the prevalent form that is presumed to result from prenatal stroke or very early postnatal stroke), results in aberrant organization of the motor system, with the damaged cortex failing to establish normal connections to the spinal cord as well as to other brain areas. Simultaneously, the undamaged CST maintains exuberant bilateral projections, invading the normal termination zone of the contralateral side. CST integrity has been examined in children with hemiplegia using **transcranial magnetic stimulation (TMS),** which activates the damaged side with weak electrical currents while the undamaged side maintains bilateral terminations in the spinal cord (Eyre et al., 2007).

The CST is capable of considerable reorganization after damage, and this reorganization of structures and networks likely underlies recovery of function (see Eyre, 2003). The contralateral (opposite-side) CST projection controls the less-affected limb, and the ipsilateral (same-side) pathway from the less-affected cortex plays a role in the control of the involved extremity (Staudt et al., 2004). Involvement of the ipsilateral CST appears to correlate with the extent of the cortical damage, suggesting that the ipsilateral pathway may mediate recovery when the contralateral pathway controlling the affected limb is severely damaged (Staudt et al., 2004). The ipsilateral pathway is not readily established until approximately age 12 months, even when the brain injury occurs at or before birth (Eyre et al., 2007), suggesting that activity-dependent competition between the two cortices during postnatal development progressively drives the organization and subsequent refinement of the CST. Therefore, recruitment of the ipsilateral pathway may promote long-term functional recovery.

Ipsilateral pathways are also implicated in the recovery of function after adult stroke, particularly during the early stages of recovery and in cases involving large brain lesions that do not spare enough motor areas to support movement (e.g., Marshall et al., 2000). Thus, tasks that recruit the ipsilateral pathways, such as symmetrical bilateral movements (e.g., Stinear & Byblow, 2004), may be beneficial. Bilateral practice may result in changes in cortical representations (Cauraugh & Summers, 2005) and excitability in the undamaged hemisphere (Stinear & Byblow, 2004) in adult stroke patients, which in turn may provide a neural basis for bimanual therapy.

One study (Kuhnke et al., 2008) investigated whether the type of corticospinal reorganization (ipsilateral vs. contralateral, determined with TMS) influences the efficacy of CIMT. Only participants with preserved contralateral projections showed improvements in dexterity as determined by the Wolf Motor Function Test (Wolf et al., 2001). These data, albeit from a small group of participants (teens to adults), may suggest that clients with ipsilateral CST may not benefit as much from CIMT as those who maintain normal contralateral CST projections.

PRACTITIONER'S DILEMMA: WHEN TO USE P–CIMT OR BIMANUAL TRAINING

To date, the research evidence cannot provide complete guidance to practitioners about exactly when or for whom bimanual training or P–CIMT should be selected. Table 13.2 presents some criteria, showing how I think individual differences could inform which approach to select (see Gordon, 2011).

For example, Gordon et al.'s (2011) results and the results of others (Facchin et al., 2011; Sakzewski, Ziviani, Abbott, et al., 2011a, 2011b; Sakzewski, Ziviani, & Boyd, 2011) have suggested that either approach could be used to elicit improvements in manual dexterity and bimanual performance (i.e., they could be used interchangeably).

Table 13.2 Suggested Criteria for Selection of CIMT or Bimanual Training

CRITERION	CIMT	BIMANUAL TRAINING
Dexterity	☐	☐
Bimanual assist quality	☐	☐
Frequency of use	☐	☐
Function (goals)		☐
Coordination of two hands		☐
Mild hemiplegia		☐
Severe hemiplegia		☐
Reduction of impairments	☐	
Behavioral problems	?	
Restraint tolerance problems		☐
Low IQ	?	
Diversity of activities		☐
Short duration	?	
Lack of 1:1 child–interventionist ratio	☐	

Note. ☐ = criterion for selecting the therapy; ? = criterion for considering the therapy; CIMT = constraint-induced movement therapy.

Bimanual training seemingly may be better for achievement of bimanual goals (de Brito Brandão et al., 2012; Gordon et al., 2011) and bimanual coordination (Hung et al., 2011) for children of certain ages with certain baseline abilities present, whereas CIMT may be better for improving unimanual goals and coordination or reducing unimanual motor impairments (e.g., wrist supination) because more control is possible over how the affected UE is used.

One can speculate that bimanual training may be better for a child with mild impairments (i.e., who already possesses good manipulation skills but shows developmental nonuse during bimanual activities), whereas P–CIMT may be preferred to help induce early success in voluntary control of the more-impaired UE if done safely and then later integrated into bimanual functions. Bimanual training may also be better for a child with an inability to grasp (when the choice of activities with CIMT would be very limited), because tasks can be graded such that the involved UE has to be used only

as a passive assist to start (e.g., stabilizing paper on the desk while drawing). It would also be a viable alternative for a child who does not tolerate the restraint. Clearly, further research and careful clinical documentation would be vital to validate these tentative criteria.

Bimanual training likely provides greater diversity of activities and is potentially less invasive than CIMT because there is no restraint, although verbal prompting can be equally invasive if not provided with care. Nevertheless, some therapists trained and experienced in bimanual training consider it much more difficult for interventionists to execute because they must continually anticipate how the child will perform the task and shape the environment accordingly (i.e., always be one step ahead). Bimanual activities are often more motivating for older children, however, because these activities do not require children to continually focus on their impaired hand in isolation. The activities are generally more salient and may be selected to maximize interest (e.g., video games). Such motivational and social aspects of types of practice need to be considered in intervention design (Ochsner & Lieberman, 2001).

Finally, these approaches are not mutually exclusive and could be performed back to back with sufficient intensity (see, e.g., Aarts et al., 2010). In fact, note that the advantages seen for HABIT in Gordon et al.'s (2011) randomized controlled trial may well be the result of the conduct of these approaches in a well-controlled scientific environment rather than a clinical environment. Although Gordon et al. maintained treatment fidelity solely within each approach for comparison reasons, the hybrid approach, in which CIMT is followed up with a bimanual transfer package (Aarts et al., 2010; Case-Smith et al., 2012; Taub et al., 2007), may eliminate the unique advantages of exclusive bimanual training. Cohen-Holzer et al. (2011) examined 1 hour of CIMT followed by 5 hours of bimanual training each day for 10 days and found significant improvements on the AHA, JTTHF, and PEDI and in grip strength that were maintained at 6-month follow-up. Whether these combined approaches are better than either treatment individually (see Gordon, 2011) has yet to be formally tested; the results of such comparative studies will be valuable to future clinical decision making and choice of therapies for individual children.

SUMMARY

The introduction and subsequent study of CIMT in the pediatric population can be credited as a milestone in thinking about the importance of treatment intensity (as well as combined use with constraint) in rehabilitation. The results of a now large number of studies suggest that children with CP benefit in a significant and enduring way from multiple types of intensive UE training. The specific ingredients that prove to be beneficial and the precise dose responses are not known. It is conceivable that the key ingredient is simply treatment intensity, although an interaction between ingredients and intensity could also be key. (See Chapter 16, "Research Priorities: Understanding and Transcending the Limits of Current Knowledge to Inform Best Practices in Pediatric CIMT.")

The results to date suggest that it is important to put the training goals first and then to choose an appropriate protocol to meet those goals. Although considerably more evidence supports the efficacy of CIMT, this chapter provides evidence that training in bimanual skills can improve bimanual function skills and may be a viable alternative with both advantages and disadvantages. My view is that they can be used interchangeably depending on the child and therapeutic goal over the long course of developmental care. Nevertheless, although large improvements can result from such intensive training, the underlying sensory and motor impairments still persist, and these approaches should be integrated with, rather than replace, other long-term pediatric care approaches.

ACKNOWLEDGMENT

This work was supported by the Thrasher Research Fund.

REFERENCES

Aarts, P. B., Jongerius, P. H., Geerdink, Y. A., & Geurts, A. C. (2011). Modified constraint-induced movement therapy combined with bimanual treatment (mCIMT–BIT) in children with unilateral spastic cerebral palsy: How are improvements in arm–hand use established? *Research in Developmental Disabilities, 24,* 509–518.

Aarts, P. B., Jongerius, P. H., Geerdink, Y. A., van Limbeek, J., & Geurts, A. C. (2010). Effectiveness of modified constraint-induced movement therapy in children with unilateral spastic cerebral palsy: A randomized controlled trial. *Neurorehabilitation and Neural Repair, 24,* 509–518.

Ahl, L. E., Johansson, E., Granat, T., & Carlberg, E. B. (2005). Functional therapy for children with cerebral palsy: An ecological approach. *Developmental Medicine and Child Neurology, 47,* 613–619.

Arnould, C., Penta, M., Renders, A., & Thonnard, J. L. (2004). ABILHAND–Kids: A measure of manual ability in children with cerebral palsy. *Neurology, 63,* 1045–1052.

Bower, E., Michell, D., Burnett, M., Campbell, M. J., & McLellan, D. L. (2001). Randomized controlled trial of physiotherapy in 56 children with cerebral palsy followed for 18 months. *Developmental Medicine and Child Neurology, 43,* 4–15.

Boyd, R., Sakzewski, L., Ziviani, J., Abbott, D. F., Badawy, R., Gilmore, R., . . . Jackson, G. D. (2010). INCITE: A randomized trial comparing constraint induced movement therapy and bimaunal training in children with congenital hemiplegia. *BMC Neurology, 10,* 4.

Carswell, A., McColl, M. A., Baptiste, S., Law, M., Polatajko, H., & Pollock, N. (2004). The Canadian Occupational Performance Measure: A research and clinical literature review. *Canadian Journal of Occupational Therapy, 71,* 210–222.

Case-Smith, J., DeLuca, S. C., Stevenson, R., & Ramey, S. L. (2012). Multicenter randomized controlled trial of pediatric constraint-induced movement therapy: 6-month follow-up. *American Journal of Occupational Therapy, 66,* 15–23. http://dx.doi.org/10.5014/ajot.2012.002386

Cauraugh, J. H., & Summers, J. J. (2005). Neural plasticity and bilateral movements: A rehabilitation approach for chronic stroke. *Progress in Neurobiology, 75,* 309–320.

Charles, J., & Gordon, A. M. (2006). Development of hand–arm bimanual intensive training (HABIT) for improving bimanual coordination in children with hemiplegic cerebral palsy. *Developmental Medicine and Child Neurology, 48,* 931–936.

Charles, J., Lavinder, G., & Gordon, A. M. (2001). The effects of constraint induced therapy on hand function in children with hemiplegic cerebral palsy. *Pediatric Physical Therapy, 13,* 68–76.

Charles, J. R., Wolf, S. L., Schneider, J. A., & Gordon, A. M. (2006). Efficacy of a child-friendly form of constraint-induced movement therapy in hemiplegic cerebral palsy: A randomized control trial. *Developmental Medicine and Child Neurology, 48,* 635–642.

Cohen-Holzer, M., Katz-Leurer, M., Reinstein, R., Rotem, H., & Meyer, S. (2011). The effect of combining daily restraint with bimanual intensive therapy in children with hemiparetic cerebral palsy: A self-control study. *NeuroRehabilitation, 29,* 29–36.

Crajé, C., Aarts, P., Nijhuis-van der Sanden, M., & Steenbergen, B. (2010). Action planning in typically and atypically developing children (unilateral cerebral palsy). *Research in Developmental Disabilities, 31,* 1039–1046.

de Brito Brandão, M. B., Gordon, A. M., & Mancini, M. C. (2012). Functional impact of constraint-therapy and bimanual training in children with cerebral palsy. *American Journal of Occupational Therapy, 66,* 672–681. http://dx.doi.org/10.5014/ajot.2012.004622

Deci, E., & Ryan, R. (2000). The "what" and "why" of goal pursuits: Human needs and the self-determination of behavior. *Psychological Inquiry, 11,* 227–268.

DeMatteo, C., Law, M., Russell, D., Pollock, N., Rosenbaum, P., & Walter, S. (1992). *QUEST: Quality of Upper Extremity Skills Test.* Hamilton, Ontario: McMaster University, Neurodevelopmental Clinical Research Unit.

Duff, S. V., & Gordon, A. M. (2003). Learning of grasp control in children with hemiplegic cerebral palsy. *Developmental Medicine and Child Neurology, 45,* 746–757. PMID: 14580130

Eliasson, A. C. (2007). Bimanual training for children with unilateral CP—Is this something new? *Developmental Medicine and Child Neurology, 49,* 806.

Eliasson, A. C., Forssberg, H., Hung, Y. C., & Gordon, A. M. (2006). Development of hand function and precision grip control in individuals with cerebral palsy: A 13-year follow-up study. *Pediatrics, 118,* 1226–1236. PMID: 17015511

Eliasson, A. C., Gordon, A. M., & Forssberg, H. (1992). Impaired anticipatory control of isometric forces during grasping by children with cerebral palsy. *Developmental Medicine and Child Neurology, 34,* 216–225. PMID: 1559601

Eliasson, A. C., Krumlinde-Sundholm, L., Rösblad, B., Beckung, E., Arner, M., Ohrvall, A. M., & Rosenbaum, P. (2006). The Manual Ability Classification System (MACS) for children with cerebral palsy: Scale development and evidence of validity and reliability. *Developmental Medicine and Child Neurology, 48,* 549–554.

Eyre, J. A. (2003). Development and plasticity of the corticospinal system in man. *Neural Plasticity, 10,* 93–106.

Eyre, J. A., Smith, M., Dabydeen, L., Clowry, G. J., Petacchi, E., Battini, R., . . . Cioni, G. (2007). Is hemiplegic cerebral palsy equivalent to amblyopia of the corticospinal system? *Annals of Neurology, 62,* 493–503.

Eyre, J. A., Taylor, J. P., Villagra, F., Smith, M., & Miller, S. (2001). Evidence of activity-dependent withdrawal of corticospinal projections during human development. *Neurology, 57,* 1543–1554.

Facchin, P., Rosa-Rizzotto, M., Visonà Dalla Pozza, L., Turconi, A. C., Pagliano, E., Signorini, S., . . . Fedrizzi, E.; GIPCI Study Group. (2011). Multisite trial comparing the efficacy of constraint-induced movement therapy with that of bimanual intensive training in children with hemiplegic cerebral palsy: Postintervention results. *American Journal of Physical Medicine and Rehabilitation, 90,* 539–553.

Fedrizzi, E., Pagliano, E., Andreucci, E., & Oleari, G. (2003). Hand function in children with hemiplegic cerebral palsy: Prospective follow-up and functional outcome in adolescence. *Developmental Medicine and Child Neurology, 45,* 85–91.

Forssberg, H., Kinoshita, H., Eliasson, A. C., Johansson, R. S., Westling, G., & Gordon, A. M. (1992). Development of human precision grip II: Anticipatory control of isometric forces targeted for object's weight. *Experimental Brain Research, 90,* 393–398. PMID: 1397153

Gordon, A. M. (2011). To constrain or not to constrain, and other stories of intensive upper extremity training for children with unilateral cerebral palsy. *Developmental Medicine and Child Neurology, 53*(Suppl. 4), 56–61. http://dx.doi.org/10.1111/j.1469-8749.2011.040066.x

Gordon, A. M., Charles, J., & Wolf, S. L. (2005). Methods of constraint-induced movement therapy for children with hemiplegic cerebral palsy: Development of a child-friendly intervention for improving upper-extremity function. *Archives of Physical Medicine and Rehabilitation, 86,* 837–844. PMID: 15827942

Gordon, A. M., Chinnan, A., Gill, S., Petra, E., Hung, Y. C., & Charles, J. (2008). Both constraint-induced movement therapy and bimanual training lead to improved performance of upper extremity function in children with hemiplegia. *Developmental Medicine and Child Neurology, 50,* 957–958. http://dx.doi.org/10.1111/j.1469-8749.2008.03166.x

Gordon, A. M., & Duff, S. V. (1999). Fingertip forces during object manipulation in children with hemiplegic cerebral palsy. I: Anticipatory scaling. *Developmental Medicine and Child Neurology, 41,* 166–175.

Gordon, A. M., Hung, Y. C., Brandao, M., Ferre, C. L., Kuo, H.-C., Friel, K., . . . Charles, J. R. (2011). Bimanual training and constraint-induced movement therapy in children with hemiplegic cerebral palsy: A randomized trial. *Neurorehabilitation and Neural Repair, 25,* 692–702. http://dx.doi.org/10.1177/1545968311402508

Gordon, A. M., & Magill, R. A. (2012). Motor learning: Application of principles to pediatric rehabilitation. In S. K. Campbell, R. J. Palisano, & M. N. Orlin (Eds.), *Physical therapy for children* (4th ed., pp. 151–174). New York: Elsevier.

Gordon, A. M., Schneider, J. A., Chinnan, A., & Charles, J. R. (2007). Efficacy of a hand–arm bimanual intensive therapy (HABIT) in children with hemiplegic cerebral palsy: A randomized control trial. *Developmental Medicine and Child Neurology, 49,* 830–838. PMID: 17979861

Gordon, A. M., & Steenbergen, B. (2008). Bimanual coordination in children with cerebral palsy. In A. C. Eliasson & P. Burtner (Eds.), *Improving hand function in children with cerebral palsy: Theory, evidence, and intervention* (pp. 160–175). London: Mackeith Press.

Gorter, H., Holty, L., Rameckers, E. E., Elvers, H. J., & Oostendorp, R. A. (2009). Changes in endurance and walking ability through functional physical training in children with cerebral palsy. *Pediatric Physical Therapy, 21,* 31–37.

Green, D., Schertz, M., Gordon, A. M., Moore, A., Margalti, T. S., Farquharson, Y., . . . Fattal-Valevski, F. (2013). A multisite study of functional outcomes following a themed approach to hand–arm bimanual intensive therapy for children with hemiplegia. *Developmental Medicine and Child Neurology, 55,* 527–533.

Haley, S. M., Coster, W. J., Ludlow, L. H., Haltiwanger, J., & Andrellos, P. (1992). *Pediatric Evaluation of Disability Inventory (PEDI).* Boston: New England Medical Center Hospitals.

Hanna, S., Law, M., Rosenbaum, P., King, G., Walter, S., Pollock, N., & Russell, D. J. (2003). Development of hand function among children with cerebral palsy: Growth curve analysis for ages 16 to 70 months. *Developmental Medicine and Child Neurology, 45,* 448–455.

Hoare, B. J., Imms, C., Rawicki, H. B., & Carey, L. (2010). Modified constraint-induced movement therapy or conventional occupational therapy following injection of botulinum toxin-A to improve bimanual performance in children with hemiplegic cerebral palsy: A randomised controlled trial methods paper. *Biomedical Central Neurology, 10,* 58–78.

Holmefur, M., Krumlinde-Sundholm, L., Bergstrom, J., & Eliasson, A. C. (2010). Longitudinal development of hand function in children with unilateral cerebral palsy. *Developmental Medicine and Child Neurology, 52,* 352–357.

Hung, Y.-C., Casertano, L., Hillman, A., & Gordon, A. M. (2011). The effect of training specificity on bimanual coordination in children with hemiplegia. *Research in Developmental Disabilities, 32,* 2724–2731.

Hung, Y. C., Charles, J., & Gordon, A. M. (2004). Bimanual coordination during a goal-directed task in children with hemiplegic cerebral palsy. *Developmental Medicine and Child Neurology, 46,* 746–753.

Hung, Y. C., Charles, J., & Gordon, A. M. (2010). Influence of accuracy constraints on bimanual coordination during a goal-directed task in children with hemiplegic cerebral palsy. *Experimental Brain Research, 201,* 421–428.

Islam, M., Gordon, A. M., Forssberg, H., Sköld, A., & Eliasson, A. C. (2011). Grip force coordination during a bimanual task in unilateral cerebral palsy. *Developmental Medicine and Child Neurology, 53,* 920–926.

Jebsen, R. H., Taylor, N., Trieschmann, R. B., Trotter, M. J., & Howard, L. A. (1969). An objective and standardized test of hand function. *Archives of Physical Medicine and Rehabilitation, 50,* 311–319.

Kantak, S. S., Sullivan, K. J., & Burtner, P. (2008). Motor learning in children with cerebral palsy: Implications for rehabilitation. In A. C. Eliasson & P. Burtner (Eds.), *Improving hand function in children with cerebral palsy: Theory, evidence and intervention* (pp. 260–275). London: MacKeith Press.

Ketelaar, M., Vermeer, A., Hart, H., van Petegem-van Beek, E., & Helders, P. J. (2001). Effects of a functional therapy program on motor abilities of children with cerebral palsy. *Physical Therapy, 81,* 1534–1545.

Kiresuk, T. J., Smith, A., & Cardillo, J. E. (1994). *Goal Attainment Scaling: Applications, theory, and measurement.* Hillsdale, NJ: Lawrence Erlbaum.

Kleim, J. A., Barbay, S., Cooper, N. R., Hogg, T. M., Reidel, C. N., Remple, M. S., & Nudo, R. J. (2002). Motor learning–dependent synaptogenesis is localized to functionally reorganized motor cortex. *Neurobiology of Learning and Memory, 77,* 63–77.

Krebs, H. I., Fasoli, S. E., Dipietro, L., Fragala-Pinkham, M., Hughes, R., Stein, J., & Hogan, N. (2012). Motor learning characterizes habilitation of children with hemiplegic cerebral palsy. *Neurorehabilitation and Neural Repair, 26,* 855–860.

Krumlinde-Sundholm, L., & Eliasson, A. C. (2003). Development of the Assisting Hand Assessment: A Rasch-built measure intended for children with unilateral upper limb impairments. *Scandinavian Journal of Occupational Therapy, 10,* 16–26.

Krumlinde-Sundholm, L., Holmefur, M., Kottorp, A., & Eliasson, A. C. (2007). The Assisting Hand Assessment: Current evidence of validity, reliability, and responsiveness to change. *Developmental Medicine and Child Neurology, 49,* 259–264.

Kuhnke, N., Juenger, H., Walther, M., Berweck, S., Mall, V., & Staudt, M. (2008). Do patients with congenital hemiparesis and ipsilateral corticospinal projections respond differently to constraint-induced movement therapy? *Developmental Medicine and Child Neurology, 50,* 898–903.

Law, M., Baptiste, S., McColl, M., Opzoomer, A., Polatajko, H., & Pollock, N. (1990). The Canadian Occupational Performance Measure: An outcome measure for occupational therapy. *Canadian Journal of Occupational Therapy, 57,* 82–87.

Law, M., Darrah, J., Pollock, N., Rosenbaum, P., Russell, D., Palisano, R., . . . Watt, J. (1998). Family-centred functional therapy for children with cerebral palsy: An emerging practical model. *Physical and Occupational Therapy in Pediatrics, 18,* 83–102.

Marshall, R. S., Perera, G. M., Lazar, R. M., Krakauer, J. W., Constantine, R. C., & DeLaPaz, R. L. (2000). Evolution of cortical activation during recovery from corticospinal tract infarction. *Stroke, 31,* 656–661.

Martin, J. H., Chakrabarty, S., & Friel, K. M. (2011). Harnessing activity-dependent plasticity to repair the damaged corticospinal tract in an animal model of cerebral palsy. *Developmental Medicine and Child Neurology, 53*(Suppl. 4), 9–13.

Martin, J. H., Choy, M., Pullman, S., & Meng, Z. (2004). Corticospinal system development depends on motor experience. *Journal of Neuroscience, 24,* 2122–2132.

Nudo, R. J. (2003). Functional and structural plasticity in motor cortex: Implications for stroke recovery. *Physical Medicine and Rehabilitation Clinics of North America, 14*(Suppl.), S57–S76.

Ochsner, K. N., & Lieberman, M. D. (2001). The emergence of social cognitive neuroscience. *American Psychologist, 56,* 717–734.

Øien, I., Fallang, B., & Østensjø, S. (2010). Goal-setting in paediatric rehabilitation: Perceptions of parents and professional. *Child Care, Health, and Development, 36,* 558–565.

Sakzewski, L. (2012). Bimanual therapy and constraint induced movement therapy are equally effective in improving hand function in children with congenital hemiplegia. *Journal of Physiotherapy, 58,* 59.

Sakzewski, L., Ziviani, J., Abbott, D. F., Macdonell, R. A., Jackson, G. D., & Boyd, R. N. (2011a). Participation outcomes in a randomized trial of 2 models of upper-limb rehabilitation for children with congenital hemiplegia. *Archives of Physical Medicine and Rehabilitation, 92,* 531–539.

Sakzewski, L., Ziviani, J., Abbott, D. F., Macdonell, R. A., Jackson, G. D., & Boyd, R. N. (2011b). Randomized trial of constraint-induced movement therapy and bimanual training on activity outcomes for children with congenital hemiplegia. *Developmental Medicine and Child Neurology, 53,* 313–320.

Sakzewski, L., Ziviani, J., & Boyd, R. N. (2011). Best responders after intensive upper-limb training for children with unilateral cerebral palsy. *Archives of Physical Medicine and Rehabilitation, 92,* 578–584.

Shumway-Cook, A., Hutchinson, S., Kartin, D., Price, R., & Woollacott, M. (2003). Effect of balance training on recovery of stability in children with cerebral palsy. *Developmental Medicine and Child Neurology, 45,* 591–602.

Sköld, A., Hermansson, L. N., Krumlinde-Sundholm, L., & Eliasson, A. (2011). Development and evidence of validity for the Children's Hand-Use Experience Questionnaire (CHEQ). *Developmental Medicine and Child Neurology, 53,* 436–442.

Sköld, A., Josephsson, S., & Eliasson, A. C. (2004). Performing bimanual activities: The experiences of young persons with hemiplegic cerebral palsy. *American Journal of Occupational Therapy, 58,* 416–425. http://dx.doi.org/10.5014/ajot.58.4.416

Staudt, M., Gerloff, C., Grodd, W., Holthausen, H., Niemann, G., & Krageloh-Mann, I. (2004). Reorganization in congenital hemiparesis acquired at different gestational ages. *Annals of Neurology, 56,* 854–863.

Steenbergen, B., Hulstijn, W., de Vries, A., & Berger, M. (1996). Bimanual movement coordination in spastic hemiparesis. *Experimental Brain Research, 110,* 91–98.

Steenbergen, B., Verrel, J., & Gordon, A. M. (2007). Motor planning in congenital hemiplegia. *Disability Research, 29,* 13–23.

Stinear, J. W., & Byblow, W. D. (2004). Rhythmic bilateral movement training modulates corticomotor excitability and enhances upper limb motricity poststroke: A pilot study. *Journal of Clinical Neurophysiology, 21,* 124–131.

Taub, E., Griffin, A., Nick, J., Gammons, K., Uswatte, G., & Law, C. R. (2007). Pediatric CI therapy for stroke-induced hemiparesis in young children. *Developmental Neurorehabilitation, 10,* 3–18.

Thorndike, E. L. (1914). *Educational psychology: Briefer course.* New York: Columbia University Press.

Uswatte, G., Giuliani, C., Winstein, C., Zeringue, A., Hobbs, L., & Wolf, S. L. (2006). Validity of accelerometry for monitoring real-world arm activity in patients with subacute stroke: Evidence from the extremity constraint-induced therapy evaluation trial. *Archives of Physical Medicine and Rehabilitation, 87,* 1340–1345.

Utley, A., & Steenbergen, B. (2006). Discrete bimanual co-ordination in children and young adolescents with hemiparetic cerebral palsy: Recent findings, implications and future research directions. *Pediatric Rehabilitation, 9,* 127–136.

Valvano, J., & Newell, K. M. (1998). Practice of a precision isometric grip-force task by children with spastic cerebral palsy. *Developmental Medicine and Child Neurology, 40,* 464–473.

Verschuren, O., Ketelaar, M., Gorter, J. W., Helders, P. J., & Takken, T. (2009). Relation between physical fitness and gross motor capacity in children and adolescents with cerebral palsy. *Developmental Medicine and Child Neurology, 51,* 866–871.

Wiesendanger, M., & Serrien, D. J. (2004). The quest to understand bimanual coordination. *Progress in Brain Research, 143,* 491–505.

Wolf, S. L, Catlin, P. A., Ellis, M., Archer, A. L., Morgan, B., & Piacentino, A. (2001). Assessing Wolf Motor Function Test as outcome measure for research in patients after stroke. *Stroke, 32,* 1635–1639.

TASOS KARAKOSTAS, MPT, PhD, and ERIK C. KING, MD, MS

14

Beyond Upper-Extremity Benefits of Pediatric CIMT: Reported Changes in Gait and Other Neuromotor Skills

CHAPTER HIGHLIGHTS

- Theoretical structure for additional benefits of pediatric CIMT
- Gait of children with hemiplegia and pediatric CIMT
- Gait of children with brachial plexus and pediatric CIMT.

KEY TERMS

Brachial plexus injury
Cortical reorganization
Corticospinal–pyramidal system
Hemiplegia
Mechanical coupling
Neural plasticity
Reticulospinal system
Vestibular system

The underlying theoretical and practical foundations of pediatric constraint-induced movement therapy (P–CIMT) to address upper-extremity (UE) motor deficits have been presented in previous chapters of this book. The body of literature and knowledge has increased sufficiently to allow randomized controlled studies involving comparisons between P–CIMT and other approaches, including intensive occupational therapy approaches (Echols, DeLuca, Ramey, & Taub, 2002; Eliasson, Krumlinde-Sundholm, Shaw, & Wang, 2005; Taub, Ramey, DeLuca, & Echols, 2004; Wallen et al., 2011).

Nearly all studies of P–CIMT, however, have focused on UE deficits secondary to learned nonuse (Crocker, MacKay-Lyons, & McDonnell, 1997; DeLuca, Echols, Ramey, & Taub, 2003; Echols et al., 2002). Moreover, the patient population that overwhelmingly appears to be the focus of the P–CIMT approach is children with hemiplegic cerebral palsy (CP; Eliasson et al., 2005; Gordon, Charles, & Wolf, 2005; Taub et al., 2004). A need is present, therefore, to explore whether other functional benefits related to P–CIMT exist and whether these benefits can be achieved for other pediatric patient populations with UE motor deficits.

THEORETICAL STRUCTURE FOR ADDITIONAL BENEFITS OF P–CIMT

In addition to the work of Taub and others (DeLuca, Case-Smith, Stevenson, & Ramey, 2012; DeLuca, Echols, Law, & Ramey, 2006; Echols et al., 2002; Taub et al., 2004), presented elsewhere in this book, other basic science–based research, both earlier and concurrent, provides a theoretical infrastructure for additional benefits that may stem from the use of P–CIMT. Findings by Illert and coworkers and by Alstermark and colleagues are worth mentioning (Alstermark, Isa, & Tantisira, 1990; Alstermark, Lindström, Lundberg, & Sybirska, 1981; Alstermark & Lundberg, 1982; Alstermark, Lundberg, Pinter, & Sasaki, 1987a; Alstermark, Lundberg, & Sasaki, 1984a, 1984b, 1984c; Alstermark, Pinter, & Sasaki, 1983, 1985; Fritz, Illert, & Reeh, 1982; Fritz, Illert, & Saggau, 1981; Gödderz, Illert, & Yamaguchi, 1990; Grant, Illert, & Tanaka, 1980; Illert, Jankowska, Lundberg, & Odutola, 1981; Illert, Lundberg, Padel, & Tanaka, 1978; Illert, Lundberg, & Tanaka, 1976a, 1976b, 1977; Illert & Wiedemann, 1984; Maier, Illert, Kirkwood, Nielsen, & Lemon, 1998). Both groups have published an extended body of literature focused on mapping the primary and alternative neural pathways involved in controlling UE function, with a focus on the C3–C5 propriospinal neurons.

Of course, alternative neural pathways are a manifestation of neural plasticity, serving to take over the continuation and restoration of function after a defect and subsequent cortical reorganization (Alstermark, Isa, Lundberg, Pettersson, & Tantisira, 1989, 1991; Alstermark, Lundberg, Pettersson, Tantisira, & Walkowska, 1987; Alstermark, Pinter, & Sasaki, 1992; Isa, Ohki, Alstermark, Pettersson, & Sasaki, 2007; Pettersson, Alstermark, Blagovechtchenski, Isa, & Sasaski, 2007; Pettersson, Lundberg, Alstermark, Isa, & Tantisira, 1997; Sasaki et al., 2004). **Neural plasticity** encompasses changes or adaptations in the structure, function, and organization of the nervous systems (neurons, or nerve cells, and neural pathways) in response to new experiences that may occur after injury or during rehabilitation and recovery. **Cortical reorganization** comprises changes in the organization and function of the brain.

What has been of further interest, however, is that the same alternative neural pathways and their respective centers of origin in the brain that have been identified as being involved in the restoration of UE function after damage are also involved in postural and lower-extremity (LE) functions. For example, the C3–C5 propriospinal neurons receive input from the corticospinal, rubrospinal, tectospinal, reticulospinal, and vestibular tracts to control UE function. The same neurons, however, project to the lumbar segments and, along with the corticospinal–pyramidal and vestibular systems, are involved

in stabilizing the trunk during UE activities (Alstermark, Lundberg, Pinter, & Sasaki, 1987b).

The importance of the corticospinal–pyramidal, reticulospinal, and vestibular systems and respective brain centers for LE function has been established (Gage, Schwartz, Koop, & Novacheck, 2009). The **corticospinal–pyramidal system** includes both the corticospinal and corticobulbar tracts; they contain mostly axons originated from the motor cortex and transmit information from the brain to the spinal cord. The **reticulospinal system** (or anterior reticulospinal tract) is an extrapyramidal subconscious motor tract that descends from the reticular formation in two tracts to supply information from the brain to the trunk and proximal limb muscles. The **vestibular system** provides a person with a sense of spatial orientation and contributes information related to body movement and balance. The vestibular system comprises two main components: the semicircular canal system, which indicates rotational movements, and the otolith organs, which indicate linear accelerations. The internal capsule, an integral component of the cortical control of the locomotor system (Gage et al., 2009), through which the corticospinal fibers pass, has been found to be involved in UE function and the control of hand movement (Wenzelburger et al., 2005). Consequently, the UE, LE, and postural neurocontrolling mechanisms appear to noticeably overlap.

The mechanical coupling between the UE and LE for a smooth, coordinated, and symmetrical gait also has been established. **Mechanical coupling** refers to the dual control by physical forces in the body of both upper- and lower-body movements. During natural walking gait, at self-selected speeds and at increased speeds, the LE generates angular momentum that is counteracted by the contralateral UE, resulting in a more energy-efficient gait (Capozzo, 1993; Donker, Mulder, Nienhuis, & Duysens, 2002).

Preliminary studies with adults who experienced a cerebrovascular accident and were treated with CIMT to address UE deficits have reported concurrent benefits to overall posture, balance, and LE function. Positive outcomes included increased loading capability of the hemiparetic LE, resulting in more symmetrical weight-bearing capabilities of the involved and uninvolved LEs, improved balance, and small gains in gait and mobility (Fritz, Pittman, Robinson, Orton, & Rivers, 2007; Taub, Uswatte, & Pidikiti, 1999; Vearrier, Langan, Shumway-Cook, & Woollacott, 2005).

Consequently, in light of this theoretical and experimental infrastructure, our group, to the best of our knowledge, was the first to investigate and report on the potential effects of P–CIMT on the LE function of children with UE deficits (Coker, Karakostas, Dodds, & Hsiang, 2010; Karakostas, Coker, & Hsiang, 2009). Our work is guided by the hypothesis that P–CIMT, either directly, through cortical reorganization and recruitment of related neurological pathways to the LE, or indirectly, by facilitating the mechanical coupling of the UE and LE as a function of improved UE motor performance secondary to P–CIMT participation, has an effect on the walking gait of children participating in a P–CIMT program.

Note that since our first set of reports and presentations, two more reports have identified a relationship between P–CIMT and gait (Gillick & Koppes, 2010; Zipp & Winning, 2012). Consequently, although the results of our studies are specific to the characteristics of our program and our approach in implementing it, the existence of two additional reports on the relationship between P–CIMT and gait supports our conclusion that participation in a P–CIMT program can exert positive effects on the walking gait of participants.

GAIT OF CHILDREN WITH HEMIPLEGIA AND P–CIMT

Our group first looked at changes in the gait characteristics of children with **hemiplegia** (i.e., weakness on one side of the body) as a function of P–CIMT and as a function of the orthotic intervention used (Coker et al., 2010; Karakostas, Coker, Bonk, & Dias, 2009; Karakostas et al., 2009). In our first study, preschool-age children with hemiplegic CP participated in a day camp in an academic setting for 5 consecutive days (Medical University of South Carolina, Charleston). Each day involved 6 hours of P–CIMT. The camp approach was similar

to that described in Chapter 10 of this volume and elsewhere (Eliasson, Bonnier, & Krumlinde-Sundholm, 2003). The uninvolved UE was constrained with a puppet mitt covering a resting hand splint.

Children who participated in this study were at Gross Motor Functional Classification System (GMFCS) Levels I to III on the basis of self-initiated movement during sitting (trunk control) and walking (Palisano, Rosenbaum, Bartlett, & Livingston, 2007; Palisano et al., 1997). The weaker hand had, at minimum, 10° of voluntary finger extension and could serve as at least a gross assist during self-care and play activities. The side of hemiparesis was equally distributed among the group of participants. Cognitively, each participant was able to follow at least two-step commands.

Although a licensed occupational therapist and physical therapist provided the overall supervision and management of the camp, each child who participated in the camp received P–CIMT from an occupational therapy student and a physical therapy student trained in the techniques of P–CIMT. These therapy camp counselors were charged with the responsibility of addressing a subset of the specific UE deficits identified for each participant during pretesting. All participating children had been involved in traditional occupational and physical therapy programs before attending the P–CIMT camp. Figure 14.1 shows a typical camp activity.

The neurokinematics of walking gait reach their adultlike patterns around age 6 or 7 years; they seem to be inconsistent before age 4 years (Sutherland, 1997; Sutherland, Olsen,

Figure 14.1   CHILD AT CAMP WORKING ON BALANCE AND REACHING WHILE COMPLETING AN OBSTACLE COURSE; A CONSTRAINT MITT IS WORN ON THE LEFT HAND.

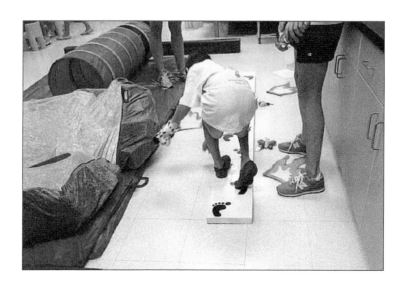

Source. P. Coker-Bolt.

Biden, & Wyatt, 1988). With appropriate normalization approaches, however, the time–distance characteristics of walking gait become stable as early as age 2 years (Hoff, 1996). Consequently, our study focused on the effects of the P–CIMT program on the time–distance characteristics of the walking gait of children with hemiplegic CP.

The temporal–spatial parameters defining walking gait include walking velocity, cadence, stride length and time, right–left step length and time, right–left single-limb stance time, double-limb stance time, right–left swing phase time, overall stance time, and base of support. On the basis of selected time–distance parameters, walking symmetry can also be assessed. The parameters defining walking symmetry are the step-time differential between the right and left steps and the step-length differential between the right and left steps. An operational definition of each of these terms appears in Appendix 14.A.

To collect all of our time–distance walking parameters, we used the GAITRite system, an 18-ft-long instrumented electronic walkway (CIR Systems, Clifton, NJ). The GAITRite contains embedded sensors that can sample at a rate up to 333 Hz. We sampled our data at 80 Hz, allowing a time resolution of 0.0125 seconds per sampled data point. The reliability of the GAITRite in accurately assessing the temporal–spatial characteristics of gait across the entire age spectrum has been found to be excellent (Bilney, Morris, & Webster, 2003; Cutlip, Mancinelli, Huber, & DiPasquale, 2000; McDonough, Batavia, Chen, Kwon, & Ziai, 2001; Menz, Latt, Tiedemann, Mun San Kwan, & Lord, 2004; van Uden & Besser, 2004; Webster, Wittwer, & Feller, 2005). Figure 14.2 shows children using the GAITRite walkway.

Although a summary of our data collection procedures has been published elsewhere (Coker et al., 2010), we must emphasize that all children were instructed to walk the length of the carpet at their natural, typical, self-selected speed. Having the children walk in this way was important to ensure that only automatic control neural pathways were involved in the walking patterns we were capturing (Egerton, Danoudis, Huxham, & Iansek, 2011). All children were tested barefoot, and children who were using ankle–foot orthoses (AFOs) were also tested with their AFOs so we could assess gait changes from the P–CIMT intervention that were not necessarily related to the AFOs. For children who were tested both with and without their AFOs, the order of testing was randomized. All children were tested within the week before the start of the P–CIMT camp (pretest) and within 3 days after the camp (posttest). (All children were also tested 6 months after they completed camp; these data will be the subject of a future report.)

Partial results for barefoot testing before and after camp have previously been published (Coker et al., 2010). The current state of our analysis demonstrates the same statistically significant trends after participation in the P–CIMT camp-based program: increases in walking velocity, cadence, step length (of both the involved and uninvolved LE), and single-limb stance time (of both the involved and uninvolved LE). We also observed statistically significant decreases in the base

Figure 14.2   CHILDREN USING THE GAITRite WALKWAY.

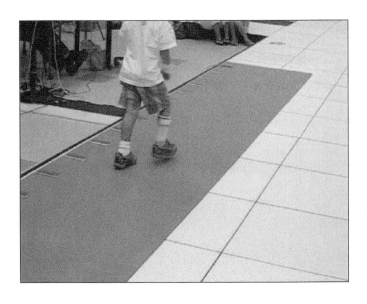
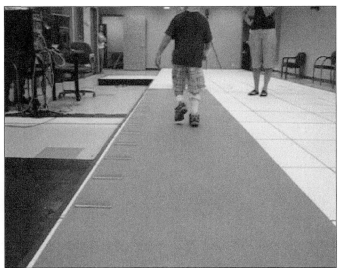

of support and double-limb stance time, as well as a decrease in the step-time difference—all important for walking ability. The reduced base of support combined with the increased single-limb stance time and decreased double-limb stance time are valuable for balance. The decreases in the step-time difference between the involved and uninvolved LEs help a child achieve a more symmetrical gait.

The most important differences between testing before and after P–CIMT camp for the children who had AFOs are shown in Table 14.1. These data provide some insight into the manner in which P–CIMT and the orthotic intervention may have contributed together and individually to improved walking patterns after the P–CIMT camp intervention (Karakostas et al., 2009). When the "Barefoot × AFO Interaction" column of Table 14.1 shows no significant interaction between the barefoot and AFO conditions, the remaining two columns demonstrate the individual contributions of either the P–CIMT camp (barefoot)

or the use of the AFO. Our data analysis suggests that P–CIMT had a direct effect on reducing the step-time difference (from 0.08 to 0.04 seconds), therefore making the gait more symmetrical. Moreover, single-limb support time, expressed as a percentage of the gait cycle time of the involved LE, increased from 34.53% to 37.32% as a result of the P–CIMT camp. With respect to the base of support, an interaction between P–CIMT camp AFO use is obvious. However, the effectiveness of the P–CIMT camp was stronger in the changes in the base of support, which decreased from an average of 11.05 cm at pretest to 9.3 cm at posttest. Consequently, increased balance appears to be related more to P–CIMT than to the use of the AFO. The data suggest that when P–CIMT and bracing are used in combination, the gait becomes even more effective. Velocity is increased because of an increase in step length for both the involved and uninvolved LE, which is related to decreased double-limb support time and increased swing time to take the next step.

Table 14.1 SUMMARY OF TEMPORAL–SPATIAL GAIT CHARACTERISTICS FOR WALKING BAREFOOT AND WITH AFOS BEFORE AND AFTER P–CIMT CAMP

PARAMETER[a]	BAREFOOT, *p*	AFO, *p*	BAREFOOT × AFO INTERACTION, *p*
Mean normalized velocity	.0017	.0001	.0092
Normalized step length (step length/leg length)			
Involved LE	**.0071**	.05	.2191
Uninvolved LE (% gait cycle)	**.0017**	<.0001	.0081
Single support			
Involved LE	**.0064**	.0997	.4308
Uninvolved LE	.014	<.0001	.0522
Double support (% gait cycle)			
Involved LE	**<.0001**	<.0001	.0622
Uninvolved LE	**<.0001**	<.0001	.0403
Swing phase			
Involved LE	.0186	.0824	.0055
Uninvolved LE	.0018	<.0001	.7676
Base of support	**<.0001**	.1327	.0018
Step-time difference	**.0436**	.8747	.8464

Note. Bolded data demonstrate the individual effect of the P–CIMT camp (Barefoot column) or of the use of the AFO. AFO = ankle–foot orthosis; LE = lower extremity; P–CIMT = pediatric constraint-induced movement therapy.
[a]For an operational definition of each term, see Appendix 14.A.

As noted earlier, Gillick and Koppes (2010) and Zipp and Winning (2012) also published findings of improved walking ability after participation in a P–CIMT camp. Gillick and Koppes conducted a qualitative study investigating the effects of a 19-day (3 hours/day) P–CIMT program on the gross motor and LE functional changes of 6 independently ambulatory children (aged 5–11 years) with spastic hemiparesis, GMFCS Level I. They reported improvements in participants' walking ability after the P–CIMT intervention. In fact, using the standing (Section D) and the walking–running–jumping (Section E) categories of the GMFCS tool, Gillick and Koppes detected improvements in both sections, reflecting overall improved LE function secondary to P–CIMT intervention. The largest improvements were in the walking–running–jumping section.

Zipp and Winning (2012) investigated the effects of a 15-day (6 hours/day) P–CIMT program on the walking and LE function of 16 children with hemiplegia (aged 4 to 12 years). Walking performance was quantified with the use of the GAITRite. However, this study was limited in scope as far as gait is concerned because the authors focused only on the velocity, cadence, and number-of-steps outcome measures of the GAITRite. The young age of some of the children potentially allowed for uncontrolled neurokinematic variability in the sample population, especially considering that the measured parameters were not normalized to account for anthropometric variability. Children were fitted with a complete cast to constrain the uninvolved UE from midhumerus down to the distal end of the extremity. Whether such an approach enforces or effectively facilitates the coupling mechanism between the UEs and LEs is doubtful, however, because of the movement constraint imposed on the elbow joint (Webb, Tuttle, & Baksh, 1994). Finally, children received a total of 90 hours of P–CIMT. The children who participated in the camp-based P–CIMT program demonstrated improvements in walking velocity and cadence.

GAIT OF CHILDREN WITH BRACHIAL PLEXUS AND P–CIMT

We also considered whether P–CIMT to treat children with **brachial plexus (BP) injury** (i.e., UE weakness related to insult or injury to nerves in the brachial plexus) that involves no apparent LE deficits would have a significant effect on LE gait function. A group of preschool-age children with BP injury participated in a 10-day P–CIMT camp in a hospital-based outpatient setting (Children's Memorial Hospital, Chicago) and were compared with a control group of children of similar age with BP injury who participated in the hospital's traditional occupational therapy program for children with BP injury.

Participation in the camp involved 3 hours per day of P–CIMT and a home exercise program for the two intervening weekends. The activities and structure of this camp were very similar to those of our previous study, including cross-site training. This camp was supervised by occupational therapy practitioners who addressed each child's UE and overall mobility deficits during the camp. Each child worked with a volunteer who was given training on the camp and basic principles of P–CIMT. All participants had received traditional occupational therapy before joining the P–CIMT camp.

Collection and reporting of the time–distance walking parameters were identical to those in our previous study. P–CIMT camp participants were tested barefoot in the week before the camp (pretesting), within 3 days after the camp (posttesting), and 6 months after completion of the camp. Control children similarly were tested at baseline and then after receiving 30 hours of traditional treatment. Because the children with BP injury who were randomized into the traditional program were seen 2 or 3 times a month, we included only 1 posttreatment testing session.

Current exploration of our data implementing discriminant analysis has been focused on the nonbilateral outcome measures of the GAITRite. These parameters include the velocity, cadence, base of support, and step-time and step-length differentials between the right and the left steps. Table 14.2 shows that the P–CIMT camp group demonstrated significantly greater velocity and cadence and smaller step-length difference during the first post-P–CIMT evaluation than did the control group, who demonstrated no significant improvements. In addition, walking symmetry (step-length difference) improved significantly as a result of P–CIMT, and when contrasted with the control group, the P–CIMT group showed significantly greater improvement.

Of perhaps greater interest is that when one observes UE performance as a function of the P–CIMT versus a traditional pediatric rehabilitation approach, both the experimental and control groups appeared to improve (Karakostas, Bednarek, Rodman, & King, 2011; Karakostas, Bednarek, Rodman, & Malas, 2011). However, when one observes the gait of the control group, a similar improvement is not detected. Our results show that the step-length difference increased for the children who participated in traditional occupational therapy treatment, whereas it decreased for the children who participated in the P–CIMT camp. Therefore, improvement in UE function in traditional pediatric rehabilitation appears to be segment specific, whereas improvement after P–CIMT is more global—that is, it expands to other functions, such as that of the LE, and other functional activities, such as walking.

Moreover, if improved LE function during gait was related only to the improved coupling mechanism as a result of improved

Table 14.2   SUMMARY OF TEMPORAL–SPATIAL GAIT CHARACTERISTICS FOR VELOCITY, CADENCE, AND STEP LENGTH BEFORE AND AFTER P–CIMT CAMP

PARAMETER	BEFORE P–CIMT, MEAN (*SD*)	AFTER P–CIMT, MEAN (*SD*)	*p*	BEFORE P–CIMT, EXPERIMENTAL VS. CONTROL, *p*	AFTER P–CIMT, EXPERIMENTAL VS. CONTROL, *p*
Normalized velocity				.24	.58
Experimental	3.57 (0.80)	3.96 (0.69)	.02*		
Control	3.95 (0.23)	4.12 (0.80)	.61		
Normalized cadence				.06	.06
Experimental	293.56 (30.22)	313.37 (27.36)	.01*		
Control	308.19 (19.38)	323.16 (39.47)	.36		
Step length, difference				.84	.04*
Experimental	0.98 (0.34)	0.50 (0.40)	.02*		
Control	0.89 (0.66)	1.92 (0.95)	.18		

Note. P–CIMT = pediatric constraint-induced movement therapy; *SD* = standard deviation.
*$p \leq .05$.

UE function, then a successful traditional occupational therapy approach to address UE deficits would also result in walking improvements. However, our results suggested that this is not the case. Therefore, it may be that the primary underlying foundation of the improved gait performance of the children with BP injury may be related to the corticoplastic changes induced as a function of the P–CIMT approach.

To date, our results have suggested that P–CIMT has a positive effect on the temporal–spatial aspects of gait. The LE base of support can improve directly as the result of P–CIMT participation. Children who participated in the P–CIMT camp program used a narrower base of support after the camp, suggesting decreased demands for postural stability. Symmetry also improved, as reflected in the decrease in the step-length differential after the camp. A more symmetrical gait can also decrease postural and energy demands during walking. Therefore, it may be that P–CIMT can be used for at least partial remediation of LE deficits or remediation of walking deficits related to UE function. Consequently, we propose that measurement of the temporal–spatial aspects of gait after P–CIMT could provide an additional means to determine the success of P–CIMT programs and begin to shift the focus of intervention to both UE and LE deficits.

Finally, we have observed that gait symmetry appears to consistently improve with P–CIMT. A more symmetrical gait is also a more rhythmical gait. An independent study suggested that improvements in rhythmical motion may be further related to cognitive improvements (Goldshtrom, Knorr, & Goldshtrom, 2010). In addition, the parents of 3 of the children who participated in our P–CIMT program commented that the children's language skills improved as the camp progressed. Consequently, it appears that P–CIMT may be related to other changes that may have social or other implications.

SUMMARY

To date, most research on P–CIMT has focused on remediation of UE deficits secondary to learned nonuse, but emerging studies are now looking at spillover or secondary effects of constraint therapy on other body systems, including gross motor function, balance, and gait. The preliminary findings of these studies and the information presented in this chapter highlight the importance of P–CIMT for overall functional abilities and participation level in daily life activities. Practitioners engaging children in P–CIMT should closely monitor any secondary effects of this intervention.

REFERENCES

Alstermark, B., Isa, T., Lundberg, A., Pettersson, L. G., & Tantisira, B. (1989). The effect of low pyramidal lesions on forelimb movements in the cat. *Neuroscience Research, 7,* 71–75.

Alstermark, B., Isa, T., Lundberg, A., Pettersson, L. G., & Tantisira, B. (1991). The effect of a low pyramidal transection following previous transection of the dorsal column in cats. *Neuroscience Research, 11*, 215–220.

Alstermark, B., Isa, T., & Tantisira, B. (1990). Projection from excitatory C3–C4 propriospinal neurones to spinocere-bellar and spinoreticular neurones in the C6–Th1 segments of the cat. *Neuroscience Research, 8*, 124–130.

Alstermark, B., Lindström, S., Lundberg, A., & Sybirska, E. (1981). Integration in descending motor pathways controlling the forelimb in the cat: 8. Ascending projection to the lateral reticular nucleus from C3–C4 propriospinal also projecting to forelimb motoneurones. *Experimental Brain Research, 42*, 282–298.

Alstermark, B., & Lundberg, A. (1982). Electrophysiological evidence against the hypothesis that corticospinal fibres send collaterals to the lateral reticular nucleus. *Experimental Brain Research, 47*, 148–150.

Alstermark, B., Lundberg, A., Pettersson, L. G., Tantisira, B., & Walkowska, M. (1987). Motor recovery after serial spinal cord lesions of defined descending pathways in cats. *Neuroscience Research, 5*, 68–73.

Alstermark, B., Lundberg, A., Pinter, M., & Sasaki, S. (1987a). Vestibular effects in long C3–C5 propriospinal neurones. *Brain Research, 404*, 389–394.

Alstermark, B., Lundberg, A., Pinter, M., & Sasaki, S. (1987b). Subpopulations and functions of long C3–C5 propriospinal neurones. *Brain Research, 404*, 395–400.

Alstermark, B., Lundberg, A., & Sasaki, S. (1984a). Integration in descending motor pathways controlling the forelimb in the cat: 10. Inhibitory pathways to forelimb motoneurones via C3–C4 propriospinal neurones. *Experimental Brain Research, 56*, 279–292.

Alstermark, B., Lundberg, A., & Sasaki, S. (1984b). Integration in descending motor pathways controlling the forelimb in the cat: 11. Inhibitory pathways from higher motor centres and forelimb afferents to C3–C4 propriospinal neurones. *Experimental Brain Research, 56*, 293–307.

Alstermark, B., Lundberg, A., & Sasaki, S. (1984c). Integration in descending motor pathways controlling the forelimb in the cat: 12. Interneurones which may mediate descending feed-forward inhibition and feed-back inhibition from the forelimb to C3–C4 propriospinal neurones. *Experimental Brain Research, 56*, 308–322.

Alstermark, B., Pinter, M., & Sasaki, S. (1983). Brainstem relay of disynaptic pyramidal EPSPs to neck motoneurons in the cat. *Brain Research, 259*, 147–150.

Alstermark, B., Pinter, M. J., & Sasaki, S. (1985). Pyramidal effects in dorsal neck motoneurones of the cat. *Journal of Physiology, 363*, 287–302.

Alstermark, B., Pinter, M. J., & Sasaki, S. (1992). Tectal and tegmental excitation in dorsal neck motoneurones of the cat. *Journal of Physiology, 454*, 517–532.

Bilney, B., Morris, M., & Webster, K. (2003). Concurrent related validity of the GAITRite walkway system for quantification of the spatial and temporal parameters of gait. *Gait and Posture, 17*, 68–74.

Capozzo, A. (1993). The forces and couples in the human trunk during level walking. *Journal of Biomechanics, 16*, 265–277.

Coker, P., Karakostas, T., Dodds, C., & Hsiang, S. (2010). Gait characteristics of children with hemiplegic cerebral palsy before and after modified constraint-induced movement therapy. *Disability and Rehabilitation, 32*, 402–408. http://dx.doi.org/10.3109/09638280903171592

Crocker, M. D., MacKay-Lyons, M., & McDonnell, E. (1997). Forced use of the upper extremity in cerebral palsy: A single-case design. *American Journal of Occupational Therapy, 51*, 824–833. http://dx.doi.org/10.5014/ajot.51.10.824

Cutlip, R. G., Mancinelli, C., Huber, F., & DiPasquale, J. (2000). Evaluation of an instrumented walkway for measurement of the kinematic parameters of gait. *Gait and Posture, 12*, 134–138.

DeLuca, S. C., Case-Smith, J., Stevenson, R., & Ramey, S. L. (2012). Constraint-induced movement therapy (CIMT) for young children with cerebral palsy: Effects of therapeutic dosage. *Journal of Pediatric Rehabilitation Medicine, 5*, 133–142. http://dx.doi.org/10.3221/PRM-2012-02.06

DeLuca, S. C., Echols, K., Law, C. R., & Ramey, S. L. (2006). Intensive pediatric constraint-induced therapy for children with cerebral palsy: Randomized, controlled, crossover trial. *Journal of Child Neurology, 21*, 931–938. PMID: 17092457

DeLuca, S. C., Echols, K., Ramey, S. L., & Taub, E. (2003). Pediatric constraint-induced movement therapy for a young child with cerebral palsy: Two episodes of care. *Physical Therapy, 83*, 1003–1013. PMID: 14577827

Donker, S. F., Mulder, T., Nienhuis, B., & Duysens, J. (2002). Adaptations in arm movements for added mass to wrist or ankle during walking. *Experimental Brain Research, 146*, 26–31.

Echols, K., DeLuca, S., Ramey, S., & Taub, E. (2002). Constraint-induced movement therapy versus traditional therapeutic services for young children with cerebral palsy: A randomized controlled trial. *Developmental Medicine and Child Neurology, 44*, 29.

Egerton, T., Danoudis, M., Huxham, F., & Iansek, R. (2011). Central gait control mechanisms and the stride length–cadence relationship. *Gait and Posture, 34*, 178–182.

Eliasson, A. C., Bonnier, B., & Krumlinde-Sundholm, L. (2003). Clinical experience of constraint induced movement therapy in adolescents with hemiplegic cerebral palsy—A day camp model. *Developmental Medicine and Child Neurology, 45,* 357–359.

Eliasson, A. C., Krumlinde-Sundholm, L., Shaw, K., & Wang, C. (2005). Effects of constraint-induced movement therapy in young children with hemiplegic cerebral palsy: An adapted model. *Developmental Medicine and Child Neurology, 47,* 266–275.

Fritz, N., Illert, M., & Reeh, P. (1982). Location of median and ulnar motornuclei in the cat. *Neuroscience Letters, 30,* 103–108.

Fritz, N., Illert, M., & Saggau, P. (1981). Location of dorsal interosseus motor nuclei in the cat. *Neuroscience Letters, 21,* 243–248.

Fritz, S. L., Pittman, A. L., Robinson, A. C., Orton, S. C., & Rivers, E. D. (2007). An intense intervention for improving gait, balance, and mobility for individuals with chronic stroke: A pilot study. *Journal of Neurologic Physical Therapy, 31,* 71–76.

Gage, J. R., Schwartz, M. H., Koop, S. E., & Novacheck, T. F. (2009). *The identification and treatment of gait problems in cerebral palsy* (2nd ed.). London: Mac Keith Press.

Gillick, B. T., & Koppes, A. (2010). Gross motor outcomes in children with hemiparesis involved in a modified constraint-induced therapy program. *Journal of Pediatric Rehabilitation Medicine, 3,* 171–175.

Gödderz, W., Illert, M., & Yamaguchi, T. (1990). Efferent pattern of fictive locomotion in the cat forelimb: With special reference to radial motor nuclei. *European Journal of Neuroscience, 2,* 663–671.

Goldshtrom, Y., Knorr, G., & Goldshtrom, I. (2010). Rhythmic exercises in rehabilitation of TBI patients: A case report. *Journal of Bodywork and Movement Therapies, 14,* 336–345.

Gordon, A. M., Charles, J., & Wolf, S. L. (2005). Methods of constraint-induced movement therapy for children with hemiplegic cerebral palsy: Development of a child-friendly intervention for improving upper-extremity function. *Archives of Physical Medicine and Rehabilitation, 86,* 837–844.

Grant, G., Illert, M., & Tanaka, R. (1980). Integration in descending motor pathways controlling the forelimb in the cat: 6. Anatomical evidence consistent with the existence of C3–C4 propriospinal neurones projecting to forelimb motornuclei. *Experimental Brain Research, 38,* 87–93.

Hoff, A. L. (1996). Scaling gait data to body size. *Gait and Posture, 4,* 222–223.

Illert, M., Jankowska, E., Lundberg, A., & Odutola, A. (1981). Integration in descending motor pathways controlling the forelimb in the cat: 7. Effects from the reticular formation on C3–C4 propriospinal neurones. *Experimental Brain Research, 42,* 269–281.

Illert, M., Lundberg, A., Padel, Y., & Tanaka, R. (1978). Integration in descending motor pathways controlling the forelimb in the cat: 5. Properties of and monosynaptic excitatory convergence on C3–C4 propriospinal neurones. *Experimental Brain Research, 33,* 101–130.

Illert, M., Lundberg, A., & Tanaka, R. (1976a). Integration in descending motor pathways controlling the forelimb in the cat: 1. Pyramidal effects on motoneurones. *Experimental Brain Research, 26,* 509–519.

Illert, M., Lundberg, A., & Tanaka, R. (1976b). Integration in descending motor pathways controlling the forelimb in the cat: 2. Convergence on neurones mediating disynaptic cortico-motoneuronal excitation. *Experimental Brain Research, 26,* 521–540.

Illert, M., Lundberg, A., & Tanaka, R. (1977). Integration in descending motor pathways controlling the forelimb in the cat: 3. Convergence on propriospinal neurones transmitting disynaptic excitation from the corticospinal tract and other descending tracts. *Experimental Brain Research, 29,* 323–346.

Illert, M., & Wiedemann, E. (1984). Pyramidal actions in identified radial motornuclei of the cat. *Pflugers Archiv: European Journal of Physiology, 401,* 132–142.

Isa, T., Ohki, Y., Alstermark, B., Pettersson, L. G., & Sasaki, S. (2007). Direct and indirect cortico-motoneuronal pathways and control of hand/arm movements. *Physiology, 22,* 145–152.

Karakostas, T., Bednarek, M., Rodman, L., & King, E. (2011, November). *Exploring corticoplasticity to treat upper extremity deficits in children with brachial plexus injury using constraint induced movement therapy: Assessment of upper and lower extremity function, gait.* Paper presented at the meeting of the Society for Neuroscience, Washington, DC.

Karakostas, T., Bednarek, M., Rodman, L., & Malas, B. (2011, October). *Brachial plexus injury: A randomized control study to address upper extremity function using modified constraint-induced movement therapy.* Paper presented at the meeting of the Illinois Occupational Therapy Association, Galena.

Karakostas, T., Coker, P., Bonk, M., & Dias, L. (2009, October). *Can a modified constraint induced movement therapy protocol affect the walking gait of children with hemiplegia?* Paper presented at the meeting of the Illinois Physical Therapy Association, Bloomington, IL.

Karakostas, T., Coker, P., & Hsiang, S. (2009, May). *Modified constrained induced movement therapy: Effects on selected gait characteristics of children with hemiplegia.* Paper presented at the meeting of the Gait and Clinical Motion Analysis Society, Denver, CO.

Maier, M. A., Illert, M., Kirkwood, P. A., Nielsen, J., & Lemon, R. N. (1998). Does a C3–C4 propriospinal system transmit corticospinal excitation in the primate? An investigation in the macaque monkey. *Journal of Physiology, 511,* 191–212.

McDonough, A. L., Batavia, M., Chen, F. C., Kwon, S., & Ziai, J. (2001). The validity and reliability of the GAITRite system's measurements: A preliminary evaluation. *Archives of Physical Medicine and Rehabilitation, 82,* 419–425.

Menz, H. B., Latt, M. D., Tiedemann, A., Mun San Kwan, M., & Lord, S. R. (2004). Reliability of the GAITRite walkway system for the quantification of temporo-spatial parameters of gait in young and older people. *Gait and Posture, 20,* 20–25.

Palisano, R., Rosenbaum, P., Bartlett, D., & Livingston, M. (2007). *GMFCS–E & R: Gross Motor Function Classification System expanded and revised.* Hamilton, Ontario: CanChild Centre for Childhood Disability Research, McMaster University. Retrieved from http://motorgrowth.canchild. ca/en/GMFCS/resources/GMFCS-ER.pdf

Palisano, R., Rosenbaum, P., Walter, S., Russell, D., Wood, E., & Galuppi, B. (1997). Development and reliability of a system to classify gross motor function in children with cerebral palsy. *Developmental Medicine and Child Neurology, 39,* 214–223.

Pettersson, L. G., Alstermark, B., Blagovechtchenski, E., Isa, T., & Sasaski, S. (2007). Skilled digit movements in feline and primate—recovery after selective spinal cord lesions. *Acta Physiologica, 189,* 141–154.

Pettersson, L. G., Lundberg, A., Alstermark, B., Isa, T., & Tantisira, B. (1997). Effect of spinal cord lesions on forelimb target-reaching and on visually guided switching of target-reaching in the cat. *Neuroscience Research, 29,* 241–256.

Sasaki, S., Isa, T., Pettersson, L. G., Alstermark, B., Naito, K., Yoshimura, K., . . . Ohki, Y. (2004). Dexterous finger movements in primate without monosynaptic cortico-motoneuronal excitation. *Journal of Neurophysiology, 92,* 3142–3147.

Sutherland, D. H. (1997). The development of mature gait. *Gait and Posture, 6,* 163–170.

Sutherland, D. H., Olsen, R. A., Biden, E. N., & Wyatt, M. P. (1988). *The development of mature walking.* London: Mac Keith Press.

Taub, E., Ramey, S. L., DeLuca, S., & Echols, K. (2004). Efficacy of constraint-induced movement therapy for children with cerebral palsy with asymmetric motor impairment. *Pediatrics, 113,* 305–312. PMID: 14754942

Taub, E., Uswatte, G., & Pidikiti, R. (1999). Constraint-induced movement therapy: A new family of techniques with broad applications to physical rehabilitation—A clinical review. *Journal of Rehabilitation Research and Development, 39,* 237–251.

van Uden, C. J., & Besser, M. P. (2004). Test–retest reliability of temporal and spatial gait characteristics measured with an instrumented walkway system (GAITRite). *BMC Musculoskeletal Disorders, 5,* 13.

Vearrier, L. A., Langan, J., Shumway-Cook, A., & Woollacott, M. (2005). An intensive massed practice approach to retraining balance post-stroke. *Gait and Posture, 22,* 154–163.

Wallen, M., Ziviani, J., Naylor, O., Evans, R., Novak, I., & Herbert, R. D. (2011). Modified constraint-induced therapy for children with hemiplegic cerebral palsy: A randomized trial. *Developmental Medicine and Child Neurology, 53,* 1091–1099.

Webb, D., Tuttle, R. H., & Baksh, M. (1994). Pendular activity of human upper limbs during slow and normal walking. *American Journal of Physical Anthropology, 93,* 477–489.

Webster, K. E., Wittwer, J. E., & Feller, J. A. (2005). Validity of the GAITRite walkway system for the measurement of averaged and individual step parameters of gait. *Gait and Posture, 22,* 317–321.

Wenzelburger, R., Kopper, F., Frenzel, A., Stolze, H., Klebe, S., Brossmann, A., . . . Deuschl, G. (2005). Hand coordination following capsular stroke. *Brain, 128,* 64–74.

Zipp, G. P., & Winning, S. (2012). Effects of constraint-induced movement therapy on gait, balance, and functional locomotor mobility. *Pediatric Physical Therapy, 24,* 64–68.

APPENDIX 14.A. OPERATIONAL DEFINITIONS OF GAIT-RELATED TERMS

Base of support—Perpendicular distance from the heel center of one footprint to the line of progression formed by two footprints of the opposite foot.

Cadence—Number of steps performed in 1 minute. In our studies, we used the approach recommended by Hoff (1996) to normalize this parameter.

Gait cycle time—Stride time.

Double-limb stance time—Time in the gait cycle in which both lower extremities (LEs) are in contact with the ground supporting the participant's body weight. In our studies, we normalized this parameter to the gait cycle time. The parameter, then, is expressed as a percentage of the gait cycle.

Overall stance time—Total time in the gait cycle that the LE spends in contact with the ground supporting the participant's body weight. In our studies, we normalized this parameter to the gait cycle time. The parameter, then, is expressed as a percentage of the gait cycle.

Right–left step length and time—*Step length* is the distance covered from the foot strike of one LE to the next foot strike of the other LE. In our studies, we normalized step length to the participant's leg length. *Step time* is the time it takes to perform one step. In our studies, we normalized step time to the gait cycle time. The parameter, then, is expressed as a percentage of the gait cycle.

Right–left single-limb stance time—Time in the gait cycle in which the LE is in contact with the ground by itself supporting the participant's body weight. In our studies, we normalized this parameter to the gait cycle time. The parameter, then, is expressed as a percentage of the gait cycle.

Right–left swing phase time—Time in the gait cycle that the LE spends swinging forward for the next foot strike. In our studies, we normalized this parameter to the gait cycle time. The parameter, then, is expressed as a percentage of the gait cycle.

Step-length differential—Difference between the distance covered with the right step and the distance covered with the left step.

Step-time differential—Difference between the time it takes to take a step with the right foot and the time it takes to take a step with the left foot.

Stride length and time—*Stride length* is the distance covered from the foot strike of one foot to the next foot strike of the same foot. In our studies, we normalized this parameter to the participant's leg length. *Stride time* is the time taken from the foot strike of one foot to the next foot strike of the same foot. Stride time is also referred to as *gait cycle time.*

Walking velocity—Distance covered per unit of time. In our studies, we used the approach recommended by Hoff (1996) to normalize this parameter.

section III

Collaboration and Coordination With Families and Other Professionals

PATTY COKER-BOLT, PhD, OTR/L; MARY REBEKAH TRUCKS, MS, OTR/L; and REGGI LUTENBACHER, MS, OTR/L

15

Working With Families and Therapy Teams to Maximize Pediatric CIMT Benefits

CHAPTER HIGHLIGHTS

- Understanding families and building successful collaborations
- Collaborating with families to set goals
- Parents administering pediatric CIMT programs
- Research on parent and child perspectives and pediatric CIMT
- Therapists from a signature pediatric CIMT program reflect on working with families
- Perspectives of four parents whose child completed pediatric CIMT programs.

KEY TERMS

ACQUIREc therapy
Bimanual intensive training
Caregiver
Component goals
Function-based goals
Task-oriented practice

This chapter explores successful collaborations between families and providers of pediatric constraint-induced movement therapy (P–CIMT) and provides specific examples from clinicians and parents on how to build therapy teams that maximize outcomes from participation in a constraint therapy program.

Successful pediatric rehabilitation approaches start with building strong relationships among the therapist, caregiver, and child. Integrated models of therapy (i.e., therapy based on two or more models) rely on child- and parent-centered goals to help drive the direction and scope of therapy services. It is important to ensure families understand key components of P–CIMT and posttherapy activities, which can be done by reviewing key features of P–CIMT (Table 15.1).

Table 15.1   KEY FEATURES OF P–CIMT TO DISCUSS WITH FAMILIES

FEATURE	IMPORTANT ASPECTS OF P–CIMT TO DISCUSS WITH FAMILIES
Constraint and wear schedule	• Describe the type of constraint and provide an example, if possible. • Discuss the constraint-wearing schedule and problem solve any daily activities that may present specific challenges while the constraint is worn (e.g., meals, naps, bedtime).
Intensity of treatment	• Discuss task-oriented practice and the amount of time the child will be engaged in repetitive activities each day.
Integration of new skills into home activities	• Discuss what occurs after the P–CIMT program ends. It is important to have parents consider how to continue building on new skills gained from the constraint program.
Maintenance of new skills over time	• A high-quality P–CIMT program can help a child demonstrate dramatic motor changes. Discuss how these new skills need to be used in everyday life to maintain a habit of use over time.
Bimanual activities	• Improving skills in the weaker UE should be transferred to improvements in two-handed activities. Discuss with parents how to encourage use of both hands in everyday tasks to help build new motor patterns.

Note. P–CIMT = pediatric constraint-induced movement therapy; UE = upper extremity.

UNDERSTANDING FAMILIES AND BUILDING SUCCESSFUL COLLABORATIONS

Anyone who spends large amounts of time with the child and is responsible for the child's well-being during the day is considered a **caregiver.** Although a child's parent seems like the most obvious caregiver for a child, children can have many caregivers, including extended family, close friends of the family, teachers, day care staff, nannies, therapists, and so on.

Each caregiver needs to know effective strategies to elicit movements and encourage functional ability for the child. It is important for the child's various caregivers to clearly understand the principles of P–CIMT and all the essential elements that will affect the program's outcomes.

The ideal therapeutic situation is for caregivers to be involved throughout the P–CIMT process. In **ACQUIREc therapy,** a signature form of P–CIMT, caregivers are expected to participate in at least one session each week of the program. However, it is understandable if caregivers cannot be present for all individual or group sessions provided by the practitioner, because of other life demands (e.g., work, other appointments). In these cases, after the session has ended, the practitioner communicates with caregivers (e.g., by phone or e-mail) regarding the best way for them to be involved in therapy.

Some caregivers sit alongside the therapist and child the entire treatment period, but this setup can create an emotional tug-of-war for young children, who may want to take direction only from the parent. This allegiance to the parent can interrupt the bonding process with the therapist and affect the overall therapeutic process. If the caregiver is comfortable with

it, the therapist requests that he or she watch therapy slightly out of the child's line of view (e.g., around a doorway, from other side of the room). This distance enables the caregiver to see what the child and therapist are doing while still allowing "alone time" for the child to bond with the therapist.

As the child feels more comfortable with the practitioner, the practitioner encourages the caregiver to be a part of therapy to facilitate successful carryover for the home program.

COLLABORATING WITH FAMILIES TO SET GOALS

P–CIMT goals are based on the child's age, developmental level, motor abilities, cognitive abilities, and motivation. Parents often do not immediately respond to a question such as "What are your goals for your child?" However, most parents come to therapy with ideas that they would like to see their child improve in use of the weaker hand for everyday activities.

These ideas are often based on the parent's observations of his or her child's abilities during attempts to complete tasks at home or school or in the community. Such observations reflect the real-world problems the child is having and should form a basis for collaboration between therapist and parent on more specific P–CIMT goals. Exhibit 15.1 provides examples of age-appropriate developmental tasks that could be used to help parents identify real-world tasks that a child is having difficulty performing.

The child (if age-appropriate), parents, and therapist establish component and function-based goals after the pretesting session and then refine them during the first few P–CIMT treatment days. **Component goals** are usually short-

Exhibit 15.1　Examples of Age-Appropriate Treatment Goals With Families

GOALS FOR CHILDREN AGES 18 MONTHS TO 2 YEARS

- Grasp and hold toys
- Increase purposeful movement of affected arm or hand with no cues from family
- Self-feeding (e.g., finger foods, spoon feeding)
- Remove clothing
- Push arms or legs through sleeves of shirt or pants
- Hold and carry a large ball with two hands

- Use affected arm as a protective response during falls
- Push a button on toy
- Turn a knob
- Pull a toy with a string
- Remove socks and shoes
- Pop bubbles (with index finger extension)
- Reach with both hands to be picked up by parent

GOALS FOR CHILDREN AGES 3 TO 5 YEARS

- Carry objects during household tasks (e.g., cups, plates)
- Catch or throw small or medium ball
- Release toys or objects into bucket or container (e.g., clean up toys)
- Stabilize paper while coloring or writing
- Hold paper while snipping or cutting with scissors
- Put on shirt using two hands

- Put on socks and shoes
- Use both hands to fasten a zipper
- Ride a tricycle (e.g., hold handle bars, steer)
- Raise and lower pants before and after toileting
- Balance and coordinate to dress self while standing

GOALS FOR CHILDREN AGES 6 TO 8 YEARS

- Cut out shapes with scissors
- Zip and unzip a backpack with affected hand holding backpack
- Tie shoes
- Cut food (using knife and fork)
- Participate in sports activities (e.g., swimming, soccer, gymnastics)
- Ride a bike or scooter (e.g., maintain balance, hold handle bars, steer)

- Play a musical instrument
- Play video games
- Carry lunch tray
- Open containers at mealtime
- Independently complete hygiene tasks (e.g., brushing teeth, bathing)

GOALS FOR CHILDREN AGES 10 YEARS AND OLDER

- Carry heavier weight required for school (e.g., book bag) or home (e.g., chores)
- Create art (e.g., pottery, making jewelry)
- Fasten seatbelt in car
- Pull hair back with hair tie (pony tail) and complete higher level grooming (e.g., applying make-up)
- Orient using smart phones and tablet computers
- Type and use a computer keyboard

- Put on jewelry (e.g., earrings, necklace, bracelet, watch)
- Prepare for driving a vehicle
- Help with setting and clearing the table
- Complete simple meal preparation
- Do laundry
- Fold clothing
- Do other household chores

term goals centered on a child's individual movements (e.g., supinating forearm to neutral to hold tray with both hands). **Function-based goals** are typically long-term goals that relate to the child's daily occupations (e.g., feeding self).

The child and family contribute to goal setting by considering areas of interest that the child finds enjoyable and motivating. Children and families usually need a certain amount of direction in goal setting. For example, the therapist might ask the child what activities are difficult in school, during dressing, or when playing with family and friends. The therapist might also ask the child to describe a favorite activity

or something he or she would like to do better with the more affected hand.

Parent goals are based on observations and can be general or specific, depending on the child's age. Parents may change their goals throughout the course of treatment as they notice their child making improvements with the more affected upper extremity (UE). Because of the intensity of treatment of P–CIMT, which produces steady changes in motor performance and function, the practitioner should discuss goals with the child and parents each day to adapt goals on the basis of the child's evolving motor progress. Exhibit 15.1 lists age-appropriate activities that can be used when collaborating to set goals with families before initiating a P–CIMT program.

PARENTS ADMINISTERING P–CIMT PROGRAMS

If the therapist expects the parent to implement P–CIMT activities at home, it is important that the child be consistently reinforced as he or she uses his or her impaired hand during **task-oriented practice,** which is motor skill practice related to a specific functional activity (e.g., catching a ball). For example, during the first week of a P–CIMT program, a child learned to independently grasp his fork, stab his food, and eat his entire meal with only verbal cues. The practitioner communicated this new skill to the parents through an end-of-day summary, so the parents could encourage the child to practice this new skill at home.

Upon arrival to a treatment session to start the second week of P–CIMT, the parent reported that the child could not accomplish the new skill at home. The child insisted his mother feed him popcorn the previous night, because he could not do this skill by himself. The therapist asked the father to observe the morning breakfast session with the child, and he could see the child navigate finger foods with his weaker hand and use a utensil and a regular cup without physical assistance.

At this time, the child admitted he was tired in the evenings and enjoyed the attention he received from his parents, which contributed to his persistence in having a family member feed him instead of practicing this new skill at home. It was important for the parents to see the child successfully complete the new skill and the child to be aware that the parents and practitioner had expectations that he would practice new skills at home, even after a therapy session has ended.

Beyond having families in actual therapy sessions, use of several strategies can improve inclusion of families in treatment and training sessions for P–CIMT. Such strategies include videotaping sessions to be viewed by all caregivers who will have a role in providing task-oriented practice or encouraging new skill use in the affected UE after the conclusion of P–CIMT. Another option is to develop a book or manual that outlines parent-, child-, and therapist-generated goals that are matched with specific therapy-based treatment suggestions.

Parents will frequently say, "I see my child assisting with dressing with you, but on the weekends, it is a huge battle and he won't try at all. What am I doing wrong?" In this situation, the therapist should take the time to help the parent problem solve by showing how to correctly and consistently cue, motivate, and reinforce the child's abilities.

Because there are different levels of caregiver involvement, communication between therapist and caregiver is crucial. It is important to talk with the parents before, during, and after P–CIMT to help reduce potential areas of frustration for the child and family. Exhibit 15.2 lists considerations for practitioners when asking parents to implement P–CIMT programs.

If the child is older (i.e., ages 5 years to adolescent), talking to parents in a location separate from the child is best. The therapist must communicate with parents the treatment plan, modifications made, and progress, and give parents advice on activity vs. resting after P–CIMT, setting the pace of therapy, and strategies to motivate the child and reduce any challenging behaviors. Parents must be aware of and comfortable with all of these areas to help children carry over new skills learned in P–CIMT to the home and school environments. The ultimate goal is to have the child be with caretakers who understand the child's functional ability and how to motivate the child to use new skills on a daily basis.

Exhibit 15.2   Considerations When Asking Parents to Implement P–CIMT Programs

- Does the parent share the same concerns as the therapy team about the child's strengths and weaknesses in regard to using the more-affected UE?
- Does the parent understand the child's current body mechanics and competing and compensatory movements? Does the parent understand how these patterns may affect task practice during P–CIMT?
- Does the parent have time during the day to implement the intensive task-oriented practice?
- How does the child respond to the parent's instruction? Will the child comply when asked to complete challenging tasks?
- Does the parent understand strategies that are used to motivate and encourage the child during task-oriented practice?
- Does the parent require training in providing P–CIMT activities and shaping of motor skills? If so, how will this training be delivered by the therapy team before starting a P–CIMT program?
- Will having the parent implement the P–CIMT affect parent–child relationship or cause stress between parent and child?
- Can parents comply with the program developed by the therapists? Some studies have found that parents could not implement P–CIMT programs as designed by therapy teams (e.g., Wallen et al., 2011).

RESEARCH ON PARENT AND CHILD PERSPECTIVES AND P–CIMT

Most P–CIMT literature has focused on outcomes related to a child's motor-skill performance and ability to complete daily functional tasks. Few studies have examined the family's perspective (caregiver or child) on participation in a P–CIMT program.

A study by Gilmore, Ziviani, Sakzewski, Shields, and Boyd (2010) reported qualitative data from 32 children enrolled in a larger study, the INCITE Trial (Boyd et al., 2010; Sakzewski et al., 2012), which compared modified pediatric constraint-induced movement therapy (mP–CIMT) with another form of intensive training. The INCITE Trial's outcomes included subjective measures of quality of life provided through parent and child questionnaires: the child version of the Cerebral Palsy Quality of Life (CPQOL–Child; University of Melbourne, n.d.) and the child–parent report KIDSCREEN–52 (KIDSCREEN Group, 2006).

Children ages 8 years and older who completed a mP–CIMT camp-based program 6 hours per day for 2 weeks answered the questionnaires, along with their mothers, before and after participation in the program. Children completing the camp-based program reported significant improvements between baseline and 3 weeks postintervention in the domains of physical well-being, psychological well-being, and moods and emotions on the KIDSCREEN–52.

These changes were maintained up to 1 year after treatment was completed. Two domains on the CPQOL–Child that demonstrated significant improvements after receiving mP–CIMT intervention included more positive feelings about overall functioning and participation in activities and improvements in overall physical health. These improvements appear to directly reflect the focus of the intervention program and specific goals identified by the child and caregiver.

For example, questions in the domain about overall function addressed how children feel about how they use their arms and hands and the ability to dress, eat, and drink independently. Almost a quarter of participation goals identified by children and caregivers that related to leisure, sports, and recreation showed significant gains, with improvements reflected in well-being across related domains of the CPQOL–Child measure. A well-designed, goal-directed, and functionally focused P–CIMT intervention could broadly affect a family's and child's sense of well-being and participation in life tasks.

Gilmore and colleagues (2010) conducted individual interviews with these 32 children. Questions focused on (1) what the child liked best about the camp-based program, (2) what he or she didn't like about the program, (3) any

differences the child noticed in the way the impaired upper limb was used after camp, and (4) what the child would like to change about the camp-based format.

Three main themes emerged from the interview data: (1) experience of wearing the glove used in the mP–CIMT intervention, (2) reaction to the camp format, and (3) views about the gains made during the camp. Children discussed some of the perceived barriers to completing the mP–CIMT program, and most complaints were about frustration from wearing the mitt during tasks that required a high level of skill, such as feeding.

Children provided suggestions for improving the therapy experience, such as adding a rest break or even a nap between training sessions. Some frustration was noted in being unable to use the stronger arm or hand during everyday tasks. The authors noted that use of a constraint mitt may reduce a child's individual choice and autonomy, and some frustration may occur in the initial phase of constraint therapy because of the loss of competence when performing everyday tasks.

The authors suggested considering including children when making activity choices and modifying activities and using a structured rewards system to maximize constraint compliance and tolerance, especially during early initiation of this approach. On the positive side, the children noted feelings of accomplishment when meeting personal goals and felt "quicker" using the weaker hand. Many daily chores were easier to complete, such as putting away dishes or fixing hair.

A recent qualitative study by Knis-Matthew and colleagues (2011) provided some insight into how families felt after their child completed a mP–CIMT program. This study provided information from interviews with four parents of children with CP who participated in a camp-based program, which was conducted for 10 children ages 4–9 years. The children participated in task-oriented practice for 6 hours per day for 5 days each week over a 3-week period.

Three themes emerged from the parent interviews, one related specifically to the P–CIMT program: (1) parents expressed how life changed when their child was diagnosed with CP and that family support was critical for coping, (2) parents felt information and support for their children were difficult to find, and (3) parents thought a group format enhanced P–CIMT for their child and also provided social benefits.

Two parents reported considering enrolling their children in clinic- and home-based P–CIMT programs but felt the lack of organization or information about the programs prevented them from actually enrolling their child. A parent stated, "I was nervous because he was only 3, and I was really fearful about it. I was very nervous about him going and so I went to meet the director and she was nervous about it too" (Knis-Matthew, 2011, p. 11). This parent statement is very revealing and reflects that parents who are asked to provide P–CIMT should participate in formal training. Ensuring that parents have a good understanding of the principles of P–CIMT and how to successfully implement a program are critical to building a relationship with families before starting P–CIMT.

When one family's orthopedist first discussed CIMT treatment with a mother, the parent initially agreed to try the treatment in her home. However, afterward the mother stated,

> His cast was like a clam shell. It was introducing this big bulky thing in the comfort of home. I know that as therapists you would want to believe that we carry over a lot of this into the home life. But there has to be some security. There has to be some safe haven where you can just be a kid and you could just do whatever . . . he needs a break, too. (Knis-Matthew, 2011, p. 11)

Although parents discussed some of the difficulties with their child's participation in P–CIMT programs, many parents also described notable gains in their child's bilateral movements, during and after the camp-based program:

> The things he can do with his right hand amaze me. It makes him more aware of it and more functional. He gets very proud of himself. That helps with his self-esteem. It is just a very positive thing. (Knis-Matthew, 2011, p. 12)

THERAPISTS FROM A SIGNATURE P–CIMT PROGRAM REFLECT ON WORKING WITH FAMILIES

Parents and their perceptions of the ACQUIREc P–CIMT program are very important to practitioners. Families often travel long distances for a month of this high-intensity, signature form of P–CIMT (see Chapter 8, "The ACQUIREc Protocol: What We Have Learned From a Decade of Delivering a Signature Form of P–CIMT"). Upon returning home, parents often share their experiences and observations about their child's progress with other parents and their local health care providers and therapists.

Most families discover the ACQUIREc programs through Internet searches, but some hear about the treatment from their community practitioners or other families. The most common reason parents give for seeking high-intensity treatment is discouragement by lack of progress with standard therapy, and they are willing to try something different that has research evidence to support it. Many parents report they did not know what to expect when they started the program, but they gained first-hand experience on how P–CIMT was provided to their child. This report was true even

for parents who had multiple conversations with ACQUIREc staff as well as with other parents who had participated in the program. First-time participants rarely know the reasonable expectations for their child and often arrive for testing with low expectations. However, once they see the immediate progress, parents' outlooks quickly improve. Parents realize that if they challenge their child with the right amount of assistance and "just-right challenge," their child can make significant gains.

Parents mention numerous qualities as beneficial aspects to the ACQUIREc program. Some parents report the one-on-one therapist-to-child interaction as a major benefit. We have heard, "The most beneficial aspect of the program is the quality and experience of the therapists. These therapists have seen it all, been successful, and always set the bar very high for your child."

The cast is also seen as an advantage in the ACQUIREc program. Although some parents arrive with an initial concern about the cast remaining on the entire time of the P–CIMT program, they quickly observe the benefits and realize that regular wear of the cast is an important part of the treatment process.

Parents describe the intensive 5-days-per-week, 6-hours-per-day, 4-week treatment protocol as another advantage to the ACQUIREc protocol. Although the 4-week intensive stay is a benefit, it is also one of the most challenging parts of participating in the program (e.g., families from out of town might have to stay in local accommodations). However, parents support the idea that working in the home-like setting helps their child focus and engage more in therapy.

Another expressed benefit to ACQUIREc therapy is receiving an extensive home program upon completion of treatment. After watching therapy over the 4-week period, parents feel they have a better knowledge of how to work with their child and continue to challenge, support, and encourage further use of the involved UE upon returning home. Most parents develop the confidence in their ability to implement the home program in a way that maintains the challenge but also provides the child with opportunities to be successful in his or her attempts. Although the parents and child cannot complete every suggestion in the home program each day, they see it as an advantage to have the information at their disposal for integrating the activities into their child's daily life.

Successful P–CIMT programs foster strong collaborations before, during, and after the program. It is critically important for practitioners to build strong relationships among the child's practitioners, caregivers, and child before implementing a new P–CIMT program. Families should feel comfortable with all aspects of the P–CIMT program and understand the essential elements of P–CIMT and posttherapy home activities. Long-term benefits of participating in the program vary from child to child. Parents who consistently implement the home program see increased long-term benefits compared with parents who do not consistently follow through with the child's home activities. One mother stated, "I think that my daughter has more confidence in herself as a result of participating in the ACQUIREc program. She has learned that there is absolutely nothing that she cannot do if she puts her mind to it. I know that she would not be able to do the monkey bars at the playground or participate on swim team without the ACQUIREc program."

PERSPECTIVES OF FOUR PARENTS WHOSE CHILD COMPLETED P–CIMT PROGRAMS

In this section, we share the experiences of four families who received different forms of P–CIMT from different clinics or universities. Tables 15.2 and 15.3 depict abbreviated versions of what two mothers wrote in response to a set of the same questions. Exhibit 15.3 contains excerpts from a parent blog where a mother shared her experiences as they unfolded with a signature form of P–CIMT offered in a clinic setting. A father who wrote a book about his child's life depicts his family's experience with another form of signature P–CIMT, ACQUIREc.

Recently, one father wrote a book about his experience seeking help for his child who suffered from prenatal stroke. The father was a physician, and the family's story was similar to many others we have known: Parents were strongly committed to finding the very best types of treatment possible for their child with special needs. Adam Wolfberg (2012) in *Fragile Beginnings: Discoveries and Triumphs in the Newborn ICU* wrote about discovering P–CIMT and what his family experienced when they contacted Stephanie DeLuca and received the full course of therapy from the Pediatric Neuromotor Clinic.

Table 15.2   RESPONSES OF A MOTHER OF A 4-YEAR-OLD CHILD WHO PARTICIPATED IN A WEEK-LONG CAMP P–CIMT PROGRAM

QUESTION	RESPONSE
Tell me about your child's CIMT experience (e.g., type of program, setting).	My son attended the program Monday to Friday from 9:00 a.m. [un]til 3 p.m. He had two therapy students with him in the morning and two therapy students with him after lunch. They followed a program outline for the summer camp. The camp had a daily theme that was a great part of making his day exciting and wanting to participate in the constraint therapy! It was also easier for him to understand his therapy, because he saw other children struggle with similar situations and knew they had to deal with the same obstacles as [him]."
How did your child respond to constraint at first and then later into the program?	I think seeing others makes it easier for any child to [participate] in P–CIMT. My son, I feel, doesn't really mind the constraint, and he knows it will help him in the end!
What was the dosage (i.e., time wearing constraint, time for task practice)?	My son was actually casted 2 weeks prior with his weaker hand in supination so it would help with the rotation of the wrist during P–CIMT. Then, while he was at camp, he wore a hand splint for 6 hours, Monday to Friday. After camp, we casted for another 2 weeks on his left arm ("good arm") to get 100% use from his right side. It still amazes me that we get so much use from the right hand after having 6 hours a day for 5 days! Even a month later (after camp has ended)!!
In your own words, what were the immediate benefits?	Immediately, he was more aware of his right hand and arm. He attempted to open the car door, but it was locked; [he] played on the iPad with his right hand while with the left hand, he [fed] himself a sandwich. Also, I didn't have to keep reminding him to use [his] right hand. He has actually started using both hands to pull his pants up and down!! The most immediate thing would be that usually he is so excited about using both hands that he says ""Look" or "Take a picture of me." He was actually just doing activities and not even aware, so that means he didn't have to think to use his right (impaired) hand—it just came naturally.
What are some of the longer term benefits?	Our son sees things now and is aware of what he can do in a different way. He does care about doing typical (everyday) activities. Camp gave him the encouragement and confidence he needs and allowed him to bond with other children who face similar difficulties. He now knows he is not alone.
How did CIMT compare to other therapy approaches your child had in the past?	CIMT was great in so many ways: (1) confidence and self-help awareness related to using his right hand are my best answers, (2) it's always nice to know you are not alone and can have a friend that shares the same struggles, (3) more rapid gains, [and] (4) not as much frustration because there were other children playing that were doing and approaching the task the same way, and then at home he was happy to show us the activities that they did at camp!

Note. CIMT = constraint-induced movement therapy; P–CIMT = pediatric constraint-induced movement therapy.

Table 15.3   RESPONSES OF A MOTHER OF A 4-YEAR-OLD CHILD WHO PARTICIPATED IN A CLINIC-BASED SIGNATURE FORM OF P–CIMT

QUESTION	RESPONSE
Tell me about your child's CIMT experience (e.g., type of program, setting).	The CIMT program we attended was within a specialized therapy unit of a special-needs school (and part of a much larger organization, including a hospital, other outpatient therapy and education programs, and other schools and day care centers). Therapy primarily took place in one room with some access to a kitchen and gym-like area. My son worked with a PT, OT, and briefly with a speech–language pathologist. One thing we felt would have been beneficial for the parents would have been an observation room [or] area for us to watch the therapy without interfering.
How did your child respond to constraint at first and then later into the program?	Initially my son was resistant to the cast and very frustrated/upset by it. Fairly quickly, however, he realized that the cast was not coming off, and he transitioned from complaining about the cast to focusing on how to go about playing and other tasks.
What was the dosage (i.e., time wearing constraint, time for task practice)?	3 weeks of wearing the cast full-time. Therapy for approximately 3–4 hours, 5 days a week. Weekends we did "homework" therapy assignments. For the 4th week of the program, the cast was removed, and bilateral skills became the therapeutic focus.
In your own words, what were the immediate benefits?	Immediately our son gained strength, use, and increased awareness of his left arm, hand, and fingers, which he retained for several months.
What are some of the longer term benefits?	The biggest long-term benefit we are observing is from the therapy, its goals and outcomes, and seeing how well it worked. Therefore, when we noticed our son's awareness and use of his affected side diminishing, after treatment, we worked with our OT to create a "mini" constraint program (we used a removable cast a few days a week for short reminder therapy sessions) at home. This immediately improved his use of the limb. We continue to use strategies taught to us by the CIMT therapists through "homework" sessions in our daily routines (e.g., we always have him reach for his gummy vitamins with his affected hand and use a pincer grasp).
How did CIMT compare to other therapy approaches?	The main difference—and I think this is the key to the success—is the duration and intensity of the therapy. More rapid and enduring gains were made and there was a greater depth of understanding of the child as an individual and therefore a more tailored approach to the program and suggested therapies and solutions to roadblocks met.

Note. CIMT = constraint-induced movement therapy; OT = occupational therapist; P–CIMT = pediatric constraint-induced movement therapy; PT = physical therapist.

"Parents will say to us, 'There is no way my child can do 6 hours of therapy a day,'" said Dr. DeLuca …"We don't accept that." What she found was that parents had more trouble watching their children struggle— even if the children ultimately succeeded—than the children had doing it.

Hour after hour, in our temporary Birmingham living room, Larissa [Wolfberg's daughter] and Reggi [the ACQUIREc therapist] worked on the same exercises, strengthening muscles, trying again and again to accomplish the pinching, grasping, reaching, and turning that would recruit neurons to the task of expanding the strength, range, and dexterity of her right hand.

We quickly adopted Reggi's phrases: "Whoa, Joe" when Larissa did something particularly impressive, like carrying a cup of water across the room. Or "Now, Larissa, you're all catywhompus" when Larissa took a disorganized approaching to opening

the refrigerator door instead of doing as Reggi had shown her: lining herself squarely up in front of the door, bringing her elbow to her side, rotating her arm, and grasping the door handle.

By far the most skilled occupational therapist Kelly [Larissa's mother] or I had ever met, Reggi never tired, never lost her patience, and never had a situation she couldn't redirect into an activity that enhanced the function of Larissa's hand.

Each day, after 6 hours without a break, during which time Larissa dressed, made breakfast and lunch, played countless games, and did strengthening exercises, Reggi said good-bye until the next morning.

A month later the cast came off, and the effect of neuroplasticity was apparent: Larissa's right hand could rotate further, lift more, and operate with more precision than it had when we arrived in the stifling heat of Birmingham. (p. 135)

Exhibit 15.3   A Parent's Reflections About the P–CIMT Process

Note. These entries are the personal reflections from a mother's blog.

NIGHT 1: NERVES

I've never vomited because of nerves until now. Brian and I both had trouble getting to sleep tonight, thinking about what tomorrow will bring, but after I finally fell asleep my arm being in an uncomfortable position woke me up. This, of course, started a torrent of thoughts, and well, here I am at 2:00 a.m. feeling better for having a bit of literal upheaval.

We've been on the waiting list for this therapy program for over a year. For all that time, just as we were looking forward to any chance of improvement for Simon, we've been dreading the hardship this would present him. He only has one good working arm and hand to work and play with (which is more than some children have and we are grateful!), but now we are going to take that away, and he won't understand why.

I remember when we first got the AFO [ankle–foot orthosis] for his leg, he cried and cried to wear it. He kept asking, "Why, Mommy?" but of course couldn't understand the answer. It broke my heart to make him uncomfortable, unhappy. And that we could take off for breaks, and it didn't impede his movement but helped it. This . . . is full-time and meant to make things more difficult.

But he got used to his "super boot." We will get used to this, too.

DAY 1: GETTING THE CAST

So, today was the "big" day we'd been most dreading—the initial casting. Getting the cast made was every bit as difficult as I'd imagined it would be. Admittedly, I've had some experience with this, since a cast is required to make AFOs, and we've been through that three times now. Each time there is screaming and crying [and] a heroic effort by Simon to escape and plead for help (in both English and Spanish thanks to Dora & Diego) matched by my equally stoic effort to soothe him, hold him down, and keep him from maiming the individual working on the cast (Figure 15.1).

This time it took four adults: myself and Brian holding onto him, and two therapists working on the arm. It was a big challenge; he's quite strong for a little guy who weighs only 30 lbs, and he is quite adept at wiggling out of tight places. Trying to get the cast on correctly was tricky, and then removing it to prep it further was even harder.

Brian and I are both a little surprised by the cast itself. From photos we'd seen of the program, we were expecting a full-on cast in our choice of rainbow color. Apparently, that isn't how it is being done now. What we have is . . . interesting. They use a waterproof material to make the cast (which is great), and then they remove it (very confusing for the small child in question), trim off the rough parts and tape up the edges with a waterproof tape, [and] finally reinser[t] the child's limb and secur[e] it with electrical tape (in our choice of rainbow colors). Practically speaking, I understand that the desire is to be able to remove the cast to check the skin and then reuse the same cast, but the result looks like I tried to set Simon's arm myself with paper mâché and duct tape.

Figure 15.1   PLACING THE CAST.

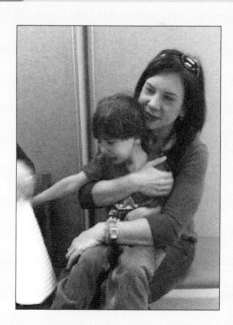

But never fear. I'm working on a cosy for it. So far, I've found a Paul Frank pirate-themed, knee-high sock I think may work, if I can trim and hem it properly . . . Heck, maybe this will lead to me opening an Etsy shop full of cast-cosies.

Yes, I am that shallow.

The BIG surprise of today is that Simon has almost immediately started adapting. As soon as he'd recovered himself somewhat, therapy began, with a walk up and down stairs while attempting to hold onto a railing and then pressing elevator buttons (a favorite task on any day). I expected a fair amount of resistance to using the "other" arm, and honestly, with me in the room there were a lot of tears and wanting Mommy to "hold you." However, after I finally accepted that I needed to go and hide (within earshot), and after a few failed attempts at getting the casted side to do anything (and a bit more crying), Simon just went with it. He is really trying to make this work, and I am amazed. But, I should have known. Is there anything like the resilience of a child? Even under the most trying circumstances, they will find a way to be a kid. To be present in the moment. To play, eat goldfish crackers, and press all the buttons on the elevator. I have so much more to learn from that.

(Continued)

Exhibit 15.3   A Parent's Reflections About the P–CIMT Process *(Cont.)*

DAY 3: A BARREL OF MONKEYS

So, we've officially been kicked out. Brian and [me], that is.

I know that this is best. [I]t is the same situation at school, at the speech clinic (though I can watch from a 2-way mirror there), and even at "You Can Do It Too," his physical therapy/gymnastics program. When Mom and Dad are around, the little guy is constantly looking to us for a way out of doing whatever it is he needs to be doing. This is true with most kids, and it isn't that we aren't welcome—we just need to let separation do its magic.

Another parenting lesson: Give the kid some space, and you will see what he can do.

What he is doing is amazing—truly. In the space of a day, he has moved past being upset about his cast (well, okay, we still hear a little complaining) to trying to find ways to make the left side do what he wants it to do. He's working very hard to isolate fingers, grasp, and turn a limb that had heretofore been nearly unresponsive except as a prop (Figure 15.2).

Brian and I did get to join in on the last few tasks of the day as we discussed the weekend "homework" with Simon's therapist. First, Simon had a snack of goldfish and juice using only his left hand to practice raking and grasping and pulling. Afterward, he hung monkeys from the Barrel of Monkeys all over the basketball net and then put them back "to bed" in the barrel. This was Simon's idea, and his therapist ran with it (Figure 15.3).

Watching the Kennedy Krieger Institute (KKI) therapist in action is really amazing. Like anyone with a special needs kid, I've seen A LOT of therapists (PT, OT, SLP. you name it) in action. They are all nice, well-intentioned people that love kids and try their best to help. However, some folks are much more effective than others.

I've been lucky to work with some wonderful people. And, from what I have observed, there are a few key traits that go into making a great therapist in any discipline. One is the ability to get down to the level of the child and engage [him or her] through language, eye contact, and physical contact. For each kid, at each stage of development, this is different but equally important. I tend to think it's like being at a cocktail party with a bunch of people you don't know. You are going to be drawn into conversation with the person that leans in when you speak, makes eye contact with you, and carries himself or herself in a way that seems happy to be there, relaxed, confident, and open.

The other really key component is the ability to be flexible. If something isn't working, if the kid isn't engaged or is simply getting too frustrated to function, stop what you are doing and try something else. I can't tell you how many times I've seen a therapist doggedly press on with whatever activity they meant to do, only to completely lose the child they were trying to help in a puddle of misery. That doesn't work for anyone. Use the cues that the child is sending, if they are interested in a particular toy, modify the play to suit the therapy you're targeting.

Figure 15.2 LEARNING TO USE THE HAND DURING PLAY ACTIVITIES.

Figure 15.3 PLAYING ON DAY 3 WITH THE BARREL OF MONKEYS GAME.

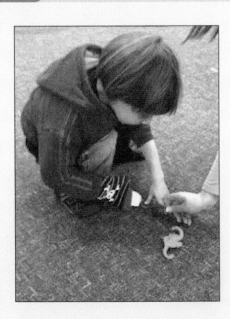

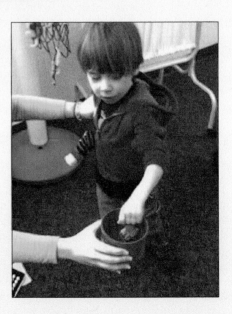

(Continued)

Exhibit 15.3 A Parent's Reflections About the P–CIMT Process *(Cont.)*

Of course, the above isn't easy and takes a considerable amount of creativity. Often getting to the point of a functional relationship like that takes a lot of time and a lot of dialogue. It is a constant work in progress. I think that is why I'm so impressed that the therapist working with Simon was able to hit the ground running, and I think that is also why we've seen such immediate progress.

She's careful not to let him get too frustrated with any task, so he keeps working. She follows his lead and lets him select the activities, which she adapts to include therapy, but he thinks it is his idea. She's on his level and talking to him constantly with praise and silly songs and laughter. The entire time Simon thinks that he is playing. I am starting to think that maybe this whole thing will work after all.

DAY 8: WITS AND WILLS

The official score is—Simon: 2, Therapists: 1, Mommy: 0.

As I mentioned earlier, Simon is starting to get a bit more frustrated. He's also starting to get a bit tired of the constant therapy—something we all could see coming, [because] he far prefers independent and self-directed play. Our infernal meddling is really starting to irk him.

Yesterday, Daddy took Simon to KKI for what we are starting to refer to as "morning school." There were some tears at separation, but they were reasonably short-lived. However, the general grouchiness persisted. The OT would pull out toy after toy, trying to spark some interest in our taciturn little guy, but he flatly refused to play.

OT: Simon, how about Potato Head!

Simon: No, no, no. (Shakes the head vehemently.) NO.

OT (dumping the pieces out onto the table): But look at all this great stuff! Let's play!

Simon: NO, NO, NO!!!!!!!!!!!!!!!

OT: You don't want to play? Ok. Let's put it away. Can you help put it away?

At this point, Simon thinks he has scored a victory. What he fails to realize is that the entire time he is satisfyingly removing the offending toy; the therapist is getting him to stretch, pull, grasp, and release the objects using his left hand and arm. In other words, he is working on therapy.

Simon: 0, Therapists: 1

Today, I took Simon. There were A LOT of tears at separation. But I kissed him good-bye and closed the door. I then proceeded to wander the halls, passing by his door every few minutes to (let's be honest) torture myself by listening to his building meltdown. About 20 minutes in, I couldn't take it anymore and knocked. The therapist cracked the door (I think she knew it was me), so Simon couldn't catch a glimpse and said she wanted to give it another 10 minutes. I told her where I'd be waiting.

Sure enough, a few minutes later, a red-faced, tear-streaked little guy came out of the room to go and "find Mommy." The deal was he had to carry a bean-bag turtle in his left hand the entire way. Finding the terms acceptable, he came to get me and tearfully fell into my arms. I'm pretty sure those final sobs were simply to punctuate how awful I was for leaving him in the first place.

Together (with the turtle), we made our way back to our classroom. While I hung out in the background, providing encouragement and an occasional cuddle-break, Simon managed to get through another hour or so of "work."

Simon: 1, Therapists: 1, Mommy: 0

However, when the PT switched with the OT, Simon took the opportunity to up the ante, and raised his price. I was still in the room with him (and, honestly, I really enjoy watching and participating—I learn so much that way, though I know I am a distraction), but he was melting down again and wasn't interested in further cooperation.

It went something like this:

Therapist: Simon, let's play with this Elmo microwave!

Simon: Moooooommmmmmmyyyyyy........

Mommy: Come on, Simon! You can play with Elmo! How fun, let's see what we can do!

Simon: Mooommmyyy, want to go? Go bye-bye in the car?

Mommy: After we finish here. Simon is a big boy, let's play!

Therapist: Look, Simon, Mommy is here! Let's make her something to eat with this fun Elmo microwave! You can push the buttons! What food should we make?

(Continued)

Exhibit 15.3   A Parent's Reflections About the P–CIMT Process *(Cont.)*

Simon (ignores therapist, looks at Mommy): Go get some food? Go bye-bye in the car? Get a BAGEL? Want some turkey bagel? Go? Get a BAGEL! In the CAR?!

Mommy (sigh): Okay, Simon. You play like a big boy and after we are ALL DONE I will take you to get a bagel.

Simon: Turkey bagel?

Mommy: Yes. Turkey bagel.

Simon: Okay!

We got through the rest of the day this way. He'd complete a task, remind me of our bargain, and then we'd get through the next task.

Repeat, bribe, repeat, bribe, repeat.

Finally, we were done for the day and, true to my word, I took the little guy out for lunch to his favorite place to get a bagel with turkey. He was thrilled, and I don't think I was imagining that he was just the tiniest bit smug about it.

DAY 9: TRAINING WHEELS ON A TRICYCLE

Daddy took Simon to KKI today, and according to both of his therapists, he did 1,000 times better. No tears, an overall happy mood, cooperation and lots of good focused work. I noticed the difference immediately when he came home for lunch. He was relaxed and pleasant and was even using his left hand—without hesitation—to grab at some grapes (um, wow!).

This morning, he rode the therapy trike all the way down the hall, something he refused to attempt yesterday! (Figure 15.4).

I'm trying to simply be happy about this positive progress without taking it personally that I am a problem. Apparently, right now I'm a major distraction. This issue has cropped up in a minor way in the past, and Simon does cry a little every time I part with him for preschool. However, since no other therapy program we have participated in has been so intense (in activity or duration), I guess that Simon's desire for an "out" hasn't been quite as strong, either.

Ultimately, this means that it is better for Daddy to take Simon to therapy the majority of the time. Though it never sat well with me, this was the loose plan from the beginning. When we were initially talking about our participation in the program, I was worried that I wouldn't have enough time to work if I was at KKI all morning, all week, all month. I'd only get about 3 "business" hours in a day (the kids get home at 4 in the afternoon from regular school), a potential problem.

As a designer, I'm fortunate enough to sustain being self-employed (aside from my teaching appointment), and therefore I have a lot of flexibility. It is because of my children that I set my business up this way (though I do occasionally entertain fantasies of growing the business, moving it out of the house, hiring staff... sigh. I digress...). Anyway, for the past 4.5 years, I've been able to wrap my work life around Simon's therapy schedule and other appointments (sometimes as many as 6 or 7 a week). Most of my real creative work happens in the "off" hours, anyway, at night and on weekends, so any business hours I am able to devote to client contact—meetings, etc. Despite my acrobatic flexibility, I knew that being gone so much would be difficult. I can't tell my clients to hold onto projects for a month, and I *do* like to give at least the vague impression of professionalism. Having office hours is key to that facade.

Fortunately, Brian has a wonderful, family-friendly employer who was willing to let him be flexible with his hours for the duration of this program. Believe me, we both know and appreciate what a gift this is, especially having had "agency" backgrounds (the exact *opposite* of family-friendly) in our past.

So, I'm very grateful for this help, and in general for the awesome, amazing co-parenting my spouse is happy to participate in. Deep down, however, I have to admit that I am also disappointed at the thought of not being there the entire time. Like I said, I've done this for 4.5 years, and stepping back does not come easy for me. What I really want is to be in the classroom, observing, learning, and being as active a participant as possible in Simon's growth and progress.

Figure 15.4   RIDING THE THERAPY TRIKE.

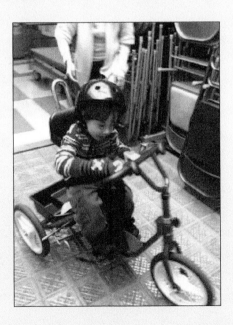

(Continued)

Exhibit 15.3   A Parent's Reflections About the P–CIMT Process *(Cont.)*

But I have to accept that me being there (heck, me being in the building) isn't helping either of us. In this situation, Mommy is a crutch and a distraction. I need to limit myself to the designated meeting times throughout the week (fortunately, that is a big part of the program) and the "homework" as the best ways to help and be involved.

Letting go. Is there anything more confusing in parenthood than knowing the difference between when to push yourself in and when to pull yourself back?

Employing this concept with my "big girl," who has excellent communication skills and is all around an overachieving, social kid, has been tough enough. Two years ago, despite the fact that I had every confidence in her ability to navigate any challenge ahead, the separation anxiety I felt when she went to elementary school was staggering.

With Simon, knowing when to let go is even more confusing. The decision is filled with trepidation, and the act almost physically painful (for both of us). He is so very vulnerable, and we have been through so very much—every cell in my being aches to protect him.

I know that holding on so tightly is not the way to help him grow, learn, and become the best he can be, whatever form that will take. But where is the distinction between holding up and holding on? Being an advocate and being a hindrance? And how on earth will I find it?

DAY 17: SUPINATION, PINCER GRASPS, AND PACK RATS

Bringing your finger to meet your thumb is referred to as a *pincer grasp*. The act of turning your wrist is called *supination*. Both of these are necessary movements for so many little daily tasks, from dressing and feeding yourself, to opening a door, or [to] turning the pages of a book.

Today was the first time Simon was able to accomplish these subtle movements. With the barest assistance—just a tiny touch to the elbow, he came that much closer to self-reliance.

A *pack rat* is what I feel I've become, after sorting through a decade's worth of paper.

Clearing up yesterday's avalanche of paperwork inspired a full-on office clean out. In my desk, I found a copy of an e-mail I saved from a dear college friend. She sent it to me the night before Simon was born, after I e-mailed to let her know that something was wrong with the baby and that he was being induced the next day.

This is what she wrote back:

> Tomorrow the luckiest baby in the world will be born. He will be blessed with coming into a fabulous family who will love and support him throughout his life. He will have the most amazing parents who will be there with him through all of his milestones and achievements. He will have a wonderful sister who will teach him everything she knows. He will be surrounded by family and friends who love him every moment of his life.

At the time, with so much scary and unknown ahead of me, I thought the words were kind and her optimism brought me comfort.

Today, with so much behind me, they bear the ring of truth. Four years later, I know we are the luckiest family in the world to be by Simon's side, witnessing the miracle of his milestones, surrounded by family and friends who love us all at every moment.

A slight turn of the hand, an old wish comes true, and little miracles happen every day.

DAY 28: CAST AWAY

Today, Simon had his cast removed. Not just for a skin check but for good this time (or at least until we repeat the program at some future date). For the rest of this week, the team will be working with Simon to practice bilateral skills, so that moving forward Simon will (hopefully) not simply revert back to using his "good side" for all tasks but will actively engage his left side as much as possible.

Weirdly, I'm a little sad to see it go. I feel that, though he has made steady progress throughout the program, it was just in the last week or so that he'd built the strength and coordination necessary to use the limb for any meaningful task. He went from simply being able to rake and swat at objects, to being able to pick things up, isolate fingers (sort of), and actually *play* with toys again. It makes me wonder what he'd be able to accomplish within another 4 weeks (yes, I am greedy!).

It is also just in the past few days that we've noticed what seems to be a slight shift in Simon's speech, or, maybe more accurately, in his ability to interact, to communicate. For the first time, ever, when I called for him, he *replied*. When his sister fell down yesterday, he *asked* her if she was alright. He said that! *"Are you alright?"* Sunday morning, I had the closest thing to a conversation I have ever had with him. He said he wanted to get tickets to go on a train. Being playful, I asked him where he wanted to go, not expecting any sort of reply. Without hesitation, he told me that he wanted to go to the beach with Mommy and Daddy. Surprised but wanting to keep it going, I asked him what we would do at the beach. He said we would have a picnic.

(Continued)

Exhibit 15.3   A Parent's Reflections About the P–CIMT Process *(Cont.)*

For years, I have longed to *talk to* my little boy. To ask him what his favorite color is. To tell him when his birthday is coming and find out where he wants to have his party. Does he want pirates or Elmo on the party bags? I want to plan a trip to Disney with him, the way we did with Olivia when she turned 5, and have him understand enough that the anticipation will keep him up at nights and drive us all a little crazy.

To comprehend and be comprehended. To begin to explore all the wonders of childhood that require communication to be fully understood and enjoyed. I want to be able to show Simon how wonderful the world can be, how beautiful and exciting and fun it is to be a kid before his childhood is over and we all have to grow up too soon.

As I write this I find that I am literally holding my breath. We're on the edge of a precipice and I want to take Simon, hold hands, and jump. Can it be that the connections we were hoping for are happening? How freeing that would be.

DAY 33: SELF-CARE

It's the little things that sometimes make the biggest difference.

This morning, *very early,* two of my oldest girlfriends met me for breakfast at a diner, because that was the only time I could find for myself this weekend. As I apologized for making them schlep out so early (one of them just got in from New York at 2:00 a.m.), they very sincerely said that they were just happy to see me, and if that meant losing a little sleep, it was no big deal.

I got enough warm fuzzies off of that to last me through the month.

Later on, Simon demonstrated his best attempt at self-care yet. **He undressed himself at bath-time, using *both* hands and needing minimal assistance.** He even put his clothes in the hamper. (Now, if I can only teach his dad that trick. . . .)

Simon was very pleased with himself, and we applauded after each garment was removed, down to his sweet little socks.

DAY 35: GRADUATION

Today, Simon graduated from the CIMT program. At times throughout the month, we felt overwhelmed by the intensity of the program—the casting was scary, the frustration tough, and the schedule challenging. We worried that we wouldn't be up to the task when it came to homework. We had anxiety over testing and evaluations and outcomes. We didn't know if we had the right tools or the right skills. We constantly questioned whether we made the right decisions, and we wonder where we should go and what we should do next.

Throughout the program, when it was tough, we took deep breaths and time outs and made priorities to make it work. We took turns, we made lists, we put things in perspective.

Now, as we are presented with choices about where to go next, about what therapy and programs to pursue, about how to alter Simon's IEP [individualized education program], about what questions to ask which doctors, I will think about where I want Simon to be 6 months from now. Thanks to this program, we've seen some of what he is capable of when we do have the right program in place and the right guidance and support.

When we needed help, it came to us in many forms and I am so grateful. Our family and friends have cheered us on at every step of the way. Simon's teachers and school therapists provided patience, support, and willingness to adapt to new ideas from an external source. Most of all, I'm grateful for the amazing staff we worked with at KKI. We have learned so much, and I feel that the door has opened to many more opportunities for Simon to grow, learn new skills, and become closer to fulfilling his expanding potential.

We will continue, of course, to research and study, to practice our skills, and [to] look for opportunities to help Simon and other families like our own. I find myself wondering if all that I've written here over the past 36 days is really the beginning of a book, a way to find other Lauras and Brians and Simons and share our knowledge and laughter and tears. Maybe.

Most of all, as I look back, I see how much Simon has accomplished. I am so proud of our little boy. Of his patience, his determination, his willingness to move forward and work within such heavy constraints. His ability to play and be happy and just be a kid day after day within such difficult and sometimes uncomfortable constraints. The mind-blowing and incredibly inspiring progress he has made. I cannot wait to see where he will go next, and I know I am privileged to be a part of it.

Today, at our last meeting of the CIMT program, we reviewed notes, and thanked and hugged our therapist, who will be in touch soon. In just a few weeks, we should be back for regular OT sessions to continue our work on self-care, prewriting, and other targeted tasks. As we left the building, they didn't hand Simon a diploma, and I didn't buy him the customary balloons or roses.

Instead, we went and got a turkey sandwich for our little miracle.

—*Laura Lebrun Hatcher*

Note. CIMT = constraint-induced movement therapy; OT = occupational therapist; PT = physical therapist; SLP = speech–language pathologist.

Wolfberg shares with readers what happened after CIMT, writing in a later chapter that Larissa returned to using her left hand after the cast was removed and

> her impaired right hand went from starring in the Birmingham hand camp to playing a decidedly supporting role. It wasn't that her right hand couldn't reach up and open the refrigerator door; it was just so much easier for her left hand. Testing at the end of the month long session showed she had made enormous gains, but we were warned that unless we kept up with her home program—a set of activities designed to reinforce and strengthen the progress she had made—those gains would be lost, at least in part. (p. 150)

Both parents tried to keep up a home program, but admitted that within a month "it was forgotten amid the demands of getting the kids to school and then bathed and to bed in the evening" (p. 150).

Three years later, the family chose to have Larissa participate in a second month-long ACQUIREc program. Larissa had the same therapist, Reggi. Although the parents worried about not keeping up the home program, Larissa had maintained and even extended the gains. She also was age 8 years. As her father noted, Larissa could now set her own goals for the therapy, which included tying her shoes, zippering her coat, and riding a bike.

What Wolfberg describes is what many ACQUIREc therapists have heard from other families: Their community therapist often struggled to decide whether to teach a child a best set of accommodations to the disability (i.e., hemiparesis) or to simply find ways of achieving everyday tasks without using the impaired arm and hand at all. For instance, Larissa's therapist at home considered teaching her to type by using just two or three fingers, or perhaps teaching only one-handed (left-handed) typing. In this case,

> Reggi disagreed with both suggestions. "I think she can use all of her fingers," Reggi said, and over 4 weeks, she showed Larissa how those fingers of her right hand could learn to independently strike the keys of both a computer and a pink Barbie piano . . . [Larissa] concentrated intensely and learned during the course of 2 weeks to pick up a Yahtzee die between her thumb and index finger, turn her hand over, and drop the cube into the palm of her hand. (p. 150)

Yet, even the second-time around, the parents sometimes found it difficult to watch their child try so hard. Larissa's mother commented, "I never hear her complain. Never. . . . And she tries so hard to do whatever Reggi tells her. But I have to tell you that it is very painful to watch her work so hard to do with her right hand what most children take for granted" (p. 150). In the final analysis, Larissa's mother said this about her daughter: "She inspires me. . . . She really does, because she's always so positive and never feels sorry for herself. But it makes me feel bad for her."

SUMMARY

Parents and children are vital to the success of any rehabilitation program. Because P–CIMT is so different from the standard forms of therapy (often once or twice a week for relatively short periods of time, usually 1 hour) that many families and children have become used to, they have a high need to understand ahead of time what the specific P–CIMT therapy will involve. They also want to know what their role will be in the therapy process and how they can help with a realistic follow-up home program.

Currently, the empirical literature on parental responses to P–CIMT is very sparse. Hopefully, future clinical and research programs will collect information from parents and children about the range of their experiences in different P–CIMT protocols. This information can help practitioners tailor programs to better meet the everyday concerns of parents and children. More personal stories could be shared with other parents and therapists deciding whether to try a P–CIMT program. We realize that the examples in this chapter reflect largely positive experiences by parents.

We look forward to seeing a more extensive and representative set of parent and child experiences as the field continues to seek answers about what types and amounts of P–CIMT protocols are effective for children at different stages in their development.

REFERENCES

Boyd, R., Sakzewski, L., Ziviani, J., Abbott, D., Badawy, R., Gilmore, R., . . . Jackson, G. (2010) INCITE: A randomized trial comparing constraint-induced movement therapy and bimanual training in children with congenital hemiplegia. *BMC Neurology, 10*(4). http://dx.doi.org/10.1186/1471-2377-10-4

Gilmore, R., Ziviani, J., Sakzewski, L., Shields, N., & Boyd, R. (2010). A balancing act: Children's experience of modified constraint-induced movement therapy. *Developmental Neurorehabilitation, 13,* 88–94.

KIDSCREEN Group. (2006). KIDSCREEN–52. Available at http://www.kidscreen.org/english/questionnaires/kidscreen-52-long-version/

Knis-Matthew, L. Falzarano, M., Baum, D., Manganiello, J., Patel, S. & Winters, L. (2011). Parents' experiences with services and treatment for their children diagnosed with cerebral palsy. *Physical & Occupational Therapy in Pediatrics,* http://dx.doi.org/10.3109/01942638.2011.566806.

Sakzewski, L., Carlon, S., Shields, N., Ziviani, J., Ware, R, & Boyd, R. (2012). Impact of intensive upper-limb rehabilitation on quality of life: A randomized trial in children with unilateral cerebral palsy. *Developmental Medicine and Child Neurology, 54,* 415–423.

University of Melbourne. (n.d.). *Cerebral Palsy Quality of Life–Child.* Available at http://cpqol.org.au/cpqolchild9_12.pdf

Wallen, M., Ziviani, J., Naylor, O., Evans, R., Novak, I., & Herbert, R. D. (2011). Modified constraint-induced therapy for children with hemiplegic cerebral palsy: A randomized trial. *Developmental Medicine and Child Neurology, 53,* 1091–1099.

Wolfberg, A. (2012). *Fragile beginnings: Discoveries and triumphs in the newborn ICU.* Boston: Beacon Press.

section IV

Future for Research, Policy, and Practice

SHARON LANDESMAN RAMEY, PhD, and
STEPHANIE C. DeLUCA, PhD

16

Research Priorities: Understanding and Transcending the Limits of Our Current Knowledge to Inform Best Practices in Pediatric CIMT

CHAPTER HIGHLIGHTS

- Research blueprint
- High-priority questions to guide future research.

Pediatric constraint-induced movement therapy (P–CIMT) has transitioned rapidly from a novel, intensive therapy applied in case studies to small- to moderate-size clinical trials. P–CIMT is now becoming part of the repertoire of treatment options widely endorsed by pediatricians, neurologists, and pediatric physiatrists. The existing scientific evidence supports the use of P–CIMT for many children; at the same time, several critical issues must be resolved to maximize our understanding of what constitutes optimal treatment for different types of children at different stages in their development. In addition, identifying the basic neurobiological mechanisms associated with P–CIMT and differential responses may contribute to further refinements and individualization in the field of pediatric rehabilitation.

This chapter identifies key topics that have surfaced in the published scientific literature, in professional meetings, and in our firsthand interactions with families and children as being of high priority for practitioners. We also include suggestions made by the other contributors to this volume and expand on excellent discussions in many of the original reports about CIMT and P–CIMT in the scientific literature. We are indebted to our colleagues for their vigilance and awareness of the current limits of our knowledge and for identifying pressing priorities for future scientific inquiry.

KEY TERMS

Accelerometry
Adjunctive supports
Alliances
Amblyopia
Botulinum toxin therapy
Cost-effectiveness
Cost-efficiency
Deep brain stimulation
Dosage
Electromyography
Environmental press
E-stim
Evidence-based practice
Fiber optics
Forced use
Goal Attainment Scaling
High-intensity P–CIMT
Implementation science
International Classification of Functioning model
Kinematics
Kinesiology taping
Lifespan databases
Mental imagining
Mitt
Neuroimaging
Operationalization
Pediatric Neuromotor Research Clinic
Return on investment
Service delivery systems research
Sling
Splint
Stem cell infusion
Therapy-induced neuroplasticity
Virtual reality

RESEARCH BLUEPRINT

This chapter presents a set of research priorities as a blueprint for collaborating and advancing the knowledge base about P–CIMT specifically and about pediatric rehabilitation more generally. The proposed research collaborations would expand knowledge about the life course development of children with cerebral palsy and other neuromotor and developmental disabilities (as defined in Chapter 4, "Motor Development and Physical Growth in Children With Cerebral Palsy") at a time when early and sustained therapies are widely available to almost all such children. We propose the creation of collaborative **lifespan databases** that are maintained and updated to allow for many years of future research efforts. These databases would include multiple indicators of quality of life and occupational participation, as well as objective measures of neuromotor competence and daily living skills. Research about P–CIMT also should include systematic exploration of whether P–CIMT could produce even greater and more enduring benefits if combined with other forms of specified treatment, enhanced natural supports (e.g., parents, community activities), or innovative technological interventions (e.g., computer-assisted games, real-time neuroimaging feedback).

Collectively, the results from implementing this research blueprint would help ensure that the therapeutic interventions provided in clinical and community settings truly reflect the best of **evidence-based practice (EBP)**—that is, interventions firmly based in sound scientific study and interpretation. In addition, these results would provide a more grounded understanding of how to effectively prepare practitioners for careers that will demand high levels of documented performance and continuing education for work within the flexible health care and educational delivery settings in which children with neuromotor challenges are served. Finally, professional practice exists within a larger policy context. The topics of cost, equity, availability, and fidelity of treatment are crucial to realizing the full benefits that P–CIMT and adjunct treatments can offer.

To support this ambitious research blueprint, mentoring and training are required for pediatric neurorehabilitation scientists from a wide array of disciplines in traditional treatment methodologies, in scientific evaluation of the older techniques, in emerging methodologies such as P–CIMT, and perhaps most importantly in the skills needed to critically evaluate the development of new treatment techniques. Ideally, a major expansion would occur in research–clinical partnerships and the creation of communities of evidence-based practitioners who work closely with active research networks supported by professional associations, competitive research funding, and private foundations and philanthropy.

We have grouped the identified research priorities and promising directions under eight major themes:

1. Resolving the critical issues of optimal P–CIMT dosage, type of constraint, and specific protocols for improving unilateral and bilateral upper-extremity (UE) functioning, with a strong focus on understanding differential responses (e.g., as a function of age, etiology, comorbidities, initial functional level) and effective strategies to adapt P–CIMT to the individual needs of a child and family at particular stages of development

2. Improving the standardized measurements (sensitivity, validity, reliability, and breadth) both for UE neuromotor functioning and for quality of life and occupational outcomes for children of different ages, strength levels, and challenges to yield an accurate, comprehensive, and sensitive-to-change profile of the child before, during, and after P–CIMT

3. Conducting longitudinal research to evaluate potential long-term P–CIMT effects (taking into account the post-P–CIMT therapy experiences and supportive environments a child receives) and identifying subsequent times or situations when children and youth may potentially benefit from additional P–CIMT or other forms of therapy

4. Evaluating the types of professional expertise and training that best support the delivery of high-quality, effective P–CIMT, including considerations in the delivery of P–CIMT such as group versus individual setting, delivery by single or multiple providers and family members, use of technology assistance, and need for formal certification for qualified P–CIMT practitioners

5. Studying the effects of P–CIMT in combination or coordination (before, during, or after) with other EBPs and new promising interventions

6. Delineating the neurobiological mechanisms—over time—that support and reflect the effects of P–CIMT for children at different stages of development, taking into account individual brain and behavioral differences (as well as treatment histories) before intervention

7. Conducting **implementation science** research to identify effective strategies for delivering P–CIMT to all children and youths who are likely to benefit from this form of therapy, encompassing research on professional learning and improvement of health service delivery systems

8. Evaluating P–CIMT in terms of **cost-effectiveness** (i.e., relative costs and outcomes of various options), **cost-efficiency** (i.e., ways to produce optimum results for a given expenditure), and **return on investment** (i.e., future cost savings from improved function and health) by conducting comparative studies that examine current practices, expenditures, and documented outcomes and that test innovative strategies for delivery of P–CIMT.

Relevant research findings are more important than ever in the current world of health care reform and increased consumer engagement for the following reasons:

- Consumers (i.e., families and their children) are more informed than ever about the full range of treatment options and relative risks.
- Third-party payers insist on evidence of the therapeutic and health benefits of treatments.
- Clinical practitioners continuously renew and refine their skills and actively document the progress of all clients they serve.
- Communities, schools, and employers cooperate to ensure that obstacles (e.g., physical, psychological) to full engagement of people with disabilities are eliminated and that appropriate, high-quality supports are readily available.

In the past, clinicians, families, and scientists often appeared to be competing for limited resources. An alternative is to form strong **alliances** that strategically identify shared goals and gaps in knowledge to prioritize research activities and afford opportunities for rapid acceleration of translation of research findings into sustainable benefits for client populations. Current examples of effective alliances include those among consumers, investigators, and practitioners in the fields that address learning disabilities, autism spectrum disorders, Down syndrome, and fetal alcohol spectrum disorders. We predict that we are on the cusp of an era of similar alliances among those concerned with children with cerebral palsy (CP) and closely related neuromotor impairments. This era will present a marked contrast to earlier times, when physicians and practitioners all too often presented information to parents as if the physicians and practitioners were the sole authorities on what is best for children and frequently concealed from families and children the extent of uncertainty and professional debate about which treatments really worked, for whom, under what conditions, and at what costs in time and money.

We hope readers of this handbook will help usher in this new era. Vital to success will be the productivity that results from an expanded research agenda that yields relevant, practical, and useful findings to support open information exchange and continued vigilance in monitoring and improving the quality, timeliness, and equity of evidence-based treatments for children and youth with neuromotor impairments.

The following sections discuss the rationale for conducting research in each of the eight high-priority areas. Each section offers some (but not all) examples of research topics, methodological approaches, study populations, and data analytic strategies that would support the research blueprint. Science, just like clinical practice, is an art that evolves from the creativity, experience, and synergy of scientists, clinicians,

and consumers (i.e., children and their families). Science can be informed by real-world challenges, just as clinical practice can be informed by the results of scientific studies.

HIGH-PRIORITY QUESTIONS TO GUIDE FUTURE RESEARCH

WHAT ARE THE OPTIMAL TREATMENT COMPONENTS AND PROTOCOLS FOR DELIVERING EFFECTIVE P–CIMT?

In the leading research reviews about pediatric rehabilitation and P–CIMT (see Chapter 2, "Pediatric CIMT: History and Definition"), almost all of the authors have concluded that the available data from studies conducted to date are not adequate to answer many critical questions. Two of the most pressing questions are

1. What is the best dosage (intensity of treatment)?
2. What are the effects of different types of constraint used part- or full-time?

Indeed, because high intensity and constraint are two of the cardinal distinguishing features of P–CIMT (see Chapter 2, on the history of P–CIMT, and Chapter 7, on operationalizing P–CIMT), direct comparisons of the differential effects of various dosages and types of constraint would provide crucial data needed by clinicians who prescribe and deliver P–CIMT.

Dosage

The topic of intensity of intervention is emerging as a major theme for therapeutic and preventive interventions for children with a broad range of developmental disabilities, including autism spectrum disorders; intellectual disabilities; and learning, attention, and behavior problems. Intensity or **dosage** of a treatment intervention includes multiple dimensions that warrant consideration in future research (and thus always should be included in reports of clinical P–CIMT studies):

- Length of each treatment session
- Total number of treatment sessions
- Spacing or density of the treatment sessions (e.g., how many per week)
- Total duration of the treatment window (from entry into treatment to treatment completion).

Although it may seem that one could simply identify the clinical trials that produced the largest magnitude of benefits and reasonably infer that the intensity and dosage used in these trials were "superior" to those used in trials that produced lesser benefits, in fact this conclusion is not possible. The reasons that the current published findings cannot provide an adequate answer are many. The magnitude of benefits (often expressed in terms of effect sizes) produced by different P–CIMT protocols cannot be directly compared across studies in which participating children differed considerably in age or initial (baseline) ability level, in which different measures were used to assess outcomes, or in which incomplete details were provided in the published reports about the exact intensity or dosage and the precise form and use of constraint. The authors of many studies devised their own outcome measures, for which evidence of strong psychometric integrity is lacking. Further, many trials had relatively small sample sizes and research design limitations, leading to limits in the ability to interpret and, perhaps most importantly, generalize the findings.

Thus, the research is not yet adequate to support conclusions about the effects of various dosages or constraint procedures. In the final analysis, studies that systematically vary the dosage of P–CIMT to ascertain minimal and maximal thresholds need to consider the characteristics of the children themselves, recognizing that optimal dosage may differ for particular subgroups (e.g., infants and toddlers, children with severe vs. mild UE impairment).

The features of intensity and constraint are not only important from a clinical perspective but also vital to developing and refining a theory of **therapy-induced neuroplasticity** (the ability of the central nervous system to reorganize its structures and networks in response to therapeutic activity; see Chapter 1, "History and Development of CIMT for Adults With Stroke," for a discussion of the theoretical foundation of CIMT). Concerning the intensity of treatment, many practitioners hold the strong opinion that **high-intensity P–CIMT,** such as 6 hours of therapy per day for 21 days over a 3- to 4-week treatment window, is too demanding or intrusive for the children and their families. Other practitioners hold the opposite view, that only highly intensive therapy can produce large and lasting benefits. Practitioners favoring high intensity hypothesize that because a child's progress is both rapid and visible, highly intensive P–CIMT is more rewarding and less frustrating than low-dosage therapy, which may not produce immediate large benefits.

Although published reports have stated that little or no attrition or dropout occurs because of perceptions of excessive burden associated with high-intensity dosage (DeLuca, Echols, Law, & Ramey, 2006; DeLuca, Echols, & Ramey, 2007; Taub, Ramey, DeLuca, & Echols, 2004), many clinicians still fear that daily treatment for several hours or more may be "too much." Parents as well are sometimes concerned about the challenges presented by the signature form of P–CIMT for family schedules, school and sports activities, and ongoing relationships with other practitioners who have been working with their child. In addition, because "standard" therapy provided by both occupational therapy and physical

therapy practitioners typically is provided in 1-hour sessions, practitioners and parents may view longer sessions as an excessive burden.

So far, only a small-scale study (Case-Smith, DeLuca, Stevenson, & Ramey, 2012), a randomized controlled trial with 18 children, directly compared two markedly different dosage levels, both of which are high relative to standard therapy practices. This recent trial, which used practitioners who received common training in a P–CIMT manualized protocol, demonstrated both significant and comparable benefits for young children (aged 3 to 6 years) who received either 3 hours of P–CIMT per day for 21 days (total = 63 treatment hours) or 6 hours per day for 21 days (total = 126 treatment hours; Case-Smith et al., 2012). Although these results are noteworthy, one small-scale study is woefully inadequate to answer the major question about what constitutes an optimal dosage and whether the dosage levels needed to produce measurable and sustained benefits differ as a function of the child's age, initial developmental skill level, or family engagement in practicing and extending the benefits that may occur during professionally administered P–CIMT. At a theoretical level, a model of the developing brain as influenced by therapeutic experiences would benefit substantially from data about dose–response curves.

Constraint

Obviously, constraint has been deemed a distinguishing feature of P–CIMT. The compelling idea is that constraint of the child's less-impaired, more-functional UE will help redirect the child's attention to using the more-impaired, less-functional side of his or her body by creating an **environmental press** (i.e., motivation to meet occupational demands placed by the environment) for the child to use this side because the more functional side is not readily available for use. In the earliest applications of P–CIMT, the constraint alone was the condition that prompted **forced use** of the other side—that is, casting without applying active therapy or using principles of learning and shaping. As reviewed in earlier chapters in this volume, the use of constraint by itself does not seem to produce significant or sustained improvement in the more-impaired side.

Currently, clinicians and scientists are engaged in a vigorous debate during professional meetings and in peer-reviewed journals about the type and duration of constraint that should be used in P–CIMT; some have even questioned whether constraint is truly advantageous if the treatment is sufficiently intensive (high dosage). The types of constraint used have varied considerably and have included a soft **mitt** applied just to the hand; a **splint** applied to just the lower part of the arm and hand; a soft **sling** for the entire UE; a rigid **cast** for the lower part of the arm; and a rigid cast for the entire arm that extends to the fingertips, sometimes placing the arm and hand in a straight line (elbow extended), but more often with the elbow bent. In addition to these variations in the type of constraint used, some P–CIMT protocols use the constraint solely during the therapy sessions, others have the child wear the constraint for many hours per day (often for most of the waking hours), and yet others have the child wear the constraint 24 hours per day throughout the entire treatment period (e.g., 3 or 4 weeks).

Table 16.1 lists many of the reasons that have been advanced to endorse different approaches to constraint. The table helps illustrate the divergent clinical and scientific perspectives that can all appear to be rational and logical; this debate can be resolved only through the collection of objective data obtained through well-designed clinical research studies. Accordingly, continued debate in the absence of new data on this topic is nonproductive. Instead, we advocate conducting timely research that directly tests the possible benefits and potential iatrogenic (negative) effects of the different forms of constraint.

For clinicians who need to make informed choices today, before the results of such research become available, it is important to note the following:

- To date, many published studies have reported that all or most children adapt quite readily to the use of constraint, with the most active monitoring taking place in studies that use full-time, full-arm constraint and that monitor weekly for possible signs of harm to the casted arm.

Table 16.1 CONTRASTING VIEWS ON PART-TIME, PART-ARM CONSTRAINT VS. FULL-TIME, FULL-ARM CASTING

TOPIC	ARGUMENT FOR PART-TIME, PART-ARM CONSTRAINT	ARGUMENT FOR FULL-TIME, FULL-ARM CASTING
Child safety	The child maintains the ability to use his or her more-functional UE for protection (e.g., during a fall) both during and outside of therapy sessions.	The child is able to raise or move the arm protectively (e.g., in a fall) with a bent elbow cast. The cast can be constructed for quick removal.
Stigmatization	The child will not be seen by others as looking different and will not need to explain "what happened."	The child who can say why he or she is wearing a cast will not be stigmatized. For a child who cannot explain, a cast worn for a short time is unlikely to be a real stigma because many children wear a cast for other reasons.
Frustration levels for the child	The child will not have to adjust to a full-time cast that prevents use of his or her better side. However, having the practitioner put on and take off a constraint may be frustrating for a child who does not like being constrained, which could make the therapy session more challenging.	Initially, a full-time cast may be frustrating because the child cannot do things in the usual ways, but after getting used to the cast, the child may enjoy seeing rapid progress with the targeted arm and hand. For some, the novelty of the cast is like a fun game.
Ability to focus on learning new unilateral skills with the more-impaired extremity	Less-intense constraint is a more natural way to promote skill acquisition and improvement. Many activities focus on unilateral skills that can be classified as helping or support skills. During therapy, the partly constrained extremity can sometimes be part of the therapy activity and feedback.	The child is "forced" to focus on use of the more-impaired side for daily activities. Competition from the better side is eliminated, so the child does not have to inhibit its use. Many children seem newly aware of the more-impaired extremity that they had previously neglected.
Ability to integrate new skills for use bimanually and bilaterally	Many P–CIMT protocols that use a part-time soft constraint have a strong focus on the child learning how to use the more-impaired side in bilateral activities that will be dominated by the less-impaired side.	Theoretically, when unilateral skills reach a certain level of competence, they can be integrated into the child's repertoire of bimanual activities. Without an adequate level of competence, the child may return to disregarding the more-impaired side after therapy ends.
Competing sensory input	Less-intense constraint does not significantly reduce sensory input from either side, which is natural for the child.	More-intense constraint reduces sensory input from the less-impaired UE and may help the child concentrate on what is happening with the more-impaired UE (sensory and motor input).

(Continued)

Table 16.1 CONTRASTING VIEWS ON PART-TIME, PART-ARM CONSTRAINT VS. FULL-TIME, FULL-ARM CASTING *(Cont.)*

TOPIC	ARGUMENT FOR PART-TIME, PART-ARM CONSTRAINT	ARGUMENT FOR FULL-TIME, FULL-ARM CASTING
Competing neuromotor input or movements	Less-intense constraint is ideal because it is more natural for the child to learn to use the less-capable UE under the same conditions that will occur after therapy is completed (i.e., neuromotor input and movements from both sides).	More-intense constraint reduces competing input and movements from the less-impaired UE, which could distract the child from focusing on the more-impaired UE. After the child experiences substantial progress in unilateral skills with the more-impaired side, he or she can learn later to adjust to input from both sides.
Total practice time (therapy plus nontherapy hours)	The child focuses on the more-impaired UE during therapy but, between therapy sessions, adapts new skills to typical everyday situations with both arms and hands available.	The child has a real reason to practice using the more-impaired UE during nontherapy times. This ecological demand created by the full-time cast promotes rehearsal and improvement across many everyday situations. Even during sleep, the child has to use the more-impaired side to make positional adjustments.
Compensatory movement strategies	The child with asymmetrical abilities is able to continue use of his or her own compensatory strategies.	More intense constraint prevents use of some of the compensatory strategies a child has developed. If progress during therapy is sufficient, these strategies may drop out of the child's repertoire.
Brain development in areas that support use of the more-impaired extremity	Areas of the brain that support bimanual and bilateral activity are particularly likely to be strengthened if there is significant progress with the more impaired side as a helper. Subsequent improvement in the areas indicative of the more-impaired arm and hand also may show changes.	Areas of the brain indicative of use of the more-impaired side are likely to show changes (structural and functional) associated with new unilateral skills. Areas reflecting bilateral use also may show changes during therapy or later.
Loss of skills and strength in the constrained extremity	Less-intense constraint is unlikely to have any negative effect on the constrained side.	Studies of typically developing children show mostly small and short-term effects of wearing a cast. Some research also reports improvements on the constrained side (although this is difficult to explain). Monitoring of full-time casting in P–CIMT has shown no negative effects thus far.
Ease for parents of caring for the child	Parents probably will not need to make any adjustments in their care of and interactions with the child. They can, however, be encouraged to promote the use of new skills shown during therapy sessions and to reinforce improved bilateral activities.	Parents are likely to learn new ways to support their child during the treatment period (sometimes 4 or more weeks) because the child cannot use the less-impaired arm and hand. Parents may feel this is a good opportunity to praise the child for making new efforts to use the more-impaired arm and hand.

Note. P–CIMT = Pediatric constraint-induced movement therapy; UE = upper extremity.

- Different types of constraint have produced measurable benefits, but the exact magnitudes cannot yet be compared.

Clinical discussions about children showing signs of noncooperation or resistance to the use of constraint mainly have related to P–CIMT protocols in which the constraint was placed only during the therapy session. As Table 16.1 illustrates, the topic of constraint is a complex one, and future findings may well reveal that certain constraint conditions are particularly favorable for very young versus older children or for children with very severe versus far milder degrees of initial impairment in UE function.

The P–CIMT clinical research community has an opportunity to learn a great deal from the years of investment in a series of thoughtfully planned, multisite randomized controlled trials supported by the National Institutes of Health's (NIH's) National Eye Institute on the topic of using patches for children with **amblyopia,** in which one eye does not function as well as the other. The clinical issues with amblyopia have much in common with those surrounding P–CIMT because the clinical treatments engage both "constraint" (i.e., patching that takes away use of the more-functional eye) and a variety of other therapies ranging from no active therapy for the targeted eye to use of refractive correction and participation by children in planned eye activities. This vigorous and exemplary program of NIH-sponsored research has used multiple clinical sites, enrolled large sample sizes, applied common baseline and outcome measures, monitored treatment fidelity, and studied both younger and older children with severe to mild forms of the condition.

For published examples that report highly informative findings generated by this amblyopia research (funded by the NIH Cooperative Agreement mechanism), see Holmes and colleagues (2011), Repka and Pediatric Eye Disease Investigator Group (2003), and Holmes and Clarke (2006). Briefly, the findings indicate that multiple factors impinge on children's positive responses to variations in patching treatment, including both the clinical protocol and the children's individual characteristics. These findings have influenced clinical practice and the refinement of theories about neuroplasticity as applied to the developing visual system.

Other Components

In addition to the central features of intensity of therapy (dosage) and use of constraint, the following components of P–CIMT and variations in its administration may also be worthy of scientific investigation:

- Whether to have the P–CIMT protocol include a full range of prespecified activities and skills that all children receive (i.e., a uniform protocol similar to that used for adults with stroke) or to individualize treatment on the basis of the child's current ability and expressed interest in certain types of activity (e.g., learning a new sports activity, being able to do fine motor activities such as writing and drawing)
- The relative value of explicit direct shaping activities during therapy sessions (with immediate feedback and demands for improved performance) versus time spent in task repetition and rehearsal (without constant monitoring and feedback); this topic has been studied directly in CIMT research on adults with stroke (Wolf et al., 2007, 2008)
- The importance of focusing on unilateral skill development in the more-impaired UE versus emphasizing its role as an "assisting hand" that mostly will be engaged in bimanual and bilateral activities when the constraint is removed and therapy has ended.

ARE ASSESSMENT TOOLS AND MEASUREMENT TECHNIQUES FOR STUDYING THE EFFECTS OF P–CIMT ADEQUATE?

Because UE skills develop rapidly in the first decade of life, how can findings about therapy-induced improvement be disentangled from those indicating natural developmental progress and related to how close to "normative" a child with neuromotor impairment is before and after treatment? To what extent should children with more severe neuromotor impairment be considered "less mature" (in terms of selecting the best measures to use for them), and should adjustments be made for expectations about their progress?

In Chapter 6, "Assessment Tools to Measure Upper-Limb Function and Impact of Therapy," Boyd and Sakzewski identify a set of assessment tools and measurement strategies that are suitable for use in P–CIMT clinical studies, noting in some detail their strengths and limitations. Chapter 6 also provides excellent, practical, and useful (although not entirely comprehensive) advice for scientists and clinicians working in this field. We particularly endorse the *International Classification of Functioning* model, which explicitly identifies participation and function measures rather than only discrete tested UE skills that do not always translate into real-world alterations in a child's life (see World Health Organization, 2001).

Methodological research is urgently needed to ensure a more comprehensive and sensitive picture of outcomes for children with neuromotor disabilities from infancy through adulthood. The methodological issues related to valid and reliable assessments are compounded when applied to conducting rehabilitation research on children with neuromotor impairments because the neuromotor performance of children can fluctuate widely over the course of the day and under various conditions of stress and fatigue. For children with CP, for example, this daily fluctuation occurs to a far greater degree than for typically developing children.

In addition, fewer age-appropriate tools for assessing UE skills and everyday use are available for infants and toddlers (ages birth to 2 years) and preschool-age children (ages 3 to 5 years) than for older children. Further, many of the UE skills that are important for later occupational engagement do not emerge until the school years, and they often continue to develop and become more sophisticated well into the adolescent years. Fine motor skill levels are related both to age and to learning and training opportunities (e.g., activities that children have learned through repeated participation). The development of skills with age creates many practical and statistical problems when conducting research that seeks to compare how well an intervention such as P–CIMT works for children of different ages because no common metric is available (nor can one be readily created). Even efforts to calculate common outcomes based on the percentage of treatment goals achieved, degree of improvement, or new skills acquired are flawed and difficult to disentangle from both the child's age and initial level of UE functioning.

Above all, assessment tools themselves differ in what they measure, so many summary scores cannot readily be placed into a common metric for estimating the relative effect sizes of treatment. In addition, some of the tools used in P–CIMT research were designed specifically for children with hemiparesis or asymmetric UE functioning, whereas others were developed for testing typically developing children or a heterogeneous group of children with developmental disabilities. Standardized tools for a general population simply score how well a child completes a given item (taking into account the child's age), but they fail to record which arm or hand a child uses for the item. Although research scoring methods can be adopted and the tests can be administered with special instructions for the child to use a given arm or hand, the scores generated from these modified procedures cannot readily be compared to age norms or attached to adaptive function and overall participation in life activities. Until further methodology research is conducted to standardize alternative ways of administering the most widely used assessment tools created for typically developing children, cross-study comparisons of children's performance will remain problematic.

Assessments should guide the clinical choices that practitioners make and help identify the best course of interventions when starting treatment, but most assessments do not do this. What skills or motor components should a practitioner focus on based on the child's presentation or current level of function? The Pediatric Evaluation of Disability Inventory, for example, on the basis of a Rasch analysis of self-care, mobility, and communication tasks, orders activities in a sequence of easy- to hard-to-perform items (combining child ability and item ability scales) to help practitioners set more specific functional goals based on the child's current abilities (Haley et al., 2011).

The field of pediatric rehabilitation in general could benefit immensely from advances in the measurement of neuromotor competence. Research teams throughout the world currently are engaged in innovative research that uses technology to record and quantify many interesting and theoretically important dimensions of movement and voluntary control. For example,

- Three-dimensional **kinematics** records movement through sensors placed at various anatomical points of the arm to measure time, distance, speed, accuracy, smoothness of arm and hand movements, and other variables.
- Multichannel **electromyography** systems measure muscle activation and synergy.
- Sophisticated wireless **accelerometry** can be applied to multiple body parts in both laboratory and everyday settings.
- **Fiber optics** embedded in special gloves uses infrared light to measure many aspects of small movements, in real time, involving the fingers, hands, and wrists.

These techniques are still being refined, and some were developed for use with children of only a narrow age or ability range. It is hoped that continued advances in these sophisticated methods will make them more readily available for standardized use in clinical and research settings.

Another major topic related to measuring the effects of P–CIMT on children is the degree to which P–CIMT exerts a lasting effect on a child's everyday occupational performance and overall quality of life. As with most topics covered in this chapter, there are strong differences of opinion. One position is that a highly focused form of therapy should achieve its specific therapy-related goals. For instance, when testing whether a new form of medical treatment helps improve a given medical condition, scientists seldom add on the expectation that the patient's quality of life will be improved overall. However, it is reasonable to think that early intervention provided for children with CP—particularly intervention that includes highly intensive forms of therapy—could have a broad effect on a child's life, especially if the child's overall competence increases rapidly in a major way. In turn, these changes permit the child to engage in a larger range of age-typical activities in the realms of social, academic, and recreational programs. The child may begin to have a more positive attitude toward taking on challenging tasks, and the child's parents and teachers may see a brighter future for the child because of the rapid improvement after an intensive therapy intervention.

Many treatment decisions for children with disabilities involve a multidisciplinary team, which often establishes multiple outcome goals for a given child. Several P–CIMT outcome studies have selected Goal Attainment Scaling (GAS) as a primary outcome measure (see Chapter 6), reflecting a clinical emphasis on the individualization of treatment goals for each child, often in partnership with the child and the parents. **Goal Attainment Scaling,** as described by Palisano, Haley, and Brown (1992), is a method devised to provide an individualized, criterion-referenced measure of change. Steenbeek, Ketelaar, Galama, and Gorter (2007) conducted a critical review of research evidence on the use of GAS in pediatric rehabilitation and summarized it as follows:

> We conclude that the literature supports promising qualities of GAS in pediatric rehabilitation. GAS

is a responsive method for individual goal setting and for treatment evaluation. However, current knowledge about its reliability when used with children is insufficient. There is a need for further development of GAS and its application for children of different ages and disabilities, across therapists of different disciplines. (p. 550)

GAS thus provides a promising technique that supports what clinicians and consumers often recognize occurs during treatment: namely, that treatment goals are individualized and that their attainment is important to measure.

Other areas that have been proposed as important to measure include engagement in activities ranging from social and recreational activities to daily living skills (e.g., Canadian Occupational Performance Measure, Law et al., 2005; Vineland Adaptive Behavior Scales, Sparrow, Cicchetti, & Balla, 2006) and quality of life, particularly for older children and adolescents. These types of measure are worthy of inclusion but do not represent the primary targets of P–CIMT. Similarly, as discussed in Chapter 14, "Beyond Upper-Extremity Benefits of Pediatric CIMT: Reported Changes in Gait and Other Neuromotor Skills," on secondary effects, P–CIMT has been reported to sometimes coincide with or contribute to changes in other dimensions of a child's life, as well as in particular areas of brain functioning. Continued research that explores hypotheses about the relationship of neuromotor competence and development in other domains will be valuable for both a clinical and theoretical understanding of the course of development in children with different types and degrees of neuromotor challenges.

WHAT ARE THE LONG-TERM EFFECTS OF P–CIMT?

How are long-term outcomes influenced by children's post-P–CIMT therapy experiences, including the subsequent types of therapy and school and family supports they receive? Also, for children who receive multiple P–CIMT treatments (sometimes spaced a year or two apart), are the long-term effects of P–CIMT significantly different than for those who receive only one P–CIMT treatment episode?

In the field of pediatric rehabilitation generally, few longitudinal treatment outcome studies extend beyond 6 or 12 months post treatment. Fortunately, most clinical trials of P–CIMT have followed the treated children for 6 months post treatment. Thus far, the data strongly support the conclusion that benefits detected at the end of treatment continue (and sometimes reach even higher levels) 6 months later. What is notably absent in the published research about children with CP is a representative portrayal of their divergent life courses and the factors that contribute to greater health, adult independence, and personal well-being throughout their adulthood. Epidemiological data clearly show that the life expectancy for children with CP is much greater today than it was in the past (see Chapter 4, "Motor Development and Physical Growth in Children With Cerebral Palsy").

The availability of multiple supports, early intervention services, and improved health management contributes to the expectation that a large proportion of children with CP will become productive citizens who can engage in a full range of adult activities, from the personal and family to the social, recreational, educational, and occupational realms. The few prospective longitudinal studies that have been conducted on people with CP thus far have not included systematic analyses of the impact of therapies and support services they receive at different times in their lives. We strongly advocate for the establishment of linked lifespan databases and perhaps of large, voluntary registries of people whose lives can be studied over many decades, offering children and their families the opportunity to share their experiences widely to increase the accuracy and representativeness of the knowledge base about the life course of children with diverse neuromotor impairments. Much care will be needed to ensure that the privacy and confidentiality of participants is protected.

The **Pediatric Neuromotor Research Clinic (PNRC)** we established at the University of Alabama at Birmingham in 1999 and led until 2012 provided us with the opportunity to offer multiple treatments of P–CIMT to more than 60 children whose parents initiated contact for a follow-up or booster course of P–CIMT. Most often, these families sought a second course of treatment about 1 year later because their child seemed more mature and ready to learn more in terms of both fine motor skills and coordination and strength, and particularly to help with sports and other physical activities the children wanted to pursue. Because we operated this clinic as a research clinical service, almost all of the families volunteered to have their children participate in the research protocol (with informed consent), which included systematic outcome measures. Our analyses indicate that second (and even third and fourth) episodes of P–CIMT continue to produce significant benefits for these children (see Chapter 8, "ACQUIREc Protocol: What We Have Learned From a Decade of Delivering a Signature Form of Pediatric CIMT," for a description of PNRC activities). Larger-scale research using a randomized controlled trial design in which children receive one, two, or even three P–CIMT treatments combined with multiyear longitudinal follow-up would provide much-needed data to inform treatment recommendations about when and for whom additional P–CIMT treatment might be indicated.

Conducting long-term studies of children is time-consuming and expensive. In countries that maintain standard health care records and tracking systems for the entire population, certain outcomes can be monitored for a representative and large cohort of children regarding their life course, including multiple health, educational, and occupational outcomes. For some populations with special needs, the creation of voluntary patient registries (often through partnerships of advocacy organizations and universities) and the establishment of clinical research networks (such as those supported by NIH) are highly productive approaches to learning about the long-term outcomes of large and diverse samples of children.

WHAT TYPES OF PROFESSIONAL EXPERTISE, TRAINING, AND TECHNOLOGY CAN BEST SUPPORT DELIVERY OF HIGH-QUALITY, EFFECTIVE P–CIMT?

Are there differences in the professional competencies needed depending on the type of P–CIMT protocol (e.g., group vs. individual treatment) and where it is delivered (e.g., clinic, school, camp, home)? Can parents and paraprofessionals serve as effective change agents by applying the principles of P–CIMT?

Most studies of traditional, or signature, P–CIMT have engaged licensed occupational or physical therapy practitioners to deliver the treatment. Several studies, however, have trained parents or teachers either as primary providers of P–CIMT or as **adjunctive supports** in the delivery of P–CIMT (see Chapter 9, "Alternative Pediatric CIMT: Understanding the How and Why of Clinical Variations in Pediatric CIMT"; Chapter 12, "Novel and Complementary Therapy Strategies: Critical Issues and Opportunities for Combining With Pediatric CIMT"; and Chapter 15, "Working With Families and Therapy Teams to Maximize Pediatric CIMT Benefits"). Further, in many studies of P–CIMT delivered in camps and other group settings, therapists and other staff and volunteers, students, paraprofessionals, and parents have been part of the planned intervention (see Chapter 10, "Group-Based Models of Pediatric CIMT: Special Camps, School-Based Treatment, and Home Environment Models"). To date, however, the implicit assumption has been that the traditional or signature form of P–CIMT is best administered under the guidance and expertise of a highly qualified professional, whereas modified forms often reach out to engage other people who are part of a child's everyday social support system.

Sound practical, scientific, and fiscal reasons exist to design studies that directly test hypotheses about the required skill sets and knowledge needed to produce significant and lasting benefits from P–CIMT. For example, studies could compare P–CIMT delivered by people with different professional backgrounds but comparable training in the specifics of a given P–CIMT protocol. Outcomes could include direct observation of how well the P–CIMT is administered (i.e., fidelity of implementation), the extent to which appropriate accommodations are made for the individual needs of the child, and changes in neuromotor competence at the componential skill and functional occupational levels. Ideally, the field needs to know which types of rehabilitation providers, along with support from others, produce the largest magnitude benefits.

Other avenues of research could test the merit of combining the delivery of high-intensity P–CIMT provided by a trained professional with group activities or extension therapies delivered by paraprofessionals and supported at home by parents. Similarly, many efforts are under way to develop innovative technology applications that will help children with hemiparesis practice and improve their UE skills. These technology supports for P–CIMT can be considered in systematic research on ways to efficiently and effectively deliver P–CIMT, discussed in the next section.

CAN THE BENEFITS OF P–CIMT BE INCREASED WHEN COMBINED WITH OTHER EVIDENCE-BASED PRACTICES OR NEW PROMISING INTERVENTIONS?

When the results of a P–CIMT trial are presented at a professional meeting, an audience member often asks the question, "Could the P–CIMT benefits have been enhanced if the children had received botulinum toxin therapy during treatment?" Currently, research on this question is under way, but the answer for clinical practice is not resolved. Many trials to date either exclude children who have been receiving botulinum toxin therapy or require the children to suspend botulinum toxin therapy while they participate in P–CIMT (Lukban, Rosales, & Dressler, 2009). **Botulinum toxin therapy** is a treatment used to reduce muscle spasms. It usually involves injections at the site of the recurring spasms to improve voluntary control of muscles. Botulinum toxin therapy could be an important adjunct to P–CIMT because it could reduce the effects of spasticity and allow children an opportunity to strengthen and learn to balance the opposing muscle groups that control involved joints.

In addition to botulinum toxin therapy, other treatments that appear worthy of considering for use before, during, or after P–CIMT include electrical stimulation or E-stim, kinesiology taping, deep brain stimulation, stem cell infusion, virtual reality, and mental imagining of neuromotor activities. **E-stim** and **kinesiology taping** are provided as adjuncts to P–CIMT and help muscles move joints into targeted positions to maximize function (see Chapter 12). E-stim has the potential to help strengthen muscles through stronger activation using electrical stimulation. Kinesiology taping is the application of slightly elastic tape designed to recoil to help with the movement of joints to which it is applied. **Deep brain stimulation** and **stem cell infusion** are more invasive procedures that could potentially help children going through

P–CIMT by mitigating the effects of severe dystonia and diffuse brain injuries. **Virtual reality** and **mental imagining** are two technology-driven therapy additions that may help children develop improved mastery through stronger neural representations of the practiced skills (Steenbergen, Crajé, Nilsen, & Gordon, 2009).

This list of potential adjunctive therapies is by no means exhaustive; rather, it underscores the fact that parents and clinicians alike are—and will continue to be—vigorous in seeking out multiple forms of therapy and interventions that could be beneficial to children. Similarly, scientists are interested in documenting whether synergistic and multiplicative benefits (i.e., more than merely additive effects) occur when therapies are combined intentionally and, alternatively, whether codelivery of certain interventions might interfere with or decrease their effectiveness. If so, understanding the likely mechanisms related to enhancing or preventing benefits of multiple therapies would be important for clinicians to know about so that the timing and sequencing of different treatments can be well informed to produce optimal, long-term progress for a child.

WHAT NEUROBIOLOGICAL MECHANISMS ARE LIKELY TO SUPPORT AND REFLECT THE EFFECTS OF P–CIMT?

What neurobiological mechanisms are involved in P–CIMT, and to what extent does P–CIMT promote compensatory or natural developmental central nervous system processes? Advances in **neuroimaging,** which provides an understanding of the central nervous system through visual images, have been exciting for the field of pediatric rehabilitation. The ability to obtain valid images of the brains of infants and young children has improved, although many complex issues still are not entirely resolved in this emerging field. Several studies have reported changes in some brain structures and brain functioning after older children have received P–CIMT (e.g., Sterling et al., 2013; Sutcliffe, Gaetz, Logan, Cheyne, & Fehlings, 2007; Sutcliffe, Logan, & Fehlings, 2009; Szaflarski et al., 2006).

In addition, pediatric research is likely to be further informed by some of the findings from neuroimaging studies (using a variety of techniques) of adults with stroke who have participated in CIMT. For instance, one recent study using both functional magnetic resonance imaging and transcranial magnetic stimulation found that changes differed as a function of stroke patients' initial level of impairment and correlated with the amount of behavioral improvement measured on a standardized clinical assessment (Könönen et al., 2012). The authors concluded that basic neuroscience research accompanying clinical studies is valuable and nominated several specific neurobiological mechanisms as potentially involved in producing and sustaining the benefits of CIMT:

The potential to enhance neurological recovery by manipulating the biological adaptability of the brain has become relevant to clinical practice. Basic neuroscience studies suggest that therapeutic interventions may enhance the restoration of motor functions by potential neurobiological mechanisms such as recovery of neuronal excitability, increased activity in neurons adjacent to injured ones and in partially spared pathways, representational adaptations in neuronal assemblies, recruitment of parallel and subcomponent pathways, altered efficacy of synaptic activity, and regeneration and sprouting from injured and uninjured axons and dendrites. (p. 585)

HOW CAN EXISTING SERVICE DELIVERY SYSTEMS BE CHANGED SO P–CIMT CAN BE PROVIDED TO ALL CHILDREN AND YOUTH WHO ARE LIKELY TO BENEFIT?

Implementation science and **service delivery systems research** involve the search for a better understanding of the barriers to making new and efficacious treatments available. When we first began to present the findings from our research on P–CIMT, we frequently encountered a highly charged reaction from practitioners and clinical administrators, who told us, "It would be both logistically and financially *impossible* for us to implement this high-intensity form of CIMT in *our* clinic!" The barriers that clinicians and administrators promptly identify relate to the administrative setup of their current clinical environment; the large numbers of children they see regularly in these clinical settings (particularly challenging for clinics with waiting lists that seek to serve everyone, offering at least a little therapy to all who seek it); and the fact that their practitioners are not used to (or prepared for) working individually with one child for an extended period, such as the 6 consecutive hours per day for 21 days (including some weekend days) that we had implemented in our first clinical trials. All of these concerns are understandable, yet they pose substantial threats to the ability to implement many of the P–CIMT protocols that have produced at least modest effect sizes.

The relatively young field of implementation science is dedicated to identifying and then testing ways to overcome the barriers that limit the implementation of EBPs in real-world settings. The goal of implementation science is to drive up the timely, effective (i.e., high quality, consistent with proven methods), affordable, and equitable delivery of evidence-based treatments across a wide array of clinical and community settings. Implementation science often involves developing and then comparing different strategies to train and support clinical staff to deliver a new treatment. Such strategies often go beyond merely the technical details of what constitutes the new treatment or intervention. That is, behavior change within the health care system often involves factors such as motivation, attitudes, working relationships with other professionals (both within and outside one's primary specialty area), and communication with clients.

An important construct identified in many studies of adult behavior change is receptivity to change. Often, clinicians are unaware of biases that may influence the care they provide; these biases range from those that affect initial diagnoses to those that influence recommendations for treatment delivery and monitoring. Mental flexibility and confidence in the results of scientific investigations also exert an influence on how readily and completely certain "new" treatments become adopted. Undeniably, almost every field has had a history of popular treatments (sometimes later labeled as "fads") that come and go and scientific and clinical discoveries that later are revealed to have been incomplete or inaccurate. For some practitioners, this fact leads to deep skepticism and high reluctance to change their own practices, particularly if they think they are doing a good job and seeing "with their own eyes" evidence of progress in the children for whom they provide treatment. Others, however, recognize that remaining open-minded and staying current with the evidence as it becomes available support their professional commitment to providing the highest quality of care, knowledge, and services to those they serve. To date, we are aware of little research related to P–CIMT that addresses the central themes of concern in implementation science. As further evidence becomes available about P–CIMT and its benefits and potential limits, we look forward to investigators and clinical providers teaming up to engage in research on how best to offer P–CIMT to large numbers of children in ways that produce benefits at least equal to those obtained under rigorous clinical trial conditions.

The challenges associated with changing the service delivery system and practitioners' knowledge and skills so that P–CIMT can be readily provided in effective ways certainly are not unique to pediatric rehabilitation. Many efficacious treatments that are well supported by multiple and rigorous clinical trials have been delayed or only partially extended to the majority of real-world clinical and educational settings where they could be used to improve client and student outcomes. We are indebted to the American Occupational Therapy Association for the support and the encouragement provided so that we could produce this volume on the state of knowledge about P–CIMT and share it with clinical practitioners from many disciplines, rehabilitation scientists, health care administrators and policymakers, and consumers (parents and their children). This volume represents an important step in promoting active dialogue about when, where, and for whom to provide P–CIMT and how best to

monitor its application in diverse clinical, educational, and community settings.

The historical and current setup of clinical environments in pediatric rehabilitation is not readily compatible with most P–CIMT protocols. Clinical environments usually are designed and operated to allow practitioners to see many clients a day, with brief periods between to enter notes (i.e., documentation), complete required forms, and perhaps reflect on a particular matter that arose. Such environments appear to maximize the potential for reimbursement from third-party payers, who historically have relied on practitioners' clinical judgments about treatment effects regarding each visit for therapeutic services that the client receives. Insurance companies rely on these clinical judgments to help determine payments and to guide the general parameters associated with services and procedures for particular conditions and types of clients.

The system is set up to regard treatment effectiveness in terms of the client's and practitioner's productivity in completing a set of activities during a given therapeutic hour rather than in terms of any real impact of therapeutic services on the functional skills and life situation of the client. This is one of the important, but often overlooked, reasons why rehabilitation therapies that have been proven via scientifically rigorous testing later fail to demonstrate efficacy. In this type of setting, therapy simply is not designed to be a type of treatment (which in most of medicine involves a set of activities in a predesigned protocol) per se; rather, most of the reimbursement structure for rehabilitation consists of payment for individual activities that a clinician documents as completed. To complicate matters, treatment interventions then are reimbursed at varying rates.

This picture is increasingly complicated in today's era of EBP. Although the system is designed as described above, the resulting failure to document strong treatment outcomes for rehabilitation becomes a double-edged sword. Third-party payers, consumers, national leaders, and even government agencies are quick to point out the need for all of medicine's treatments to be based on sound principles that can be scientifically tested and that have demonstrated efficacy. Rehabilitation researchers have responded and have begun to systematically examine the field's techniques and treatments, but the system in many ways is inherently designed to fail in this regard, and, in turn, third-party payers have quickly embraced these failures to justify cutting covered services and number of treatment sessions.

Rehabilitation clinicians and researchers must advocate for treatments to become recognized as protocol based. An emphasis on protocol does not take away from the clinician's ability to individualize services. Rather, we suggest recognizing and defining the broad principles that already are often used across clients, activities, and treatments; rehabilitation professionals will benefit by becoming more skilled in operationalizing these broader principles. This process of **operationalization,** or precise definition of protocols, in turn allows the field to demonstrate through documentation the validity of these principles. We believe that operationalization, along with the development of stronger outcome measures, will lead to a better understanding of what is truly effective in therapeutic settings and, more importantly, will lead the field to an era in which these newly developed treatment protocols easily demonstrate their efficacy and effectiveness when subjected to scientific testing. It is our firm belief and hope that P–CIMT can serve as a model for many other rehabilitation treatments to usher in this new approach. Even though many and varied P–CIMT protocols have been described in the literature, one of the biggest advantages (in terms of demonstrating efficacy) of P–CIMT over other rehabilitation approaches is that it is based on core principles that, at least in part, have been built into most protocols.

Another major difficulty that clinicians point out when talking about how they might build P–CIMT into their clinical settings is that they see too many children to be able to maintain its intensity. This point is indeed difficult to address. The numbers of children being referred for rehabilitation services have grown steadily throughout the years. Advances in medicine have resulted in many children living with chronic diseases and consequences of injuries that they would not have survived in previous times. In addition, parents are more aware of and more willing to seek available services for many reasons, including the passage of proactive legislation to help children who are at risk for any type of developmental delay obtain services. All of these factors are positive for children, but rather than approaching them as reasons for the difficulty of implementing EBPs such as P–CIMT, we should approach them as a call to implement the best EBPs. Although the task of implementing best EBPs is difficult, it is not insurmountable. The first place to begin to address this issue is by firmly understanding the impact of the many potential protocol variations listed in the questions discussed in this chapter. What we do not want is for the field to respond to this point with such reactivity that the core principles and points of P–CIMT are diluted and definably lost through increasingly divergent clinical protocols. Understanding the effect of various P–CIMT protocols on varying ages and etiologies is crucial to understanding how we can correctly overcome this hurdle (e.g., through less intensity or the use of paraprofessionals).

Another area of concern regarding implementation science is the impact of the intensity of P–CIMT services on practitioners. This point was briefly addressed earlier in this chapter, but it is not trivial. Many professionals who work in the field of pediatric rehabilitation seem to have a common set of characteristics that enhance their individual ability to work with children. The same good pediatric skill set applies to and helps with implementing many treatments such as P–CIMT. The work environment for practitioners in P–CIMT protocols requires them to remain focused on a limited set of techniques with the same child for many hours every day for an extended period of time. They also are often required to work and think independently without the aid of colleagues in the immediate vicinity of treatment. This type of work will not be successfully accomplishable by all practitioners, and even if accomplishable, will not be enjoyed by all. Understanding how practitioners can maintain the efficacy of P–CIMT protocols while maximizing the therapeutic experience from their own perspective is an area that must be studied in future research.

WHAT DO WE KNOW ABOUT THE COST-EFFECTIVENESS, COST-EFFICIENCY, AND RELATIVE RETURNS ON INVESTMENT FROM P–CIMT COMPARED WITH USUAL AND CUSTOMARY FORMS OF THERAPY?

The need for cost-effectiveness and cost-efficiency research is on the rise in medicine. Historical difficulties in demonstrating efficacy, however, have made this type of research virtually nonexistent in the pediatric rehabilitation field, even for usual and customary forms of therapy. Regardless, cost-effectiveness and cost-efficiency have been a common discussion point among professionals regarding P–CIMT. As mentioned earlier in this chapter, we simply do not know the long-term effects of P–CIMT. Are increased motor abilities maintained or even built on? If so, do these skills enhance the child's (and ultimately the adult's) ability to accomplish a greater number of functional and daily occupations? Could increased motor abilities limit the need for other services, social stigma, or secondary injuries and conditions? All of these issues need to be addressed to truly understand the return on investment that might occur from P–CIMT and are worthy of study, but to be effectively studied, these questions need to be built into a longitudinal battery of research studies.

In the absence of any understanding about the longitudinal implications for cost-effectiveness and cost-efficiency, it is usually quickly pointed out that P–CIMT is very labor-intensive and, therefore, a very costly treatment process. This point has been raised by many practitioners as a reason why P–CIMT cannot be implemented clinically. It is our position, however, that cost-effectiveness and cost-efficiency cannot be separated from the many other points brought forth in this chapter. No one would suggest that usual and customary therapeutic services should not occur, even though they often fail to demonstrate treatment efficacy despite their costs. Rather, there is, at some level, an inherent recognition that therapeutic services have the potential to provide benefit. This chapter provides points that readily suggest that cost–benefit ratios need to be developed for both the short- and long-term effects of a variety of rehabilitation treatments, including P–CIMT protocols. This research is crucial and will serve to enhance what we should be doing as a field: providing both efficacious and effective treatments that enhance and alter the lives of our clients in a positive manner.

SUMMARY

The research blueprint provided in this chapter, although expansive, is by no means all inclusive. It has been the sincere pleasure of the authors to be part of the developing field surrounding P–CIMT, both because of the impact we have seen this treatment approach have on many children and families and because of the many implications this treatment approach has for the entire pediatric rehabilitation field. We hope that this research blueprint will inspire and further promote pediatric rehabilitation through the development of new, efficacious treatments that can enhance the abilities and lives of the children we serve. We also hope that it can help clinicians, scientists, families, and advocates for the field in advocating for funding for pediatric rehabilitation. We are on the cusp of a new era in pediatric rehabilitation, and we encourage its leaders to benefit from lessons that have already been provided by research on P–CIMT and to take them to other areas of pediatric rehabilitation. Collaboration among all the vested parties—clinicians, scientists, and, most importantly, clients and families—will be crucial as we move forward.

REFERENCES

Case-Smith, J., DeLuca, S. C., Stevenson, R., & Ramey, S. L. (2012). Multicenter randomized controlled trial of pediatric constraint-induced movement therapy: 6-month follow-up. *American Journal of Occupational Therapy, 66*, 15–23. http:/dx.doi.org/10.5014/ajot.2012.002386

DeLuca, S. C., Echols, K., Law, C., & Ramey, S. (2006). Intensive pediatric constraint-induced therapy for children with cerebral palsy: Randomized, controlled, crossover trial. *Journal of Child Neurology, 21*, 931–938. PMID: 17092457

DeLuca, S. C., Echols, K., & Ramey, S. L. (2007). *ACQUIREc therapy: A training manual for effective application of pediatric constraint-induced movement therapy.* Hillsborough, NC: MindNurture.

Haley, S. M., Coster, W. J., Dumas, H. M., Fragala-Pinkham, M. A., Kramer, J., Ni, P. S., . . . Ludlow, L. H. (2011). Accuracy and precision of the Pediatric Evaluation of Disability Inventory Computer-Adaptive Tests (PEDI–

CAT). *Developmental Medicine and Child Neurology, 53*, 1100–1106.

Holmes, J. M., & Clarke, M. P. (2006). Amblyopia. *Lancet, 367*, 1343–1351.

Holmes, J. M., Lazar, E. L., Melia, B. M., Astle, W. F., Dagi, L. R., Donahue, S. P., . . . Weise, K. K.; Pediatric Eye Disease Investigator Group. (2011). Effect of age on response to amblyopia treatment in children. *Archives of Ophthalmology, 129*, 1451–1457.

Könönen, M., Tarkka, I. M., Niskanen, E., Pihlajamäki, M., Mervaala, E., Pitkänen, K., & Vanninen, R. (2012). Functional MRI and motor behavioral changes obtained with constraint-induced movement therapy in chronic stroke. *European Journal of Neurology, 19*, 578–586.

Law, M., Baptiste, S., Carswell, A., McColl, M., Polatajko, H., & Pollock, N. (2005). *Canadian Occupational Performance Measure* (3rd ed.). Ottawa: CAOT Publications ACE.

Lukban, M. B., Rosales, R. L., & Dressler, D. (2009). Effectiveness of botulinum toxin A for upper extremity and lower limb spasticity in children with cerebral palsy: A summary of evidence. *Journal of Neural Transmission, 111*, 319–331.

Palisano, R. J., Haley, S. M., & Brown, D. A. (1992). Goal Attainment Scaling as a measure of change in infants with motor delays. *Physical Therapy, 72*, 432–437.

Repka, M. X., & Pediatric Eye Disease Investigator Group. (2003). Amblyopia in children less than seven years of age: Experience of the amblyopia treatment study 1. In J.-T. de Faber (Ed.), *9th Meeting of the International Strabismological Association* (pp. 163–166). Sydney, Australia: Swets & Zeitlinger.

Sparrow, S. S., Cicchetti, D. V., & Balla, D. A. (2006). *Vineland Adaptive Behavior Scales* (2nd ed.). Bloomington, MN: AGS Assessments.

Steenbeek, D., Ketelaar, M., Galama, K., & Gorter, J. W. (2007). Goal Attainment Scaling in paediatric rehabilitation: A critical review of the literature. *Developmental Medicine and Child Neurology, 49*, 550–556.

Steenbergen, B., Crajé, C., Nilsen, D. M., & Gordon, A. M. (2009). Motor imagery training in hemiplegic cerebral palsy: A potentially useful therapeutic tool for rehabilitation. *Developmental Medicine and Child Neurology, 51*, 690–696.

Sterling, C., Taub, E., Davis, D., Rickards, T., Gauthier, L. V., Griffin, A., & Uswatte, G. (2013). Structural neuroplasticity change after constraint-induced movement therapy in children with cerebral palsy. *Pediatrics, 4*, e1664–e1669.

Sutcliffe, T. L., Gaetz, W. C., Logan, W. J., Cheyne, D. O., & Fehlings, D. L. (2007). Cortical reorganization after modified constraint-induced movement therapy in pediatric hemiplegic cerebral palsy. *Journal of Child Neurology, 22*, 1281–1287.

Sutcliffe, T. L., Logan, W. J., & Fehlings, D. L. (2009). Pediatric constraint-induced movement therapy is associated with increased contralateral cortical activity on functional magnetic resonance imaging. *Journal of Child Neurology, 24,* 1230–1235.

Szaflarski, J. P., Page, S. J., Kissela, B. M., Lee, J. H., Levine, P., & Strakowski, S. M. (2006). Cortical reorganization following modified constraint-induced movement therapy: A study of 4 patients with chronic stroke. *Archives of Physical and Medical Rehabilitation, 87,* 1052–1058.

Taub, E., Ramey, S. L., DeLuca, S. C., & Echols, K. (2004). Efficacy of constraint-induced movement therapy for children with cerebral palsy. *Pediatrics, 113,* 305–312. PMID: 14754942

Wolf, S. L., Newton, H., Maddy, D., Blanton, S., Zhang, Q., Winstein, C. J., . . . Light, K. (2007). The EXCITE trial: Relationship of intensity of constraint induced movement therapy to improvement in the Wolf Motor Function Test. *Restorative Neurology and Neuroscience, 25,* 549–562.

Wolf, S. L., Winstein, C. J., Miller, J. P., Thompson, P. A., Taub, E., Uswatte, G., . . . Clark, P. C. (2008). Retention of upper limb function in stroke survivors who have received constraint-induced movement therapy: The EXCITE randomised trial. *Lancet Neurology, 7,* 33–40.

World Health Organization. (2001). *International classification of functioning, disability and health.* Geneva: Author.

SHARON LANDESMAN RAMEY, PhD; STEPHANIE C. DeLUCA, PhD;
TERESSA GARCIA REIDY, MS, OTR/L; DORY AINSWORTH WALLACE, MS,
OTR/L; and MARY REBEKAH TRUCKS, MS, OTR/L

Appendix A

Key Findings From Original Research Articles With Functional and Occupational Outcomes of Pediatric CIMT and Related Componential Interventions

HOW THIS APPENDIX IS ORGANIZED

This appendix provides a detailed listing of published articles that present original findings about a wide range of therapy interventions designated as constraint-induced movement therapy (CIMT) or variations of CIMT that usually include at least two and often more key components of CIMT (see Chapter 7, "Operationalizing CIMT: Transforming Basic Principles and Scientific Evidence Into Clinical Practice for Individual Children"). The table lists articles chronologically corresponding to their year of publication.

We included only articles published in English that present original data about functional outcomes related to the hemiparetic upper extremity (UE). Articles were omitted if the description of the treatment intervention was insufficient to classify the dosage or the type of constraint used. Similarly, articles were excluded if they presented data solely about outcomes other than UE (e.g., only about lower extremity outcomes, changes in brain functioning) or looked only at differential benefits within a study sample for which primary outcomes were previously reported. Finally, articles that were available only in a pre-publication, online, conference abstract, or self-published format (i.e., not peer-reviewed) were excluded.

A list of the abbreviations used for standardized outcome measures follows the table. For full details about these measures, refer to the study publication. (Many of these measures are described in Chapter 6, "Assessment Tools to Measure Upper-Limb Function and the Impact of Therapy.")

The full list of references corresponding to each entry in the appendix is provided using standard alphabetical listing.

METHOD FOR DESIGNATING THE TYPE OF P–CIMT TREATMENT

In a post hoc manner, we classified each of the treatment interventions using a standard set of criteria, consistent with the recommendations in Chapter 7, "Operationalizing Pediatric CIMT: Guidelines for Transforming Basic Principles and Scientific Evidence Into Clinical Practice for Individual Children." It is important to note that there have been no consistent publication guidelines for identifying a P–CIMT protocol as qualifying for the designation of a "modified" or "alternative" form. Rather, these terms have been self-selected by the authors of each study. Accordingly, we have been guided by the general model developed and now in use for categorizing forms of CIMT for adults with stroke (for more details, see Chapters 1, "History and Development of CIMT," and 7, "Operationalizing Pediatric CIMT: Guidelines for Transforming Basic Principles and Scientific Evidence Into Clinical Practice for Individual Children"). This model delineates three major forms of CIMT:

1. The *signature* or *traditional* form is the highest intensity, with a minimum dosage of 3 hours per day for at least 5 days per week for a minimum of 2 weeks. To qualify as signature P–CIMT, therapy must include active shaping and repetitive practice, be provided in homelike or natural settings, and use the constraint during at least the majority of the therapy sessions. Ideally, a transfer package is included as well.

2. *Modified* P–CIMT is highly similar to the signature form but usually has a lower dosage or other distinctive features. The minimum dosage for P–CIMT to be designated is 2 hours per day for at least 5 days per week for a minimum of 2 weeks.

3. *Alternative* P–CIMT often contains most but not all of the elements of the signature and modified forms. For example, a high-intensity camp-based model offered for only 1 week would be designated as alternative P–CIMT because it did not meet the minimum criteria of 2 weeks. Similarly, treatment provided entirely in an inpatient hospital setting would be considered alternative, because it did not provide therapy in an environment that is natural, such as a home, home-like, or typical school or child care setting. Therapy that is offered only a few days a week or for much briefer sessions (e.g., 1.0 or 1.5 hours) would fall below the threshold for modified P–CIMT. If the therapy provided did not emphasize shaping and repetitive practice but merely increased the time of play or regular (usual and customary) therapy, then it also would fall into this category of being an alternative form of P–CIMT.

Because the history of P–CIMT has overlapped with interest in the therapeutic effects of casting or constraining the non-affected or less-affected UE, we have included publications that address use of "constraint only" (often these permit the standard once or twice a week therapy with no modifications to this at all).

A major challenge in this rapidly emerging area of evidence-based practice is that there have been many inconsistencies and omissions related to how a treatment intervention is described in a given publication. In preparing this appendix, for example, we note that many publications did not precisely describe where the treatment was provided or whether the intervention included a parent education component or a formal transition plan to promote maintenance of new and improved UE skills (unilateral and bilateral). We hope that, in the future, a standard method for describing the key elements of P–CIMT will be adopted widely to permit more systematic comparisons of treatment protocols across studies and different clinical populations.

Finally, we recognize there remains a highly urgent set of questions that still are not resolved about the optimal dosage, constraint, and mix of providers (e.g., specialists, parents, teachers) and ways to combine different forms of supports and therapies to improve a child's functional outcomes over the course of his or her life (see Chapter 16, "Research Priorities: Understanding and Transcending the Limits of Current Knowledge to Inform Best Practices in Pediatric CIMT"). Accordingly, the current proposed guidelines for classifying P–CIMT into three groups may change and become even more evidence-backed as new evidence becomes available to assist in distinguish treatment protocols of the multi-component P–CIMT interventions. Above all, the purpose of including this appendix in this handbook is to provide information that will lead to a practically useful synthesis of what has been learned from research and clinical studies, so clinical providers and parents alike can be as well informed as possible in their decision making about what treatment protocols are likely to produce the best results for an individual child at a given stage in his or her development.

AUTHOR/YEAR STUDY DESIGN	STUDY POPULATION: N, AGE RANGE, DIAGNOSIS	INTERVENTION TYPE OF P–CIMT OR OTHER INTERVENTION	KEY FINDINGS AND COMMENTS
Yasukawa (1990) Case study	N = 1, 15 mo, CP (hemi)	*Constraint* Cast, 2 hr/wk with conventional OT × 18 mo.	Cast was used in several ways as adjunct to OT. Shows promise as a component.
Crocker, MacKay-Lyons, & McDonnell (1997) Case study	N = 1, 2 yr, CP (hemi)	*Constraint* Resting hand splint worn majority of waking hours × 3 wk with no additional therapy provided (usual therapy allowed).	Child showed increased spontaneous use. Gains in assistive use for bimanual activities via video observations and PDMS. (*Note:* Effort with a 3-yr-old failed due to poor adjustment to splint.)
Charles, Lavinder, & Gordon (2001) Case study	N = 3, 8–13 yr, CP (hemi)	*Signature P–CIMT* Cotton sling worn during 6 hr of therapy per day (play and functional activities guided by investigator for 2 hr and child for 4 hr) × 14 consecutive days.	Types of gains and maintenance varied for each child. Overall, intervention approach is highly promising. Authors recommended including home practice program as part of intervention.
Glover, Mateer, Yoell, & Speed (2002) Case study	N = 2 Case #1. 18 mo, CP (hemi) Case #2. 38 mo, CP (hemi)	*mP–CIMT* Case #1. Forearm splint worn majority of waking hours with 2 hr/day of OT or PT × 11 days Case #2. Same as above except added a 1.5 hr/day home practice component and then another 2 wk of OT/PT.	Both cases improved on multiple outcomes. Case #1 varied in cooperation or frustration on some days. Identified importance of parent engagement as feature of CIMT.
Pierce, Daly, Gallagher, Gershkoff, & Schaumburg (2002) Case Study	N = 1, 12 yr, CP (hemi)	*Alternative P–CIMT* Restraining hand mitt worn in hourly therapy sessions, 2 1-hr PT sessions and 2 1-hr OT sessions per week × 3 wk.	Child showed large gains on WMFT, grip strength, and activities of daily living. Many gains but not all maintained at 8 mo. postintervention.
Willis, Morello, Davie, Rice, & Bennett (2002) Randomized controlled trial	N = 25, 1–8 yr, "static brain lesion" (hemi) (12 treatment, 13 control)	*Constraint* Cast worn continuously × 4 wk (standard OT or PT permitted).	Cast treatment group but not controls showed large gains on PDMS at end and at 6 mo postintervention.
DeLuca, Echols, Ramey, & Taub (2003) Case study with repeat P–CIMT	N = 1 Intervention #1. 15 mo, CP (quad) Intervention #2. 21 mo, CP (quad)	*Signature P–CIMT* Intervention #1. Full-arm cast worn continuously with 6 hr/ day of shaping and repetitive practice × 15 days (5 days/ wk) Intervention #2. Same as above except provided for 21 consecutive days.	Child adjusted well to cast and high-dosage therapy. Large gains on PDMS Gross Motor, many new skills, increased daily use of UE. Gains maintained from Intervention #1 to #2. Also improved in weight bearing, social, and ambulation skills.
Eliasson, Bonnier, & Krumlinde-Sundholm (2003) Case study series	N = 9, 8–18 yr, CP (hemi)	*Alternative P–CIMT* Forearm splint with hand mitt worn for 7 hr/day in group camp that encouraged daily recreational activities and manipulative exercises, 5 days/wk × 2 wk.	Significant gains on Jebson–Taylor and Bruinincks–Oseretsky lasting to 5 mo. (*Note:* This was a letter to the editor.)
Karman, Maryles, Baker, Simpser, & Berger-Gross (2003) Case study series	N = 7, 7–17 yr, acquired brain injury (hemi)	*Signature P–CIMT* Hand mitt worn during all waking hours (in hospital) with 6 hr/day of shaping and repetitive practice (provided by multiple people) × 14 days.	All 7 showed large improvements in amount and quality of UE use, but variation occurred in individual gains (i.e., type, amount).
Taub, Ramey, DeLuca, & Echols (2004) Randomized controlled trial	N = 18, 7–96 mo, CP (mixed hemi and asymmetrically involved) (9 treatment, 9 control)	*Signature P–CIMT* Full-arm cast worn continuously with 6 hr/day shaping and massed practice × 21 days in child's home.	All adapted well to cast and high dosage. Significant gains in amount and quality of UE use (PMAL). Large increase in new behaviors. Gains maintained at 6 mo. "Spillover effects" (e.g., language, social) detected (observation and parent report). Controls did not change.

(Continued)

AUTHOR/YEAR STUDY DESIGN	STUDY POPULATION: N, AGE RANGE, DIAGNOSIS	INTERVENTION TYPE OF P–CIMT OR OTHER INTERVENTION	KEY FINDINGS AND COMMENTS
Eliasson, Krumlinde-Sundholm, Shaw, & Wang (2005) Two-group comparison	N = 41, 18 mo–4 yr, CP (hemi) (21 treatment, 20 controls who lived outside clinical area)	*Alternative P–CIMT* Restraint glove 2 hr/day while parent encouraged UE activities plus 1 hr/wk therapist supervision × 2 mo.	Children showed significant gains at both the end (large effect size) and 6 mo later (medium effect size) on newly developed AHA. Controls did not improve.
Miller & Hale (2005) Case study	N = 1, 20 yr, CP (quad)	*Alternative P–CIMT* Constraint was the therapist holding the young adult's hand during 1-hr sessions, 4 times/wk × 30 wk.	Large gains detected by 10 wk into intervention and even larger gains by end of 30 wk on AART.
Naylor & Bower (2005) Case study series	N = 9, 18–60 mo, CP (hemi)	*Alternative P–CIMT* Constraint was the therapist holding the child's hand during 1-hr sessions offered 2 times/wk by therapist and 5 times/wk by parent for 4 wk.	UE function improved significantly on the QUEST for all 9 cases. Five cases rated as good compliance and 4 as "variable compliance" with intervention protocol.
Sung et al. (2005) Randomized controlled trial	N = 31, infants–8 yr, CP (hemi) (18 treatment, 13 control)	*Alternative P–CIMT* Short-arm cast worn continuously for 6 wk while child received conventional OT for 30 min for 2 sessions/wk. Controls had 30 min OT for 2 sessions/wk.	Intervention group showed significant gains in the BBT and Erhard as well as the self-care score on the WeeFIM. Controls did not show gains.
Charles, Wolf, Schneider, & Gordon (2006) (a) Randomized controlled trial	N = 22, 4–8 yr, CP (hemi) (11 CIMT, 11 control)	(a) *Signature P–CIMT* Sling worn on noninvolved UE for 6 hr/day for 10 of 12 treatment days with last 2 days bilateral treatment days. All treatment days had guided shaping and repetitive practice.	(a) Improvements seen in speed and dexterity and functional use measures after P–CIMT but no changes in the measures of impairment level. Controls did not show added speed benefits.
Deluca, Echols, Law, & Ramey (2006) Randomized controlled trial with crossover group	N = 17, 7–96 mo, CP (hemi and quad) (9 CIMT, 8 control/cross-over 8)	*Signature P–CIMT* See Taub et al. (2004) cited earlier.	(*Note:* Same children as in Taub et al., 2004). All children who crossed over made large, significant gains on the QUEST, PMAL, and emerging new behaviors comparable to original treatment group effects. Spillover effects mentioned.
Gordon, Charles, & Wolf (2006) (b) Clinical combined group (added an older age treatment group)	N = 8 new cases, 9–13 yr, CP (hemi)	(b) *Signature P–CIMT* Same as above.	(b) Significant and similar improvements seen in the older age group at 1 wk, 1 mo, and 6 mo posttreatment on Jebson–Taylor and Bruininks–Oseretsky. Both younger and older groups made benefits. No significant group differences overall.
Assis, Massaro, Chamlian, Silva, & Ota (2007) Case study	N = 1, 11 yr, CP (hemi)	*Signature P–CIMT* Sling worn 70% waking hours, 3 hr daily exercise with PT for 2 wk with task practice and shaping.	Improved dexterity, shoulder stabilization. Decreased associated reactions, and improved position of paretic limb.
Bollea et al. (2007) Case study	N = 1, 7 mo, stroke	*Complex P–CIMT* Therapy varied over 12 mo, often using full-arm cast for 4 hr/day with 2 hr OT shaping and repetitive task activities included. Twice had 2-mo intervals with no constraint.	During intervention, the child developed reaching and grasping and other new motor behaviors. In parallel, he also exhibited a decrease of neglect of hemiparetic side.
Charles & Gordon (2007) Case series with repeat P–CIMT	N = 8, 5–11 yr, CP (hemi)	*Signature P–CIMT* See Charles et al. (2006) cited earlier. Children received second intervention at least 12 mo later.	Initial improvements were maintained up to 1 yr. Second intervention resulted in further significant improvement.

(Continued)

AUTHOR/YEAR STUDY DESIGN	STUDY POPULATION: N, AGE RANGE, DIAGNOSIS	INTERVENTION TYPE OF P–CIMT OR OTHER INTERVENTION	KEY FINDINGS AND COMMENTS
Dickerson & Brown (2007) Case study	N = 1, 24 mo, CP (hemi)	*Signature P–CIMT* Splint worn most waking hours plus 6 hr/day of OT × 21 days followed by extra therapy post-CIMT (5 1-hr sessions in 2 wk).	Major gains in reach, grasp and release, push, pull, sustained grasp, finger feeding, and bilateral use. Showed new spontaneous use of hemiparetic UE in unilateral and bilateral activities, and self-confidence and awareness of hemiparetic side improved.
Gordon et al. (2007) Case series	N = 6, 6–15 yr, chronic hemiparesis	*Alternative P–CIMT* Resting hand with OT shaping and repetitive practice 2 hr/day, 5 days/wk × 4 wk in a clinic.	No significant improvement in sensory motor function or quality of upper-limb movement. All improved in individual functional goals. Children and parents were positive about treatment.
Juenger et al. (2007) Case series	N = 10, 10–30 yr, congenital hemiparesis	*Alternative P–CIMT* Glove with sling for 10 hr/day inpatient day camp with therapy 2 hr/day × 12 days. Shaping and repetition in individual therapy plus group therapy with peers.	Large and significant functional improvement on the WMFT. Increased brain activation in primary sensorimotor cortex of affected hemisphere.
Sutcliffe, Gaetz, Logan, Cheyne, & Fehlings (2007) Case study	N = 1, 8 yr, CP (hemi)	*Alternative P–CIMT* Continuous casting with 1 hr/wk OT (standard practice management of CP aimed at meeting family's functional goals) × 3 wk.	Demonstrated cortical reorganization that was maintained 6 mo following intervention.
Cope, Forst, Bibis, & Liu (2008) Case study	N = 1, 12 mo, CP (hemi)	*Alternative P–CIMT* Full-arm cast worn continuously with 8 hr/wk of OT and PT × 2 wk.	Improved in many areas on TAUT, PMAL, and PDMS up to 6 mo posttreatment. Spillover effects in language and gross motor areas.
Fergus et al. (2008) Case study	N = 1, 13 mo, CP (hemi)	*Alternative P–CIMT* Hand mitt used and parents given suggestions for shaping behaviors. Phase 1 = 6 hr/day × 21 days of constraint and parent intervention. Phase 2 = decreased constraint time for 5 consecutive wk. Phase 3 = 4 hr/day × 21 days. Then additional phases.	Beneficial long-term effects of P–CIMT, including decreased flexion posturing and increasing reaching and grasp. Increased awareness and spontaneous use of hemiparetic UE.
Kuhnke et al. (2008) Case series	N = 16, 11–30 yr, congenital hemiparesis (9 ipsilateral and 7 contralateral projections)	*Modified P–CIMT* Individually tailored glove worn 10+ hr/day × 12 days with 2 hr/day of individual shaping and repetitive practice, 6 days/wk × 2 wk plus 6–8 hr/day of group therapy activities in a camp setting.	Significant improvements in WMFT immediately and 6 mo posttreatment, for both ipsi- and contralateral groups. Children with contralateral lesions showed increased speed, and those with ipsilateral took longer but showed improvements.
Martin, Burtner, Poole, & Phillips (2008) Case study	N = 1, 35 mo, CP (hemi)	*Signature P–CIMT* Full-arm cast worn during 4 hr/day therapy plus 3–5 hr/day extra.	Improved grip strength, PEDI, Melbourne, and *ICF* activity and participation. Spillover with improved speech and intelligibility.
Wallen, Ziviani, Herbet, Evans, & Novak (2008) Single clinical group	N = 9, 6 mo–8 yr, CP (hemi)	*Alternative P–CIMT* Custom mitt worn 2 hr/day every day for 8 wk while parent provided "adjunct" intervention (promoting UE use) and once a week OT session at home.	Mixed pattern of findings. Motly no or small changes on AHA, parent questionnaire, and spasticity at immediate and 6 mo posttreatment (described as feasibility study).

(Continued)

AUTHOR/YEAR STUDY DESIGN	STUDY POPULATION: N, AGE RANGE, DIAGNOSIS	INTERVENTION TYPE OF P–CIMT OR OTHER INTERVENTION	KEY FINDINGS AND COMMENTS
Coker, Lebkicher, Harris, & Snape (2009) Case study with repeat P-CIMT	N = 1, 9 mo (when CIMT began), CP (hemi)	*Alternative P–CIMT* Intervention #1. Resting hand splint with mitt with 4 1 hr/day sessions from OT/PT/student × 4 days/wk × 4 wk. Parents trained and provided with home program 3 days/wk with 1 hr written activity plan. Intervention #2. Same as above.	#1. Large gains in grasp, visual–motor skills, PDMS Fine and Gross Motor, spontaneous use of hemiparetic UE. #2. Improvements in all areas above plus other benefits (e.g., increased awareness, weight bearing, transitions, walking). Some declines noted by 6 mo posttreatment, but many skills maintained or further improved.
deBode, Fritz, Weir-Haynes, & Mathern (2009) Case series	N = 4, 12–22 yr, hemiparesis secondary to hemispherectomy	*Signature P–CIMT* Resting hand splint worn 90% of waking hours × 11 days with 3 hr/day therapy × 10 days.	Improvements found on AAUT and BBT but no differences on the FM. An fMRI showed subtle shifts in location of activations, but activation remained within primary sensorimotor and supplementary motor areas.
Park, Rha, Lee, Yoo, & Chang (2009) Two-group comparison	N = 32, 1–9 yr, CP (hemi) (14 CIMT plus botulinum toxin, 15 only botulinum toxin injections)	*Alternative P–CIMT* Group receiving P–CIMT wore an orthosis during waking hours with 1 hr/day PT and OT × 3 wk with parents given individualized instructions for how to practice (shape) activities.	Children receiving both BoNT-A injections plus CIMT had significant changes in the Modified Group receiving P–CIMT had more improvements in tone than the group only receiving botulinum toxin injections on the MAS ratings and greater functional improvement ratings on the PMAL.
Smania et al. (2009) Randomized controlled trial with crossover	N = 10, 1–9 yr, CP (hemi) (5 CIMT, 5 control)	*Alternative P–CIMT* Hand mitt worn 8 hr/day × 5 wk with 1 hr therapy × 2 days/wk × 5 wk. Controls received same amount of therapy but no restraint.	On study-specific use and function test, children in CIMT showed more improvements then controls in unimanual and bimanual function, but benefits did not last at 4 wk posttreatment.
Stearns, Burtner, Keenan, Qualls, & Phillips (2009) Case series	N = 6, 5–8 yr, CP (hemi)	*Signature P–CIMT* Bivalve cast worn 8–12 hr/day with 4 hr/day therapy × 5 days/wk × 14 days.	Significant improvements in all strength and dexterity measures. Increases in muscle activation on pinch measures and grip.
Aarts, Jongerius, Geerdink, van Limbeek, & Geurts (2010) Randomized controlled trial	N = 52, 2.5–8 yr, CP (hemi) (26 CIMT, 26 controls)	*Alternative P–CIMT* Sling worn during 3-hr therapy sessions with shaping and repetitive task practice × 3 days/wk × 8 wk, followed by 2 wk of bimanual therapy.	Increased spontaneous use of the more affected upper limb. CIMT group showed a 13% improvement of AHA in comparison to U&C group and 36% improvement over U&C on the ABILHAND–Kids, but pre- to posttreatment changes in either group were significant.
de Brito Brandão, Mancini, Vaz, Pereira de Melo, & Fonseca (2010) Randomized controlled trial	N = 16, 5–8 yr, CP (hemi) randomized to intervention (8 CIMT, 8 controls)	*Signature P–CIMT* Resting hand splint worn for 10 hr/day with 3 hr/day therapy including structured activities × 2 wk. Followed by 1 wk bimanual training.	Significant improvement at posttreatment on the Jebson–Taylor and the PEDI for those in the P-CIMT group but not in the controls.
Psychouli, Burridge, & Kennedy (2010) Case series	N = 9, 5–11 yr, CP (hemi)	*Constraint* Each child received all 3 constraints: mitt, short-arm splint, and long-arm splint. Each worn in random order for a minimum of 1 hr daily (no upper limit set) × 4 days.	Long-arm splint was the most effective in promoting arm use of the affected UE whereas the short-arm splint had greatest acceptance rating by children. Outcomes based on analysis of videotaped play sessions.
Suskauer, Trovato, Zabel, & Comi (2010) Case study	N = 1, 4 yr, Sturge–Weber syndrome	*Alternative P–CIMT* Full-time cast × 20 days with 6 hr/day therapy × 14 days in a day rehabilitation center.	Improved active range of motion, reach, and grasp and release and decreased spasticity. At 2 yr posttreatment, spasticity still reduced, but functional gains were not maintained.

(Continued)

AUTHOR/YEAR STUDY DESIGN	STUDY POPULATION: N, AGE RANGE, DIAGNOSIS	INTERVENTION TYPE OF P–CIMT OR OTHER INTERVENTION	KEY FINDINGS AND COMMENTS
Vaz et al. (2010) Case study	N = 1, 2 yr, brachial plexus injury	*Alternative P–CIMT* Elastic band used at home during ½ hr/day × 2 wk. Parent was instructed in how to progress activities.	Improved in functional skills on the TAUT across quality, participation, willingness, and performance.
Al-Oraibi & Eliasson (2011) Randomized controlled trial	N = 20, 22–105 mo, CP (hemi) (7 CIMT, 7 neurodevelopmental treatment)	*Constraint* Customized glove worn 2 hr/day × 6 days/wk with 1 day/wk therapy session × 8 wk.	Significant improvements on AHA were made by CIMT group compared with no changes in the NDT group.
Eliasson, Shaw, Berg, & Krumlinde-Sundholm (2011) Randomized controlled trial with crossover	N = 25, 18 mo–5 yr, CP (hemi) (12 CIMT, 13 controls then crossed over to receive CIMT)	*Modified P–CIMT* Hand glove and splint worn during therapy session of 2 h/day, 5 day/wk × 8 wk. Treatment provided by parent or preschool teachers supervised by OT once a week.	AHA scores in CIMT group improved more than control group, with an effect size of 1.16. Similar benefits detected for the crossover group.
Lin et al. (2011) Randomized controlled trial	N = 21, 48–19 mo, CP (hemi) (10 CIMT, 10 control)	*Alternative P–CIMT* Elastic bandage and hand glove worn for 3.5–4.0 hr/day for 4 consecutive wk when engaged in exercises and daily activities plus child received 3.5–4.0 hr of therapy twice per wk × 4 wk at home from physical therapist focused on shaping and repetitive task.	CIMT group improved significantly more than the controls on the PDMS gross motor section and on the Bruininks–Oseretsky. Parent stress was also rated higher in the CIMT group on the dysfunctional interaction scale of the PSI.
Wallen et al. (2011) Randomized clinical trial comparing two treatments Post hoc analyses and responses, see Ramey et al., DeLuca, Case-Smith, & Stevenson (2012) Author reply, see Wallen et al. (2012)	N = 50, 19 mo–7yr, CP (hemi) (25 CIMT, 25 intensive OT)	*Alternative P–CIMT* Custom mitt worn 2 hr/day every day × 8 wk while parent provided "adjunct" intervention (promoting UE use) plus once a week OT session at home. Intensive OT group received OT once a week and 20 min/day of home program by parents.	No clinically significant differences were found between groups at posttreatment or 6 mo later; however, neither group showed statistically significant gains on objective measures according to Ramey et al.'s (2012) post hoc analyses. Both groups showed some improvements.
DeLuca, Case-Smith, Stevenson, & Ramey (2012) and Case-Smith, DeLuca, Stevenson, & Ramey (2012) Randomized controlled trial	N = 18, 3–6 yr, CP (hemi) (9 received 6 hr/day ACQUIREc and 9 received 3 hr/day)	*Signature P–CIMT* Full-arm cast worn continuously with shaping and massed practice provided by therapist (ACQUIREc protocol) for 5 days/wk × 4 wk. The daily dosage differed for the 2 groups: 6 hr/day therapy vs. 3 hr/day therapy.	Both groups significantly improved after CIMT on the AHA, PMAL, QUEST, and SHUEE at immediate and 6 mo posttreatment. The higher dosage did not produce better outcomes than the 3 hr/day dosage at either time period. Gains were maintained at 6 mo.
Haynes & Phillips (2012) Case series	N = 2, 9 & 28 mo, CP (hemi)	*Alternative P–CIMT* Long-arm cast worn during NDT-based play session for 2 hr/day × 7 days/wk × 2 mo. Sessions were delivered by a combination of people (i.e., occupational and physical therapists, rehabilitation specialists, and parents).	Improvements seen on PDMS on one child corresponding to 5 mo developmental gain. The other child had a 32-point gain on the QUEST. On the ACQUIRE Therapy Motor Patterns, one child gained 10 points and the other 11 points.

(Continued)

AUTHOR/YEAR STUDY DESIGN	STUDY POPULATION: N, AGE RANGE, DIAGNOSIS	INTERVENTION TYPE OF P–CIMT OR OTHER INTERVENTION	KEY FINDINGS AND COMMENTS
Hsin et al. (2012) Randomized controlled trial	N = 22, 6–8 yr, CP (hemi) (11 CIMT, 11 controls)	*Alternative P–CIMT* Elastic bandage and hand glove worn (for 3.5–4.0 hr/day for 4 consecutive wk when engaged in exercises and daily activities plus child received 3.5–4.0 hr therapy twice per wk × 4 wk at home from physical therapist focused on shaping and repetitive task practice. Controls received same dosage of PT per week, but therapy focused on function-oriented activities and NDT and motor learning.	CIMT group showed large effect size benefits at immediate and 3 mo posttreatment on UE efficiency on Bruininks–Oseretsky as well as improved PMAL quality and quantity of use and quality of life in social well-being, participation and physical health, emotional well-being, and other areas compared with controls who received same dosage (about 8 hr/wk) but had different therapy content and used no constraint.
Chen et al. (2013) Randomized controlled trial	N = 47, 6–12 yr, CP (hemi) (24 CIMT, 23 controls)	*Alternative P–CIMT* Elastic bandage and restraint mitt 3.5–4.0 hr/day every day plus therapy of 3.5–4.0 hr for 2 days/wk × 4 wk at home focused on shaping and repetitive practice. Controls received same dosage of therapy, but content was traditional positioning, strengthening, unilateral and bilateral activities with NDT, and no constraint used.	CIMT produced significant gains on PDMS, PMAL quality and amount of use, temporal and spatial–temporal movement efficiency, and smoothness based on kinematics.
Rocca et al. (2013) Clinical study	N = 14, 5–18 yr, congenital or acquired brain injury (hemi)	*Alternative P–CIMT* Hand splint and glove for 3 hr/day for 3 days/wk × 10 wk at a clinic. Treatment was 1.5 hr/day by therapist and 1.5 hr/day by parent. For remaining 4 days/wk, parent provided 3 hr/day of similar therapy activities.	Significant gains on QUEST for 12 of 14 cases and on GMFM for 11 of 14 cases. Further improvement detected at 6 mo posttreatment for 9 of 14. Lesion volume and severity of damage not associated with functional motor improvement after CIMT; only predictor of clinical improvement was higher baseline average lesion FA.

Note. Articles are listed in chronological order.
AART = Action Arm Research Test; ACQUIREc = Acquisition of new motor skills through Continuous practice and shaping to produce Quality movement of the Upper extremity through Intensive therapy and Reinforcement in Everyday patterns and places; AAUT = Actual Amount of Use Test; AHA = Assisting Hand Assessment; BBT = Block and Box Test; BoNT-A = botulinum neurotoxin type A; CIMT = constraint-induced movement therapy; CP = cerebral palsy; FA = functional activities; FM = fine motor; fMRI = functional magnetic resonance imaging; GMFM = Gross Motor Function Measure; ICF = *International Classification of Functioning, Disability and Health*; MAS = Modified Ashworth Scale; mP–CIMT = modified pediatric constraint-induced movement therapy; NDT = neurodevelopmental treatment; OT = occupational therapy; P–CIMT = pediatric constraint-induced movement therapy; PDMS = Peabody Developmental Motor Scale; PEDI = Pediatric Evaluation of Disabilities Inventory; PMAL = Pediatric Motor Activity Log; PSI = Perceived Stress Index; PT = physical therapy; QUEST = Quality of Upper Extremity Skills Test; SHUEE = Shriners Hospital for Children Upper Extremity Evaluation; TAUT = Toddler Arm Use Test; U&C = usual and customary care or treatment; UE = upper extremity; WMFT = Wolf Motor Function Test.

REFERENCES

Aarts, P. B., Jongerius, P. H., Geerdink, V. A., van Limbeek, J., & Geurts, A. C. (2010). Effectiveness of modified constraint-induced movement therapy in children with unilateral spastic cerebral palsy: A randomized controlled trial. *Neurorehabilitation and Neural Repair, 24*(6), 509–518. http://dx.doi.org/10.1177/1545968309359767

Al-Oraibi, S., & Eliasson, A. (2011). Implementation of constraint-induced movement therapy for young children with unilateral cerebral palsy in Jordan: A home-based model. *Disability and Rehabilitation, 33*(21), 2006–2012.

Assis, R. D., Massaro, A. R., Chamlian, T. R., Silva, M., & Ota, S. M. (2007). Constraint-induced movement therapy for a child with hemiplegic cerebral palsy: Case report. *Acta Fisiátrica, 14*(1), 62–65.

Bollea, L., Di Rosa, G., Gisondi, A., Guidi, P., Petrarca, M., Giannarelli, P., & Castelli, E. (2007). Recovery from hemiparesis and unilateral spatial neglect after neonatal stroke: Case report and rehabilitation of an infant. *Brain Injury, 21*(1), 81–91. http://dx.doi.org/10.1080/02699050601148882

Case-Smith, J., DeLuca, S. C., Stevenson, R., & Ramey, S. L. (2012). Multicenter randomized controlled trial of pediatric constraint-induced movement therapy: 6-month follow-up. *American Journal of Occupational Therapy, 66*, 15–23. http://dx.doi.org/10.5014/ajot.2012.002386

Charles, J. R., & Gordon, A. M. (2007). A repeated course of constraint-induced movement therapy results in further improvement. *Developmental Medicine and Child Neurology, 49*, 770–773. http://dx.doi.org/10.1111/j.1469-8749.2007.00770.x

Charles, J., Lavinder, G., & Gordon, A. M. (2001). The effects of constraint induced therapy on hand function in children with hemiplegic cerebral palsy. *Pediatric Physical Therapy, 13*, 68–76.

Charles, J. R., Wolf, S. L., Schneider, J. A., & Gordon, A. M. (2006). Efficacy of a child-friendly form of constraint-induced movement therapy in hemiplegic cerebral palsy: A randomized control trial. *Developmental Medicine and Child Neurology, 48*, 635–642. http://dx.doi.org/10.1111/j.1469-8749.2006.tb01332.x

Chen, C., Kang, L., Hong, W.-H., Chen, F.-C., Chen, H.-C., & Wu, C. (2013). Effect of therapist-based constraint-induced therapy at home on motor control, motor performance and daily function in children with cerebral palsy: A randomized controlled study. *Clinical Rehabilitation, 27*(3), 236–245. http://dx.doi.org/10.1177/0269215512455652

Coker, P., Lebkicher, C., Harris, L., & Snape, J. (2009). The effects of constraint-induced movement therapy for a child less than one year of age. *NeuroRehabilitation, 24*(3), 199–208. PMID: 19458426

Cope, S. M., Forst, H. C., Bibis, D., & Liu, X. C. (2008). Modified constraint-induced movement therapy for a 12-month-old child with hemiplegia: A case report. *American Journal of Occupational Therapy, 62*, 430–437. http://dx.doi.org10.5014/ajot.62.4.430

Crocker, M. D., MacKay-Lyons M., & McDonnell, E. (1997). Forced use of the upper extremity in cerebral palsy: A single-case design. *American Journal of Occupational Therapy, 51*, 824-833.

de Bode, S., Fritz, S. L., Weir-Haynes, K., & Mathern, G. W. (2009). Constraint-induced movement therapy for individuals after cerebral hemispherectomy: A case series. *Physical Therapy, 89*(4), 361–369.

de Brito Brandão, M., Mancini, M. C., Vaz, D. V., Pereira de Melo, A. P., & Fonseca, S. T. (2010). Adapted version of constraint-induced movement therapy promotes functioning in children with cerebral palsy: A randomized controlled trial. *Clinical Rehabilitation, 24*(7), 639–647. http://dx.doi.org/10.1177/0269215510367974

DeLuca, S. C., Case-Smith, J., Stevenson, R., & Ramey, S. L. (2012). Constraint-induced movement therapy (CIMT) for young children with cerebral palsy: Effects of therapeutic dosage. *Journal of Pediatric Rehabilitation Medicine, 5*, 133–142. http://dx.doi.org/10.3233/PRM-2012-0206

DeLuca, S. C., Echols, K., Law, C. R., & Ramey, S. L. (2006). Intensive pediatric constraint-induced therapy for children with cerebral palsy. *Journal of Child Neurology, 21*, 931–938. http://dx.doi.org/10.23107/7010.2006.00201

DeLuca, S. C., Echols, K., Ramey, S. L., & Taub, E. (2003). Pediatric constraint-induced movement therapy for a young child: Two episodes of care. *Physical Therapy, 83*, 1003–1013. PMID: 1477827

Dickerson, A. E., & Brown, L. E. (2007). Pediatric constraint-induced movement therapy in a young child with minimal active arm movement. *American Journal of Occupational Therapy, 61*(5), 563–573. http://dx.doi.org/10.5014/ajot.61.5.563

Eliasson, A. C., Bonnier, B., & Krumlinde-Sundholm, L. (2003). Clinical experience of constraint induced movement therapy in adolescents with hemiplegic cerebral palsy: A day camp model. *Developmental Medicine and Child Neurology, 45*, 357–360. http://dx.doi.org/10.1111/j.1469-8749.2003tb00409.x

Eliasson, A. C., Krumlinde-Sundholm, L., Shaw, K., & Wang, C. (2005). Effects of constraint-induced movement therapy in young children with hemiplegic cerebral palsy: An adapted model. *Developmental Medicine and Child Neurology, 47*, 266–275. http://dx.doi.org/10.1111/j.1469-8749.2005tb01132.x

Eliasson, A. C., Shaw, K., Berg, E., & Krumlinde-Sundholm, L. (2011). An ecological approach of constraint induced movement therapy for 2–3-year-old children: A randomized control trial. *Research in Developmental Disabilities, 32*(6), 2820–2828. http://dx.doi.org/10.1016/j.ridd.2011.05.024

Fergus, A., Buckler, J., Farrell, J., Isley, M., McFarland, M., & Riley, B. (2008). Constraint-induced movement therapy for a child with hemiparesis: A case report. *Pediatric Physical Therapy, 20*(3), 271–283. http://dx.doi.org/10.1097/PEP.0b013e318181e569

Glover, J. E., Mateer, C. A., Yoell, C., & Speed, S. (2002). The effectiveness of constraint induced movement therapy in two young children with hemiplegia. *Pediatric Rehabilitation, 5*(3), 125–131. http://dx.doi.org/10.1080/1363849021000039326

Gordon, A. M., Charles, J., & Wolf, S. L. (2006). Efficacy of constraint-induced movement therapy on involved upper-extremity use in children with hemiplegic cerebral palsy is not age-dependent. *Pediatrics, 117,* 363–373. http://dx.doi.org/10.1542/peds.2005-1009

Gordon, A., Connelly, A., Neville, B., Vargha-Khadem, F., Jessop, N., Murphy, T., & Ganesan, V. (2007). Modified constraint-induced movement therapy after childhood stroke. *Developmental Medicine and Child Neurology, 49,* 23–27. PMID: 17209972

Haynes, M. P., & Phillips, D. (2012). Modified constraint induced movement therapy enhanced by a neuro-development treatment-based therapeutic handling protocol: Two case studies. *Journal of Pediatric Rehabilitation Medicine, 5*(2), 117–124. http://dx.doi.org/10.3233/PRM-2012-0203

Hsin, Y., Chen, F.-C., Lin, K., Kang, L., Chen, C., & Chen, C. (2012). Efficacy of constraint-induced therapy on functional performance and health-related quality of life for children with cerebral palsy: A randomized controlled trial. *Journal of Child Neurology, 27*(8), 992–999. http://dx.doi.org/10.1177/0883073811431011

Juenger, H., Linder-Lucht, M., Walther, M., Berweck, S., Mall, V., & Staudt, M. (2007). Cortical neuromodulation by constraint-induced movement therapy in congenital hemiparesis: An fMRI study. *Neuropediatrics, 38*(3), 130–136. http://dx.doi.org/10.1055/s-2007-985904

Karman, N., Maryles, J., Baker, R.W., Simpser, E., & Berger-Gross, P. (2003). Constraint-induced movement therapy for hemiplegic children with acquired brain injuries. *Journal of Head Trauma Rehabilitation, 18*(3), 259–267.

Kuhnke, N., Juenger, H., Walther, M., Berweck, S., Mall, V., & Staudt, M. (2008). Do patients with congenital hemiparesis and ipsilateral corticospinal projections respond differently to constraint-induced movement therapy? *Developmental Medicine and Child Neurology,* 50(12), 898–903. http://dx.doi.org/10.1111/j.1469-8749.2008.03119.x

Lin, K., Wang, T., Wu, C., Chen, C., Chang, K., Lin, Y., & Chen, Y. (2011). Effects of home-based constraint-induced therapy versus dose-matched control intervention on functional outcomes and caregiver well-being in children with cerebral palsy. *Research in Developmental Disabilities, 32*(5), 1483–1491. http://dx.doi.org/10.1016/j.ridd.2011.01.023

Martin, A., Burtner, P. A., Poole, J., & Phillips, J. (2008). Case report: ICF-level changes in a preschooler after constraint-induced movement therapy. *American Journal of Occupational Therapy, 62,* 282–288. http://dx.doi.org/10.5014/ajot.62.3.282

Miller, R., & Hale, L. (2005). Constraint-induced movement therapy for a youth with a chronic traumatic brain injury. *New Zealand Journal of Physiotherapy, 33*(3), 85–90.

Naylor, C. E., & Bower, E. (2005). Modified constraint-induced movement therapy for young children with hemiplegic cerebral palsy: A pilot study. *Developmental Medicine and Child Neurology, 47,* 365–369.

Park, E. S., Rha, D.-W., Lee, J. D., Yoo, J. K., & Chang, W. H. (2009). The short-term effects of combined modified constraint-induced movement therapy and botulinum toxin injection for children with spastic hemiplegic cerebral palsy. *Neuropediatrics, 40*(6), 269–274. PMID: 20446220

Pierce, S. R., Daly, K., Gallagher, K. G., Gershkoff, A. M., & Schaumburg, S. W. (2002). Constraint-induced therapy for a child with hemiplegic cerebral palsy: A case report. *Archives of Physical Medicine and Rehabilitation, 83,* 1462–1463.

Psychouli, P., Burridge, J., & Kennedy, C. (2010). Forced use as a home-based intervention in children with congenital hemiplegic cerebral palsy: Choosing the appropriate constraint. *Disability and Rehabilitation Assistive Technology, 5*(1), 25–33. http://dx.doi.org/10.3109/17483100903121489

Ramey, S. L., Deluca, S. C., Case-Smith, J., & Stevenson, R. (2012). Caution is warranted in interpreting data from a recent trial of modified constraint-induced therapy. *Developmental Medicine and Child Neurology, 54*(5), 477–479; author reply 479–481. http://dx.doi.org/10.1111/j.1469-8749.2012.04240.x

Rocca, M. A., Turconi, A. C., Strazzer, S., Absinta, M., Valsasina, P., Beretta, E., ... Filippi, M. (2013). MRI predicts efficacy of constraint-induced movement therapy in children with brain injury. *Neurotherapeutics.* Advance online publication. http://dx.doi.org/10.1007/s13311-013-0189-2

Smania, N., Aglioti, S. M., Cosentino, A., Camin, M., Gandolfi, M., Tinazzi, M., . . . Faccioli, S. (2009). A modified constraint-induced movement therapy (CIT) program improves paretic arm use and function in children with cerebral palsy. *European Journal of Physical and Rehabilitation Medicine, 45*(4), 493–500. PMID: 20032907

Stearns, G. E., Burtner, P., Keenan, K. M., Qualls, C., & Phillips, J. (2009). Effects of constraint-induced movement therapy on hand skills and muscle recruitment of children with spastic hemiplegic cerebral palsy. *NeuroRehabilitation, 24*(2), 95–108. PMID: 19339749

Sung, I. Y., Ryu, J. S., Pyun, S. B., Yoo, S. D., Song, W. H., & Park, M. J. (2005). Efficacy of forced-use therapy in hemiplegic cerebral palsy. *Archives of Physical Medicine and Rehabilitation, 86*, 2195–2198.

Suskauer, S. J., Trovato, M. K., Zabel, T. A., & Comi, A. M. (2010). Physiatric findings in individuals with Sturge–Weber syndrome. *American Journal of Physical Medicine and Rehabilitation, 89*(4), 323–330.

Sutcliffe, T. L., Gaetz, W. C., Logan, W. J., Cheyne, D. O., & Fehlings, D. L. (2007). Cortical reorganization after modified constraint-induced movement therapy in pediatric hemiplegic cerebral palsy. *Journal of Child Neurology, 22*, 1281–1287. PMID: 18006957.

Taub, E., Ramey, S. L., DeLuca, S. C., & Echols, K. (2004). Efficacy of constraint-induced movement therapy for children with cerebral palsy with asymmetric motor impairment. *Pediatrics, 113*, 305–312. PMID: 14754942

Vaz, D. V., Mancini, M. C., do Amaral, M. F., de Brito Brandão, M., de França Drummond, A., & da Fonseca, S. T.

(2010). Clinical changes during an intervention based on constraint-induced movement therapy principles on use of the affected arm of a child with obstetric brachial plexus injury: A case report. *Occupational Therapy International, 17*, 159–167. http://dx.doi.org/10.1002/oti.295

Wallen, M., Ziviani, J., Herbert, R., Evans, R., & Novak, I. (2008). Modified constraint-induced therapy for children with hemiplegic cerebral palsy: A feasibility study. *Developmental Neurorehabilitation, 11*(2), 124–133. http://dx.doi.org/10.1080/17518420701640897

Wallen, M., Ziviani, J., Naylor, O., Evans, R., Novak, I., & Herbert, R. D. (2011). Modified constraint-induced therapy for children with hemiplegic cerebral palsy: A randomized trial. *Developmental Medicine and Child Neurology, 53*, 1091–1099. http://dx.doi.org/10.1111/j.1469-8749.2011.04086.x

Wallen, M., Ziviani, J., Naylor, O., Evans, R., Novak, I., & Herbert, R. D. (2012). Author reply: Caution is warranted in interpreting data from a recent trial of modified constraint-induced therapy. *Developmental Medicine and Child Neurology, 54*(5), 479–481.

Willis, J. K., Morello, A., Davie, A., Rice, J. C., & Bennett, J. T. (2002). Forced use treatment of childhood hemiparesis. *Pediatrics, 110*, 94–96.

Yasukawa, A. (1990). Upper-extremity casting: Adjunct treatment for a child with cerebral palsy hemiplegia. *American Journal of Occupational Therapy, 44*, 840–846. http://dx.doi.org/10.5014/ajot.44.9.840

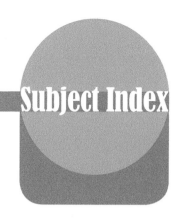

Subject Index

Note. Page numbers in *italics* indicate exhibits, figures, and tables.

Citation Index

Note. Page numbers in *italics* refer to exhibits, figures, and tables.